D1062605

The Art, Science, and Technology of Pharmaceutical Compounding

FIFTH EDITION

Notices

The author, editors, and publisher have made every effort to ensure the accuracy and completeness of the information presented in this book. However, the author, editors, and publisher cannot be held responsible for the continued currency of the information, any inadvertent errors or omissions, or the application of this information. Therefore, the author, editors, and publisher shall have no liability to any person or entity with regard to claims, loss, or damage caused or alleged to be caused, directly or indirectly, by the use of information contained herein.

The inclusion in this book of any product in respect to which patent or trademark rights may exist shall not be deemed, and is not intended as, a grant of or authority to exercise any right or privilege protected by such patent or trademark. All such rights or trademarks are vested in the patent or trademark owner, and no other person may exercise the same without express permission, authority, or license secured from such patent or trademark owner.

The inclusion of a brand name does not mean the author, the editors, or the publisher has any particular knowledge that the brand listed has properties different from other brands of the same product, nor should its inclusion be interpreted as an endorsement by the author, the editors, or the publisher. Similarly, the fact that a particular brand has not been included does not indicate the product has been judged to be in any way unsatisfactory or unacceptable. Further, no official support or endorsement of this book by any federal or state agency or pharmaceutical company is intended or inferred.

The Art, Science, and Technology of Pharmaceutical Compounding

FIFTH EDITION

Loyd V. Allen Jr., PhD

EDITOR IN CHIEF
International Journal of Pharmaceutical Compounding
Edmond, Oklahoma

and

PROFESSOR EMERITUS
College of Pharmacy
University of Oklahoma
Oklahoma City, Oklahoma

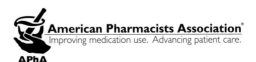

American Pharmacists Association®
Improving medication use. Advancing patient care.
APhA

Washington, D.C.

Acquisition Editor	Julian I. Graubart
Production Editor	Mary-Ann B. Moalli, Publications Professionals LLC
Proofreader	Nora Mara, Publications Professionals LLC
Cover Design	Scott Neitzke, APhA Integrated Design and Production Center
Composition	Circle Graphics
Indexing	Mary Coe

Published by the
American Pharmacists Association
2215 Constitution Avenue, NW
Washington, DC 20037-2985

APhA was founded in 1852 as the American Pharmaceutical Association.

To comment on this book via e-mail, send your message to the publisher at aphabooks@aphanet.org.

Library of Congress Cataloging-in-Publication Data

Names: Allen, Loyd V., Jr., author. | American Pharmacists Association, issuing body.
Title: The art, science, and technology of pharmaceutical compounding / Loyd V. Allen Jr.
Description: Fifth edition. | Washington, D.C. : American Pharmacists Association, [2016] | Includes bibliographical references and index.
Identifiers: LCCN 2016018808 | ISBN 9781582122632
Subjects: | MESH: Drug Compounding | Dosage Forms
Classification: LCC RS200 | NLM QV 779 | DDC 615/.19—dc23 LC record available at https://lccn.loc.gov/2016018808

How to Order This Book

Online: www.pharmacist.com/shop
By phone: 800-878-0729 (770-280-0085 from outside the United States)
VISA®, MasterCard®, and American Express® cards accepted

Contents

APPENDIXES

Sample Formulations

Sample formulations included in this edition of *The Art, Science, and Technology of Pharmaceutical Compounding*, grouped primarily by dosage form, are listed in the order in which they appear in the book.

Powders and Granules

Capsules

Tablets

Lozenges, Troches, and Films

Emulsions

Foams

Ointments, Creams, and Pastes

Gels

Veterinary Preparations

Preface to the Fifth Edition

Compounding is constantly changing, and compounding today is not the same as it was yesterday! Just since the fourth edition, the Drug Quality and Security Act (H.R. 3204) was passed, resulting in a new "category" of compounding pharmacy. The section 503A traditional compounding pharmacies are now accompanied by the new section 503B outsourcing pharmacies designed to address the issue of drug shortages.

On any given day in recent years, 200 to 300 or even more drugs may be in short supply. They range from drug products to sterile vehicles, including 0.9% sodium chloride injection. In many cases, compounding pharmacies have been able to fill the gap when a drug product is unavailable because of shortages. Also, compounding pharmacies continue to fill in for the many thousands of drug products that have been discontinued for economic reasons but are still needed by physicians and patients.

In this fifth edition, numerous changes and additions are as follows:

1. All chapters have been updated and several significantly revised.
2. Three new chapters have been added:
   - Chapter 20, Foams
   - Chapter 28, Compounding with Special Ingredients
   - Chapter 33, Pharmaceutical Compounding Errors
3. Information on the new law affecting compounding, the Drug Quality and Security Act, is incorporated throughout the book, especially in Chapter 1.
4. Chapter 3, Compounding with Hazardous Drugs, has been extensively updated.
5. Information on compounding films has been added to Chapter 14, Lozenges, Troches, and Films.
6. Uses for the individual ingredients are provided in the sample formulations.
7. References to the *United States Pharmacopeia/National Formulary (USP/NF)* now state the "current edition" and not a specific year, page number, and so on. The rationale for this change is that the current edition is the only official edition and must be used.

In summary, pharmaceutical compounding continues to grow. However, proper training is vitally important. One should not enter into compounding without it because errors will occur and may result in harm to patients. A compounding pharmacist brings clinical pharmacy to reality because of the requirements of working hand in hand with a physician and a patient to provide individualized medications for complete pharmaceutical care.

April 2016

Preface to the Fourth Edition

The practice of pharmacy compounding continues to grow. Factors contributing to the expanding role of the compounding pharmacist in health care include drug shortages, the discontinuation of drug products, the lack of pediatric formulations, hospitals' outsourcing of compounding through contracts with independent and specialty pharmacies, veterinary compounding, the need for alternative drug delivery and for dosage adjustment, and the use of short-dated (unstable) drugs.

Recent court decisions have upheld previous rulings that the Food and Drug Administration has no authority over compounding pharmacies that practice in compliance with state laws and regulations; pharmacy compounding is governed by the laws of the individual states through the state boards of pharmacy. More state boards of pharmacy are integrating *United States Pharmacopeia (USP)* General Chapters <795> and <797> either by reference or by direct incorporation into their regulations.

At a recent International Society of Pharmaceutical Compounding seminar in Tampa, Florida, speakers from around the world explained in detail the compounding activities in their countries. In addition, the regulatory, political, and social framework in which compounding is done was presented. Compounding is truly a worldwide activity that involves individualizing patient care with personalized medications.

In recent years, some colleges and schools of pharmacy have been enhancing their offerings in the area of compounding. Some are developing centers for compounding to train undergraduate and graduate pharmacists, provide continuing education, and conduct research. In some universities, this is being financially supplemented by alumni who have been successful in compounding pharmacy.

To the profession and those involved in compounding, the needs are quite evident:

1. Stability studies on several thousand compounded formulations need to be conducted to enable the publication of uniform formulations in the *United States Pharmacopeia/National Formulary* for continuity and uniformity of compounded preparations.
2. Continuing-education courses with laboratory experience need to be developed for pharmacists in practice who did not receive adequate training in compounding or wish to enhance their skills. Many pharmacists desire to incorporate compounding into their practices but lack the basic or advanced skills to do so.

3. The curriculum of many colleges of pharmacy needs to be modified to incorporate additional pharmaceutical and medicinal chemistry, pharmaceutics, pharmacy calculations, and other activities directly related to compounding.

4. Political and social issues need to be addressed by all the major professional pharmacy organizations to enable pharmacists to be reimbursed for compounded preparations so they can provide the needed care for their patients.

5. *USP* Chapters <795> and <797> need to be fully implemented in all pharmacies nationwide, regardless of whether individual state boards of pharmacy require that.

6. Use of the Biopharmaceutical Classification System (BCS classification) in compounding to identify and resolve potential problem areas of drug bioavailability should be considered.

7. Clinical pharmacokinetic studies need to be conducted on numerous compounded formulations that are widely used.

8. It needs to be recognized that the development of standardized *USP* monographs with stability studies is the fastest way to resolve the pediatric formulation situation.

New in this fourth edition are a chapter on ingredients and the factors required to ensure use of the proper quantity of drug so the proper dose will be administered; additional information on compounding for special population groups, including patients with ketogenic diets, allergies, and nasogastric tubes; information on hazardous drugs; and a discussion of accreditation standards. In addition, the text has been updated throughout.

December 2011

Preface to the Third Edition

Much has happened in pharmaceutical compounding during the past 5 years. Two court decisions have supported pharmacists' right to compound; many state boards of pharmacy have updated and strengthened their regulations concerning compounding; the United States Pharmacopeial Convention (USP) has introduced new standards; and opportunities for the compounding pharmacist have expanded.

On April 29, 2002, the U.S. Supreme Court decided in favor of a group of pharmacists who had challenged Section 503a of the Food and Drug Administration Modernization Act relating to compounding—specifically, the part of the act restricting advertising. The high court found this portion of the act to be nonseverable from the rest of the section, so the entire section of 503a related to compounding was thrown out. In addition, in the *Midland* decision, a U.S. district court found in favor of a group of pharmacists who had filed a lawsuit against the Food and Drug Administration stating that the agency had no jurisdiction over the practice of pharmacy compounding as long as it complied with the laws and regulations of the individual state.

As a result of new USP standards related to compounding, many states are rewriting and expanding their laws and regulations related to compounding. Additional quality initiatives and standards are likely to be developed for several years to come in response to the new USP standards.

Furthermore, new opportunities for compounding continue to arise as manufacturers discontinue products; few new drug products are marketed in pediatric dosage forms; home health care, the geriatric population, and veterinary compounding continue to expand; and currently compounded dosage forms undergo modifications to enhance patient compliance and meet the requirements of prescribers.

Presentations on compounding at national meetings of both pharmacy and medical organizations also reflect the growth of compounding. It appears that most physicians do prescribe compounded medications.

Other areas of growth are reflected in the new chapters included in this edition: Compounding for Terrorist Attacks and Natural Disasters, Compounding with Hazardous Drugs, and Cosmetics for Special Populations and for Use as Vehicles. The chapter on terrorist attack and natural disasters describes how compounding can play an important role during events that disrupt the routine supply of medications. The cosmetics compounding chapter reflects the growing need for cosmetics that do not contain allergens that may be present in commercially available products.

A noteworthy occurrence over the past 5 years has been the establishment and implementation of the Pharmacy Compounding Accreditation Board. With the involvement and support of eight national pharmacy organizations, this group surveys and accredits select pharmacies that have worked to meet the new, enhanced compounding standards.

The expansion of pharmacy compounding is also evidenced by the growth of companies providing support, equipment, supplies, and material for compounding pharmacies. Furthermore, many pharmacy journals are increasing their coverage of compounding.

Pharmacy compounding is growing not only in the United States but throughout the world. The International Society of Pharmaceutical Compounding held its first symposium at the International Pharmaceutical Federation (FIP) meeting in Salvador Bahia, Brazil, in 2006, with great attendance and presentations on compounding in many countries. Future meetings in Spain, the United States, and other countries are planned.

Compounding pharmacists continue to be leaders in the implementation of pharmaceutical care. New models are being developed, refined, and shared in meetings and through other means of communication. Computerized databases now provide compounding pharmacists throughout the world with thousands of formulas, physicochemical data, and standard operating procedures. A daily list server enables pharmacists to share their questions and ideas related to compounding.

The technological, pharmaceutical, medical, and social aspects of pharmaceutical compounding will continue to change. As pharmacogenomics becomes a more important part of medical practice, compounding pharmacists should be able to meet the specific needs of individual patients—a longtime goal of pharmacy and medicine.

September 2007

Preface to the Second Edition

The phenomenal growth of pharmaceutical compounding in recent years has been spurred by several simultaneous events. First, the number of discontinued drug products continues to increase. A number of reasons contribute to this increase, including low profits on certain products that are ultimately discontinued, difficulty in manufacturing and formulation processes that lead to a decision to discontinue the product, and the difficulty in obtaining—including importing—certain raw materials used in some commercial products. Despite the reason for discontinuing a product, patients still need the medication; fortunately, in most cases, pharmacists can compound these preparations.

Second, physicians are becoming more aware of use in other parts of the world of various drugs and dosage forms that are not produced and marketed here in the United States. To obtain these preparations, U.S. physicians turn to pharmacists in many cases.

Third, many physicians have patients who can benefit from new drugs or new drug applications. The physicians work with compounding pharmacists to formulate the preparations.

Fourth, the incidence of drug shortages has been increasing in recent years. This increase may be caused by several factors, including just-in-time manufacturing, miscalculations of actual drug usage rates, and difficulty in obtaining some imported raw materials.

We are now in an era of increased emphasis on quality and documentation of compounded formulations. Therefore, it is incumbent on all pharmacists who compound to be intimately familiar with General Chapter <795>, Pharmacy Compounding, of the *United States Pharmacopeia 25/National Formulary 20*. Pharmacists—as well as all personnel involved in compounding—should be trained in the principles outlined in this chapter and should practice within its guidelines.

Colleges and schools of pharmacy are beginning to reinstate laboratory classes in the curriculum; these classes are important as pharmacy compounding requires a strong scientific base in inorganic and organic chemistry, physical pharmacy, pharmaceutics, natural products chemistry, biochemistry, and other physical and life sciences. Approximately 75% of the colleges and schools of pharmacy now have some students who receive specialized training from the compounding support industry.

Compounding of sterile products also continues to grow and should be done only by pharmacists who have been properly trained and validated in aseptic processing. Some states already require specific annual training by pharmacists involved in compounding sterile preparations. Recent activities related to the Food and Drug Administration Modernization Act of 1997 have served to document the importance of pharmacy compounding and the need for it. The Food and Drug Administration (FDA) recognizes the importance of and supports the ability of pharmacists to compound specific preparations for individual patients. FDA is working closely with the United States Pharmacopeia in continuing to enhance the quality of compounded preparations.

In summary, as this second edition is prepared, pharmacy compounding has regained a place of prominence and importance in the overall provision of pharmaceutical products, patient services, and pharmaceutical care. After all, individualization of individual prescriptions through pharmacy compounding is the actualization of providing total pharmaceutical care.

May 2002

Preface to the First Edition

Historically, compounding has been an integral part of pharmacy practice, as shown by the following definitions and references to pharmacy.

- Pharmacy is the art or practice of preparing and preserving drugs, and of compounding and dispensing medicines according to the prescriptions of physicians.[1]
- Pharmacy is (1) the art, practice, or profession of preparing, preserving, compounding, and dispensing medical drugs and (2) a place where medicines are compounded or dispensed.[2]
- Pharmacy is the science, art, and practice of preparing, preserving, compounding, and dispensing medicinal drugs and of giving instructions for their use.[3]

Compounding is a professional prerogative that pharmacists have performed since the beginning of the profession. Even today, definitions of pharmacy include the "preparation of drugs."[4,5]

The heritage of pharmacy, spanning some 5000 years, has centered on providing pharmaceutical products for patients. Pharmacists are the only health professionals who possess the knowledge and skill required to compound and prepare medications to meet the unique needs of patients.

Compounding Yesterday

The apothecary is listed in the Bible as one of the earliest trades or professions. As one reads through the Bible, it is evident that people experienced pain, disease, and suffering and that they used medicines of various types for healing:

> "And thou shalt make it an oil of holy ointment, an ointment compound after *the art of the apothecary:* it shall be an holy anointing oil." Exodus 30:25 [emphasis added]

> "Dead flies cause *the ointment of the apothecary* to send forth a stinking savour; so doth a little folly him that is in reputation for wisdom and honour." Ecclesiastes 10:1 [emphasis added]

"From the sole of the foot even unto the head there is no soundness in it, *but wounds, and bruises, and putrifying sores;* they have not been closed, neither bound up, neither mollified with ointment." Isaiah 1:6 [emphasis added]

"And by the river upon the bank thereof, on this side and on that side, shall grow all trees for meat, whose leaf shall not fade, neither shall the fruit thereof be consumed; it shall bring forth new fruit according to his months, because their waters they issued out of the sanctuary; and the fruit thereof shall be for meat, and *the leaf thereof for medicine.*" Ezekiel 47:12 [emphasis added]

In many cases, the medicines used were either topical ointments or products such as wines and plant extracts that were taken internally. The apothecary was noted for the mixing of perfumes, ointments, and some medicines, and the physician was noted for taking care of the sick. In some cases, the same individual performed both functions. The heritage of the compounding pharmacist is well documented throughout history as one involved in preparing products used for treatment of disease and for cosmetic purposes.

Compounding Today

Prescription compounding is a rapidly growing component of pharmacy practice. This change can be attributed to a number of factors, including individualized patient therapy, lack of commercially available products, home health care, intravenous admixture programs, total parenteral nutrition programs, and problem solving for the physician and patient to enhance compliance with a specific therapeutic regimen. Pharmacists are creative and should have the ability to formulate patient-specific preparations for providing pharmaceutical care.

An article by Angel d'Angelo, RPh, editor of the *U.S. Pharmacist,* explains that compounding is our heritage. There is no other professional license that allows for the extemporaneous compounding of therapeutic agents. Complete pharmaceutical care must involve the dosage form, which might necessitate compounding a patient-specific form not available commercially—possibly the compounding of a preparation without a preservative or a specific allergy-producing excipient that must be removed from the formulation. With pharmacokinetic services, the need for individualized dosage units will be required more frequently to meet these patient-specific needs. Pharmacists who compound have a desirable and needed skill.[6]

Pharmacy is united in the sense that pharmacists have a responsibility to serve their patients and to compound an appropriately prescribed product in the course of their professional practice. It is the right and responsibility of pharmacists to compound medications to meet the specific needs of patients. Pharmacists are ultimately responsible for the integrity of the finished product prepared by them or under their immediate supervision.

Pharmacists are the only health professionals formally trained in the art and science of compounding medications. Consequently, they are expected to possess the knowledge and skills necessary to compound extemporaneous preparations. In 1995, compounded prescriptions represented approximately 11% of all prescriptions dispensed,[7] which is a fivefold to tenfold increase in the percentage of such prescriptions dispensed in the 1970s and 1980s. It is evident that the need for individualized drug therapy for patients has been realized and is resulting in patient-specific prescriptions and the compounding of medications that are not commercially available.

The purpose of this book is (1) to provide a basic foundation of knowledge that will enable pharmacists to sharpen their skills in compounding pharmacy, (2) to serve as an educational tool for those pharmacists who did not receive instruction in compounding in colleges or schools of pharmacy, and (3) to become a textbook for current pharmacy students taking courses in pharmaceutical compounding. This first edition of the book serves as a basic text; it will be revised and developed in greater depth with future editions.

The support of Paddock Laboratories in developing some of the materials used in this book is gratefully acknowledged. Some material was originally published or adapted from materials published in the *Secundum Artem* series by Paddock Laboratories, Inc., of Minneapolis, Minnesota. Other material, including the cover design, has been adapted from the *International Journal of Pharmaceutical Compounding* (*IJPC*), a bimonthly professional and scientific journal devoted to pharmaceutical compounding and published in Edmond, Oklahoma. Photographs of compounding equipment were graciously supplied by the Professional Compounding Centers of America, Inc. The use of these materials is sincerely appreciated.

1998

References

1. *Webster's Revised Unabridged Dictionary of the English Language.* Springfield, Mass: G & C Merriam Co; 1913:1075.
2. *Webster's Tenth New Collegiate Dictionary.* Springfield, Mass: Merriam Webster, Inc; 1993:871.
3. *International Dictionary of Medicine and Biology.* Vol. III. New York: John Wiley and Sons; 1986.
4. *The Compact Oxford English Dictionary.* 2nd ed. New York: Oxford University Press Inc; 1991.
5. *American Heritage Dictionary of the English Language.* 3rd ed. 1992, in electronic form in Microsoft Bookshelf '95. 1995.
6. Angel d'Angelo. Compounding: our heritage. *Int J Pharm Compound.* 1997;1(4):286.
7. Ray Gosselin. Pharmaceutical care: part of TQM? *Drug Topics.* July 10, 1995;139(13):10.

Introduction

Pharmacists are unique professionals who are well trained in the natural, physical, and medical sciences and aware that a single mistake in the daily practice of their profession may potentially result in patient harm and even death. However, because of their demonstrated expertise, their demeanor, and the manner in which they have practiced their profession over the years, pharmacists continue to be ranked among the most respected individuals in our society. In general, pharmacists have the reputation of being available to residents of the local community in times of need, interacting with and providing needed medications for patients, and working with patients to regain or maintain a certain standard of health or quality of life.

Pharmacists possess knowledge and skills that are not duplicated by any other profession. Their roles can include dispensing and compounding medications, counseling patients, minimizing medication errors, enhancing patient compliance, monitoring drug therapy, and minimizing drug expenditures.

Pharmacy activities that individualize patient therapy include clinical and compounding functions. The functions are related and equally important to the success of such activities. A pharmacist's expertise must be used to adjust dosage quantities, frequencies, and even dosage forms for enhanced compliance. All pharmacists should be aware of the drug therapy options provided by compounding. Members of the pharmacy profession are united in the belief that they have a responsibility to serve their patients and compound an appropriately prescribed product in the course of professional practice. Pharmacists have both the right and the responsibility to compound medications (sterile and nonsterile) to meet the specific needs of patients.

What Is Compounding?

The definition of compounding has been the subject of much discussion and has been addressed by the United States Pharmacopeia, the standards-setting body for pharmaceuticals in the United States.

Compounding is defined in Chapter <795> of the *United States Pharmacopeia* as follows:

> The preparation, mixing, assembling, altering, packaging, and labeling of a drug, drug-delivery device, or device in accordance with a licensed practitioner's prescription, medication order, or initiative based on the

practitioner/patient/pharmacist/compounder relationship in the course of professional practice. Compounding includes the following:

- Preparation of drug dosage forms for both human and animal patients
- Preparation of drugs or devices in anticipation of prescription drug orders based on routine, regularly observed prescribing patterns
- Reconstitution or manipulation of commercial products that may require the addition of one or more ingredients
- Preparation of drugs or devices for the purposes of, or as an incident to, research (clinical or academic), teaching, or chemical analysis
- Preparation of drugs and devices for prescriber's office use where permitted by federal and state law[1]

The Drug Quality and Security Act (H.R. 3204) defines compounding as "the combining, admixing, mixing, diluting, pooling, reconstituting, or otherwise altering of a drug or bulk drug substance to create a drug."

Compounding may hold different meanings for different pharmacists. It may mean the preparation of suspensions, topicals, and suppositories; the conversion of one dose (e.g., oral to rectal, injection to oral) or dosage form into another; the preparation of select dosage forms from bulk chemicals; the preparation of intravenous admixtures, parenteral nutrition solutions, and pediatric dosage forms from adult dosage forms; the preparation of radioactive isotopes; or the preparation of cassettes, syringes, and other devices with drugs for administration in the home setting.

Compounding occurs in all different types of pharmacies, including the following:

- Independent community pharmacies
- Chain pharmacies
- Hospital pharmacies
- Mail-order pharmacies
- *Compounding-only* pharmacies
  - Independent (human and veterinary)
  - Specialty (home health care, hospital contract, etc.)
- Nuclear pharmacies

Compounding is especially important to select patient-group populations, including those with needs related to pediatrics, geriatrics, bioidentical hormone replacement therapy, pain management, dentistry, environmental and cosmetic sensitivities, sports injuries, and veterinary compounding (small and large animals, herds, exotic and companion animals).

Reasons for the increase in compounding can be related to the following:

- Limited dosage forms
- Limited strengths
- Home health care
- Hospice
- Unavailable drug products and combinations
  - Discontinued drugs
  - Drug shortages
- Orphan drugs
- Veterinary compounding

- New therapeutic approaches
- Special patient populations
- Biotechnology-derived drug products

A pharmacist plays an important role on the hospice team and can greatly enhance quality of life for hospice patients. Pediatric patient compliance is a challenge, because children either do not want or are unable to take tablets or capsules and manufacturers do not provide liquid dosage forms for many medications; this is where a pharmacist steps in. Compounding for the geriatric patient can be a much greater challenge than for almost any other group of patients. Physical, emotional, and social difficulties often affect compliance, and many geriatric health problems are chronic rather than acute. Pharmacists have also become intimately involved in working with veterinarians in the treatment of animals (companion, herd, recreational, food, and exotic).

Compounding has always been a basic part of pharmacy practice; today it continues to be a rapidly growing area, and many pharmacists in all types of practice are becoming involved in compounding sterile and nonsterile preparations. Newly evolving dosage forms and therapeutic approaches suggest that compounding of pharmaceuticals and related products specifically for individual patients will become more common in pharmacy practice in the years ahead.

Approximately 75% of community pharmacists, virtually all hospitals, many chain store and mail-order pharmacies, and many specialty pharmacies compound. Nonsterile or sterile compounding is involved in about 10% of all prescribed and ordered medications today, and compounding is valued up to about $25 billion to $30 billion a year.

Compounding pharmacy is unique because it allows pharmacists to use more of their scientific, mathematical, and technology background than do some other types of practices. Compounding pharmacists develop a unique relationship with the patients they serve. They work hand in hand with physicians to solve clinical problems not addressed by commercially available dosage forms. Ironically, as we in health care become more aware that patients are individuals, respond as individuals, and must be treated as individuals, some health care providers appear to be grouping patients into categories for treatment, for reimbursement from third-party payers, or for a determination of levels of care in managed care organizations. Similarly, the trend toward using pharmaceutical manufacturers' fixed-dose products, which are available just because the marketing demand is sufficiently high to justify their manufacture and production, seems inappropriate. Since when should the availability, or lack of availability, of a specific commercially available product dictate the therapy of a patient?

Should Every Pharmacist Compound?

Only properly trained pharmacists should be involved in pharmaceutical compounding. If pharmacists wish to compound but do not possess the required techniques and skills, they should participate in continuing education programs that have been designed to provide the proper training, including the scientific basis and practical skills necessary for sound, contemporary compounding. Today, any pharmacist is legally qualified to compound, but not all are technically qualified and trained to be a compounding pharmacist. To be capable of meeting the special or advanced needs of today's patients, whether human or animal, a compounding pharmacist must

- Have access to the most recent information available,
- Maintain an inventory and provide for proper storage of drugs and flavoring agents and be capable of obtaining any chemical within a reasonable time,

- Be dedicated to pharmacy and willing to put forth the necessary financial and time investment,
- Have the appropriate physical facilities and equipment to do the job properly (the extent and type of compounding may be determined or limited by the facility),
- Be committed to lifelong learning and continuing education, because a major advantage of compounded prescriptions is their provision of treatments that are new, undeveloped, and often not commercially available, and
- Have a willingness to tear down walls and build bridges to share experiences with others for the good of all.

Should You Compound?

When considering whether or not to compound, pharmacists should consider the technical aspects and economic effect of the service. A new chapter has been added to this edition of the text, "Pharmaceutical Compounding Errors," Chapter 33. The purpose of this chapter is to assist in making one aware of potential errors that can occur in compounding.

Technical Considerations

There are three types of compounded prescriptions: isolated, routine, and batch prepared. An isolated prescription is one that a pharmacist is not expecting to receive and does not expect to receive again. A routine prescription is one that a pharmacist may expect to receive on a routine basis in the future; there may be some benefit in standardizing such preparations (maintaining preparation protocols on file) to ensure product quality. A batch-prepared prescription is one that is prepared in multiple identical units as a single operation in anticipation of the receipt of future prescriptions.

Pharmacists must consider not only their technical qualifications to compound a preparation, but also the technical validity of the prescription. Box I-1 presents a series of questions designed to aid in evaluating the technical considerations for compounding. The batch compounding of sterile preparations, especially in the hospital and home health care environments, has increased noticeably. There are a number of reasons for this increase, including the following:

- The changing patterns of drug therapy, such as home parenteral therapy and patient-controlled parenteral administration
- The use in hospitals of injectable drugs that are not commercially available to meet individual patient needs or the prescriber's clinical investigational protocols
- Cost containment, whereby a pharmacy batch produces drug products that are intended to be similar to commercially available products

Batch compounding can reduce the cost of a medication that must be taken over a long period or continuously for a chronic condition. This process allows a patient to store the preparation at home and reduce the number of pharmacy visits. Pharmacists who choose to perform batch compounding should be capable and willing to do it properly, particularly when sterile drug products are involved (see Box I-2).

Economic Considerations

Several economic considerations must be weighed when making the decision to compound prescriptions, including a pharmacist's compensation for the service and the effect of the service on health care costs. Both factors are equally important.

BOX I-1 Technical Considerations for Compounding a Prescription

The following are technical considerations for compounding a prescription:

- Is the preparation commercially available in the exact dosage form, strength, and packaging?
- Is the prescription rational concerning the ingredients, intended use, dose, and method of administration?
- Are the physical, chemical, and therapeutic properties of the individual ingredients consistent with the expected properties of the ordered preparation?
- Will this compounded preparation satisfy the intent of the prescribing physician and meet the needs of the patient?
- Is there an alternative (e.g., different dosage form, different route of administration) by which the patient will receive a benefit?
- Is there a bona fide prescriber–pharmacist–patient relationship?
- Can ingredient identity, quality, and purity be assured?
- Does the pharmacist have the training and expertise required to prepare the prescription?
- Are the proper equipment, supplies, and chemicals or drugs available?
- Is there a literature reference that might provide information on use, preparation, stability, administration, and storage of the compounded preparation?
- Can the pharmacist perform the necessary calculations to compound the preparation?
- Can the pharmacist project a reasonable and rational beyond-use date for the prescription?
- Is the pharmacist willing to complete the necessary documentation to compound the preparation?
- Can the pharmacist do some basic quality control to check the preparation before dispensing (e.g., capsule weight variation, pH, visual observations)?
- What procedures are in place for investigating and correcting failures?
- How long will the patient be using the preparation, and is the expected duration of therapy consistent with an appropriate expiration date? Alternatively, should the preparation be compounded in small quantities and dispensed to the patient at short intervals?
- Does the patient have the necessary storage facility, if required, to ensure the potency of the preparation until its beyond-use date?

Pharmaceutical compounding is a cognitive service; therefore, appropriate reimbursement is justified. The pricing of a compounded prescription should account for pharmacodynamic and pharmacotherapeutic decision making, formulation expertise, time involved, and reimbursement for materials. Compounding prescriptions can be attractive for a pharmacist both professionally and financially. Historically, compounding has been said to be an act whereby the professional and scientific knowledge of a pharmacist can find its expression. For those pharmacists dedicated to performing quality compounding, the professional, psychological, and financial rewards can be substantial.

Compounding prescriptions can be one way of lowering the cost of drug therapy. In some cases, a pharmacist's preparation of a specific prescription for a patient may be less

---

BOX I-2 Technical Considerations for Batch Compounding

The following are technical considerations for batch compounding:

- Will the processes, procedures, compounding environment, and equipment used to prepare this batch produce the expected qualities in the finished preparation?
- Will all the critical processes and procedures be carried out exactly as intended so that every batch produces the same high-quality preparation?
- Will the finished preparation have all the qualities as specified on completion and packaging of each batch?
- Will each batch retain all the qualities within the specified limits until the labeled expiration date?
- Will pharmacy personnel be able to monitor and trace the history of each batch, identify potential sources of problems, and institute appropriate corrective measures to minimize the likelihood of their occurrence?

---

expensive than a manufactured version, which may mean that the patient may actually obtain the drug rather than have to do without it. If compounding a prescription will enable a patient to afford the drug therapy, it must be considered.

Another way in which compounding may lower drug costs concerns the economic use of very expensive drug products that may have short shelf lives. If a patient does not need the entire contents of a vial or dosage unit, the remaining drug product is often discarded and wasted. In numerous instances, however, a pharmacist can divide the commercial product into smaller usage units, store it properly, and dispense the required quantity on individual prescriptions.

A related economic question involves the commercialization of compounded preparations. Over the years, many compounded preparations have eventually become commercially available. Table I-1 lists commercial products recently introduced to the market. Inevitably, a pharmaceutical manufacturer will produce a product when it becomes economically profitable to do so.

Summary

Compounding pharmacists are interested in and excited about their practice. In fact, many pharmacists intimately involved in pharmaceutical care have come to realize the importance of providing individualized patient care through the compounding of patient-specific preparations. As compounding pharmacy continues to grow, it will provide an opportunity for more pharmacists to use their innovative skills to solve patients' drug problems.

Pharmaceutical compounding provides pharmacists with a unique opportunity to practice their time-honored profession. It will become an even more important part of pharmacy practice in the future, particularly for those involved in community, hospital, long-term care, home health care, veterinary care, and specialty practices.

Although pharmacists should not hesitate to become involved in pharmacy compounding, they should be aware of the requirements for and uniqueness of formulating a specific drug product for a specific patient. This service is an important component in

TABLE I-1 Compounded Preparations That Are Now Commercially Manufactured

Aminopyridine (4-) capsules (fampridine)

Bevacizumab (Avastin—new packaging to Lucentis)

Buffered hypertonic saline solution

Buprenorphine nasal spray

Clindamycin topical solution

Colchicine injection

Colchicine tablets (Colcrys)

Dalfampridine (Ampyra) tablets

Dextromethorphan hydrobromide with quinidine sulfate capsules (Nuedexta)

Diazepam rectal gel (Diastat)

Erythromycin topical solution

Estradiol topical gel

Fentanyl lozenges

Fentanyl sublingual spray

Hydroxyprogesterone caproate injection (Makena)

Minoxidil topical solution

Nitroglycerin rectal ointment

Nystatin lozenges

Omeprazole and sodium bicarbonate liquid (Zegerid)

Premixed intravenous solutions (select ones)

Progesterone vaginal gel (Crinone)

Quinine sulfate capsules

Testosterone topical gel (Androgel)

Tetracaine–adrenalin–cocaine (TAC) solution

---

providing pharmaceutical care. After all, without the pharmaceutical product, there is no pharmaceutical care.

Reference

1. National Association of Boards of Pharmacy. Model State Pharmacy Act and Model Rules of the National Association of Boards of Pharmacy. Available at: www.nabp.net/publications/model-act. Accessed: September 22, 2015.

Abbreviations and Approximate Solubility Descriptors

Container Specifications

Tightly closed	T
Well-closed	W
Light-resistant	LR

Solubility Parameters

Very soluble	VS
Freely soluble	FS
Soluble	Sol
Sparingly soluble	SpS
Slightly soluble	SlS
Very slightly soluble	VSS
Partially soluble	PartSol
Practically insoluble	PrIn
Insoluble	IS
Miscible	Misc
Immiscible	Immisc
Partially miscible	PartMisc
Dispersible	Disp
Swells	Swells

Approximate Solubility Descriptors

Descriptive Term	Parts of Solvent Required for 1 Part of Solute
Very soluble	Less than 1
Freely soluble	From 1 to 10
Soluble	From 10 to 30
Sparingly soluble	From 30 to 100
Slightly soluble	From 100 to 1000
Very slightly soluble	From 1000 to 10,000
Practically insoluble or insoluble	10,000 and greater

Source: United States Pharmacopeial Convention. General Notices. In: *United States Pharmacopeia/National Formulary*. Rockville, MD: United States Pharmacopeial Convention.

Chapter 1

Laws, Regulations, Standards, and Guidelines for Compounding Practices

Compounding is an integral part of pharmacy practice and is essential to the provision of health care. Compounding is defined in the Introduction to this book according to Chapter <795> of the *United States Pharmacopeia (USP)*[1] and the definitions in the Drug Quality and Security Act (H.R. 3204, 113th Cong., 2013).

Compounding can be as simple as the addition of a liquid to a manufactured drug powder or as complex as the preparation of a multicomponent parenteral nutrition solution. In general, compounding differs from manufacturing in that compounding involves a specific practitioner–patient–pharmacist relationship, the preparation of a relatively small quantity of medication, and different conditions of sale (i.e., specific prescription orders). The section, "Distinguishing Compounding from Manufacturing," later in this chapter, more fully defines compounding and manufacturing and provides guidelines for differentiating the two activities.

A pharmacist is responsible for compounding preparations of acceptable strength, quality, and purity, with appropriate packaging and labeling in accordance with good pharmacy practices, official standards, and current scientific principles. Pharmacists should continually expand their compounding knowledge by participating in seminars, studying current literature, and consulting with colleagues.

Regulatory Framework

In general, professions such as medicine and pharmacy are established as legal entities within a state by the professional practice acts of that state that are enacted by the state lawmakers (legislature). Once a profession is established, the state legislatures enact laws to govern its practice. The lawmakers also establish a governing board to oversee the practice of the profession in their state. In some states, the governing board may oversee more than one profession. Usually, the board creates regulations to govern the practice. Although a state's laws must be changed by the legislature, regulations can be changed by the state boards.

Physicians are regulated by state boards of medicine that govern practice by enacting and enforcing regulations and disciplining practitioners who do not abide by the laws and regulations. Similarly, state boards of pharmacy govern pharmacy practice by enacting and enforcing regulations and disciplining practitioners who do not abide by the laws and regulations. In addition to state laws and regulations, pharmacists must comply with various standards of practice, including those in *USP* Chapter <795>, Pharmaceutical Compounding—Nonsterile Preparations, and *USP* Chapter <797>, Pharmaceutical Compounding—Sterile Preparations, when these standards are addressed by the individual state board of pharmacy.

Since 1820, a nongovernmental organization, the United States Pharmacopeial Convention (USP), has established some of the standards of quality for compounded and manufactured pharmaceuticals and published them in its compendium, the *United States Pharmacopeia*. In the 1906 Federal Food and Drugs Act, both the *USP* and the *National Formulary (NF)* were designated as official compendia of the United States, and this designation has been reaffirmed since that time. The state boards of pharmacy can be responsible for enforcing these standards, because the USP has no enforcement powers.

The 1906 Federal Food and Drugs Act prohibited the sale of adulterated or misbranded drugs, but it did not require that drugs be approved by any agency. The U.S. Food and Drug Administration (FDA) was formally organized in 1938 under the Federal Food, Drug, and Cosmetic Act; this law required FDA to approve marketed drugs on the basis of safety. In 1962, the Kefauver-Harris Amendments required that marketed drugs (those approved by FDA) also be effective. Thus, FDA is responsible for ensuring the safety and effectiveness of manufacturers' marketed drugs.

FDA was established in part to monitor the relatively young pharmaceutical industry, which had no enforceable standards at the time. The Federal Food, Drug, and Cosmetic Act does not refer to pharmaceutical compounding. Court decisions have stated that FDA lacks authority over a pharmacy's compounding that is performed in compliance with the pharmacy practice laws of the state. However, some specific criteria of the Drug Quality and Security Act must be met as described later in this chapter; if not, then FDA may become involved.

Compounding has long been recognized as a legal and vitally important core component of traditional pharmacy practice. In 1938, the *USP* had already been providing compounding instructions for 118 years. Compounding occupied such an important role in U.S. pharmacy practice in the early 20th century that a number of state pharmacy practice acts not only regulated compounding, but also specifically included the term *compounding*. Before 1938, states considered every location where compounding occurred and where drugs, medications, or chemicals were sold or dispensed to be a pharmacy. In other words, wherever compounding took place, the facility was termed a pharmacy and thus was subject to that state's pharmacy practice act.[2]

Furthermore, before 1938, states and the District of Columbia restricted the compounding, dispensing, or selling of drugs, medications, or poisons and the compounding of physicians' prescriptions to pharmacists or assistant pharmacists registered or licensed by the state board of pharmacy. However, a number of jurisdictions, while restricting pharmacy compounding (and other pharmacy practices) to registered or licensed pharmacists (or, in some cases, assistant pharmacists under the personal supervision of registered pharmacists), expressly noted that such restrictions did not apply to licensed medical practitioners compounding their own prescriptions. The states restricted persons who could engage in the activity to specific state-registered or state-licensed health professionals.

As further evidence of the importance of compounding to pharmacy practice, by 1938 a number of states required applicants for pharmacist registration and licensure to prove they had spent specific amounts of time gaining practical experience in locations where drugs, medications, and poisons were compounded, dispensed, and retailed and medical practitioners' prescriptions were compounded. The jurisdictions sought to ensure that a pharmacist had a certain amount of experience in compounding.

At that time, a number of jurisdictions allowed only licensed or registered pharmacists to operate pharmacies for retailing, dispensing, or compounding of drugs, medications, or poisons or for compounding of physicians' prescriptions. In addition, before 1938 the owner or manager of a pharmacy could not legally permit anyone but a licensed pharmacist to engage in pharmacy compounding.

Clearly, registered pharmacists were compounding drugs as part of their practice in 1938, and they have continued to do so since then. In 1938, pharmacists were compounding more than 250 million prescriptions annually, or approximately two prescriptions for every person in the United States. In 1940, the federal government recognized the importance of compounding in the practice of pharmacy within the armed forces and civil service. This began with the Durham-Reynolds Bill of 1943 (Public Law 130) establishing the Pharmacy Corps in the U.S. Army. Compounding was the norm at large military posts; a number of products, such as cough syrups, irrigating solutions, and ointments, were routinely compounded.

The intent of the Federal Food, Drug, and Cosmetic Act had nothing to do with compounding. At the time of the act's passage, the state boards of pharmacy, pharmacists, and other health care professionals would have opposed any measure that attempted to ban pharmacy compounding. Congress did not intend to outlaw compounding any more than it intended to prohibit dispensing and selling of drugs, medications, and poisons, the other traditional pharmacy practices that were then, and are still, regulated by the states.

Unapproved Drugs

FDA looks at all unapproved drug products that are being marketed in the United States. This is of interest to compounding pharmacists because FDA has determined that compounded preparations are now considered "unapproved new drugs." In fact, any modification to a drug outside the approved labeling of a drug can be considered to be compounding.

The Federal Food and Drugs Act of 1906 first brought drug regulation under federal law. That act prohibited the sale of adulterated or misbranded drugs. The Federal Food, Drug, and Cosmetic Act of 1938 required that new drugs be approved for safety. As discussed below, the active ingredients of many drugs currently on the market were first introduced, at least in some form, before 1938.

Under the 1938 grandfather clause, a drug product that was on the market before passage of the 1938 act and that contained in its labeling the same representations concerning the conditions of use as it did before passage of that act was not considered a *new drug*. Therefore, it was exempt from the requirement of having an approved new drug application.

FDA estimates that several thousand unapproved drug products are currently being commercially manufactured and marketed. It also considers all compounded preparations as unapproved drugs; these include all intravenous admixtures in hospitals, pediatric oral liquids, pain management injections, and other preparations that are compounded. Thus, other agencies of the federal government—including the U.S. Department of Veterans Affairs, the Indian Health Service, all branches of the armed services, and the Federal Bureau of Prisons—are involved in compounding unapproved drugs. Many state agencies (e.g., hospitals, prisons, and welfare programs) also are involved in compounding unapproved drugs. In addition, most of the commercially manufactured veterinary drug products are not FDA approved; they are unapproved drugs. Nonprescription drug products are not FDA approved but follow the over-the-counter (OTC) monograph system that allows them to be manufactured if they comply with the OTC monographs.

Examples of drugs marketed before 1938 that were grandfathered and allowed to stay on the market as unapproved drugs are shown in Table 1-1.

Distinguishing Compounding from Manufacturing

Compounding is defined in the Introduction of this book. *Manufacturing* is the production, preparation, propagation, conversion, and processing of a drug or device, either directly or indirectly, through extraction from substances of natural origin or independently through means of chemical or biological synthesis; the term includes any packaging or repackaging of the substance(s) or labeling or relabeling of its container and the promotion and marketing of such drugs or devices. Manufacturing also includes the preparation and promotion

TABLE 1-1 Examples of Pre-1938 Drugs That Remained on the Market as Unapproved Drugs

Acetaminophen, codeine phosphate, and caffeine capsules and tablets	Levothyroxine sodium for injection
Amobarbital sodium capsules	Morphine sulfate oral solution and tablets
Amyl nitrate inhalant	Nitroglycerin sublingual tablets
Chloral hydrate capsules, syrup, and suppositories	Opium tincture
Codeine phosphate injection, oral solution, and tablets	Oxycodone tablets
	Oxycodone hydrochloride oral solution
Codeine sulfate tablets	Paregoric
Colchicine injection and tablets	Phenazopyridine hydrochloride tablets
Digitoxin tablets	Phenobarbital capsules, elixir, and tablets
Digoxin elixir and tablets	Phenobarbital sodium injection
Ephedrine sulfate capsules and injection	Pilocarpine hydrochloride ophthalmic solution
Ergonovine maleate injection and tablets	Potassium bicarbonate effervescent tablets for oral solution
Ergotamine tartrate tablets	Potassium chloride oral solution
Hydrocodone bitartrate tablets	Potassium gluconate elixir and tablets
Hydrocodone bitartrate, aspirin, and caffeine tablets	Potassium iodide oral solution
	Salsalate capsules
Hydromorphone hydrochloride suppositories	Sodium fluoride oral solution and tablets
	Thyroid tablets

of commercially available products from bulk compounds for resale by pharmacies, practitioners, or other persons.

Guidelines for distinguishing between compounding and manufacturing are as follows:

- Under certain situations (drug shortages, presence of excipients patients cannot tolerate, etc.), pharmacists may compound, in reasonable quantities, drug preparations that are commercially available in the marketplace if a pharmacist–patient–prescriber relationship exists and a valid prescription is presented.
- Pharmacists may compound nonprescription medications in commercially available dosage forms or in alternative dosage forms to accommodate patient needs as allowed by individual state boards of pharmacy.
- Pharmacists may compound drugs in limited quantities before receiving a valid prescription, on the basis of a history of receiving valid prescriptions that have been generated solely within an established pharmacist–patient–prescriber relationship, and provided that the prescriptions are maintained on file for all such preparations dispensed at the pharmacy.
- Pharmacists should not offer compounded medications to other pharmacies for resale. However, a practitioner may obtain compounded medication to administer to patients if allowed by state law, but it should be labeled with the following: "For Office Use Only"; date compounded; use-by date; and name, strength, and quantity of active ingredients. An exception to this may be the outsourcing of some compounded preparations by hospitals to contract compounding pharmacies.
- Compounding pharmacies and pharmacists may advertise or otherwise promote the fact that they provide prescription-compounding services.

FDA Modernization Act of 1997

In 1997, the efforts of many organizations, including FDA, politicians, and pharmacists resulted in section 503A of the Food and Drug Administration Modernization Act of 1997 (FDAMA97) (Public Law 105-115, § 127), supporting pharmacists' right to compound.

The purpose of section 127 of Public Law 105-115 was to ensure patient access to individualized drug therapy and prevent unnecessary FDA regulation of health professional practice. This legislation exempted pharmacy compounding from several regulatory requirements, but did not exempt drug manufacturing from the act's requirements. The legislation also set forth conditions that must be met in order to qualify for exemption from the act's requirements. Thus, compounding, according to FDAMA97, would exempt pharmacists from having to meet the *new drug* requirements for each preparation compounded.

In November 1998, the solicitation and advertising provisions of section 503A were challenged by seven compounding pharmacies as an impermissible regulation of commercial speech. The U.S. District Court for the District of Nevada ruled in the plaintiffs' favor. FDA appealed to the U.S. Court of Appeals for the Ninth Circuit. On February 6, 2001, the Court of Appeals declared section 503A invalid in its entirety (*Western States Medical Center v Shalala*, 238 F.3rd 1090 [9th Cir. 2001]). The U.S. Supreme Court affirmed the Court of Appeals decision that found section 503A of the act invalid in its entirety because it contained unconstitutional restrictions on commercial speech (i.e., prohibitions on soliciting of prescriptions for and advertising of specific compounded drugs). The Court did not rule on, and therefore left in place, the holding of the Court of Appeals that the unconstitutional restrictions on commercial speech could not be severed from the rest of section 503A. Thus, section 503A was removed from FDAMA97.

Generally, FDA continued to defer to state authorities regarding less significant violations of the act related to pharmacy compounding of human drugs. FDA anticipated that, in such cases, cooperative efforts between the states and the agency would result in coordinated investigations, referrals, and follow-up actions by the states.

However, when the scope and nature of a pharmacy's activities raise the kinds of concerns normally associated with a drug manufacturer and result in significant violations of the new drug, adulteration, or misbranding provisions of the act, FDA determined that it should seriously consider enforcement action. In determining whether to initiate such an action, the agency considered whether the pharmacy was engaged in any of the following acts:

1. Compounding drugs in anticipation of receiving prescriptions, except in very limited quantities in relation to the amounts of drugs compounded after receiving valid prescriptions.
2. Compounding drugs that have been withdrawn or removed from the market for safety reasons. Appendix I provides a list of such drugs that will be updated in the future, as appropriate.
3. Compounding finished drugs from bulk active ingredients that are not components of FDA-approved drugs without an FDA-sanctioned Investigational New Drug application in accordance with 21 U.S.C. § 355(i) and 21 C.F.R. 312.
4. Receiving, storing, or using drug substances without first obtaining written assurance from the supplier that each lot of the drug substance has been made in an FDA-registered facility.
5. Receiving, storing, or using drug components that are not guaranteed or otherwise determined to meet official compendial requirements.
6. Using commercial-scale manufacturing or testing equipment for compounding drug products.
7. Compounding drugs for third parties who resell to individual patients or offering compounded drug products at wholesale to other state-licensed persons or commercial entities for resale.
8. Compounding drug products that are commercially available in the marketplace or that are essentially copies of commercially available FDA-approved drug products. Certain circumstances may be appropriate for allowing a pharmacist to compound a small quantity of a drug that is only slightly different than a commercially available FDA-approved drug. In these circumstances, FDA will consider whether there is documentation of the medical need for the particular variation of the compound for the particular patient.
9. Failing to operate in conformance with applicable state law regulating the practice of pharmacy.

The foregoing list of factors is not intended to be exhaustive. Other factors may be appropriate for consideration in a particular case.

Events Leading Up to the Drug Quality and Security Act

The following example involves a pharmacy that was actually manufacturing under the guise of compounding. In 2012, an outbreak of fungal meningitis in the United States was traced to fungal contamination in three lots of compounded methylprednisolone suspension for epidural steroid injections. Doses from those three lots were administered to 14,000 patients. The New England Compounding Center (NECC) case was a tragedy for the 64 individuals who died, the hundreds who were sickened, and their families and loved ones. The case is discussed in detail in Chapter 33, "Pharmaceutical Compounding Errors," of this book.

The tragic events associated with NECC are a stark lesson in what can happen when quality assurance, quality control, and legal requirements are not followed. The quality assurance and quality control requirements of *USP* Chapter <797>, *USP* Chapter <71>, and other applicable *USP* chapters are designed to establish systems that ensure sterile medications are safe and that verify the medications' quality through sterility testing and other tests. These standards establish a redundant system of processes to ensure the quality of compounded sterile preparation. However, when these processes are not performed properly or their results are ignored, as is alleged in the NECC case, serious injury or death to patients can occur.

For many years, pharmacists have been reminded that *USP* <797> requirements are legally enforceable in all states. The prosecution of NECC personnel based on noncompliance with *USP* standards may set a precedent for future civil and criminal cases alleging that patients were injured as a result of noncompliance with *USP* standards. The tragic case of NECC is a call for all sterile-compounding pharmacists to scrutinize their operations to ensure full compliance with regulatory, quality, and safety standards.

The new Drug Quality and Security Act (DQSA) (H.R. 3204, 113th Cong., 2013), a direct result of the NECC tragedy, specifically prohibits traditional compounding pharmacies from dispensing for non-patient-specific office use. However, FDA is afforded flexibility in enforcement discretion. Sterile compounding facilities that register as outsourcing facilities under H.R. 3204, section 503B, may dispense non-patient-specific medications provided they meet several requirements, including compliance with Current Good Manufacturing Practices.

H.R. 3204: Drug Quality and Security Act

The new law—DQSA (H.R. 3204)—incorporates and brings up to date the court decisions regarding FDAMA97. A summary of the law is as follows:[3]

- "Drug Quality and Security Act - **Title I: Drug Compounding** - Compounding Quality Act - (Sec. 102) Amends the Federal Food, Drug, and Cosmetic Act (FFDCA) with respect to the regulation of compounding drugs. Exempts compounded drugs from new drug requirements, labeling requirements, and track and trace requirements if the drug is compounded by or under the direct supervision of a licensed pharmacist in a registered outsourcing facility and meets applicable requirements."
- Establishes requirements for pharmacies under section 503A.
- Establishes requirements for outsourcing facilities under section 503B.
- "Requires the Secretary to: (1) publish a list of drugs presenting demonstrable difficulties for compounding that are reasonably likely to lead to an adverse effect on the safety or effectiveness of the drug, taking into account the risk and benefits to patients; and (2) convene an advisory committee on compounding before creating the list."
- "(Sec. 103) Prohibits the resale of a compounded drug labeled 'not for resale,' or the intentional falsification of a prescription for a compounded drug. Deems a compounded drug to be misbranded if its advertising or promotion is false or misleading in any particular."
- "(Sec. 105) Requires the Secretary to receive submissions from state boards of pharmacy: (1) describing any disciplinary actions taken against compounding pharmacies or any recall of a compounded drug, and (2) expressing concerns that a compounding pharmacy may be violating the FFDCA."

- "(Sec. 106) Revises compounding pharmacy requirements to repeal prohibitions on advertising and promotion of compounded drugs by compounding pharmacies and repeal the requirement that prescriptions filled by a compounding pharmacy be unsolicited."
- "(Sec. 107) Requires the Comptroller General ([Government Accountability Office]) to report on pharmacy compounding and the adequacy of state and federal efforts to assure the safety of compounded drugs."

H.R. 3204, Section 503A: Pharmacies

Section 503A of H.R. 3204 likely affects more than an estimated 98% to 99% of the pharmacies in the United States, most of which do some traditional compounding. The law is summarized as follows:[4]

- "FDA expects State boards of pharmacy to continue their oversight and regulation of the practice of pharmacy, including traditional pharmacy compounding."
- "FDA also intends to continue to cooperate with State authorities to address pharmacy activities that may be violative of the [Federal Food, Drug, and Cosmetic] Act, including section 503A."
- A drug must be "compounded for an identified individual patient based on the receipt of a valid prescription order, or a notation, approved by the prescribing practitioner, on the prescription order that a compounded product is necessary for the identified patient."
- "The compounding of the drug product is performed:
  - "By a licensed pharmacist in a State licensed pharmacy or a Federal facility, or by a licensed physician on the prescription order for an individual patient . . . or
  - "By a licensed pharmacist or licensed physician in limited quantities before the receipt of a valid prescription order for such individual patient when" there is documentation of need."
- "The drug is compounded in compliance with the [USP] chapters on pharmacy compounding using bulk drug substances [active pharmaceutical ingredients (APIs)] that comply with the standards of an applicable USP or National Formulary (NF) monograph, if one exists."
  - "If such a monograph does not exist, the drug substance(s) must be a component of an FDA-approved human drug product."
  - "If a monograph does not exist and the drug substance is not a component of an FDA-approved human drug product, it must appear on a list of bulk drug substances for use in compounding developed by FDA through regulation."
- The drug product is compounded using bulk drug substances that are
  - "manufactured by an establishment that is registered . . . (including a foreign establishment)."
  - "accompanied by valid certificates of analysis for each bulk drug substance."
- "The drug product is compounded using [excipients] that comply with the standards of an applicable USP or NF monograph, if one exists, and the USP chapters on pharmacy compounding."
- "The drug product does not appear on the list [of] drug products that have been withdrawn or removed from the market because [they] have been found to be unsafe or not effective."
- Drug products "that are essentially copies of commercially available drug products" are not compounded "regularly or in inordinate amounts."

- Drug products listed by FDA that present "demonstrable difficulties for compounding that reasonably demonstrate an adverse effect on the safety or effectiveness of that drug product" are not compounded.
- "The drug product is compounded in a State that has entered into a memorandum of understanding (MOU) with FDA that addresses the distribution of inordinate amounts of compounded drug products interstate and provides for appropriate investigation by a State agency of complaints relating to compounded drug products distributed outside such State; or in States that have not entered into such an MOU with FDA, the licensed pharmacist, licensed pharmacy, or licensed physician does not distribute, or cause to be distributed, compounded drug products out of the State in which they are compounded, more than 5% of the total prescription orders dispensed or distributed by such pharmacy or physician."

H.R. 3204, Section 503B: Outsourcing Facilities

Some highlights of section 503B of H.R. 3204 include the following.

Section 503B defines an outsourcing facility as follows:

a facility at one geographic location or address that—

(i). is engaged in the compounding of sterile drugs;
(ii). has elected to register as an outsourcing facility; and
(iii). complies with all of the requirements of this section.

In addition, an outsourcing facility does not have to be a licensed pharmacy and may or may not acquire prescriptions for identified individual patients. A "sterile drug" is one that "is intended for parenteral administration, an ophthalmic or oral inhalation drug in aqueous format, or a drug that is required to be sterile under Federal or State law."

A facility that elects or chooses to register with FDA as an outsourcing pharmacy involved with sterile compounding is required to use bulk drug substances that

- appear on a list established by FDA.
- appear on the drug shortage list in effect at the time of compounding, distribution, and dispensing.
- comply with monographs in the *USP/NF* or other compendium or pharmacopeia recognized by FDA.
- are manufactured by an establishment registered with FDA.
- are accompanied by valid certificates of analysis.

The facility must comply with the following:

- Use other ingredients that comply with standards of the *USP/NF* if such monograph exists, or of another compendium or pharmacopeia recognized by FDA.
- Do not use drugs that have been withdrawn or removed by FDA because they have been found to be unsafe or ineffective.
- Do not prepare drugs that are essentially copies of one or more approved drugs (except in the case of an approved drug that appears on the drug shortage list).
- Do not prepare drugs that present demonstrable difficulties for compounding.
- Comply with FDA requirements if preparing any drugs that are the subject of a risk evaluation and mitigation strategy.

- Do not sell drugs for resale.
- Pay all applicable fees.
- Adhere to the requirements for the label, containers, and any other required information.
- Register with FDA between October 1 and December 31 of each year.
- Provide reports during June and December of each year to FDA of the drugs compounded during the previous six months.
- Comply with Good Manufacturing Practices.
- Be subject to FDA inspections.
- Submit adverse event reports.

At the time of the publication of this book, approximately 50 facilities were registered as human drug compounding outsourcing facilities under section 503B of the Federal Food, Drug, and Cosmetic Act.

The Triad

The DQSA states that a compounded product is exempt from meeting the *new drug* requirements if the drug product is compounded for an individual patient on the basis of the unsolicited receipt of a valid prescription order or a notation, approved by the prescribing practitioner, on the prescription order indicating that a compounded product is necessary for the specific patient—if the product meets certain requirements. A pharmacist may compound a drug when a prescription clearly requires compounding (because the drug is not commercially available in the form needed or a physician authorizes compounding). Also, a pharmacist may compound a drug if—with the physician's approval—the pharmacist determines that a compounded drug is necessary and notes that information on the prescription. This method allows pharmacists to suggest therapeutic switches to a compounded drug, just as they do for other types of medications. The physician, the patient, and the pharmacist form the legal compounding "triad."

Licensed Pharmacist or Physician

The product must be compounded by a licensed pharmacist—in a state-licensed pharmacy or federal facility—or by a licensed physician or other licensed practitioner authorized by state law to prescribe drugs.

Anticipatory Compounding

Limited quantities of products can be compounded in advance—if there is a history of receiving valid prescription orders for the product, generated by an established relationship between the licensed pharmacist and individual patients for whom the prescriptions are provided. An established relationship with the physician or other licensed professional who wrote the prescription must also exist.

Substances That May Be Used in Compounding

Substances that may be used for compounding include the following:

- Bulk drug substances that have monographs in the *USP/NF,* and comply with *USP* Chapter <795>
- Drug substances that are components of FDA-approved drugs or drug products, including any ingredient that is contained in commercially available FDA-approved drug products

- Bulk drug substances that appear on a list of approved bulk-drug substances developed by FDA
- Substances that are manufactured by facilities registered with FDA—including foreign facilities—and comply with standards of any monograph in the *USP/NF* (if a monograph exists), as well as with the *USP* Chapter <795>. Table 1-2 describes the chemical grades of substances.

Substances That May *Not* Be Used in Compounding

Compounding should not be performed using substances or involving products that are in the following categories:

- Products listed in Appendix I should not be used in compounding, because they are on the list of drug products withdrawn or removed from the market (because they have been found to be unsafe or ineffective).
- Inordinate amounts of commercially available drug products (not including drug products in which a change has been made for an individual patient, such as omitting a dye, flavor, sweetener, preservative, or the like) to which the patient may be sensitive should not be compounded. According to the DQSA, pharmacists are allowed to compound copies of commercially available drug products included in the FDA definition. In other words, the quantity described as "inordinate amounts" has yet to be defined. Much latitude is given to a prescribing practitioner in this area. One should note, however, that a small variation in strength, such as from 50 mg to 45 mg, would likely not be determined a significant difference.

Memorandum of Understanding

Section 503A(b)(3)(B) of H.R. 3204 established that to qualify for the exemptions in section 503A, the drug product must be compounded in accordance with either of the following:

1. It was compounded in a state that had entered into an MOU with FDA that addressed the interstate distribution of inordinate amounts of compounded drug products and provided for investigation by a state agency of complaints related to compounded drug products distributed outside such state; or
2. It was compounded in a state that had not entered into such an MOU, but the licensed pharmacist, pharmacy, or physician distributes (or causes to be distributed) compounded drug products outside of the state in which they were compounded—in quantities not exceeding 5 percent of the total prescription orders dispensed or distributed by the pharmacy or physician.

TABLE 1-2 Description of Chemical Grades

Grade	Description
USP/NF	Meets the minimum purity standards; conforms to tolerances set by the *United States Pharmacopeia/National Formulary* (USP/NF) for contaminants dangerous to health
ACS reagent	High purity; conforms to minimum specifications set by the Reagent Chemicals Committee of the American Chemical Society (ACS)
CP (chemically pure)	More refined than technical or commercial grade but still of unknown quality
Technical or commercial	Indeterminate quality

Implementation of DQSA: Draft Guidances

FDA has issued five documents related to drug compounding and repackaging that will help entities comply with important public health provisions. The documents are applicable to pharmacies, federal facilities, outsourcing facilities, and physicians.

The documents are as follows:

- Guidance: For Entities Considering Whether to Register as Outsourcing Facilities under Section 503B of the Federal Food, Drug, and Cosmetic Act[5]
- Draft Guidance for Industry: Repackaging of Certain Human Drug Products by Pharmacies and Outsourcing Facilities[6]
- Draft Guidance for Industry: Mixing, Diluting, or Repackaging Biological Products Outside the Scope of an Approved Biologics License Application[7]
- Draft Guidance for Industry: Adverse Event Reporting for Outsourcing Facilities under Section 503B of the Federal Food, Drug, and Cosmetic Act[8]
- Draft Memorandum of Understanding Addressing Certain Distributions of Compounded Human Drug Products Between the State of [insert STATE] and the U.S. Food and Drug Administration[9]

The above documents are the latest in a series of policy documents related to FDA oversight of drugs produced by state-licensed pharmacies, federal facilities, and outsourcing facilities.

Implementation of DQSA: Organization and Lists

The provisions of section 503A require rulemaking or other action by FDA. Some of these actions require decisions regarding the following.

Organization and Formation of the Pharmacy Compounding Advisory Committee
H.R. 3204, section 503B(c)(2) states the following: "Before issuing regulations to implement subsection (a)(6), the Secretary shall convene and consult an advisory committee on compounding. The advisory committee shall include representatives from the National Association of Boards of Pharmacy, the United States Pharmacopeia, pharmacists with current experience and expertise in compounding, physicians with background and knowledge in compounding, and patient and public health advocacy organizations." FDA, in consultation with the Pharmacy Compounding Advisory Committee, will make decisions regarding the following lists to be developed.

Lists to Develop: FDA, in Consultation with the Pharmacy Compounding Advisory Committee
In consultation with the Pharmacy Compounding Advisory Committee, FDA will make decisions regarding the following.

The Negative List
The first committee developed and approved a negative list consisting of drugs that have been removed from the market for safety reasons. The DQSA Pharmacy Compounding Advisory Committee reviews and recommends modifications to this list of drug products that may not be compounded as a result of having been withdrawn or removed from the market because they have been found to be unsafe or not effective. See Appendix I. To obtain the current list, visit www.accessdata.fda.gov/scripts/cdrh/cfdocs/cfcfr/cfrsearch .cfm?fr=216.24.

The Positive List of APIs
The FDA Pharmacy Compounding Advisory Committee evaluates bulk drug substances that (1) do not contain a *USP* or *NF* monograph, (2) are not components of FDA-approved drug products, or (3) do not contain a monograph in another compendium or pharmacopeia recognized by FDA to determine their suitability for use in compounding.

Demonstrable Difficulties in Compounding
The FDA Pharmacy Compounding Advisory Committee evaluates drug products that present demonstrable difficulties for compounding and that reasonably demonstrate an adverse effect on the safety or effectiveness of the drug product.

A major problem involving implementation of the law is FDA's actions in going well beyond what the law states and extending its reach into the authority of the individual state boards of pharmacy. Also, FDA is extending the law to include veterinary drug compounding and broadening the scope of section 503B compounding facilities to allow them to compound both nonsterile and sterile preparations.

United States Pharmacopeia

In 1990, the United States Pharmacopeial Convention approved the appointment of an Expert Advisory Panel on Pharmacy Compounding Practices. Initially, the panel's activities were (1) to prepare a chapter on compounding for the *USP/NF* and (2) to begin the process of preparing monographs of compounded products for inclusion in the *NF*.

The prepared chapter, <1161>, "Pharmacy Compounding Practices," was published and became official in 1996. With the mention of this chapter in FDAMA97, the chapter was renumbered as Chapter <795>; subsequently, its title was also changed to "Pharmaceutical Compounding—Nonsterile Preparations."[1] (One should note that *USP* chapters with numbers greater than <1000> are informational, whereas numbers less than <1000> are enforceable.)

The first of the compounding monographs became official in November 1998, and these monographs are published in the *USP* section of the *USP/NF*. Each published monograph involves a considerable amount of work, including a detailed, validated stability study. Some monographs that were previously published in the *USP/NF* are being reintroduced into the compendia. A second chapter related to compounding in the *USP/NF* was Chapter <1206>, "Sterile Drug Products for Home Use"; it was renumbered as <797> and was extensively revised and rewritten and then retitled as "Pharmaceutical Compounding—Sterile Preparations."[1]

Three additional *USP* chapters were written: <1075>, "Good Compounding Practices"; <1160>, "Pharmaceutical Calculations in Prescription Compounding"; and <1163>, "Quality Assurance in Pharmaceutical Compounding." Thereafter, Chapters <795>, "Pharmacy Compounding—Nonsterile Preparations," and <1075>, "Good Compounding Practices," were combined and expanded into a new General Chapter—<795>, Pharmacy Compounding—Nonsterile Preparations. In addition, Chapter <797>, Pharmacy Compounding—Sterile Preparations, has been updated.

Certification and Accreditation

An exciting recent development is the opportunity for a compounding pharmacy to obtain accreditation; other health care organizations have had that opportunity for years. Compounding pharmacies now have an external standard-setting entity to which they can apply for accreditation, the Pharmacy Compounding Accreditation Board (PCAB).[10] PCAB is now administered by the Accreditation Commission for Health Care (ACHC). ACHC also accredits (1) community retail pharmacies, (2) home infusion therapy pharmacies, (3) long-term care pharmacies, and (4) specialty pharmacies. In addition, it accredits (1) behavioral health organizations, (2) durable medical equipment providers, (3) home health agencies, (4) hospices, (5) private duty nursing services, and (6) sleep centers. PCAB-ACHC can now provide services whereby multiple-service pharmacies can obtain their accreditation from a single organization.

The mission of PCAB is to serve the public good by serving patients, prescribers, and the pharmacy profession. The comprehensive accreditation program is completely voluntary and is structured to improve quality and safety through standard practices. PCAB carries out its mission through two main tools: PCAB Principles of Compounding and PCAB Standards. A core concept of the principles is that compounding is the result of a practitioner's prescription drug order based on a valid practitioner–patient–pharmacist relationship. The principles state, moreover, that compounding is a part of the practice of pharmacy subject to regulation and oversight by the state boards of pharmacy. The PCAB Standards cover several core areas of both sterile and nonsterile compounding, including training of personnel, storage of chemicals, proper equipment usage, beyond-use dating, packaging, labeling, patient education, and quality assurance. PCAB uses two methods to determine compliance: an extensive review of the standard operating procedures (SOPs) of the facility and an on-site survey of the pharmacy.[11]

PCAB requires that a facility seeking accreditation have a set of comprehensive SOPs for use by the pharmacy staff. PCAB looks at whether SOPs (1) are in writing, (2) reflect the organization's actual activities, and (3) are being implemented as written. Well-written purchased or downloaded SOPs usually include reference information such as USP requirements, the FDA negative list (i.e., list of substances not to be used in compounding), and SOPs that should be followed throughout the industry. Some organizations purchase or download the prewritten SOPs available from various sources, whereas others develop their own SOPs. Either approach can be used, but both require extensive work.

PCAB places considerable emphasis on SOPs because testing every compounded preparation before dispensing is not possible. Compounders can rely on a set of consistent, uniform procedures that, if followed, ensure the preparation is made correctly each time and the appropriate documentation is generated. SOPs are designed to ensure that methods are standardized and documented to provide consistency and continuity.

A general approach to developing an SOP manual involves (1) reviewing the PCAB standards and creating a list of required SOPs, (2) assessing whether an organization has SOPs that address the PCAB requirements, and (3) conducting another review of the written SOPs to determine whether the SOP and the actual procedure match.[12]

Today, pharmacy and other professions are increasingly emphasizing quality assurance and the need for continuing competence of practitioners. In many areas of practice, certification is used to recognize individuals who rise to meet a certain standard. Certification likely will not be required in the future for the compounding of simple preparations, but it may be required for the compounding of complex preparations, such as high-risk sterile compounding and the compounding of biotechnology preparations and those used in nuclear pharmacy. We need to begin preparing for such requirements now. Currently, accreditation is required for some types of insurance reimbursement for third-party companies.

An important difference exists between *certification* (and *certified practitioners*) and programs that award a *certificate* for completion of a prescribed course of study. A *certificate program* may involve simply attending a seminar, reading a book, or viewing an audiovisual course. For certification, the standard must be high. Certified practitioners must have experience in the specialized field and must demonstrate an advanced level of practice. Usually, they must pass an examination and demonstrate mastery of core knowledge. In the past, they might have been called "masters" of their disciplines or trades.

Compounding Personnel

Only personnel authorized by the responsible pharmacist should be in the immediate vicinity of the drug-compounding operation. Any person with an apparent illness or open lesion that may adversely affect the safety or quality of a drug preparation being compounded should be excluded from direct contact with components, drug preparation containers, closures, in-process materials, and drug preparations until the condition is corrected or competent medical personnel determine the condition does not jeopardize the safety or quality of the preparation being compounded. All personnel who assist in compounding procedures should be instructed to report to the responsible pharmacist any health condition that may adversely affect drug preparations.

Duties

A pharmacist has (1) the responsibility and authority to inspect and approve or reject all components, drug preparation containers, closures, in-process materials, and labeling and (2) the authority to prepare and review all compounding records to ensure that no errors have occurred in the compounding process. In addition to compounding, a pharmacist provides other services, such as the following:

- Publicizes the availability of both prescription and nonprescription compounding services, which may involve chemicals, devices, and alternative dosage forms
- Provides drug searches on specific chemicals in different dosage forms, strengths, bases, and the like to accommodate specific needs of physicians and patients
- Provides follow-up information in response to a practitioner's request for information regarding a compounded medication
- Consults with practitioners regarding a particular dosage form when discussing services with a health care provider

Qualifications

Pharmacists should possess the education, training, and proficiency necessary to properly and safely perform compounding duties at the level at which they are involved. All pharmacists who engage in the compounding of drugs should be proficient in the art and science of compounding and should maintain that proficiency through current awareness and training.

Instruction for compounding pharmacists should cover the following:

- Proper use of state-of-the-art compounding equipment such as balances and measuring devices, including guidelines for selecting proper measuring devices, limitations of weighing equipment and measuring apparatus, and the importance of accuracy in measurements
- Current pharmaceutical techniques needed to prepare compounded dosage forms (i.e., comminution, trituration, levigation, pulverization by intervention, and geometric dilution)
- Properties of dosage forms to be compounded and related factors, such as stability, storage considerations, and handling procedures

- Literature regarding stability, solubility, and other physicochemical properties of the ingredients
- Handling of nonhazardous and hazardous materials in the work area, including protective measures for avoiding exposure, emergency procedures to follow in the event of exposure, and the location of material safety data sheets (MSDSs) (also called safety data sheets [SDSs]) in the facility (see Chapter 5 of this book for a discussion of MSDSs and SDSs)
- Use and interpretation of chemical and pharmaceutical symbols and abbreviations in medication orders and in formulation directions
- Review of pharmaceutical calculations

Attire
Personnel engaged in the compounding of drugs should wear clean clothing appropriate to the operation being performed. Protective apparel, such as coats or jackets, aprons, or hand or arm coverings, should be worn as necessary to protect drug preparations from contamination. A clean laboratory jacket usually is considered appropriate attire for nonsterile compounding procedures. Work with hazardous materials, such as chemotherapeutic agents, may require the use of goggles, gloves, masks or respirators, double gowns, and foot covers, and showers and eyewash stations should be provided. Clean room apparel is required for the compounding of sterile preparations in a controlled environment (clean room).

Compounding Process

Before the first step in the compounding process is taken, the following questions should be considered:

- What are the physical and chemical properties and medicinal and pharmaceutical uses of the drug substance?
- Are the quantity and quality of each active ingredient identifiable?
- Given the purpose of the prescription, will the preparation and route of administration provide adequate absorption, either locally or systemically?
- Are excipients present from any source (manufactured products) that may be expected to cause an allergic reaction, irritation, toxicity, or an undesirable organoleptic response by the patient?
- For preparations that are to be administered orally, are the active ingredients stable in the normal gastric pH range, or are they subject to extensive hepatic first-pass metabolism?

The steps to be followed before, during, and after compounding can be grouped into five categories: preparation, compounding, final check, sign-off, and cleanup steps. These are summarized here.

General Steps in the Compounding Process
Preparation
1. Judge the suitability of the prescription in terms of its safety and intended use and the dose for the patient.
2. Perform the calculations to determine the quantities of the ingredients needed.
3. Select the proper equipment, and ensure it is clean.
4. Don the proper attire, and wash hands.

5. Clean the compounding area and the equipment, if necessary.
6. Assemble all the necessary materials and ingredients to compound, and package the prescription.

Compounding

7. Compound the prescription according to the formulary record or the prescription, using techniques according to the art, science, and technology of pharmacy.

Final Check

8. Check, as indicated, the weight variation, adequacy of mixing, clarity, odor, color, consistency, and pH.
9. Enter the information in the compounding log.
10. Label the prescription.

Sign-Off

11. Sign and date the prescription, affirming that all of the indicated procedures were carried out to ensure uniformity, identity, strength, quantity, and purity.

Cleanup

12. Clean and store all equipment.
13. Clean the compounding area.

Packaging, Storage, and Labeling

A pharmacist should inspect and approve all components, drug preparation containers, closures, labeling, and other materials involved in the compounding process. These materials should be handled and stored in a manner that will prevent contamination.

Packaging

Compounded preparations should be packaged according to the specifications in the current *USP/NF*. The selection of a container depends on the physical and chemical properties of the compounded preparation and the intended use of the preparation.

To maintain potency of the stored drug, packaging materials should not interact physically or chemically with the preparation. Materials that are reactive, additive, or absorptive can alter the safety, identity, strength, quality, or purity of the compounded drug beyond the specifications for an acceptable preparation. Container characteristics of concern include inertness, visibility, strength, rigidity, moisture protection, ease of reclosure, and economy of packaging.

Plastic containers have become increasingly popular because they are less expensive and lighter in weight than glass. Only plastic containers that meet current *USP/NF* standards should be used.

Storage

Chemicals should be stored according to either the manufacturers' directions or the appropriate current *USP/NF* monographs. In general, compounding chemicals should be stored in tightly closed, light-resistant containers at room temperature; some chemicals, however, require refrigeration. Chemicals should be stored off the floor, preferably on shelves in a clean, dry environment. Commercial drugs to be used in the compounding process should be removed from cartons and boxes before they are stored in the compounding area.

Temperature requirements for storage of substances are detailed in the appropriate current *USP/NF* monographs. The temperatures of the storage areas, including refrigerators and freezers, should be monitored and recorded at least weekly.

Flammable or hazardous products should be stored appropriately in safety storage cabinets and containers, which are available from many laboratory suppliers.

Labeling

Labeling should be done according to state and federal regulations. Usually, labeling information includes the (1) generic or chemical names of the active ingredients, (2) strength or quantity, (3) pharmacy lot number, (4) beyond-use date, and (5) any special storage requirements.

When a commercial drug product has been used as a source of a drug, the generic name of the drug product, not the proprietary name, should be placed on the label. Inactive ingredients and vehicles should also be listed on the label as required. If no expiration date is provided on the chemicals or materials that are used, a system of monitoring should be established (e.g., placing the date of receipt of the materials on the label of the container or following any requirement of the individual state board of pharmacy). Monitoring expiration dates will ensure that materials, ingredients, and supplies are rotated so that the oldest stock is used first.

The use of specially coined names or short names for convenience should be discouraged. Such names can cause difficulty in emergency departments if an overdose or accidental poisoning has occurred or if health care professionals treating the patient need to know what the patient has been taking. If batch quantities of a preparation are compounded, a lot number should be assigned and placed on the labels. Surplus prepared labels should be destroyed.

If excess preparation is compounded or additional quantities are prepared in anticipation of future requests for the preparation, a pharmacist should have written procedures for the proper labeling of the excess preparation. Labeling should include (1) a complete list of ingredients, (2) a preparation date, (3) an assigned beyond-use date, (4) an appropriate testing and published data, and (5) control numbers. The preparation should then be entered into the inventory record and stored appropriately to help ensure its strength, quality, and purity. When the compounding process is completed, the excess preparation should be reexamined for correct labeling and contents.

Office-Use Compounding

Physicians and institutions occasionally ask pharmacists to compound non-patient-specific medications that are not commercially available and that must be administered by the prescriber. For example, FDA requires certain medications to be administered by the prescriber. In other cases, preparations for office use must be compounded in advance and immediately available for a physician to use in emergencies.

For these medications, the International Academy of Compounding Pharmacists (IACP) recommends language to be included on the primary label of each package. If space limitations or clinical reasons preclude inclusion on primary labeling, the information may be affixed through auxiliary labeling (e.g., if a label applied directly to the primary container could affect the quality of the medication, the label and statement should instead be applied to exterior packaging). In either case, the statement should be prominently displayed in the medication labeling. IACP recommends the following statement to help ensure (1) that the medication is administered properly and (2) that the prescriber and the patient are aware that the medication has been compounded: "This medicine was compounded in our pharmacy for use by a licensed professional only."

IACP encourages pharmacists to consider the following when dispensing a compounded preparation to an authorized prescriber for office use:

1. In the judgment of the dispensing pharmacist, the quantity being compounded and dispensed for office use is consistent with accepted practice.
2. All compounds dispensed on an office-use prescription or medication order should be labeled "For Institutional or Office Use Only—Not for Resale" or as otherwise required by state pharmacy practice acts.
3. For each dispensing of an office-use compounded preparation, a pharmacist should provide to the authorized prescriber the name and strength of the preparation or a list of active ingredients and strengths, the pharmacy's lot number, a beyond-use expiration date as determined by the pharmacist using appropriate documented criteria, and any necessary and appropriate ancillary instructions or cautionary statements.
4. A pharmacy should have written procedures for notifying each authorized prescriber or facility to which the office-use compounded preparation was dispensed in the event of a recall.

IACP encourages pharmacists to advise prescribers that the resale or redispensing of any office-use compounded product may lead to violations of practice acts or other state regulations involving labeling and record keeping.

In addition, IACP supports state regulations that require the following information be placed on the labels of office-use compounds: (1) name, address, and telephone number of the pharmacy preparing the medication; (2) lot number; (3) established or distinct common name of the medication; (4) strength; (5) statement of quantity; (6) date prescription is filled; (7) beyond-use date; (8) storage instructions; and (9) any other state labeling requirements.

Reference Library

Regarding nonsterile preparations, *USP* Chapter <795> states: "The compounder is responsible for compounding preparations of acceptable strength, quality, and purity with appropriate packaging and labeling in accordance with good compounding practices, official standards, and relevant scientific data and information."[1]

The compounding of quality preparations requires access to up-to-date, reliable drug information as well as pharmacy compounding information. Compounding pharmacists must have ready access to reference materials on all aspects of compounding. These materials may include on-site books, reprints, and journals; access to information from a compounding or drug information center; and Internet access to compounding databases.

The contents of a reference library at a particular practice site will depend in part on the type of compounded formulations being prepared. For example, references on aseptic compounding practices are needed if the site compounds sterile preparations. The following references should be a part of every pharmacy reference library and consist of the most current editions:

- Allen LV Jr. *Remington: The Science and Practice of Pharmacy*. London: Pharmaceutical Press.
- Allen LV Jr., Popovich NG. *Ansel's Pharmaceutical Dosage Forms and Drug Delivery Systems*. Baltimore: Lippincott Williams & Wilkins.

- Ansel HC, Stockton SJ. *Pharmaceutical Calculations.* Baltimore: Lippincott Williams & Wilkins.
- *AHFS Drug Information.* Bethesda, MD: American Society of Health-System Pharmacists.
- *The Merck Index.* Rahway, NJ: Merck and Co.
- *Martindale: The Complete Drug Reference.* London: Pharmaceutical Press.
- Rowe RC, Sheskey PJ, Cook WG, Fenton ME. *Handbook of Pharmaceutical Excipients.* Washington, DC: American Pharmacists Association.
- *Secundum Artem.* Minneapolis, MN: Paddock Laboratories [quarterly journal].
- Shrewsbury R. *Applied Pharmaceutics in Contemporary Compounding.* Englewood, CO: Morton Publishing Co.
- *United States Pharmacopeia–National Formulary.* Rockville, MD: United States Pharmacopeial Convention.

Some editions of these references should also be retained in a "previous editions" section of the reference library because they contain valuable information that was not carried forward to new editions; examples include *Remington: The Science and Practice of Pharmacy* and *Martindale: The Complete Drug Reference.* Older editions of some references should be discarded, however, if new research has shown that previously published information is incorrect; examples include the *United States Pharmacopeia/National Formulary, Handbook on Injectable Drugs* (L. A. Trissel; American Society of Health-System Pharmacists, Bethesda, MD), and *King Guide to Parenteral Admixtures* (King Guide Publications, Napa, CA).

Establishing a Reference Library

1. Determine the books required by the state board of pharmacy.
2. Determine the scope of practice, or breadth, required for the pharmacy.
3. Determine the depth of the scope of practice.
4. Select core books that will be required (both paper and electronic).
5. Select supplemental books that will be required (both paper and electronic).
6. Create a list of the core and supplemental books; mark with an asterisk those required by the board of pharmacy.

Maintaining a Reference Library

1. Annually (e.g., the first week in January), review the reference library and order updates (new book editions or supplements) and recently published references as required (see step 2).
2. As new editions of pharmacy references are announced, check the edition on hand to determine whether to order the latest edition.
3. Mark the books that should be retained in a previous-editions section of the reference library.
4. Mark the books that should be discarded when replaced by a new edition.

References

1. United States Pharmacopeial Convention. Chapter <795>, Pharmaceutical compounding—nonsterile preparations. In: *United States Pharmacopeia/National Formulary.* Rockville, MD: United States Pharmacopeial Convention; current edition.
2. Houck LK. Compounding: a well-established practice in 1938. *Int J Pharm Compound.* 2005; 9(5):364–7.

3. Congress.gov. Summary: H.R. 3204—113th Congress (2013–2014). Available at: www.congress .gov/bill/113th-congress/house-bill/3204.

4. U.S. Food and Drug Administration. Draft guidance: pharmacy compounding of human drug products under section 503A of the Federal Food, Drug, and Cosmetic Act. Available at: www.fda .gov/downloads/AboutFDA/CentersOffices/CDER/ucm118050.pdf.

5. U.S. Food and Drug Administration. Guidance: for entities considering whether to register as outsourcing facilities under section 503B of the Federal Food, Drug, and Cosmetic Act. Available at: www.fda.gov/downloads/Drugs/GuidanceComplianceRegulatoryInformation /Guidances/UCM434171.pdf.

6. U.S. Food and Drug Administration. Draft guidance for industry: repackaging of certain human drug products by pharmacies and outsourcing facilities. Available at: www.fda.gov/downloads /Drugs/GuidanceComplianceRegulatoryInformation/Guidances/UCM434174.pdf.

7. U.S. Food and Drug Administration. Draft guidance for industry: mixing, diluting, or repackaging biological products outside the scope of an approved biologics license application. Available at: www.fda.gov/downloads/Drugs/GuidanceComplianceRegulatoryInformation /Guidances/UCM434176.pdf.

8. U.S. Food and Drug Administration. Draft guidance for industry: adverse event reporting for outsourcing facilities under section 503B of the Federal Food, Drug, and Cosmetic Act. Available at: www.fda.gov/ucm/groups/fdagov-public/@fdagov-drugs-gen/documents/document /ucm434188.pdf.

9. U.S. Food and Drug Administration. Draft memorandum of understanding addressing certain distributions of compounded human drug products between the state of [insert STATE] and the U.S. Food and Drug Administration. Available at: www.fda.gov/downloads/Drugs /GuidanceComplianceRegulatoryInformation/PharmacyCompounding/UCM434233.pdf.

10. Cabaleiro J. Obtaining accreditation by the Pharmacy Compounding Accreditation Board, part 4: tips for "last minute" preparations. *Int J Pharm Compound.* 2008;12(5):432–3.

11. Murry T. Accreditation by the Pharmacy Compounding Accreditation Board: raising the bar for patient care. *Int J Pharm Compound.* 2008;12(2):174–5.

12. Cabaleiro J. Obtaining accreditation by the Pharmacy Compounding Accreditation Board, part 2: developing essential standard operating procedures. *Int J Pharm Compound.* 2007;11(5):397–9.

Chapter 2

Compounding Ingredient Considerations

Throughout history, pharmacists have used natural products, chemicals, and other materials for prescription compounding. In the past, these chemicals and materials were obtained from natural preparations, raw materials, and household ingredients. Today, compounding pharmacists use chemicals from various sources, depending on availability.

Chapter <795>, Pharmaceutical Compounding—Nonsterile Preparations, of the *United States Pharmacopeia (USP)* states: "The compounder is responsible for compounding preparations of acceptable strength, quality, and purity and in accordance with the prescription or medication order. The compounder is also responsible for dispensing the finished preparation, with appropriate packaging and labeling, and in compliance with the requirements established by the applicable state agencies, state boards of pharmacy, federal law, and other regulatory agencies where appropriate."[1] The compounding of quality preparations must involve the use of high-quality chemicals. If *USP* and *National Formulary (NF)* grade ingredients are used to prepare compounded formulations, the ingredients must meet the requirements of compendial monographs.

USP Chapter <795> also states the following:[1]

A USP or an NF grade substance is the preferred source of ingredients for compounding all other preparations. If that is not available, or when food, cosmetics, or other substances are or must be used, the use of another high-quality source, such as analytical reagent (AR), certified American Chemical Society (ACS), or Food Chemicals Codex (FCC) grade, is an option for professional judgment. For any substance used in compounding not purchased from a registered drug manufacturer, the compounder should establish purity and safety by reasonable means, which may include lot analysis, manufacturer reputation, or reliability of source.

In addition to the USP, NF, AR, ACS, and FCC grades mentioned above, other high-purity chemical grades include high-performance liquid chromatography, spectroscopic grade, and primary standard. These grades are used primarily in the analytical chemistry and pharmaceutical analysis field.

Manufactured drug products such as injectables, tablets, or capsules may be sources of active ingredients. If such a product is the source of the active ingredient used in the compounding of a prescription, only a manufactured drug from a container labeled with a batch control number and a future expiration date is acceptable. If a manufactured drug product is used, consideration of all the ingredients in the drug product relative to the intended use and the potential effect on the overall efficacy (strength, quality, purity, stability, compatibility) of the compounded preparation is important.

Some drug substances and products have been withdrawn or removed from the market because of safety or efficacy concerns. According to the U.S. Food and Drug Administration (FDA), preparing compounded formulations of any of these products will be subject to enforcement action.

For consistent quality in compounded preparations, use of high-quality suppliers of chemicals for compounding is important. Using the same suppliers also helps ensure consistent quality. If different suppliers are used, variations in physicochemical characteristics, such as particle size, may alter the expected response of drug preparations. Having a secondary supplier available in the event of unexpected shortfalls in supply is wise.

Knowing the purity and form of all ingredients used in compounding, especially active pharmaceutical ingredients, is important. A number of factors must be considered to ensure that the final compounded preparation falls within the strength requirements (e.g., 90%–110%) for compounded preparations or within the requirements of the *USP* monograph.

The form of the drug (base, salt, or ester) can be determined from the *USP* monograph or from the manufacturer's package insert in the case of a commercially manufactured product. Another source of information is the *United States Pharmacopeia/National Formulary (USP/NF)* monographs for bulk products.

For example, albuterol sulfate tablets USP are based on the albuterol content (present as the sulfate form). The *USP* monograph for albuterol sulfate tablets states, "Albuterol Tablets USP contain an amount of albuterol sulfate equivalent to not less than 90.0 percent and not more than 110.0 percent of the labeled amount of albuterol ($C_{13}H_{21}NO_3$)." In contrast, diphenhydramine hydrochloride capsules USP are based on the total molecule (i.e., diphenhydramine hydrochloride). The *USP* monograph states, "Diphenhydramine Hydrochloride Capsules USP contain not less than 90.0 percent and not more than 110.0 percent of the labeled amount of diphenhydramine hydrochloride ($C_{17}H_{21}NO \cdot HCl$)." Examples of drugs in the ester form are discussed later in this chapter.

Also, some drugs are either obtained as an aliquot or dilution or prepared as aliquots or dilutions to be weighed or measured later for compounding purposes. Finally, a number of drugs are available with labeled potency designations; for example, the *USP* monograph states that gentamicin sulfate USP "has a potency equivalent to not less than 590 µg of gentamicin per mg, calculated on the dried basis."

So, where do practitioners turn to obtain information on whether a drug is a salt, base, acid, ester, hydrate, solvate, or other type of substance? Most commonly, they look at the *USP/NF*, certificates of analysis (COAs), and the chemical structure or the empirical formula of the drug (for solvates and hydrates). COAs are discussed in Chapter 5 of this book; Figure 2-1 shows an example of a COA.

CERTIFICATE OF ANALYSIS

Morphine Sulfate, USP   CAS 62111-15-0

$(C_{17}H_{19}NO_3)_2 \cdot H_2SO_{44} \cdot 5H_2O$ Lot No.___XYZ_____

MW   758.83

TEST	LIMIT		RESULTS
	Min.	Max.	
Assay	98.0%	102.0% (anhydrous basis)	100.5%
Identification	To pass test		Passes test
Specific rotation	−107°	−109.5°	−108.1°
Acidity	To pass test		Passes test
Water	10.4%	13.4%	12.5%
Residue on ignition	nmt 0.1%		0.06%
Chloride	To pass test		Passes test
Ammonium salts	To pass test		Passes test
Limit of foreign alkaloids	To pass test		Passes test
Physical appearance: White, feathery, silky crystals, cubical masses of crystals, or white, crystalline powder.	To pass test		Passes test

Manufacturer name
Manufacturer address
Manufacturer telephone

Signature of Certificate of Analysis Coordinator _____

FIGURE 2-1 Example of a certificate of analysis.

Compounding with Hydrates and Solvates

Figure 2-2 shows a portion of a *USP/NF* monograph. A hydrate is apparent because the chemical structure contains water. The more molecules of water that are present in a molecule of the substance, the greater is the amount of chemical that must be weighed to obtain the actual active drug. Table 2-1 lists drugs commonly used in compounding and their allowable water content as specified in the *USP/NF*.

Let's look at different forms of dexamethasone as an example of a drug that is available with different amounts of water. Dexamethasone contains less than 0.5% of its weight in water. Dexamethasone acetate has one molecule of water of hydration and contains between 3.5% and 4.5% water; the anhydrous form contains less than 0.4% water. Dexamethasone sodium phosphate contains a sum of water and alcohol that may be up to 16.0%.

Another example is lidocaine hydrochloride. Lidocaine hydrochloride occurs as a monohydrate and as the anhydrous form. The water content may be between 5% and 7%.

Calculations

How much adjustment should be made if using lidocaine hydrochloride monohydrate in place of lidocaine hydrochloride anhydrous for a compounded prescription?

Lidocaine HCl monohydrate $C_{14}H_{22}N_2O \cdot HCl \cdot H_2O$ MW 288.81
Lidocaine HCl anhydrous $C_{14}H_{22}N_2O \cdot HCl$ MW 270.80

A comparison of the molecular weights reveals that a factor of 1.066 can be used for the adjustment because 288.81/270.80 = 1.066.

Example: If a prescription for lidocaine hydrochloride 2% gel (100 g) is to be made, then 2 g of anhydrous lidocaine HCl could be used:

$2 \text{ g} \times 1.066 = 2.132$ g of lidocaine HCl monohydrate

Also, a direct comparison of the molecular weights and the physical quantity required can be used, as follows:

$$\frac{\text{MW hydrate}}{\text{MW anhydrous}} = \frac{\text{Weight of hydrated form}}{\text{Weight of anhydrous form}}$$

$$\frac{288.81}{270.80} = \frac{x}{2 \text{ g}}$$

$x = 2.133$ g

Further, the *USP* monograph for lidocaine hydrochloride jelly USP states, "It contains not less than 95.0 percent and not more than 105.0 percent of the labeled amount of lidocaine hydrochloride ($C_{14}H_{22}N_2O \cdot HCl$)." Note that this is the anhydrous form.

Checking the COA for the lidocaine hydrochloride being used to determine the water content is also important. Fortunately, most pure powders (anhydrous) contain only 0.2%–0.5% moisture, which can be insignificant; nevertheless, it needs to be checked.

Packaging, Storage, and Weighing

Solvates and hydrates must be packaged in tight containers to prevent the loss or gain of moisture. In fact, all chemicals used in compounding are best stored in tight containers

Morphine Sulfate
(mor' feen sul' fate)

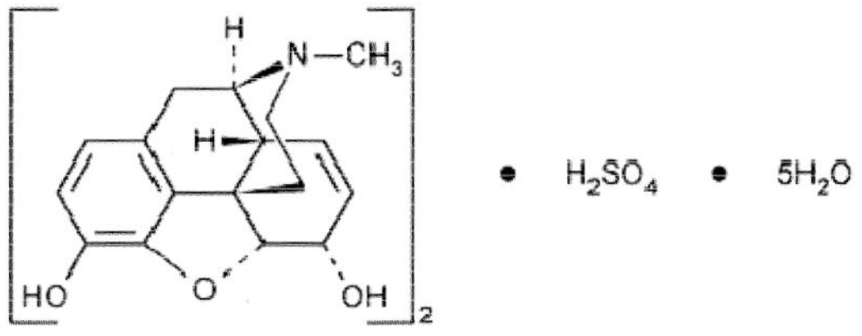

(C$_{17}$H$_{19}$NO$_3$)$_2$·H$_2$SO$_4$·5H$_2$O   758.83
Morphinan-3,6-diol, 7,8-didehydro-4,5-epoxy-17-methyl, (5α,6α)-, sulfate (2:1) (salt), pentahydrate.
7,8-Didehydro-4,5α-epoxy-17-methylmorphinan-3,6α-diol sulfate (2:1) (salt) pentahydrate [6211-15-0].

Anhydrous 668.77 [64-31-3].
» Morphine Sulfate contains not less than 98.0 percent and not more than 102.0 percent of (C$_{17}$H$_{19}$NO$_3$)$_2$·H$_2$SO$_4$, calculated on the anhydrous basis.

Packaging and storage—Preserve in tight, light-resistant containers. Store up to 40° as permitted by the manufacturer.

USP REFERENCE STANDARDS ⟨ 11 ⟩—
USP Morphine Sulfate RS

Identification—
A: *Infrared Absorption* ⟨ 197K ⟩: dried at 145° for 1 hour.
B: To 1 mg in a porcelain crucible or small dish add 0.5 mL of sulfuric acid containing, in each mL, 1 drop of formaldehyde TS: an intense purple color is produced at once, and quickly changes to deep blue-violet *(distinction from codeine, which gives at once an intense violet-blue color, and from hydromorphone, which gives at first a yellow to brown color, changing to pink and then to purplish red)*.
C: To a solution of 5 mg in 5 mL of sulfuric acid in a test tube add 1 drop of ferric chloride TS, mix, and heat in boiling water for 2 minutes: a blue color is produced, and when 1 drop of nitric acid is added, it changes to dark red-brown *(codeine and ethylmorphine give the same color reactions, but hydromorphone and papaverine do not produce this color change)*.
D: A solution (1 in 50) responds to the tests for *Sulfate* ⟨ 191 ⟩

SPECIFIC ROTATION ⟨ 781S ⟩: between –107° and –109.5°.
Test solution: the equivalent of 20 mg per mL, in water.

Acidity— Dissolve 500 mg in 15 mL of water, add 1 drop of methyl red TS, and titrate with 0.020 N sodium hydroxide: not more than 0.50 mL is required to produce a yellow color.

WATER, *Method I* ⟨ 921 ⟩: between 10.4% and 13.4% is found.

RESIDUE ON IGNITION ⟨ 281 ⟩: not more than 0.1%, from 500 mg.

Chloride—To 10 mL of a solution (1 in 100) add 1 mL of 2 N nitric acid and 1 mL of silver nitrate TS: no precipitate or turbidity is produced immediately.

Ammonium salts—Heat 200 mg with 5 mL of 1 N sodium hydroxide on a steam bath for 1 minute: no odor of ammonia is perceptible.

Limit of foreign alkaloids—Dissolve 1.00 g in 10 mL of 1 N sodium hydroxide in a separator, and shake the solution with three successive portions of 15, 10, and 10 mL of chloroform, passing the chloroform solutions through a small filter previously moistened with chloroform. Shake the combined chloroform solutions with 5 mL of water, separate the chloroform layer, and carefully evaporate on a steam bath to dryness. To the residue add 10.0 mL of 0.020 N sulfuric acid, and heat gently until dissolved. Cool, add 2 drops of methyl red TS, and titrate the excess acid with 0.020 N sodium hydroxide: not less than 7.5 mL is required (1.5%).

Assay—
Mobile phase—Dissolve 0.73 g of sodium 1-heptanesulfonate in 720 mL of water, add 280 mL of methanol and 10 mL of glacial acetic acid, mix, filter, and degas. Make adjustments if necessary (see *System Suitability* under *Chromatography* ⟨ 621 ⟩).

Standard preparation—Dissolve an accurately weighed quantity of USP Morphine Sulfate RS in *Mobile phase,* and dilute quantitatively, and stepwise if necessary, with *Mobile phase* to obtain a solution having a known concentration of about 0.24 mg per mL. Prepare a fresh solution daily.

System suitability preparation—Dissolve suitable quantities of USP Morphine Sulfate RS and phenol in *Mobile phase* to obtain a solution containing about 0.24 and 0.15 mg per mL, respectively.

Assay preparation—Transfer about 24 mg of Morphine Sulfate, accurately weighed, to a 100-mL volumetric flask, dissolve in and dilute with *Mobile phase* to volume, and mix.

Chromatographic system (see *CHROMATOGRAPHY* ⟨ 621 ⟩)—The liquid chromatograph is equipped with a 284-nm detector and a 3.9-mm × 30-cm column that contains packing L1. The flow rate is about 1.5 mL per minute. Chromatograph the *Standard preparation* and the *System suitability preparation,* and record the peak responses as directed for *Procedure:* the relative retention times are about 0.7 for phenol and 1.0 for morphine sulfate; the resolution, *R,* between phenol and morphine sulfate is not less than 2.0; the tailing factor for the morphine sulfate peak is not more than 2.0; and the relative standard deviation for replicate injections of the *Standard preparation* is not more than 2.0%.

Procedure—Separately inject equal volumes (about 25 µL) of the *Standard preparation* and the *Assay preparation* into the chromatograph, record the chromatograms, and measure the responses for the major peaks. Calculate the quantity, in mg, of (C$_{17}$H$_{19}$NO$_3$)$_2$·H$_2$SO$_4$ in the portion of Morphine Sulfate taken by the formula:

$$100C(r_u / r_s)$$

in which *C* is the concentration, in mg per mL, of anhydrous morphine sulfate in the *Standard preparation,* as determined from the concentration of USP Morphine Sulfate RS corrected for moisture content by a titrimetric water determination; and r_u and r_s are the peak responses obtained from the *Assay preparation* and the *Standard preparation,* respectively.

FIGURE 2-2 Portion of a *USP/NF* monograph.

TABLE 2-1 Maximum Allowable Water Content for Selected Substances

Drug	Maximum Water Content (%)	Drug	Maximum Water Content (%)
Acetylcysteine	1.0	Estriol	0.5
Acyclovir	6.0	Estrone	0.5
Albuterol	0.5	Fluconazole	0.5
Albuterol sulfate	0.5	Gentamicin sulfate	18.0
Ammonium alum	48.0	Glycopyrrolate	0.5
Potassium alum	46.0	Heparin sodium	5.0
Amikacin	8.5	Homatropine hydrobromide	1.5
Aminophylline	7.9	Hydrocodone bitartrate	12.0
Amitriptyline hydrochloride	0.5	Hydrocortisone	1.0
Amoxapine	0.5	Hydrocortisone sodium phosphate	5.0
Amoxicillin	14.5		
Aspartic acid	0.5	Hydromorphone hydrochloride	1.5
Aspirin	0.5	Hydroxyzine hydrochloride	5.0
Atenolol	0.5	Ibuprofen	1.0
Atropine sulfate	4.0	Ipratropium bromide	4.4
Azathioprine	1.0	Ketorolac tromethamine	0.5
Azithromycin	6.5	Labetalol hydrochloride	1.0
Beclomethasone dipropionate	3.8	Levothyroxine sodium	11.0
Hydrous benzoyl peroxide	26.0	Lidocaine hydrochloride	7.0
Benztropine mesylate	5.0	Lincomycin hydrochloride	6.0
Betamethasone acetate	4.0	Liothyronine sodium	4.0
Betamethasone sodium phosphate	10.0	Lithium carbonate	1.0
Bupivacaine hydrochloride	6.0	Lithium citrate	28.0
Buprenorphine hydrochloride	1.0	Morphine sulfate	13.4
Calcium carbonate	2.0	Nalorphine hydrochloride	0.5
Capsaicin	1.0	Nifedipine	0.5
Captopril	1.0	Nystatin	5.0
Cephalothin sodium	1.5	Ondansetron hydrochloride	10.5
Chloramphenicol sodium succinate	5.0	Papaverine hydrochloride	0.5
		Phentolamine mesylate	0.5
Citric acid, anhydrous	1.0	Prednisolone	7.0
Citric acid, monohydrate	9.0	Progesterone	0.5
Cocaine hydrochloride	1.0	Saccharin sodium	15.0
Codeine phosphate	3.0	Scopolamine hydrobromide	13.0
Codeine sulfate	7.5	Sodium chloride	0.5
Colchicine	2.0	Dibasic sodium phosphate	64.0
Cyanocobalamin	12.0	Monobasic sodium phosphate	26.5
Desmopressin acetate	6.0	Testosterone	1.0
Dexamethasone sodium phosphate	16.0	Tetracycline	13.0
Dextroamphetamine sulfate	1.0	Tetracycline hydrochloride	2.0
Dextromethorphan	0.5	Thyroid	6.0
Dextromethorphan hydrobromide	5.5	Tobramycin	8.0
Dextrose	9.5	Tobramycin sulfate	2.0
Edetate disodium	11.4	Vancomycin hydrochloride	5.0
Estradiol	3.5	Zinc gluconate	11.6

that are kept thoroughly closed at all times except for the short time during a weighing step. Storing chemicals at the indicated temperatures and minimizing exposure to very high humidity are also important.

Hygroscopic, Deliquescent, and Efflorescent Powders

Hygroscopic powders are those that will tend to absorb moisture from the air. Deliquescent powders are those that will absorb moisture from the air and even liquefy. Efflorescent powders are those that may give up their water of crystallization and may even become damp and pasty. Extra care must be taken in working with these powders; storage in tight containers will generally prevent difficulties. The *USP* description of a powder usually states whether it has hygroscopic, deliquescent, or efflorescent properties.

If a hygroscopic or deliquescent powder is being weighed on a balance and the compounder leaves for a short time and then returns, the powder may have absorbed moisture from the air and may therefore weigh heavier than it should. Weighing should be done quickly after opening the bulk chemical containers, and the containers should then be resealed.

Water and Solvent Content of Powders

If the chemical structure or the empirical formula does not show water in the molecule, checking the *USP* monograph for tests that may be related to water content of powders, such as "Loss on Drying" and "Residual Solvents," is important.

USP Chapter <731>, Loss on Drying, concerns the amount of volatile matter, including water, of any kind that is driven off under the conditions specified in the monograph. For substances appearing to contain water as the only volatile constituent, the test procedure is given in *USP* Chapter <921>, Water Determination, and the allowable range is specified in the individual monograph. The loss on drying may be significant; it should be detailed on the COA, and necessary calculations should be undertaken for adjustments.

Whereas loss on drying involves any volatile matter, many substances in the *USP/NF* are hydrates or contain water in adsorbed form. Consequently, water content is important in demonstrating compliance with the *USP/NF* standards. As detailed in *USP* Chapter <921>, water content is generally determined by titrimetric, azeotropic, or gravimetric methods.

All substances used in drug products or preparations are subject to standards related to the amount of residual solvents that are likely to be present. These standards are designed to ensure that the amounts of residual solvents in pharmaceuticals are acceptable for the safety of the patient. For our purposes, residual solvents are organic volatiles (including alcohol) that are used in the preparation of drug substances, products, or preparations. Residual solvents generally are not completely removed by practical and ordinary techniques. However, residual solvent content should be evaluated and justified, as described in *USP* Chapter <467>, Residual Solvents.

Compounding with Organic Salts

Knowing the form of a drug being used in determining the dose for administration is important. Many drugs are salts, and the dose may be based on the total salt form or just the base form of the drug. In the albuterol example given earlier in this chapter, *USP* states, "Albuterol Tablets USP contain an amount of albuterol sulfate equivalent to not less than 90.0 percent and not more than 110.0 percent of the labeled amount of albuterol $(C_{13}H_{21}NO_3)$." In other words, sufficient albuterol sulfate is present to provide the labeled amount of the albuterol base.

Example: A prescription calls for 10 mL of fentanyl 50 µg/0.1 mL (as the citrate) topical gel. How much fentanyl citrate will be required?

1. 50 µg/0.1 mL = x/10 mL x = 5 mg
2. Fentanyl MW = 336.47
    Fentanyl citrate MW = 528.59
3. 336.47/5 mg = 528.59/x x = 7.85 mg
4. Each milligram of fentanyl equals 528.59/336.47 = 1.57 mg fentanyl citrate

In the diphenhydramine example earlier in this chapter, diphenhydramine hydrochloride capsules USP are based on the total molecule—diphenhydramine hydrochloride. The weight of the hydrochloride is considered in the dose of the drug.

Example: A prescription calls for 30 capsules of diphenhydramine hydrochloride 35 mg each. How much diphenhydramine hydrochloride will be required?

Because the total salt molecule is part of the dose:

30 × 35 mg = 1.05 g of diphenhydramine hydrochloride

Advantage of the Salt Form

Most people are familiar with the following reaction, in which an acid reacts with a base by double decomposition to produce a salt and water:

$$NaOH + HCl \rightarrow NaCl + HOH$$

This reaction is also called a neutralization reaction. However, most drugs are weak acids or weak bases, not strong acids and strong bases.

Because many drugs are either weak acids or weak bases and have limited water solubility, they are often used in their salt forms to increase their aqueous solubility. For example, sodium salts are often made from weak acids; sodium salicylate is the salt of the weak acid salicylic acid and the strong base sodium hydroxide. A salt can also be made from a weak base and a strong acid; ephedrine hydrochloride can be prepared from the weak base ephedrine and the strong acid hydrochloric acid. The combination of a weak base and a weak acid can also be used; an example is codeine phosphate made from the weak base codeine and the weak acid phosphoric acid.

When salts are placed in an aqueous environment, they will dissolve to some extent, depending on their solubility in the aqueous medium and the pH of the medium. A portion of the drug will be dissolved, and some may remain undissolved. Of the dissolved portion, a part will be ionized and the remainder will be unionized, depending on the pH of the medium. Usually, the unionized portion of the drug in solution will be absorbed for systemic effect. The portion that is either ionized or unionized is described by the dissociation constant, or pK_a of the drug, and the pH of the medium.

Thus, the purpose of the salt form is usually to enhance the solubility of the drug. Use of the salt form may also enhance the drug's stability and change other attributes to make the drug easier to manipulate for producing dosage forms.

Only the unionized portion of the drug will ultimately exert its effect in the body. Some of the remainder of the salt molecule may no longer follow the base, or unionized, form of the drug to its site of action in the body.

Determining Which Form to Use

Why are some drugs dosed according to their base form (whether they be weak acids or weak bases) and some according to the total weight of their salt form? A review of revisions to the *USP* over many years reveals no apparent basis for determining which way the salts are dosed. Both the official monographs and the package insert information on FDA-approved drugs appear to be inconsistent in how they determine which way a drug is dosed. Pharmacists involved in compounding must be aware of the correct use of the terminology.

USP XII (1942) listed about 20 tablet monographs, all based on the salt form of the drug; for example, "Morphine Sulfate Tablets USP contain not less than 93 per cent and not more than 107 per cent of the labeled amount of morphine sulfate [$(C_{17}H_{19}O_3N)_2 \cdot H_2SO_4 \cdot 5H_2O$]." In that time period, monograph names were quite clear; if the salt was to be used, the salt name was part of the official name. For example, "Barbital Tablets USP" was based on the labeled amount of barbital ($C_8H_{12}N_2O_3$), but "Barbital Sodium Tablets" was based on the labeled amount of barbital sodium ($C_8H_{11}N_2O_3Na$).

The *USP XVI* (1960) monograph for amodiaquine hydrochloride tablets USP stated, "Amodiaquine Hydrochloride Tablets contain an amount of amodiaquine hydrochloride ($C_{20}H_{22}ClN_3O \cdot 2HCl \cdot 2H_2O$) equivalent to not less than 93% and not more than 107% of the labeled amount of amodiaquine base ($C_{20}H_{22}ClN_3O$)." This monograph shows that the dose is calculated on the base form of the drug.

The formulator (the compounding pharmacist) is responsible for determining whether the base/acid or salt form of the drug is to be used in calculating the amount of the active pharmaceutical ingredient. When receiving a prescription, a compounder should follow a routine procedure to correctly determine whether the salt or the base/acid form of the drug is to be used as the basis for the dose. Information can be obtained from the *USP* monograph, the product package insert, or a call to the manufacturer or the physician as necessary. Table 2-2 shows the forms (salts and bases/acids) to be used for various dosage forms of drugs from *USP/NF*. Note that whereas the drugs listed in Table 2-2 are those with official *USP* monographs, many drug products on the market do not have *USP* monographs.

TABLE 2-2 Form (Salt or Base/Acid) Used as Basis of Label Content

Substance	Capsules	Liquids[a]	Injections	Suppositories
Amikacin sulfate			B/A	
Amitriptyline hydrochloride			S	
Doxycycline		B/A		
Doxycycline calcium		B/A		
Doxycycline hyclate	B/A			
Erythromycin estolate	B/A	B/A		
Erythromycin ethylsuccinate		B/A	B/A	
Erythromycin lactobionate			B/A	
Morphine sulfate	S		S	S
Oxycodone hydrochloride		S		
Scopolamine hydrobromide		S	S	
Tetracycline hydrochloride	S	S	S	
Thiamine hydrochloride		S	S	

B/A = base or acid; S = salt.
[a]Liquids include oral solutions, suspensions, emulsions, elixirs, syrups, ophthalmics, nasal solutions, and otic solutions.

Compounding with Esters

Some drugs (e.g., atropine, cocaine, many local anesthetics) are esters by virtue of their internal chemical structure. Others are esters because a moiety has been added to form an ester for certain purposes. Only the latter are discussed here; those that are esters because of their basic molecular structure are not included.

An ester is a compound of the general formula R–C–O–R1, where R and R1 may be the same or different and may be either aliphatic or aromatic. The term *aliphatic* refers to an acyclic or cyclic, saturated or unsaturated carbon compound, excluding aromatic compounds. The term *aromatic* was originally used to describe compounds that smelled; these were later found to contain either benzene or a fused benzene ring in the structure. The term *aromatic* has been generalized to include aromatic heterocyclic structures.

An ester can be formed through the dehydration of a molecule of an alcohol and a molecule of an organic acid. For example, ethanol reacts with acetic acid to form ethyl acetate, an ester:

$$C_2H_5OH + CH_3COO \rightarrow CH_3CH_2-O-CO-CH_3$$

Advantages of the Ester Form

After salts, esters are the most important acid derivatives used in pharmacy. Esters may be prepared for a number of reasons, including solubility, stability, resistance to degradation after administration, and use as prodrugs.

Some drugs are very soluble but tend to degrade rapidly when in solution. One approach to increasing their stability and shelf life is to prepare esters that are poorly soluble. This results in a suspension dosage form instead of a solution dosage form. A drug in suspension degrades much more slowly than a drug in solution. After oral administration, the ester is cleaved and the active drug moiety is released for absorption.

Some drugs may cause pain at the site of injection, especially if they precipitate and damage the surrounding tissue. This can be overcome by preparing a drug with increased solubility. Chloramphenicol has low water solubility, but the succinate ester is formed to increase the drug's water solubility and facilitate parenteral administration. The succinate ester is inactive but is hydrolyzed to release the active chloramphenicol moiety.

The use of esters is an important means of preparing prodrugs, because esterases present in various parts of the body will cleave the ester linkage, releasing the active moiety. Carboxylic acid esters are common in pharmacy; they are neutral liquids or solids that can be hydrolyzed slowly by water and rapidly by acids or alkalies into their components.

Some of the simple esters are soluble in water, but those with more than four carbon atoms are practically insoluble in water.

One cannot simply look at the name of a compound and determine whether that drug is a salt or an ester. For example, *acetate salts* include calcium acetate, chlorhexidine acetate, desmopressin acetate, flecainide acetate, gonadorelin acetate, guanabenz acetate, leuprolide acetate, lysine acetate, mafenide acetate, and zinc acetate, and *acetate esters* include cortisone acetate, desoxycorticosterone acetate, dexamethasone acetate, fludrocortisone acetate, fluorometholone acetate, hydrocortisone acetate, isoflupredone acetate, medroxyprogesterone acetate, megestrol acetate, melengestrol acetate, methylprednisolone acetate, norethindrone acetate, paramethasone acetate, prednisolone acetate, trenbolone acetate, and betamethasone acetate. Further, *succinate salts* include sumatriptan succinate, doxylamine succinate, loxapine succinate, and metoprolol succinate, and *succinate esters* include chloramphenicol sodium succinate, hydrocortisone sodium succinate, hypromellose acetate succinate, methylprednisolone sodium succinate, and prednisolone sodium succinate.

Let's look at cefuroxime axetil as an example of an ester that is dosed according to the base form.

1. Cefuroxime axetil is $C_{20}H_{22}N_4O_{10}S$, with a molecular weight of 510.47. Cefuroxime axetil is described as a mixture of the diastereoisomers of cefuroxime axetil and contains the equivalent of not less than 745 µg and not more than 875 µg of cefuroxime ($C_{16}H_{16}N_4O_8S$) per milligram, calculated on the anhydrous basis.
2. Cefuroxime axetil tablets USP contain the equivalent of not less than 90.0% and not more than 110.0% of the labeled amount of cefuroxime ($C_{16}H_{16}N_4O_8S$).
3. Ceftin tablets (cefuroxime axetil tablets) provide the equivalent of 250 mg or 500 mg of cefuroxime as cefuroxime axetil.
4. Ceftin for oral suspension (cefuroxime axetil powder for oral suspension) provides the equivalent of 125 mg or 250 mg of cefuroxime as cefuroxime axetil per 5 mL of suspension.
5. After oral administration, cefuroxime axetil is absorbed from the gastrointestinal tract and rapidly hydrolyzed by nonspecific esterases in the intestinal mucosa and blood to cefuroxime; the axetil moiety is metabolized to acetaldehyde and acetic acid.
6. The molecular weight of cefuroxime axetil is 510.47. The molecular weight of cefuroxime is 424.39. Therefore, 1 mg of cefuroxime is contained in 510.47/424.39 = 1.2 mg of cefuroxime axetil. A 250 mg cefuroxime tablet will contain 250 × 1.2 = 300 mg of cefuroxime axetil.
7. Therefore, if the compounder is using a commercial product in preparing a dosage form, no conversion should be required. However, if a bulk active ingredient is used, the required amount of cefuroxime axetil that is equivalent to the desired dosage of cefuroxime must be calculated.

Labeling of Official Monographs

Let's look again at the example of dexamethasone. Labeled strengths of dexamethasone pose an interesting problem because they do not consistently name either the base or the ester form. "Dexamethasone" dosage form monographs are based on the labeled amount of dexamethasone. The "dexamethasone acetate" dosage form monograph is based on the labeled amount of dexamethasone. "Dexamethasone sodium phosphate" dosage form monographs are based on the labeled amount of dexamethasone phosphate.

Because some drugs may occur as salt forms, ester forms, or salt–ester forms, documenting which form is being used and whether it is a salt, ester, or combination is important. An example of a drug that occurs as both salt and ester forms is erythromycin. Erythromycin estolate is a salt; erythromycin ethylsuccinate is an ester; erythromycin gluceptate is a salt; erythromycin lactobionate is a salt; and erythromycin stearate is a salt.

Table 2-3 lists *USP*-monographed drugs that occur as esters and whether dosing for various dosage forms is based on the ester or the base form of the drug. Checking each formula for confirmation before making any necessary calculations is always best.

Compounding with Inorganic Salts

Characteristics of inorganic salts that can affect their physical and chemical properties, including particle size, tendency to absorb or give off water, and pH, are of interest for compounding pharmacists. When exposed to air, a hygroscopic powder will absorb moisture, a deliquescent powder will absorb moisture to the point of liquefaction, and an efflorescent powder will give off its water of crystallization. These effects are associated with the humidity in the immediate

TABLE 2-3 Form (Ester or Base) Used as Basis of Label Content

Drug	Topical	Capsules/ Tablets	Liquids[a]	Injections	Suppositories
Betamethasone benzoate	E				
Betamethasone dipropionate	B (Cr/Oint/Lot)		B		
Betamethasone valerate	B (Cr/Lot/Oint)				
Hydrocortisone acetate	E (Cr/Lot/Oint)		E	E	
Hydrocortisone sodium succinate				B	
Hydroxyprogesterone caproate				E	
Medroxyprogesterone acetate		E		E	
Megestrol acetate		E	E		
Methylprednisolone acetate	E (Cr)			E	
Methylprednisolone sodium succinate				B	
Prednisolone acetate			E	E	
Prednisolone sodium succinate				B	

E = ester; B = base; Cr = cream; Lot = lotion; Oint = ointment.
[a]Liquids include oral solutions, suspensions, emulsions, elixirs, syrups, ophthalmics, nasal solutions, and otic solutions.

environment. Some powders will either absorb or liberate water, depending on the humidity. These effects are especially important during pharmaceutical processes such as weighing and may result in incorrect quantities of materials being weighed. Eutectic formation is another phenomenon that results when certain materials are mixed together and become pasty or even liquefy. Eutectic mixtures can be advantageous or deleterious, depending on how they are used. Pharmacists can use numerous methods to overcome these occurrences.

Incompatibilities

Incompatibility is defined as the inability of a substance to maintain its identity or to exercise its inherent properties when brought into contact with or into the sphere of influence of another substance or a physical force. For pharmacists, incompatibilities can be either desirable or undesirable. An example of a desirable incompatibility is the addition of effervescent salts to water. An example of an undesirable incompatibility is a pH change resulting in hydrolysis and drug degradation.

Incompatibilities can be physical, chemical, or physiologic; the chemical and physical incompatibilities are of interest to compounding pharmacists. Physical incompatibilities include insolubility, immiscibility, heat, pressure, cold, light, and percussion (violent reactions). Chemical incompatibilities commonly include hydrolysis, condensation, oxidation, reduction, precipitation, gas evolution, heat liberation, and heat absorption. Some of these characteristics are mentioned in Table 2-4.

TABLE 2-4 Properties of Selected Inorganic Salts

Name	Formula	MW	H$_2$O Solubility	Use	Notes[a]
Potassium alum	AlK(SO$_4$)$_2$ · 12H$_2$O	474.39	FS	Astringent Styptic	With phenol, salicylates, or tannic acid, a green or gray color owing to traces of iron in the alum may be developed.
Ammonium carbonate	(NH$_4$HCO$_3$) and (NH$_2$COONH$_4$)		FS	Alkalizing agent Buffer	Consists of ammonium bicarbonate and ammonium carbamate in varying proportions. Contains between 30% and 34% NH$_3$. Is alkaline to litmus. Acids and acid salts decompose ammonium carbonate. Resorcinol gives a brown color that changes to blue.
Boric acid	H$_3$BO$_3$	61.83	Sol	Buffer Weak germicide	With sodium bicarbonate and moisture, liberation of carbon dioxide occurs. Traces of iron have sometimes caused discoloration in powders with phenol.
Calamine	ZnO with Fe$_2$O$_3$		IS	Astringent Protectant	Contains zinc oxide with a small amount of ferric oxide. Reacts slowly with fatty acids in oils and fats to produce lumpy masses of zinc oleate or stearate. Vanishing creams tend to dry out and crumble. Levigate with mineral oil to a smooth paste before incorporation into ointments.
Calcium chloride	CaCl$_2$ · 2H$_2$O	147.01	FS	Desiccant Diuretic	pH 4.5–9.2. Deliquescent.
Calcium hydroxide	Ca(OH)$_2$	74.09	SlS	Protectant Astringent	Is precipitated by borates, carbonates, citrates, oxalates, phosphates, sulfates, and tartrates. Precipitates most alkaloids and metals (as the hydroxide).
Magnesium carbonate			PrIn	Antacid Cathartic	Liberates carbon dioxide when mixed with acids. Precipitates free alkaloids from alkaloidal salt solutions. *(continued)*

TABLE 2-4 Properties of Selected Inorganic Salts *(Continued)*

Name	Formula	MW	H₂O Solubility	Use	Notesᵃ
Magnesium sulfate	$MgSO_4 \cdot xH_2O$	138.36 (Monohydrate)	FS	Cathartic Soak or compress for skin disorders	Efflorescent. pH 5.0–9.2.
Potassium bromide	KBr	119	FS	Sedative	Is alkaloidal precipitant. Strong oxidizing agents liberate bromine.
Potassium chloride	KCl	74.55	FS	Electrolyte source	Is neutral to litmus. Forms precipitates by reaction with lead and silver salts.
Potassium hydroxide	KOH	56.11	FS	Alkalizing agent Caustic	Deliquescent. Reacts with acids; liberates alkaloids from aqueous solutions of alkaloidal salts.
Potassium iodide	KI	166	VS	Expectorant Iodine source Antifungal therapy	Hygroscopic. Is decomposed with acids. Oxidizing agents liberate iodine.
Sodium bicarbonate	NaHCO₃	84.01	Sol	Alkalizing agent Antacid Antipruritic	Is alkaline to litmus. Is decomposed by acids and salts; acid reaction liberates carbon dioxide. Intensifies the darkening with solutions of salicylates. Precipitates some alkaloids. May react with atmospheric moisture or water of crystallization from other ingredients.
Sodium chloride	NaCl	58.44	FS	Electrolyte Tonicity-adjusting agent	Precipitates form with lead and silver salt solutions. Strong oxidizing agents liberate chlorine from acidified solutions.
Sodium hydroxide	NaOH	40	FS	Alkalizing agent Caustic	Hygroscopic. Absorbs carbon dioxide and is converted to sodium carbonate. Forms soluble soaps with fats and fatty acids.

Name	Formula	Molecular weight	Solubility	Uses	Comments
Sodium hypochlorite	NaClO	74.44	FS	Disinfectant Germicidal Dissolves necrotic tissue Deodorant	In solution. pH 7.8–8.2 (0.3% solution).
Sodium dibasic phosphate	$Na_2HPO_4 \cdot xH_2O$	141.96 (anhy)	FS	Buffer Cathartic	Hygroscopic. Produces alkaline reaction. Precipitates heavy metals.
Sodium monobasic phosphate	$NaH_2PO_4 \cdot xH_2O$	119.98	FS	Buffer Urinary acidifier	pH 4.1–4.5. Deliquescent. Is incompatible with carbonates and alkalies in general.
Sodium tribasic phosphate	Na_3PO_4	163.94 (anhy)	FS	Ingredient in detergents, buffers, water softening	Forms strongly alkaline solutions.
Zinc oxide	ZnO	81.39	IS	Mild astringent, protectant, and antiseptic	Reacts slowly with fatty acids in oils and fats to produce lumpy masses of zinc oleate or stearate. Vanishing creams tend to dry out and crumble. Levigate with mineral oil to a smooth paste prior to incorporation into ointments.
Zinc sulfate	$ZnSO_4 \cdot xH_2O$	161.46 (anhy)	FS	Astringent, emetic, and weak antiseptic	Efflorescent. Acid to litmus. Precipitates with lead, barium, strontium, and calcium salts. May dehydrate methylcellulose suspensions, leading to precipitation. Acacia, proteins, and tannins may precipitate.

anhy = anhydrous.
[a] pH values are provided in aqueous solutions. Check *USP* for concentrations used for these descriptions.

Solubility of Inorganic Salts

Some general rules regarding the solubility of inorganic salts are of interest:

1. If both the cation and the anion of an ionic compound are monovalent, the solute–solute attractive forces are usually easily overcome; therefore, these compounds are generally water soluble (e.g., NaCl, LiBr, KI, NH_4NO_3, $NaNO_2$).
2. If only one of the two ions in an ionic compound is monovalent, the solute–solute interactions also are usually easily overcome, and the compounds are water soluble (e.g., $BaCl_2$, MgI_2, Na_2SO_4, Na_3PO_4).
3. If both the cation and the anion are multivalent, the solute–solute interaction may be too great to be overcome by the solute–solvent interaction, and the compound may have poor water solubility (e.g., $CaSO_4$, $BaSO_4$, $BiPO_4$) (exceptions: $ZnSO_4$, $FeSO_4$).
4. Common salts of alkali metals (e.g., Na, K, Li, Cs, Rb) are usually water soluble (exception: Li_2CO_3).
5. Ammonium and quaternary ammonium salts are water soluble.
6. Nitrates, nitrites, acetates, chlorates, and lactates generally are water soluble (exceptions: silver and mercurous acetate).
7. Sulfates, sulfites, and thiosulfates generally are water soluble (exceptions: calcium and barium salts).
8. Chlorides, bromides, and iodides are water soluble (exceptions: salts of silver and mercurous ions).
9. Acid salts corresponding to an insoluble salt will be more water soluble than the original salt.
10. Hydroxides and oxides of compounds other than alkali metal cations and the ammonium ion generally are water insoluble.
11. Sulfides are water insoluble except for their alkali metal salts.
12. Phosphates, carbonates, silicates, borates, and hypochlorites are water insoluble except for their alkali metal salts and ammonium salts.

If these factors are not addressed before compounding, the effectiveness, stability (physical and chemical), and elegance of a prescription compounded with inorganic salts may be adversely affected. Properties of some inorganic salts are given in Table 2-4.

Compounding with Potency-Designated Ingredients

For some active pharmaceutical ingredients (APIs), including some antibiotics, endocrine products, biotechnology-derived products, and biological agents, the potency is based on *activity* and expressed in terms of units of activity, micrograms per milligram, or other standard terms of measurement. Table 2-5 includes examples of these substances with the *USP* description of their potency.

Regarding biologicals, the following is found in the *USP* General Notices:

5.50.10 Units of Potency (Biological):

For substances that cannot be completely characterized by chemical and physical means, it may be necessary to express quantities of activity in biological units of potency, each defined by an authoritative, designated reference standard.

Units of biological potency defined by the World Health Organization (WHO) for International Biological Standards and International Biological Reference Preparations are termed International Units (IU). Monographs refer to the units defined by USP

TABLE 2-5 Potency Designations as Described in *USP*

Active Pharmaceutical Ingredient	Potency Designation
Amikacin sulfate	Contains the equivalent of not less than 674 µg and not more than 786 µg of amikacin per mg, calculated on the dried basis
Amoxicillin	Contains not less than 900 µg and not more than 1050 µg of amoxicillin per mg, calculated on the anhydrous basis
Amphotericin B	Has a potency of not less than 750 µg of amphotericin B per mg, calculated on the dried basis
Ampicillin	Contains not less than 900 µg and not more than 1050 µg of ampicillin per mg, calculated on the anhydrous basis
Ampicillin sodium	Contains not less than 845 µg and not more than 988 µg of ampicillin per mg, calculated on the anhydrous basis.
Calcitonin salmon	One mg of acetic acid-free, anhydrous calcitonin salmon is equivalent to 6000 USP calcitonin salmon units
Cefuroxime sodium	Contains the equivalent of not less than 855 µg and not more than 1000 µg of cefuroxime, calculated on the anhydrous basis
Cephalexin	Has a potency of not less than 950 µg and not more than 1030 µg of cephalexin per mg, calculated on the anhydrous basis
Cephalexin hydrochloride	Contains the equivalent of not less than 800 µg and not more than 880 µg of cephalexin per mg
Cephalothin sodium	Contains the equivalent of not less than 850 µg of cephalothin per mg, calculated on the dried basis
Colistin sulfate	Has a potency equivalent to not less than 500 µg of colistin per mg
Gentamicin sulfate	Has a potency equivalent to not less than 590 µg of gentamicin per mg, calculated on the dried basis
Heparin sodium	Has a potency of not less than 140 USP heparin units in each mg, calculated on the dried basis
Insulin	Has a potency of not less than 26.5 USP insulin units in each mg, calculated on the dried basis; insulin labeled as purified contains not less than 27.0 USP insulin units in each mg, calculated on the dried basis
Insulin human	Has a potency of not less than 27.5 USP insulin human units in each mg, calculated on the dried basis
Insulin lispro	Has a potency of not less than 27.0 USP insulin lispro units per mg, calculated on the dried basis
Neomycin sulfate	Has a potency equivalent to not less than 600 µg of neomycin per mg, calculated on the dried basis
Nystatin	Has a potency of not less than 4400 USP nystatin units per mg, or, where intended for use in the extemporaneous preparation of oral suspensions, not less than 5000 USP nystatin units per mg
Oxytocin	Has oxytocic activity of not less than 400 USP oxytocin units per mg
Streptomycin sulfate	Has a potency equivalent to not less than 650 µg and not more than 850 µg of streptomycin per mg
Tobramycin	Has a potency equivalent to not less than 900 µg of tobramycin per mg, calculated on the anhydrous basis
Tobramycin sulfate	Has a potency of not less than 634 µg and not more than 739 µg of tobramycin ($C_{18}H_{37}N_5O_9$) per mg
Vancomycin hydrochloride	Has a potency equivalent to not less than 900 µg of vancomycin per mg, calculated on the anhydrous basis
Vasopressin	Has vasopressor activity of not less than 300 USP vasopressin units per mg

Reference Standards as "USP Units." For biological products, units of potency are defined by the corresponding U.S. Standard established by FDA, whether or not International Units or USP Units have been defined.

There is no relationship between the units of potency of one drug and those of another drug. In the case of potency-designated drugs, there must be a reference standard for comparison. In actual usage, the potency specifications often include a range or "not less than __" and "not more than ___." In some cases, only a lower range is given, and in a few cases, there is no upper limit.

The determinations of potency are generally done on the dried or anhydrous basis. In the case of hygroscopic APIs, precautions must be taken to maintain the substance in a dried state in tight containers. In some cases, solvent-free conditions are specified.

In the case of dihydrostreptomycin, there are different potencies depending on the use of the API. The potency may be not less than 450 µg, 650 µg, or 725 µg, depending on its form or usage (route of administration).

In some cases, as in erythromycin ethylsuccinate and erythromycin stearate, the potency is based on the sum of the percentages of three different erythromycins that make up the API. Usually, the potency designation is determined on the base of the drug, but in a few instances the salt or ester form is used.

The potency of antibiotics is commonly expressed as micrograms of activity per milligram of substance. Obviously, there will be different equivalents for the base versus the salt form of the drug. For example, as shown in Table 2-5, tobramycin has a potency of not less than 900 µg of tobramycin per milligram, and tobramycin sulfate has a potency of not less than 634 µg of tobramycin per milligram, all on the anhydrous basis. In another example, ampicillin contains not less than 900 µg and not more than 1050 µg of ampicillin per milligram, and ampicillin sodium contains not less than 845 µg and not more than 988 µg of ampicillin per milligram, both calculated on the anhydrous basis. Because of these differences, checking the labels accompanying each batch of each API for the necessary values to be used in calculations is extremely important.

In some drugs (e.g., heparin, insulin), the actual dose may be expressed in units instead of milligrams. Other examples include enzymes (pancreatin, pancrelipase, papain) and antibiotics.

Each container must be labeled with the actual potency, and this information must be used in calculations involving dosing that occur before compounding activities. These calculations must be done, checked, and documented, because different lots of the same API may have different potencies.

Example: A formula calls for 500 mg of neomycin sulfate. The label on the API shows 650 µg of neomycin activity per milligram of powder. How much of this powder is required to provide the 500 mg of neomycin sulfate?

$$\frac{650 \text{ µg}}{1000 \text{ µg}} = \frac{500 \text{ mg}}{x}$$

$x = 769$ mg of the powder is required to provide 500 mg of actual neomycin sulfate.

Compounding with Complex Organic Molecules

Most complex molecules and biotechnology products are proteins; however, some may be smaller, peptide-like molecules. Proteins are inherently unstable molecules and require special handling; furthermore, their degradation profiles can be quite complex. Pharmacists involved in compounding with biologically active proteins must be interested in their stabilization, formulation, and delivery to the site of action.

In working with complex molecules, one must be cognizant of both the active drug constituent and the total drug formulation in which it is contained. This is true when converting a commercial product into a compounded preparation. Protein drugs are very potent and are generally used in quite low concentrations. The bulk of many manufactured products and compounded preparations may be the excipients, including the vehicle, buffers, and stabilizers that are often incorporated into these products.

A number of different stabilizers from different chemical classes can be used; these include surfactants, amino acids, polyhydric alcohols, fatty acids, proteins, antioxidants, reducing agents, and metal ions. Table 2-6 describes agents that may be used as stabilizers in complex molecule and protein formulations.

TABLE 2-6 Stabilizing Agents for Complex Molecule and Protein Preparations

Class	Agent	Action
Amino acids	Alanine	Solubilizer
	Arginine	Buffer
	Aspartic acid	Inhibits isomerism
	Glycine	Stabilizer
	Glutamic acid	Thermostabilizer
	Leucine	Inhibits aggregation
Antioxidants	Ascorbic acid, cysteine hydrochloride, glutathione, thioglycerol, thioglycolic acid, thiosorbitol	Help stabilize protein conformation
Chelating agents	Ethylenediaminetetraacetic acid salts	Inhibit oxidation by removing metal ions, glutamic acid, and aspartic acid
Fatty acids	Choline, ethanolamine, phosphatidyl	Stabilizers
Proteins	Human serum albumin	Prevents surface adsorption; stabilizes protein conformation; serves as a complexing agent and cryoprotectant
Metal ions	Ca^{++}, Ni^{++}, Mg^{++}, Mn^{++}	Help stabilize protein conformation
Polyhydric alcohols	Ethylene glycol	Stabilizer
	Glucose	Strengthens conformation
	Lactose	Stabilizer
	Mannitol	Cryoprotectant
	Propylene glycol	Prevents aggregation
	Sorbitol	Prevents denaturation and aggregation
	Sucrose	Stabilizer
	Trehalose	Stabilizer
Polymers	Polyethylene glycol, povidone	Prevent aggregation
Surfactants	Poloxamer 407	Prevents denaturation and stabilizes cloudiness
	Polysorbate 20 and polysorbate 80	Retard aggregation

Stabilization

A key factor in formulating a stable preparation is pH. The optimal pH range can be achieved through the selection of appropriate physiologic buffers, usually in buffer concentration ranges of 0.01 M to 0.1 M. In general, an increase in the buffer concentration means an increase in pain on injection, so the concentration is usually kept as low as is reasonable.

Chelating agents are incorporated to bind trace metals such as copper, iron, calcium, and manganese and minimize rates of degradation. Ethylenediaminetetraacetic acid (EDTA) is commonly used at a concentration of about 0.01% to 0.05%.

Because oxidation is one of the major factors in protein degradation, antioxidants are often incorporated. Examples include ascorbic acid, sodium disulfide, monothioglycerol, and α-tocopherol.

Especially in preparation of multidose vials, preservatives are usually necessary if compatible with the active ingredient. Examples of preservatives include phenol (0.3% to 0.5%), chlorobutanol (0.3% to 0.5%), and benzyl alcohol (1% to 3%).

Other excipients may include the polyols, which are good stabilizers and are commonly used in concentrations from 1% to 10%, and tonicity-adjusting agents, which include sodium chloride and dextrose in concentrations necessary to achieve isotonicity of approximately 290 mOsm/L.

Preparation

Formulations and procedures with complex molecules should be kept as simple as possible. Sterility must be achieved and maintained in many preparations, and because most do not contain a preservative, preparation of only one dose from each vial or container is recommended in order to minimize contamination. Sometimes this is not practical, and specific manipulations are needed to meet patient needs. The standards of *USP* Chapter <797>, Pharmaceutical Compounding—Sterile Preparations, should be met while working with these sterile preparations. Two special considerations in working with biotechnologically derived preparations are the use of filters and the sorption of these drugs to containers.

The use of filters in manipulating biotechnology products can cause sorption, resulting in loss of some of the drug available to the patient. Sorption is "sticking," by either absorption into the filter or adsorption onto the surface of the filter. Special filters have been prepared to minimize this problem. For example, muromonab-CD3 (Orthoclone OKT3) injection should be filtered with a low-protein-binding filter of 0.2 to 0.22 μm. Many biotechnology products should not be filtered at all. If a filtration device is part of the intravenous administration apparatus, large-molecule drugs generally should be administered distal to the site of the filter. Filters that have been shown to minimize protein adsorption are those made from polyvinylidene difluoride, polycarbonate, polysulfone, and regenerated cellulose. As a precaution, low-protein-binding filters should be used.

Drug loss through sorption of proteins to containers (glass or plastic) can be minimized either by the use of albumin or by siliconization. Adding about 0.1% albumin to the product can decrease the sorption of proteins to containers. If glass containers are used, the albumin solution should be added and manipulated to coat the interior surface before the drug is added. If siliconization is used, one can prepare a silicone solution or emulsion and soak or rinse the glass vials in it. The drained vials should then be placed in an oven at about 250°C for 5 to 6 hours. This procedure will minimize protein adsorption to glass; it can be used for both the preparation equipment and the packaging containers.

Physicochemical Considerations

Several considerations can help ensure retention of a large-molecule drug's activity up to the time of administration to the patient. These include selecting an appropriate vehicle for drug delivery, individualizing dosages, administering drugs through novel drug-delivery systems, preparing drugs for delivery through these systems, monitoring their efficacy, and counseling patients on their use. Information on specific products is given in Table 2-7.

Physicochemical issues relevant to large-molecule drugs include the following:

- Effect of agitation or frothing on a preparation's stability
- High molecular weight and potential for aggregation (i.e., a small change in structure can result in a change in activity)
- Assignment of potency to the reference standards (whereas traditional pharmaceuticals are about 98% pure, these materials may be only 0.1% to 1% active, with their activity assigned by potentially variable assays)
- Use of micropipets, which can require frequent calibration
- Stability potentially less than with lyophilized preparations
- Interaction of the product with the inner wall of the glass vial and with the elastomeric closure
- Effectiveness of the preservative if a multidose product is mixed with other products
- Immunogenic potential, because some are produced by a fermentation-type process and proteins can co-purify with proteins

Physicochemical factors to be considered in compounding protein drug products also include the structure of the protein drug, isoelectric point, molecular weight, solubility and factors affecting solubility (e.g., surfactants, salts, metal ions, pH), stability and factors affecting stability (e.g., pH, temperature, light, oxygen, metal ions, freeze–thaw cycles, mechanical stress), polymorphism, stereoisomers, filtration media compatibility, shear, and surface denaturation.

Solubility can vary with changes in chemical structure, pH, and temperature. Proteins are generally more soluble in their native environment or medium or in a matrix that is similar to their native environment, which may include sodium chloride, trace elements, lipids, and other proteins in an aqueous medium. One must consider the ingredients' effects on the solubility of the active drug, especially because most of the products are currently administered parenterally. This is critical because the actual drug is present in a small quantity and can go unnoticed if it precipitates. Sterile water for injection and 0.9% sodium chloride solution usually are good vehicles for use in a formulation.

The pH of the compound should be maintained close to the pH of the original approved, manufactured product. Changes in pH can affect proteins in numerous ways and result in altered activity. Chemical degradation rate constants are related to pH, and the hydrogen ion concentration can affect the actual structure of proteins (i.e., quaternary structure). Buffer systems may be needed in compounding; they should be prepared at the minimum buffer strength required to produce the most stable drug product.

Chemical and physical instability must be considered and addressed appropriately. *Chemical instability* of proteins is the modification of protein structures by bond formation or cleavage to yield a new compound. *Physical instability* generally involves changes in structure, conformation, or behavior in a particular environment. Stability, both chemical and physical, depends on pH, temperature, and agitation, as well as on the overall environment in which the drug is contained.

Sorption is a problem with colony-stimulating factors and with aldesleukin (Proleukin) at low concentrations. To minimize sticking of the protein to the glass, the addition of about 0.1% albumin to the product to occupy the potential binding sites in the container is often helpful. Pharmacists must consider this problem before making any changes in packaging.

TABLE 2-7 *USP* Monograph Information on Selected Complex Molecules

Generic Name	Trade Name	Strength Designation	pH of Solution	Notes
Alteplase	Activase	Units	7.1–7.5	Endotoxins: <1 per mg
				Reconstitute by directing stream of SWFI directly into lyophilized cake. It is preservative free, because it is incompatible with preservatives.
				Use within 8 hours.
				Dilute further if necessary with equal volume of NS or D5W.
				Alteplase may also contain arginine, polysorbate 80, and phosphoric acid and/or sodium hydroxide to adjust pH.
Insulin injection, human	Humulin	Units		Endotoxins: nmt 80 per 100 USP insulin human units
				Humulin may also contain glycerin, metacresol, zinc oxide, and sodium hydroxide and/or hydrochloric acid to adjust pH.
Sargramostim	Leukine	Units	7.1–7.7	Endotoxins: nmt 50 per mg
				Avoid foaming during dissolution.
				Do not shake or vigorously agitate.
				If final concentration is less than 10 µg/mL, 0.1% human albumin should be added to the saline before adding the sargramostim. Do not use an in-line membrane filter.
				Sargramostim may also contain mannitol, sucrose, and tromethamine.
Somatropin	Genotropin, Humatrope, Norditropin	Units		Endotoxins: nmt 20 per mg
				Genotropin 5 mg also contains glycine, mannitol, sodium dihydrogen phosphate anhydrous, disodium phosphate anhydrous, m-cresol, and SWFI.

SWFI = sterile water for injection; NS = 0.9% sodium chloride injection; D5W = 5% dextrose injection; nmt = not more than.

Agitation resulting in frothing can create difficulties in two ways. First, frothing can cause difficulties in using a syringe to withdraw the required amount of drug from a vial. To avoid this problem, the formulator should mix the product by rolling the vial in the hands or gently swirling it. Second, excessive agitation can cause changes in a protein's quaternary structure that often reduce or eliminate a drug's therapeutic activity. Some products, such as filgrastim (Neupogen) and sargramostim (Leukine), are reconstituted by directing a soft stream of diluent against the inside of the container wall. Others, such as recombinant tissue plasminogen activator (tPA; alteplase), are reconstituted by directing a stream of diluent directly into the product at the bottom of the vial.

Packaging

The container used for packaging and storage after compounding must be chosen carefully. For example, the manufacturer's directions for interleukin-2 (aldesleukin) suggest the use of a plastic bag because that type of dilution container enhances consistent drug delivery. Unless otherwise specified, USP type I glass should be used for packaging when storage for extended time periods is indicated. A pharmacist should be aware of the potential for sorption of the drug to the glass walls. Closures and stoppers should be selected that are compatible and flexible; have low levels of particulates; and experience few problems with adsorption, absorption, and permeation.

Storage and Labeling

The recommended storage temperature depends on the specific preparation and may include room temperature (15°C–25°C), refrigerator temperature (2°C–8°C), or frozen (−20°C) or ultrafrozen temperature (down to −80°C). Freezing does affect the activity of certain products; for instance, the activity of filgrastim decreases if it is frozen. Some products can retain potency at room temperature after reconstitution. Sargramostim retains potency for up to 30 days at 25°C. However, most manufacturers recommend refrigeration at 2°C to 8°C, regardless of the product's potency at room temperature.

The short shelf life of these products after reconstitution can be due to chemical, physical, or microbiological instability. The manufacturer's recommendations or recommendations validated by the published literature should be followed for products after they are reconstituted and manipulated. One example is tPA, which has been used in treating intraocular fibrin formation after a vitrectomy and in managing subconjunctival hemorrhage after glaucoma filtration surgery. The prepared solution is stable in a pH range of 5 to 7.5 and is incompatible with bacteriostatic agents. To prepare a compounded preparation, a pharmacist reconstitutes the commercial product according to the manufacturer's directions, using sterile water for injection without preservatives to yield a concentration of 1 mg/mL. This solution is further diluted with 0.9% sodium chloride injection to yield a concentration of 25 μg/100 μL. Aliquots of 0.3 mL are withdrawn into 1-mL tuberculin syringes and capped. The syringes are stored in an ultrafreezer at −70°C. This product has been shown, by both bioassay and clinical use, to retain its activity for at least 1 year. This type of specific product information is not included in the manufacturer's label information and is usually obtained from the literature or by asking the manufacturer directly.

Stability

Physical stability can involve degradation by aggregation, denaturation, and precipitation. Aggregation can be the result of covalent or noncovalent processes and can be either physical or chemical in nature. Aggregate formation can actually begin when primary particles are formed from protein molecules as a result of Brownian movement.

Denaturation can result from heat, cold, extreme pH values, organic solvents, hydrophilic surfaces, shear, agitation, mixing, filtering, shaking, freeze–thaw cycles, ionic strength, and other factors. Denaturation can be quite complex and can be either reversible or irreversible.

Precipitation can result from shaking, heating, filtration, pH, and chemical interactions. The first step in a precipitation process usually is aggregation. When the aggregates gain a sufficient size, they precipitate out of solution and are clearly evident. Precipitation can occur on membrane filters, in equipment, in tubing, and in contact with other equipment and supplies.

Compounding with Aliquots, Dilutions, and Concentrates

Substances are available as aliquots, dilutions, and concentrates for a number of reasons. First, the quantities required for dosing or compounding may be so small they cannot be accurately weighed, so dilutions are prepared, assayed, and used. Second, some items, such as nitroglycerin, are explosive and must be diluted in order to be safely handled. Third, many substances, such as acids and bases, are commercially available in percentage strengths that vary from one acid to another and depend on the solubility and stability of the solute in water and on the manufacturing process. The diluted acids are aqueous solutions, usually 10% weight-in-volume (w/v), although diluted acetic acid is 6% w/v. The concentrations of the official undiluted acids are expressed as percentages weight in weight (w/w), but the strengths of official diluted acids are expressed as percentages weight in volume. Therefore, a pharmacist must consider the specific gravities of the concentrated acids when calculating the volume required to make a given quantity of diluted acid.

Triturations, Dilutions, and Concentrates

Triturations or dilutions were, at one time, official and consisted of diluting one part by weight of the drug with nine parts of finely powdered lactose; they were 10% mixtures of the drug. These dilutions were a means of conveniently obtaining small quantities of a drug for compounding purposes. Many aqueous concentrates are available and are convenient to use; a notable example in compounding is benzalkonium chloride solutions. Table 2-8 lists examples of other substances available as triturations, dilutions, and concentrates.

Example: How many milliliters of a benzalkonium chloride 17% solution would be required to prepare 4000 mL of a 1:10,000 solution?

$1 : 10,000 :: x : 4000$

$10,000x = 4000$

$x = 0.4$ g of benzalkonium chloride substance is required.

17 g $: 100$ mL $:: 0.4$ g $: x$

$17x = 40$

$x = 2.35$ mL of the benzalkonium chloride 17% solution is required.

TABLE 2-8 Examples of Substances (Official and Nonofficial) Available as Triturations, Dilutions, and Concentrates

Substance	Strength (%)	Comments
Acetic acid NF	36.0%–37.0% w/w	
Acetic acid, diluted NF	5.7%–6.3% w/v	
Alcohol, USP	94.9%–96.0% v/v; 92.3%–93.8% w/w	Sp gr 0.812–0.816
Alcohol, diluted NF	48.4%–49.5% v/v	Sp gr 0.935–0.937
Ammonia solution, strong NF	27%–31% w/w	
Ammonium lactate 70% solution	70%	
Ammonium lauryl sulfate 28%	28%	
Formaldehyde solution USP	Nlt 34.5% w/w	
Glutaraldehyde 25% aqueous solution	25%	
Glycolic acid 70%	70%	
Hydrochloric acid NF	36.5%–38.0% w/w	
Hydrochloric acid, diluted NF	9.5%–10.5% w/v	
Hydrogen peroxide concentrate USP	29.0%–32.0% w/w	Strong oxidant
Hydrogen peroxide topical solution USP	2.5%–3.5% w/v	
Hypophosphorous acid NF	30.0%–32.0%	
Isopropyl rubbing alcohol USP	68.0%–72.0%	Sp gr 0.872–0.883
Lactic acid USP	88.0%–92.0% w/w	
Nitroglycerin, diluted USP	10% usually w/w	
Phenol, liquefied USP	90% w/w	
Phosphoric acid NF	85.0%–88.0% w/w	
Phosphoric acid, diluted NF	9.5%–10.5% w/v	
Sodium hypochlorite solution USP	4.0%–6.0% w/w	
Sorbitol solution	Nlt 64.0%	
Zinc pyrithione 48% (min) aqueous dispersion	48%	

Nlt = not less than.

Methods of calculation using dilutions or triturations can include ratio and proportion, allegation alternate, and allegation medial. These procedures are described in pharmacy calculation textbooks.

Nitroglycerin
Diluted nitroglycerin contains the following cautionary labeling:

> Caution—Taking into consideration the concentration and amount of nitroglycerin ($C_3H_5N_3O_9$) in Diluted Nitroglycerin, exercise appropriate precautions when handling this material. Nitroglycerin is a powerful explosive and can be detonated by percussion or excessive heat. Do not isolate nitroglycerin ($C_3H_5N_3O_9$).

Isosorbide dinitrate and isosorbide mononitrate have similar warnings.

Example: To obtain 40 mg of nitroglycerin to prepare 100 nitroglycerin 0.4 mg dosage units:

A 10% nitroglycerin trituration contains 1 g of nitroglycerin per 10 g of mixture.

40 mg = 0.04 g

1 g : 10 g :: 0.04 g : *x* g

x g = 400 mg of the dilution would be required.

Acids and Bases

Checking the label of each lot of concentrated acid or base used for a prescription or procedure is always best, because lots can sometimes vary. The following relationship can be used:

$$\frac{\text{Strength of diluted acid} \times 1000}{\text{Strength of undiluted acid} \times \text{sp gr of undiluted acid}}$$

Example: To make 1000 mL of diluted HCl USP, using HCl assayed at 37.5% HCl with sp gr of 1.18, the amount required is

$$\frac{10 \times 1000}{37.5 \times 1.18} = 226 \text{ ml is required}$$

Dilution concentrations can be done by allegation, ratio and proportion, or other calculation methods described in pharmacy calculation textbooks.

Compounding with Commercial Products

In compounding prescriptions for humans, pharmacists can use either bulk drug substances or commercial preparations. With a few exceptions, veterinary compounding requires the use of commercial products.

The Federal Food, Drug, and Cosmetic Act recognizes the *USP/NF* as the official compendia of the United States. Compounded drugs prepared pursuant to a practitioner's prescription must meet compendial requirements if the prescription uses the compendial name. According to *USP* Chapter <795>, a USP or an NF grade substance is the preferred source of ingredients for compounding all preparations. If that is not available, or when food, cosmetics, or other substances are or must be used, then use of another high-quality source, such as analytical reagent, certified American Chemical Society, or Food Chemicals Codex grade is an option for professional judgment. A manufactured drug product may also be a source of active ingredient.

Commercial Products as Source of Active Drugs

Is the use of commercial products in compounding wise? When doing so, can a pharmacist be assured of a quality preparation? Can the standards of *USP* Chapter <795>; Chapter <797>; and Chapter <1075>, Good Compounding Practices, be met by using commercial products as the source of drugs? The answer to these questions is "sometimes, but not always." Pharmacists are placed in an interesting position: although the federal government dictates that commercial products be used in compounding veterinary preparations, doing so sometimes results in preparations that are outside *USP* standards and specifications. Box 2-1 describes an example of out-of-specification compounding.

BOX 2-1 Example: Out-of-Specification Compounding

In compounding for human patients, pharmacists have the choice of using bulk chemicals or commercial products. When using commercial products as the source of active drugs, a pharmacist does not know whether the final compounded preparation meets USP standards. An example is a relatively simple intravenous admixture containing gentamicin injection 80 mg in 50 mL of 5% dextrose injection. To prepare this, a pharmacist adds 2 mL of Garamycin injection (40 mg/mL) to an empty piggyback bag and adds 48 mL of 5% dextrose injection to make a final volume of 50 mL. The finished compounded preparation is allowed a variance of 90.0% to 110.0% of the labeled potency. The USP specification for gentamicin injection is not less than 90.0% and not more than 125.0% of the labeled amount of gentamicin. If the specific batch analyzed at the manufacturer was at 120%, then it met the USP specifications and entered the marketplace distribution system. A pharmacist who adds 2 mL of that gentamicin injection to 48 mL of 5% dextrose injection has just compounded a drug preparation that does not meet the USP compounding specifications of 90.0% to 110.0% of the labeled quantity; that is, 2 mL of 40 mg/mL at 120% of labeled quantity equals 96 mg of gentamicin present. The acceptable range would be 72 to 88 mg of gentamicin, so the preparation with 96 mg of drug does not meet the USP standard for compounding. If this solution were selected for analysis by a regulatory agency, it would be found to be beyond specifications and superpotent. This is the current regulatory situation, and it must be followed until such time that most compounding can be done using compendial standard (*USP/NF*) or other high-quality bulk drug substances.

Historically, pharmacists have used commercially available medications to prepare different dosage forms. The most common examples are the use of oral tablets and capsules to prepare oral liquids (solutions and suspensions) for pediatric patients and the use of injectable drugs to prepare intravenous admixtures. Even though FDA-approved commercial products are used, the final compounded preparation does not have FDA approval.

Considerations concerning commercial product use include the following:

1. Using commercial products as a source of active drugs usually will result in a higher prescription cost to the patient than would using bulk drug substances. This is especially true when injectables are used as the drug source.
2. All the excipients present in the commercial dosage form must be considered for their effects on the efficacy, safety, stability, and assay potency of the final compounded preparation.
3. When using solutions as the source of drugs, a pharmacist must be aware of the pH of the solution and the pH of the compounded preparation. If there is a significant difference in pH (i.e., 2 to 3 pH units), the solubility and stability of the drug and formulation may change. If the pH of the final solution is insufficient to keep the drug in solution, the preparation may be a suspension rather than a solution.
4. The presence of buffers in the commercial drug product can affect the pH of the final compounded preparation.
5. Before a pharmacist uses a commercial product to compound large batches, assaying the product for potency may be advisable. An assay is especially important

if the USP allowable range for the commercial product exceeds the 90%–110% potency range acceptable for compounded preparations. For most commercial drugs, the potency range is 95%–105% or 90%–110% of the labeled quantity; for some, the range is 80%–120%. Some *USP* monographs for commercial products go as high as 165% of the labeled quantity; although this is unusual, it is a variable a pharmacist must consider. Even if the compounding pharmacist performed every step correctly, the final preparation could fail to meet specifications because wide variability was allowed in the commercial product.

6. Some dosage forms should not be used in compounding. Modified-release dosage forms (e.g., extended release, delayed release, repeat action, targeted release) should not be used unless their suitability for use in compounding has been documented.

7. When commercial products are used in compounding, listing their manufacturer and lot number is important. This is especially important in the case of multisource generic drugs, because different excipients may be used by different manufacturers.

8. A limiting factor can be the quantity of commercial product that must be used to provide the required amount of active drug. Often, the required quantity makes use of the commercial product impractical.

In addition to these factors, some commercial dosage forms are inappropriate for use in compounding particular dosage forms, as summarized in Table 2-9. The reasons are discussed in the following sections.

Excipients in Various Dosage Forms

Powders and granules generally consist of the active drug and diluents. Medicated powders for external use may use cornstarch or talc as a diluent and adherent and may also contain water-repelling agents. Those for internal use may be intended for local effects (laxatives) or systemic effects; they may use a water-soluble or dispersible diluent, anticaking agent, coating agents, flavors or perfumes, sweeteners, and solubilizing agents.

Capsules usually consist of the active drug and diluent and may also contain lubricants, disintegrating agents, glidants, and coating agents. Some of these ingredients are water soluble and some are not.

Tablets contain the active drug and possibly diluents or fillers, disintegrating agents, glidants, lubricants, binders, antiadherents, colorants, sweeteners, and flavorants. In some cases, coating materials and plasticizers may need to be considered.

Ointments may be of the oleaginous, absorption, water-removable, or water-soluble type. The oleaginous bases consist primarily of hydrocarbon vehicles, such as petrolatum and mineral oil. Absorption bases may have, in addition, water-in-oil emulsifying agents, such as lanolin and cholesterol. Water-removable bases usually contain emulsifying agents or surfactants, and water-soluble bases are usually polymer based. Additional materials may include flavors or perfumes, stiffening agents, and water-repelling additives.

Creams generally are oil-in-water emulsions or water-in-oil emulsions and contain the aqueous and oil phases along with surfactants or emulsifying agents and possibly preservatives. Some may also contain perfumes, antioxidants, buffering agents, chelating agents, humectants, and stiffening agents.

Gels are semisolid systems usually containing a polymeric gelling agent and preservative; they may contain acidifying or alkalizing agents, antioxidants, buffering agents, chelating agents, flavors or perfumes, humectants, and sweeteners.

Suppositories and *inserts* are solid forms that usually consist of a base that melts at body temperature or dissolves in body fluids. (Compressed-tablet inserts are covered under tablets,

TABLE 2-9 Compounded Dosage Forms and Potential Commercial Drug Sources

Source of Dosage Form	Form to Be Compounded												
	Pwdrs Grans	Caps	Tabs	Oints	Crms	Gels	Solns	Susps	Emuls	Parens	Ophths	Nasal Solns	Otic Solns
Powders and granules	+	+	+	+	+	+	?	+	+	–	–	–	+
Capsules	+	+	+	+	+	+	–	+	+	–	–	–	+
Tablets	+	+	+	+	+	+	–	+	+	–	–	–	+
Ointments	–	–	–	+	+	–	–	–	?	–	–	–	+
Creams	–	–	–	?	+	?	–	–	+	–	–	–	+
Gels	–	–	–	+	+	+	+	+	+	–	+	+	+
Solutions	?	?	?	+	+	+	+	+	+	–	+	+	+
Suspensions	?	?	?	+	+	+	?	+	+	–	–	–	+
Emulsions	–	–	–	?	+	+	?	+	+	–	–	–	+
Parenterals	+	+	+	+	+	+	+	+	+	+	+	+	+
Ophthalmics	+	?	?	?	+	+	+	+	+	–	+	+	+
Nasal solutions	+	?	?	?	+	+	+	+	+	–	–	+	+
Otic solutions	–	?	?	?	+	+	+	+	+	–	–	+	+

+ = Generally okay to use; ? = Possible; use only if necessary; – = Generally not to be used

above.) The suppository bases may be complex mixtures of fatty acids to achieve a certain melting range or may be water soluble. These dosage forms may also contain stiffening agents or softening agents.

Solutions may contain the active ingredient, vehicle, solvents, preservative, sweetener, flavors, tonicity-adjusting agents, viscosity-adjusting agents, buffers, pH-adjusting agents, antifoaming agents, antioxidants, chelating agents, humectants, and wetting or solubilizing agents.

Suspensions may contain the active ingredient, vehicle, preservative, surfactants, sweetener, flavors, viscosity-adjusting agents, buffers, pH-adjusting agents, antifoaming agents, antioxidants, chelating agents, humectants, and wetting agents.

Emulsions may contain the active ingredient, vehicle, preservative, sweetener, surfactants or emulsifying agents, buffers, pH-adjusting agents, antifoaming agents, antioxidants, chelating agents, flavors, humectants, viscosity-increasing agents, and sweeteners.

Injectables (parenterals) may contain the active drug, vehicle, preservative, solvents, tonicity-adjusting agents, antioxidants, chelating agents, buffers, pH-adjusting agents, antifoaming agents, and wetting or solubilizing agents.

Ophthalmics may contain the active drug, vehicle, preservative, solvents, tonicity-adjusting agents, antioxidants, chelating agents, buffers, pH-adjusting agents, and viscosity-increasing agents.

Nasal solutions may contain the active drug, vehicle, preservative, solvents, tonicity-adjusting agents, antioxidants, chelating agents, buffers, pH-adjusting agents, antifoaming agents, flavors, humectants, and wetting or solubilizing agents.

Otic solutions may contain the active drug, vehicle, preservative, solvents, antioxidants, chelating agents, buffers, pH-adjusting agents, acidifying or alkalizing agents, humectants, and viscosity-increasing agents.

Compounded Dosage Forms and Potential Commercial Drug Sources

Powders and Granules

Powders and granules generally can be made from commercial dosage forms such as powders, granules, capsules, and tablets. Particle size is important, and pulverization and sieving should be considered to produce uniform and physically stable mixtures. Ointments, creams, gels, suppositories, and inserts are not practical to use in compounding powders and granules. Solutions and suspensions may be considered if they can be evaporated to dryness to obtain the desired quantity of active drug. Emulsions are not practical to use. Parenterals may be used if they are powders for reconstitution or can be evaporated to dryness. Ophthalmics, nasal solutions, and otic solutions are usually not practical.

Capsules

For compounding capsules, both powders and granules may serve as a source, depending on the quantity of powder present and the size of the capsule to be prepared. Granules may require pulverization before blending and encapsulation. Capsules can be used under the same conditions; pulverizing the contents before blending may be necessary. Immediate-release tablets can be pulverized with the other ingredients required to make a capsule. Ointments, creams, gels, suppositories, and inserts are not appropriate as a drug source for capsules, unless a suitable quantity of an oleaginous-based ointment can be placed in a hard-gelatin capsule to prepare a semisolid-filled capsule. Solutions and suspensions can be used only if the solvent systems are evaporated to provide the drug. Parenterals may be appropriate if they are lyophilized powders or powders for reconstitution. Liquid parenterals would require evaporation, as would ophthalmics, nasal solutions, and otic preparations.

Tablets

Powders, granules, capsules, and tablets can be used if pulverized uniformly and blended to form tablets. Most compounded tablets are of the molded type, and these sources of drug work well if the volume of powder is not too great. Ointments, creams, gels, suppositories, and inserts do not work well for this category. Solutions and suspensions would require evaporation of the solvent, as would parenterals, ophthalmics, nasal solutions, and otic solutions, if aqueous based. Lyophilized powders or powders for reconstitution for injection may work well.

Ointments

Powders, granules, capsules, and tablets may work well if the powders are thoroughly pulverized and the bulk volume of the powders is not too great. If excess powders are used, the ointment may become too thick to be used effectively. Ointments and creams may be appropriate if the phases are compatible (i.e., water and oil phases). Gels may be used in absorption, oil-in-water, and water-soluble-based ointments. Suppositories and inserts may be appropriate if the phases are compatible (i.e., oleaginous). Some inserts are actually tablets and could be considered, as previously discussed.

Solutions and suspensions may be appropriate for absorption, emulsion, and to some degree, water-soluble ointments. Care must be exercised to retain the viscosity of the preparation. Emulsions can be used if they are compatible with the final preparation (i.e., water-in-oil or oil-in-water). Oil-in-water emulsions may be incorporated into oil-in-water emulsions, absorption bases, and water-soluble bases. Water-in-oil emulsions may be incorporated into absorption bases and water-in-oil emulsion bases. Parenterals, ophthalmics, nasal solutions, and otic solutions may be satisfactory depending on compatibility considerations.

Creams

Powders, granules, capsules, and tablets may be satisfactory if the bulk volume of the excipients is not too great. Ointments and creams can be used if consideration is given to the compatibility of the different aqueous and lipophilic phases. Gels can usually be incorporated into oil-in-water creams.

Suppositories and inserts are not good choices as drug sources for creams. Solutions, suspensions, and emulsions may be suitable if the required volume is not excessive. If the volume is too large, evaporation to a suitable volume may be needed. Parenterals, ophthalmics, nasal solutions, and otic solutions may be suitable.

Gels

Powders, granules, capsules, and tablets usually are not suitable to produce clear gels. If a clear gel is not required, then they may be suitable. In an aqueous-based gel, many of the water-soluble excipients will dissolve. Ointments usually are not suitable, except for water-soluble ointments; the oil-in-water emulsion ointments (creams) may be miscible, however. The oleaginous, absorption, and water-in-oil emulsion (creams) type of ointments will not work well. Gels should work satisfactorily if there are no problems with differing pH or gelling agents. Suppositories and inserts generally will not work well. Solutions, suspensions, and oil-in-water emulsions may be satisfactory, depending on the volume to be incorporated. Parenterals, ophthalmics, nasal solutions, and aqueous otic solutions may be used if the volume is not too great.

Suppositories and Inserts

Powders, granules, capsules, and tablets generally can be used as a source of active drug in compounding suppositories and inserts, provided the volume of powder required to obtain the active drug is not excessive. Ointments and creams can sometimes be used in small quantities if the bases are compatible. Gels are not recommended unless the base is a polyethylene glycol or glycerinated gelatin base that would be compatible with gels. Suppositories and inserts can be used as appropriate if the bases are compatible. Solutions and suspensions in very small quantities can often be incorporated into suppository vehicles, but concentrating the active drug by evaporation of the water, either partially or to complete dryness, may be necessary. Emulsions may be suitable if the suppository base will take up the phases and be stable. Parenterals may be used if they are highly concentrated or if they are powders for injection. Ophthalmics, nasal solutions, and aqueous otic solutions can be used only if they are sufficiently concentrated or can be evaporated to meet the required volume limitations. Otic solutions that are oil based may be miscible with many suppository and insert bases.

Solutions

A primary consideration in preparing solutions is whether they are for internal or external use. Powders and granules may or may not be suitable, depending on whether all the excipients are soluble in the vehicle or insoluble excipients can be appropriately removed by filtration. Similarly, capsules and tablets may be suitable when they can be pulverized, placed into solution, and filtered, provided that all the excipients are soluble in the vehicle.

Oleaginous and absorption ointment bases are suitable only for nonaqueous solutions. Generally, emulsion bases are not suitable without a specific solvent blend to dissolve both phases. Active drugs contained in water-soluble ointment bases can be used to prepare aqueous solutions. Gels can often be used to prepare solutions, because the process is actually one of diluting the gel and maintaining a clear solution.

Suppositories and inserts are not suitable for solutions in most circumstances. If nonaqueous solutions are desired, then oleaginous suppository bases may be considered. If aqueous solutions are desired, then polyethylene glycol suppository–based active drugs may work.

Solutions are obviously fine to use to compound other solutions. Suspensions and emulsions can be used only if the solvent system in the compounded formulation will dissolve the suspended or emulsified materials.

Parenterals, ophthalmics, nasal solutions, and otic solutions may be appropriate, depending on the concentration required and solubility. Parenteral powders for reconstitution may be appropriate.

Suspensions

Powders, granules, capsules, and tablets usually work well. The quantity of powders and granules may need to be considered. Ointments and creams generally do not work well unless the solvent system is nonaqueous or a blend of solvents. Gels usually can be used if their base is miscible with the suspension vehicle.

Suppositories and inserts are usually not appropriate unless they are of a water-soluble base (polyethylene glycol or glycerinated gelatin) for an aqueous suspension. Nonaqueous vehicles may be satisfactory for oleaginous suppositories and inserts. Solutions and other suspensions generally are appropriate. Emulsions can be used only if the vehicle in the compounded suspension can dissolve both phases of the emulsion; otherwise, a suspension emulsion would result. Parenterals, ophthalmics, nasal solutions, and aqueous-based otic solutions or suspensions usually can be used with little difficulty.

Emulsions

Powders, granules, capsules, and tablets generally can be used as the drug source for preparing emulsions; however, emulsion suspensions can result because of the excipients present in the commercial dosage form. Ointments and creams may be appropriate, depending on the presence of additional emulsifying agents and the quantity of commercial product that must be incorporated. Gels can easily be used with oil-in-water emulsions, because they will blend into the external phase. Suppositories and inserts are not generally advisable, but using heat to melt the suppositories or inserts and incorporating them into the heated emulsion vehicle, possibly with additional surfactant and with shearing, potentially may result in a suitable emulsion.

Solutions are a good source of active drugs for preparing emulsions. Suspensions may be appropriate, and the final preparation may be an emulsion suspension. Emulsions can often be blended to form a new or even a multiple emulsion. Parenterals, ophthalmics, nasal solutions, and aqueous otic solutions may be appropriate to use. If oil-based otic solutions are used, incorporating an additional emulsifying agent or surfactant for oil-in-water emulsions may be necessary; in water-in-oil emulsions, the oil-based otic solution may be readily miscible.

Parenterals

Nonsterile commercial dosage forms of powders, granules, capsules, and tablets usually should not be used for compounding parenterals. Ointments, creams, gels, suppositories, and inserts are likewise inappropriate. Nonsterile solutions, suspensions, and emulsions should not be used even if sterilized, because of the potential endotoxin load and the presence of inappropriate excipients for parenteral administration. Parenterals can be used. In general, using ophthalmics, nasal solutions, and otic solutions would be inappropriate because of the potential endotoxin load and the presence of inappropriate excipients for parenteral administration.

Ophthalmic Preparations

Powders, granules, capsules, and tablets generally are inappropriate sources of active drugs for ophthalmic products because of the presence of excipients. Ointments may be used only if sterilization and other processes would not adversely affect the preparation of an ophthalmic ointment. Creams are not appropriate. Gels generally are not appropriate except under certain circumstances. Suppositories and inserts are inappropriate. Solutions may be considered if they are appropriate for the specific situation and the requirements for ophthalmics can be met. Suspensions and emulsions are not appropriate because of the particle size and irritant properties of these dosage forms. Parenterals are generally appropriate to use in compounding ophthalmic preparations. Nasal solutions and aqueous otic solutions should be used only if necessary and with due consideration of the excipients they contain.

Nasal Preparations

Powders, granules, capsules, and tablets generally are not suitable because of the presence of insoluble excipients. Ointments are generally not appropriate unless they have water-soluble bases. Creams are not usually suitable. Gels may work satisfactorily. Suppositories and inserts are not suitable. Solutions and suspensions may be considered if the quantity to be used is reasonable. Generally, emulsions should not be used. Parenterals, ophthalmics, and aqueous otic solutions usually can be used satisfactorily.

Otic Preparations

Powders, granules, capsules, and tablets should be used only if the presence of the excipients is considered. The insoluble excipients tend to build up in the ear canal and mix with cerumen, which can cause problems. Generally, ointments, creams, and gels should be considered as a source of active drug if small quantities can be incorporated into a liquid otic preparation. Suppositories and inserts are not appropriate. Solutions, suspensions, and emulsions may be appropriate sources. Parenterals, ophthalmics, and nasal solutions can often be used; in some cases, all that is needed is to add viscosity-enhancing agents.

Disposing of Expired Ingredients and Medications

Daily, weekly, and monthly, compounding pharmacists face the challenge of responsibly disposing of expired medications and chemicals. In years past, pharmacists avoided accumulating out-of-date drugs by incinerating them on the premises, washing them down the sink, flushing them down the toilet, or attempting to return them indirectly (via sales representatives) or directly to the manufacturer.[1]

We now know that the on-site incineration of expired drugs pollutes the air and that discarding medications in the dumpster or trash bin can result in drug diversion or in accidental poisoning because many pharmaceutical agents are hydrophilic, biologically active, and persistent and often resist wastewater treatment. Drugs currently detected in environmental samples include lipid regulators, hormones, antidepressants, beta-blockers, antibiotics, oral contraceptives, antiepileptics, antineoplastics, tranquilizers, nonopioid analgesics, and anti-inflammatory agents. Medications can remain unused for many reasons, including noncompliance, death of the patient, expiration dates, low utilization, overstocking because of a one-time use for a patient, special needs, a change in prescribing practices, and withdrawal of the drug from the U.S. market. Regardless of the reason for disposal, compounding pharmacists, like their institutional and retail colleagues, are increasingly pressured to find environmentally friendly and affordable methods of disposing of expired products.

When disposing of pharmaceutical waste, pharmacists must comply with all pertinent state and federal regulations according to the U.S. Environmental Protection Agency. Specific chemicals are listed as hazardous waste in the Resource Conservation and Recovery Act (RCRA). RCRA has classified hazardous pharmaceutical waste into three categories: the "P" list, the "U" list, and the "D" list. All RCRA hazardous waste must be managed and disposed of according to specific guidelines and cannot be discarded in sewers or landfills. Over the past decade, the disposal of hazardous pharmaceutical waste has become a science, and companies with expertise in that specialty are increasing in number.[2,3]

References

1. United States Pharmacopeial Convention. Chapter <795>, Pharmaceutical compounding—non-sterile preparations. In: *United States Pharmacopeia/National Formulary*. Rockville, MD: United States Pharmacopeial Convention; current edition.
2. Vail J. Disposing of expired drugs and chemicals: new options for compounders. *Int J Pharm Compound*. 2008;12(1):38–47.
3. Vail J. Consumer options for the disposal of unused medications. *Int J Pharm Compound*. 2008;12(1):87.

Compounding with Hazardous Drugs

In addition to ensuring safe use of medications by patients and clients, health care workers preparing and handling medications must protect themselves from danger. Traditionally, the term *hazardous drugs* was used in reference to cytotoxic agents. Current recommendations are for many other types of drugs to be handled as hazardous. Also, the *United States Pharmacopeia (USP)* has General Chapter <800>, Hazardous Drugs—Handling in Healthcare Settings, scheduled to become enforceable July 1, 2018, that will be discussed later in this chapter.

Regulatory Framework

In 1970, the Occupational Safety and Health Act created the Occupational Safety and Health Administration (OSHA) as an agency of the U.S. Department of Labor. OSHA's authority extends to employees in most nongovernmental workplaces; in general, state and local government workers are excluded. The same act also created the National Institute for Occupational Safety and Health (NIOSH), a research agency charged with identifying major hazards in the workplace and ways of controlling them. A primary consideration for these agencies is the cost of regulations and enforcement versus the actual benefit in reduced worker injury, illness, and death.

In 2004, NIOSH issued an alert[1] to increase awareness of health risks involved in working with hazardous drugs and protective measures that should be taken. The alert is aimed at personnel who prepare or administer hazardous drugs and who work in areas where these drugs are handled and therefore may be exposed to these agents in the air, on work surfaces and other surfaces, on contaminated clothing, on medical equipment, or in patient excreta. According to the alert, workplace exposure to hazardous drugs has resulted in health effects such as skin rashes and adverse reproductive outcomes (including infertility, spontaneous abortions, and congenital malformations) and possibly leukemia and other cancers.

Definition of "Hazardous"

Drugs are classified as hazardous if studies in animals or humans indicate that exposure to them has a potential for causing cancer, developmental or reproductive toxicity, or harm to organs. According to the NIOSH Working Group on Hazardous Drugs, a drug is considered hazardous if it exhibits one or more of the following characteristics in humans or animals:

1. Carcinogenicity (in animal models or the patient population, or both)
2. Teratogenicity or other developmental toxicity (or fertility impairment in animal studies or in treated patients)
3. Reproductive toxicity
4. Organ toxicity at low doses (evidence of serious organ or other toxicity at low doses in animal models or treated patients)
5. Genotoxicity (i.e., mutagenicity and clastogenicity in short-term test systems)
6. Structure and toxicity profiles of new drugs that mimic existing drugs determined hazardous by the above criteria

NIOSH updates its list of drugs that should be handled as hazardous substances (Table 3-1).[1] The reasons for including cytotoxic drugs are clear, but understanding why some of the other drugs are included is more difficult. No single approach can adequately cover the diverse potential occupational exposures to hazardous drugs. The current NIOSH approach involves three different groups of drugs, as follows:

- *Group 1: Antineoplastic drugs.* Note that many of these drugs may also pose a reproductive risk for susceptible populations.
- *Group 2:* These nonantineoplastic drugs meet one or more of the NIOSH criteria for a hazardous drug. Note that some of these drugs may also pose a reproductive risk for susceptible populations.
- *Group 3:* These drugs primarily pose a reproductive risk to men and women who are actively trying to conceive and women who are pregnant or breast feeding, because some of these drugs may be present in breast milk.

TABLE 3-1 Examples from the NIOSH List of Drugs That Should Be Handled as Hazardous Substances[a]

Group 1 Antineoplastic Drugs

Abiraterone	Floxuridine	Oxaliplatin
Arsenic trioxide	Gemcitabine	Paclitaxel
Azacitidine	Hydroxyurea	Procarbazine
Bacillus calmette Guerin (BCG)	Ifosfamide	Romidepsin
Bleomycin	Leuprolide	Streptozocin
Busulfan	Lomustine	Tamoxifen
Carboplatin	Mechlorethamine	Thioguanine
Carmustine	Megestrol	Thiotepa
Chlorambucil	Mercaptopurine	Vinblastine
Cisplatin	Methotrexate	Vincristine
Doxorubicin	Mitomycin	
Etoposide	Nilotinib	

TABLE 3-1 Examples from the NIOSH List of Drugs That Should Be Handled as Hazardous Substances[a] *(Continued)*

Group 2 Nonantineoplastic Drugs

Abacavir	Estrogens, conjugated	Progestins
Apomorphine	Estrogens, esterified	Propylthiouracil
Azathioprine	Estropipate	Sirolimus
Carbamazepine	Fosphenytoin	Spironolactone
Chloramphenicol	Ganciclovir	Tacrolimus
Cyclosporine	Medroxyprogesterone acetate	Thalidomide
Diethylstilbestrol	Mycophenolate mofetil	Uracil mustard
Divalproex	Oxcarbazepine	Valganciclovir
Estradiol	Phenytoin	Zidovudine
Estrogen/progesterone combinations	Progesterone	

Group 3 Drugs Posing a Reproductive Risk to Men and Women

Acitretin	Fluconazole	Testosterone
Alitretinoin	Gonadotropin, chorionic	Topiramate
Choriogonadotropin	Methyltestosterone	Tretinoin
Clonazepam	Mifepristone	Valproate/Valproic acid
Colchicine	Misoprostol	Voriconazole
Dinoprostone	Oxytocin	Warfarin
Ergonovine/methylergonovine	Paroxetine	Ziprasidone
Finasteride	Ribavirin	Zonisamide

[a]NIOSH adapted this list from lists used by four health care facilities (National Institutes of Health Clinical Center, Bethesda, Maryland; Johns Hopkins Hospital, Baltimore, Maryland; Northside Hospital, Atlanta, Georgia; and University of Michigan Hospitals and Health Centers, Ann Arbor) and the Pharmaceutical Research and Manufacturers of America.

Facility-Specific Hazardous Drug List

The NIOSH alert emphasized that each facility should develop its own list of hazardous drugs. Drugs that might be placed on the list include those known or suspected to cause adverse health effects from exposure in the workplace, drugs used in cancer chemotherapy, antiviral drugs, hormones, and some bioengineered drugs. The current NIOSH list is available at www.cdc.gov/niosh/docs/2014-138/pdfs/2014-138_v3.pdf.

The original list was published in 2004 and updated in 2010, 2012, and 2014. Drugs are periodically added to and removed from the list on the basis of experience and input. Each organization's list should reflect the drugs considered to be hazardous that are used in that specific workplace. Also, the physical characteristics of the drugs (such as liquid versus solid or water versus lipid solubility) need to be considered in determining the potential for occupational exposure. The list will change as new drugs are added and drugs that are no longer used are removed. The list may exclude some drugs that might be hazardous if the risk of direct exposure to those drugs is minimal. For example, if tablets or capsules of a drug are coated, a worker will not be directly exposed. However, if the coated dosage form is modified by crushing the tablets or emptying the capsules to make solutions or suspensions, then it must be considered for the list.

BOX 3-1 FDA Pregnancy Categories

A: Controlled studies in pregnant women have failed to demonstrate a risk to the fetus in the first trimester, and there is no evidence of risk in later trimesters. The possibility of fetal harm appears remote.

B: Either animal-reproduction studies have not demonstrated a fetal risk and there are no controlled studies in pregnant women, or animal-reproduction studies have shown an adverse effect (other than a decrease in fertility) that was not confirmed in controlled studies in women in the first trimester and there is no evidence of a risk in later trimesters.

C: Either studies in animals have revealed adverse effects on the fetus (teratogenic or embryocidal effects or other) and there are no controlled studies in women, or studies in women and animals are not available. Drugs should be given only if the potential benefits justify the potential risk to the fetus.

D: There is positive evidence of human fetal risk, but the benefits from use in pregnant women may be acceptable despite the risk (e.g., if the drug is needed in a life-threatening situation or for a serious disease for which safer drugs cannot be used or are ineffective).

X: Studies in animals or humans have demonstrated fetal abnormalities or there is evidence of fetal risk based on human experience, or both, and the risk of the use of the drug in pregnant women clearly outweighs any possible benefit. The drug is contraindicated in women who are or may become pregnant.

Resources for information on drug toxicity include material safety data sheets (MSDSs); product labeling (package inserts) approved by the U.S. Food and Drug Administration (FDA); special health warnings from drug manufacturers, FDA, and professional organizations; reports and case studies published in professional medical and health care journals; and evidence-based recommendations from other facilities that have successfully defined hazardous drugs and prepared a list. Also useful in preparing the list are FDA pregnancy categories (Box 3-1), which indicate the potential of a systemically absorbed drug to cause birth defects.

Limiting of Exposure

Although all drugs have toxic side effects, some exhibit toxicity at low doses. Toxicity becomes a concern when it is exhibited at doses of a few milligrams or less. The pharmaceutical industry has used a daily therapeutic dose of 10 mg/day or a dose of 1 mg/kg per day in laboratory animals that produces serious organ toxicity, developmental toxicity, or reproductive toxicity to develop occupational exposure limits of less than 10 μg/m³ after applying appropriate uncertainty factors.

The NIOSH alert notes that health risk is influenced by the extent of exposure and by the potency and toxicity of the hazardous drug. In general, no recommended exposure limits have been set by NIOSH, OSHA, or the American Conference of Governmental Industrial Hygienists (ACGIH). OSHA has permissible exposure limits (PELs), and ACGIH has threshold limit values (TLVs) for soluble platinum salts; both determinations are based on sensitization and not on the potential to cause cancer. For inorganic arsenic compounds, which include arsenic trioxide, these groups have established PELs, TLVs, and recommended exposure limits (NIOSH).[1] A workplace environmental exposure level has been established for some antibiotics, including chloramphenicol. MSDSs are a potential source of guidance on exposure limits.

Employers should implement necessary administrative and engineering controls, ensure that workers follow sound procedures for handling hazardous drugs, and supply proper protective equipment in order to provide employees with the greatest protection. The NIOSH alert does not apply to workers in the drug manufacturing sector (companies develop their own recommendations), but it does apply to pharmacy personnel, nursing personnel, physicians, operating room personnel, environmental services workers, workers in research laboratories, veterinary care workers, and shipping and receiving personnel.

Many situations occur during pharmaceutical compounding in which an employee may be exposed to hazardous drugs. Factors that can affect exposure include the amount of hazardous drug used, the frequency and duration of handling of hazardous drugs, personal protective equipment, potential for hazardous drug absorption (inhalation or skin absorption), use of ventilated cabinets, and an employee's work practices. In general, the likelihood that an employee will experience adverse effects from hazardous drugs increases with greater and more frequent exposure, inadequate equipment, and poor work practices.

Sources of Exposure

Workers in any pharmacy or health care facility, including hospitals, community pharmacies, home care settings, clinics, and physician offices, have the potential to be exposed to hazardous drugs. Although workers are aware of some sources of exposure, they may be unaware of other, inadvertent exposures. Pharmacists, pharmacy technicians, and other health care workers can be exposed to hazardous drugs when manipulations create aerosols or generate dust or when the workers come in contact with contaminated surfaces or clean up spills.

For example, in 2005 a report stated that pharmacy technicians had been exposed to cancer chemotherapeutic agents through contaminated outside surfaces of drug vials.[2] In one facility, detectable chemotherapy residues were found in the urine of two technicians who had prepared drug doses, despite their use of isolation cabinets and PhaSeal isolation units. A third technician, who had never entered the prescription area, showed significantly higher contamination; this technician had unpacked the medication as it arrived from the wholesaler and had not worn gloves. The exterior of the vials and the packing they were shipped in were all contaminated. Three studies have shown that contamination of outside surfaces of chemotherapy drug vials is a common occurrence. This danger can be reduced easily by extra washing and by wrapping the vials in plastic sleeves during the manufacturing process.

Until the pharmaceutical industry accepts responsibility for delivering contamination-free prescription medications, the burden falls on pharmacists to safeguard workers handling these materials. On receipt, containers should be decontaminated as soon as possible by personnel trained in handling hazardous drugs. Staff wearing gloves and gowns should rinse off the containers before the product enters the compounding area.

Another example of harm occurred a number of years ago to a worker who was using a now-obsolete technique. A 39-year-old pharmacist suffered two episodes of painless hematuria and was found to have cancer (grade II papillary transitional cell carcinoma). Twelve years before her diagnosis, she had worked full time for 20 months in a hospital routinely preparing cytotoxic agents, including cyclophosphamide, fluorouracil, methotrexate, doxorubicin, and cisplatin. She had used a horizontal laminar-airflow hood that directed the airflow toward her. Because she was a nonsmoker and had no other known occupational or environmental risk factors, her cancer was attributed to her antineoplastic drug exposure at work, although a cause-and-effect relationship has not been established in the literature.[1]

Hazardous drug waste is a ubiquitous source of exposure. Workers may be exposed to waste through packaging materials; disposable equipment; used syringes and related administration equipment; paper towels, 4×4 gauze, or lint-free wipes (especially those used in cleaning residue from hoods); wash and rinse water; partially filled vials; undispensed products; unused intravenous (IV) admixtures; needles and syringes; gloves; gowns; underpads; soiled materials from spill cleanup; used IV bags or drug vials that contain more than trace amounts of hazardous drugs; weigh boats and papers; disposable straw spatulas; and shoe covers (a worker who has stepped in something that was spilled should wear gloves to remove the shoe covers).

Pharmacy-Specific Sources of Exposure

Specific pharmacy activities that may expose workers to hazardous drugs are listed below.

Receipt of Materials
- Commercial products received from drug manufacturers: All bottles, vials, bags, and packages received directly from drug manufacturers or wholesalers
- Packaged bulk powders received from pharmaceutical compounding suppliers, especially those that have been repackaged
- Tanks of gases (nitrous oxide, nitrogen, and nuclear tagging material)
- Compounded radionuclides for use with imaging equipment
- Powder in gloves

Prescription Dispensing
- Counting of individual, uncoated oral doses and tablets during dispensing
- Packaging of uncoated tablets in unit dose packages or blister packages
- Broken tablets in commercial bottles
- Broken capsules or capsules that have separated in commercial bottles and emptied their contents in the container
- Reconstitution of containers of oral powders into liquids, especially injectable hazardous drugs that may cause backspray, drops, or aerosol formation
- For hazardous drugs handled the same as less hazardous substances, likely contamination of the individual and the work environment
- Buildup of tablet and capsule residue on counting trays and machines
- Accidental spillage of oral liquids while being poured into smaller bottles

Prescription Compounding
- Touching surfaces of containers of drugs on the hazardous drugs list
- Working in an uncontrolled environment with drugs on the hazardous drugs list
- Handling equipment in which drugs on the hazardous drugs list have been used
- Washing equipment in which drugs on the hazardous drugs list have been used
- Packaging and labeling containers of drugs on the hazardous drugs list
- Crushing tablets and emptying capsules to make oral liquid dosage forms for patients who cannot swallow oral solids
- Compounding capsules, troches, oral liquids, ointments, creams, gels, suppositories, injectables, and other forms

- Generating aerosols during reconstitution of commercial vials
- Expelling air from syringes that have contained hazardous drugs
- Obtaining hazardous drugs from vials or ampuls during the compounding of an IV admixture or other sterile or nonsterile dosage form
- Experiencing touch contamination of drugs present on drug vials, work surfaces, floors, and final drug preparations (vials, bottles, bags, cassettes, syringes, tubes)
- Priming an IV administration set or pump device

Patient Counseling

- Handling any container of a drug on the hazardous drugs list
- Opening a container of a drug on the hazardous drugs list and demonstrating to a patient

Transporting Hazardous Drugs

- Handling any container returned to the pharmacy by a patient, patient's family, or nursing staff member
- Transporting hazardous drugs and hazardous waste materials via local delivery vehicle
- Transporting hazardous drugs via commercial freight vendors
- Transporting hazardous drugs via pneumatic tube systems in hospitals

Cleanup and Disposal

- Handling and discarding unused, returned byproducts or portions of hazardous drugs and contaminated equipment, such as devices that have been used for administering hazardous drugs; contaminated wastes resulting from any step in the dispensing, compounding, or administration process; and unused hazardous drugs that remain in vials, bags, or cassettes or are outdated
- Decontaminating hazardous drug containers or work areas where hazardous drugs are handled
- Removing and disposing of personal protective equipment after handling hazardous drugs or waste materials
- Disposing of cleanup materials used for hazardous drugs

Route, Time, and Extent of Exposure

Exposure to hazardous drugs can occur via inhalation, skin contact, skin absorption, ingestion, or injection. The most likely routes are inhalation and skin contact with absorption. Unintentional ingestion may result from hand-to-mouth contact, and accidental injection can occur in a needle-stick or *sharps* injury.

The likelihood that a worker will experience adverse effects from exposure to hazardous drugs increases with the amount and frequency of exposure and the degree to which improper procedures are followed. Other factors that affect exposure include the purpose of handling drugs (receipt, dispensing, compounding, administration, or disposal), the quantity of drug involved, and the potential for inhalation and absorption. For example, dispensing a single tablet to a patient poses little to no risk to the health care worker. A single pair of gloves is adequate. However, repeatedly counting, cutting, or crushing tablets may pose a higher risk of worker exposure and contamination to the workplace if proper precautions are not in place. If a containment device such as a Class II biological safety cabinet (BSC) or compounding aseptic containment isolator (CACI) is not available, then double gloves, a protective gown, respiratory protection, and a disposable pad to protect the work surface should be used. Also, preparing a number of IV doses of an antineoplastic drug typically poses a higher potential risk to the worker. In addition to double gloving and a protective gown, an engineering control such as a BSC or CACI, possibly supplemented with a closed-system transfer device (CSTD), is required to protect the drug, environment, and health care worker.

Work practices and procedures that affect exposure include the use of exhaust and ventilated cabinets and the filtration level used; appropriate use of personal protective equipment; and proper cleanup procedures for personnel (e.g., showers) and the facility. Access to hazardous drug storage areas should be restricted; pass-through windows may help minimize traffic flow through these areas. Touch contamination can be minimized by using voice-activated intercoms and telephones.

Pharmacy Safety Program

The safety program used in a compounding pharmacy to protect pharmacists and technicians handling hazardous drugs should consist of activities for which efficacy and cost-effectiveness have been documented. The safety program should include use of the appropriate equipment (e.g., BSCs; see Box 3-2 for types of BSCs) to protect personnel, as well as a facility-specific list of hazardous drugs.

BOX 3-2 Types of Biological Safety Cabinets

Class I BSC. A Class I biological safety cabinet (BSC) protects personnel and the work environment but does not protect the product. It is a negative-pressure, ventilated cabinet usually operated with an open front and a minimum face velocity at the work opening of at least 75 ft/min. A Class I BSC is similar in design to a chemical fume hood except that all of the air from the cabinet is exhausted through a high-efficiency particulate air (HEPA) filter either into the laboratory or to the outside.

Class II BSC. A Class II BSC is a ventilated BSC that protects personnel, product, and the work environment. A Class II BSC has an open front with inward airflow for personnel protection, downward HEPA-filtered laminar airflow for product protection, and HEPA-filtered exhausted air for environmental protection.

Type A1 (formerly, type A). These Class II BSCs maintain a minimum inflow velocity of 75 ft/min, have HEPA-filtered downflow air that is a portion of the mixed downflow and inflow air from a common plenum, may exhaust HEPA-filtered air back into the laboratory or to the environment through an exhaust canopy, and may have positive-pressure contaminated ducts and plenums that are not surrounded by negative-pressure plenums. They are not suitable for use with volatile toxic chemicals and volatile radionuclides.

Type A2 (formerly, type B3). These Class II BSCs maintain a minimum inflow velocity of 100 ft/min, have HEPA-filtered downflow air that is a portion of the mixed downflow and inflow air from a common exhaust plenum, may exhaust HEPA-filtered air back into the laboratory or to the environment through an exhaust canopy, and have all contaminated ducts and plenums under negative pressure or surrounded by negative-pressure ducts and plenums. If these cabinets are used for minute quantities of volatile toxic chemicals and trace amounts of radionuclides, they must be exhausted through properly functioning exhaust canopies.

BOX 3-2 Types of Biological Safety Cabinets (Continued)

Type B1. These Class II BSCs maintain a minimum inflow velocity of 100 ft/min; have HEPA-filtered downflow air composed largely of uncontaminated, recirculated inflow air; exhaust most of the contaminated downflow air through a dedicated duct exhausted to the atmosphere after passing the air through a HEPA filter; and have all contaminated ducts and plenums under negative pressure or surrounded by negative-pressure ducts and plenums. If these cabinets are used for work involving minute quantities of volatile toxic chemicals and trace amounts of radionuclides, the work must be done in the directly exhausted portion of the cabinet.

Type B2 (total exhaust). These Class II BSCs maintain a minimum inflow velocity of 100 ft/min, have HEPA-filtered downflow air drawn from the laboratory or the outside, exhaust all inflow and downflow air to the atmosphere after filtration through a HEPA filter without recirculation inside the cabinet or return to the laboratory, and have all contaminated ducts and plenums under negative pressure or surrounded by directly exhausted negative-pressure ducts and plenums. These cabinets may be used with volatile toxic chemicals and radionuclides.

Class III BSC. A Class III BSC has a totally enclosed, ventilated cabinet of gas-tight construction in which operations are conducted through attached rubber gloves and observed through a nonopening view window. This BSC is maintained under negative pressure of at least 0.5 inch of water gauge, and air is drawn into the cabinet through HEPA filters. The exhaust air is treated by double HEPA filtration or single HEPA filtration and incineration. Passage of materials in and out of the cabinet is generally performed through a dunk tank (accessible through the cabinet floor) or a double-door pass-through box (such as an autoclave) that can be decontaminated between uses.

Source: Reference 1.

Four general principles established by the American Society of Health-System Pharmacists[3] for handling hazardous drugs are as follows:

1. Protect and secure packages of hazardous drugs.
2. Inform and educate all involved personnel about hazardous drugs, and train them in the safe handling procedures relevant to their responsibilities.
3. Do not let the drugs escape from containers when they are manipulated (i.e., dissolved, transferred, administered, or discarded).
4. Estimate the possibility of inadvertent ingestion or inhalation and direct skin or eye contact with the drugs.

NIOSH Recommendations for Employees

The NIOSH alert suggests many precautions workers can take to protect themselves from exposure to hazardous drugs:

- Read all information, including MSDSs, on the hazardous drugs you will be handling.
- Attend all training sessions that are offered by your employer or reasonably available that relate to handling hazardous drugs.

- Be able to recognize potential sources of exposure to hazardous drugs, including receiving, unpacking, cleaning, manipulating, compounding, packaging, labeling, packing, and shipping procedures, as well as potential exposure in patient-care settings.
- Compound hazardous drugs in an area that is designed for that purpose and is restricted to only authorized personnel.
- Compound hazardous drugs only in a ventilated cabinet designed to protect workers from exposure.
- Use double-gloving procedures as appropriate; the inner gloves should be placed under the gown cuff, and the outer gloves should cover the gown cuff. Use non-powdered gloves.
- Avoid skin contact by using a disposable nonlinting, nonabsorbent gown made of polyethylene-coated polypropylene. The gown should have a closed front, long sleeves, and elastic or knit closed cuffs. Gowns should not be reused.
- Use a face shield in those cases when splashes to the eyes, nose, or mouth may occur.
- Wash hands with soap and water immediately before donning and after removing personal protective clothing.
- Use Luer-Lok fittings when preparing and administering hazardous drugs; do not use slip-tip fittings.
- Use sharps containers for disposal of all drug-contaminated syringes and needles.
- Use CSTDs, glove bags, and needleless systems during compounding, if available and appropriate.
- Keep hazardous waste trash separate from other wastes.
- Clean and decontaminate the work areas involving hazardous drugs before and after each compounding activity, as well as at the end of each shift.
- Clean up spills immediately, using proper safety precautions and personal protective equipment. If large spills occur, notify the pharmacist in charge immediately.
- If using ampuls of a hazardous drug, gently tap down from the neck and top of the ampul before opening. Wipe the ampul with alcohol before opening. Place a sterile gauze pad around the neck of the ampul during opening to protect from spray.
- Avoid situations that may create substantial positive or negative pressure within drug vials and syringes.
- Use venting devices containing 0.2-μm filters or 5-μm filter needles, as appropriate.
- Wipe the outside of vials, bottles, bags, and administration sets before releasing, using an alcohol-moistened sterile gauze pad.
- Minimize exposure of a patient or caregiver by presenting the final preparation in a ready-to-use form if possible.
- Place final preparations in sealable containers (zippered plastic bags), if reasonable, to minimize risk of exposure of other personnel.
- Return excess drug to the drug vial or discard into a closed container (empty sterile vial), as appropriate.
- Place all contaminated materials in leakproof, puncture-resistant containers while in the contained environment. Then, place these containers in larger containers outside the contained environment for disposal.
- Do not place tablet or capsule dosage forms of hazardous drugs in automated counting machines.
- For routine handling (not compounding) of hazardous drugs and contaminated equipment, wear one pair of gloves of good quality and thickness.

- Carefully follow prescribed procedures, using dedicated equipment, for counting and pouring hazardous drugs. After use, clean the contaminated equipment with water and then detergent, and rinse with water thereafter. Both water and gauze (if used) need to be disposed of as contaminated waste.
- Wear low-permeability gowns and double gloves when compounding with hazardous drugs (e.g., weighing, crushing, dissolving, levigating, mixing). The compounding work area should be protective and away from drafts and traffic, and appropriate respiratory protection should be worn. If a plastic bag is used for crushing tablets or mixing powders, use caution to prevent breaking the plastic bag.
- Dispose of unused or wasted dosage forms of hazardous drugs in the same manner as other hazardous wastes.
- Be familiar with the protocol for emergency first aid after direct contact with hazardous drugs, as well as the follow-up procedures. Post these protocols in areas where hazardous drugs are handled.
- Attach an appropriate label, according to state laws and regulations, to hazardous drug preparations.

NIOSH Recommendations for Employers

The NIOSH alert suggests the following approaches for employers:

- Provide written and enforced standard operating procedures covering all aspects of activities involving hazardous drugs; these include receipt, storage, preparation, administration, housekeeping, decontamination, cleanup, disposal, contaminated spills, and patient wastes.
- Attend training or participate in educational activities to become familiar with all aspects of hazardous drugs that may be in the facility. Provide training that covers all aspects of handling hazardous drugs, including relevant techniques and procedures and proper use of protective equipment and materials.
- Provide employees with information regarding hazardous drugs, especially MSDSs.
- Train employees to recognize opportunities for exposure to hazardous drugs and the way to monitor and control them. Provide a safety program and information on toxicity, treatment of acute exposure, chemical inactivators, solubility, and stability of hazardous drugs used in the workplace.
- Provide a separate, isolated area for receipt and opening of containers of hazardous drugs.
- Maintain a perpetual inventory of all hazardous drugs in a facility, or at least update the inventory at regular intervals.
- Provide a work area dedicated to storage and compounding of hazardous drugs, with access limited to authorized personnel.
- Provide bins and shelving with a barrier on the front edge to minimize the chance of drugs falling off the shelf.
- Do not allow employees to compound hazardous drugs in a horizontal laminar-airflow cabinet.
- Direct employees to use appropriate laminar-airflow cabinets, biological safety cabinets, or containment isolators designed to prevent hazardous drugs from escaping into the work environment.
- Exhaust all work environments appropriately for the compounding being conducted.

- Provide respiratory protection for all employees if a containment environment is not used. Surgical masks provide no respiratory protection against powdered or liquid aerosols of hazardous drugs.
- Provide employees with all the necessary protective clothing and equipment required to work safely, and provide training in their use.
- Establish and oversee appropriate work practices for compounding hazardous drugs.
- Provide syringes and sets with Luer-Lok fittings for compounding and administering hazardous drugs. Also provide proper containers for their disposal.
- Provide CSTDs, as appropriate.
- Periodically evaluate equipment, training, standard operating procedures, and hazardous drugs to determine how exposure can be reduced to a minimum.
- Confirm that a facility and all personnel comply with local, state, and federal regulations related to handling, storage, and transportation of hazardous drugs.
- Have job-specific medical evaluations performed on appropriate employees at the following times:
  - Before job placement
  - Periodically during employment (e.g., annual blood tests)
  - Following acute exposures
  - At the time of job termination or transfer

Training

All staff who will be compounding hazardous drugs must be trained in the proper techniques necessary for working with hazardous drugs. Once trained, staff must demonstrate competence by an objective method, and competency must be reassessed on a regular basis.

All personnel who work with or around hazardous drugs must be trained to appropriately perform their jobs following standard operating procedures and using the established precautions and required personal protective equipment. Training must include appropriate procedures for personal protection and prevention of contamination. Hazardous drugs should be compounded in a controlled area where access is limited to authorized personnel trained in handling requirements. Because of the hazardous nature of these preparations, a contained environment that has air pressure negative to the surrounding areas or is protected by an airlock or anteroom is preferred; pass-through windows are desired.

In addition, the ability to recognize potential sources of exposure to hazardous drugs—receiving, unpacking, cleaning, manipulating, compounding, packaging, labeling, packing, and shipping procedures—and potential exposure in the patient-care settings is critical. Training shall include, among other items, safe manipulations, use of MSDSs, negative-pressure techniques, correct use of CSTDs, containment, cleanup, spill abatement, disposal procedures for breakages and spills, and treatment of personnel contact and inhalation exposure.

Facility and General Work Procedures

Proper air-handling engineering controls designed to eliminate or reduce worker exposure to chemical, biological, radiological, ergonomic, and physical hazards are critical. Ventilated cabinets and engineering controls must be designed for the purpose of worker protection.

Hazardous drugs should be compounded in an area restricted to authorized personnel. The work areas should be cleaned and decontaminated before and after each compounding activity, as well as at the end of each shift.

Distinctive labels should be used to indicate drug packages, bins, shelves, and storage areas for hazardous drugs as those requiring special handling precautions. Hazardous drugs should be protected from potential breakage during storage by use of bins that have high fronts and are placed on shelves that have guards to prevent accidental falling. Segregation of hazardous drug inventory improves control and reduces the number of staff members potentially exposed to the danger. Staff members must wear double gloves when stocking and inventorying these drugs and selecting hazardous drug packages for further handling. Transport of hazardous drug packages must be done in a manner to reduce environmental contamination in the event of accidental dropping.

Carts or other transport devices must have guards to protect against containers falling and breaking. Handling final preparations and transport bags with gloves contaminated with hazardous drugs will result in the transfer of the contamination to other workers. Fresh gloves should be donned whenever there is a doubt as to the cleanliness of the inner or outer gloves.

Policies and procedures to prevent spills and to govern cleanup of hazardous drug spills must be developed and implemented. Written procedures must specify who is responsible for spill management and must address the size and scope of the spill. Spills must be contained and cleaned up immediately by trained workers.

Personnel Protection

Gloves

- Wash hands before donning and after removing gloves.
- Wear powder-free, high-quality gloves made of latex, nitrile, polyurethane, neoprene, or other materials that meet the American Society for Testing Materials (ASTM) standard for chemotherapy gloves.
- Wear double gloves for all activities involving hazardous drugs.
- Before and after donning gloves, inspect for visible defects.
- Sanitize gloves with sterile 70% alcohol or other appropriate disinfectant before performing any aseptic compounding activity.
- Change gloves every 30 minutes during compounding or immediately when damaged or contaminated.
- Remove outer gloves after wiping down final preparation but before labeling or removing the preparation from the isolator.
- Outer gloves must be placed in a containment bag while in the isolator.
- In an isolator, wear a second glove inside the fixed-glove assembly.
- In an isolator, surface clean fixed gloves or gauntlets after compounding is completed to avoid spreading hazardous drug contamination to other surfaces.
- Wear clean gloves (e.g., the clean inner gloves) to surface decontaminate the final preparation, place the label on the final preparation, and place it into the pass-through.
- Don fresh gloves to complete the final check, place preparation into a clean transport bag, and remove the bag from the pass-through.
- Remove gloves with care to avoid contamination. Establish and follow detailed procedures for removal.
- Dispose of contaminated gloves as contaminated waste.

Gowns

- Select disposable gowns of material tested to be protective against the hazardous drugs to be used (low permeability).
- Wear gowns during compounding, during administration, when handling waste from patients recently treated with hazardous drugs, and when cleaning up spills of hazardous drugs.
- Wear coated gowns no longer than three hours during compounding, and change immediately when damaged or contaminated.

- Avoid skin contact by using a disposable nonlinting, nonabsorbent gown made of polyethylene-coated polypropylene material. The gown should have a closed front, long sleeves, and elastic or knit closed cuffs. Gowns should not be reused.
- Remove gowns with care to avoid spreading contamination. Specific procedures for removal must be established and followed.
- Dispose of gowns immediately upon removal.
- Contain and dispose of contaminated gowns as contaminated waste.
- Wash hands after removing and disposing of gowns.
- Wear shoe and hair coverings during the sterile compounding process to minimize particulate contamination of the critical work zone and the preparation.

Eye and Face Protection

Eye and face protection should be used whenever there is a possibility of exposure from splashing or uncontrolled aerosolization of hazardous drugs (e.g., when containing a spill or handling a damaged shipping carton). In these instances, a face shield, rather than safety glasses or goggles, is recommended.

Circumstances may warrant the use of a respirator. All workers who may use a respirator must be fit tested and trained to use the appropriate respirator according to the OSHA Respiratory Protection Standard. A respirator of correct size and suitability to the aerosol size, physical state (i.e., particulate or vapor), and concentration of the airborne drug must be available at all times. Surgical masks do not provide respiratory protection.

Nonsterile Compounding with Hazardous Drugs

Although nonsterile dosage forms of hazardous drugs contain varying proportions of drug to nondrug (nonhazardous) components, there is the potential for personnel exposure to and environmental contamination with the hazardous components if hazardous drugs are handled (e.g., packaged) by pharmacy staff. Although most hazardous drugs are not available in liquid formulations, such formulations are often prescribed for small children and for adults with feeding tubes. Formulas for extemporaneously compounded oral liquids may start with the injection or they may require that tablets be crushed or capsules opened. Tablet trituration has been shown to cause fine dust formation and local environmental contamination.

Careful, prescribed procedures, using dedicated equipment, for counting and pouring of hazardous drugs should be followed. After use, the contaminated equipment should be cleaned with water and then detergent and rinsed with water thereafter. Both water and gauze (if used) need to be disposed of as contaminated waste.

Recommendations for compounding and handling noninjectable hazardous drug dosage forms are as follows:

- Compounding should occur in a ventilated cabinet, or a large plastic glove-bag may be appropriate to use in some instances.
- Hazardous drugs should be labeled or otherwise identified for prevention of improper handling.
- Bulk containers of liquid hazardous drugs, as well as specially packaged commercial hazardous drugs, must be handled carefully to avoid spills. These containers should be dispensed and maintained in sealable plastic bags to contain any inadvertent contamination.

- During routine handling of noninjectable hazardous drugs and contaminated equipment, workers should wear two pairs of gloves that meet the ASTM standard for chemotherapy gloves.
- Counting and pouring of hazardous drugs should be done carefully, and clean equipment should be dedicated for use with these drugs.
- Tablet and capsule forms of hazardous drugs should not be placed in automated counting machines, which subject them to stress and may introduce powdered contaminants into the work area.
- Contaminated equipment should be cleaned initially with gauze saturated with sterile water; further cleaned with detergent, sodium hypochlorite solution, and neutralizer; and then rinsed with water. The gauze and rinse should be contained and disposed of as contaminated waste.
- Crushing tablets or opening capsules should be avoided, if possible; liquid formulations should be used whenever possible.
- During the compounding of hazardous drugs (e.g., crushing, dissolving, or preparing a solution or an ointment), workers should wear nonpermeable gowns and double gloves.
- Hazardous drugs should be dispensed in the final dose and form whenever possible.
- Disposal of unused or unusable noninjectable dosage forms of hazardous drugs should be performed in the same manner as for hazardous injectable dosage forms and waste.

Sterile Compounding with Hazardous Drugs

Working with Compounding Aseptic Containment Isolators

An isolator is a device that is sealed or is supplied with air through a microbial retentive filtration system (high-efficiency particulate air [HEPA] minimum) and may be reproducibly decontaminated. When closed, an isolator uses only decontaminated interfaces (when necessary) or transfer ports for materials movement. When open, it allows for the ingress and/or egress of materials through defined openings that have been designed and validated to preclude the transfer of contaminants or unfiltered air to adjacent environments. An isolator can be used for aseptic processing, containment of potent compounds, or simultaneous asepsis and containment. Some isolator designs allow operations within the isolator to be conducted through attached rubber gloves without compromising asepsis or containment.

- *Aseptic isolator:* A ventilated isolator designed to exclude external contamination from entering the critical zone inside the isolator
- *Aseptic containment isolator:* A ventilated isolator designed to meet the requirements of both an aseptic isolator and a containment isolator
- *Containment isolator:* A ventilated isolator designed to prevent the toxic materials processed inside it from escaping to the surrounding environment

A compounding aseptic containment isolator is designed to provide for worker protection from exposure to undesirable levels of airborne drug throughout the compounding and material transfer processes and to provide an aseptic environment for compounding sterile preparations. Air exiting a CACI is first passed through a microbial retentive filter (HEPA minimum) capable of containing airborne concentration of the physical size and state of the drug being compounded. If volatile, the hazardous drugs are removed in the exhaust air from the isolator by properly designed building ventilation.

The use of a CACI must be accompanied by a stringent program of work practices, including operator training and demonstrated competence, contamination reduction, and decontamination:

- Gather all needed supplies before beginning compounding. Avoid exiting and reentering the work area of the isolator.
- Do not place unnecessary items in the work area of the cabinet or isolator where hazardous drug contamination from compounding may settle on them or they may overcrowd the isolator.
- Handle the preparation in the pass-through of the isolator properly, including spraying or wiping with sterile 70% alcohol or another appropriate disinfectant, to ensure aseptic compounding.
- Reduce the hazardous drug contamination burden in the isolator by wiping down hazardous drug vials before placing them in the isolator.
- Do not place transport bags in the isolator work chamber during compounding to avoid inadvertent contamination of the outside surface of the bag.
- Wipe down the outside of the isolator opening and the floor in front with detergent, sodium hypochlorite solution, and neutralizer at least daily.
- Decontaminate the work surface of the isolator before and after compounding and at the end of the shift or day according to the manufacturer's recommendations or with detergent, sodium hypochlorite solution, and neutralizer.
- Decontaminate final preparations within the isolator and place them into the transport bags in the isolator pass-through, taking care not to contaminate the outside of the transport bag.
- Seal and then decontaminate surfaces of waste and sharps containers before removing from the isolator.
- Decontaminate the isolator after any spill during compounding.
- Seal all contaminated materials (e.g., gauze, wipes, towels, wash or rinse water) in bags or plastic containers and discard as contaminated waste.
- Decontaminate the isolator before replacing gloves or gauntlets.

Technique and Working Procedures

Only supplies and drugs essential to compounding a dose or batch should be placed in the work area of the main chamber of the isolator. Luer-Lok syringes and connections must be used whenever possible for manipulating hazardous drugs, because they are less likely to separate during compounding. Spiking an IV set into a solution containing hazardous drugs or priming an IV set with hazardous drug solution in an uncontrolled environment must be avoided.

In reconstituting hazardous drugs in vials, one must be certain to avoid pressurizing the contents of the vial because pressurization may cause the drug to spray out around the needle or through a needle hole or a loose seal, thereby aerosolizing the drug into the work zone. Pressurization can be avoided by creating a slight negative pressure in the vial. Too much negative pressure, however, can cause leakage from the needle when it is withdrawn from the vial. Small amounts of diluent should be transferred slowly as equal volumes of air are removed. The needle should be kept in the vial, and the contents should be swirled carefully until dissolved. With the vial inverted, the proper amount of drug solution should be gradually withdrawn while equal volumes of air are exchanged for solution. The exact volume needed must be measured while the needle is in the vial; any excess drug should remain in the vial. With the vial in the upright position, the plunger should be withdrawn past the original starting point to again induce a slight negative pressure before removing the needle. The needle hub should be clear before the needle is removed. If a hazardous drug is transferred to an IV bag, care must be taken to puncture only the septum of the injection port and avoid puncturing the sides of the port or bag. After the drug solution is injected into the IV bag, the IV port, container, and set (if attached by the pharmacy in the isolator) should be surface decontaminated. The final preparation should be labeled, including an auxiliary warning, and the injection port covered with a protective shield.

To withdraw hazardous drugs from an ampul, the neck or top portion should be gently tapped. After the neck is wiped with alcohol, a 5-μm filter needle or straw should be attached to a syringe that is large enough to be not more than three-fourths full when holding the drug. The fluid should then be drawn through the filter needle or straw and cleared from the needle and hub. Afterward, the needle or straw is exchanged for a needle of similar gauge and length; any air and excess drug should be ejected into a sterile vial (leaving the desired volume in the syringe); aerosolization should be avoided. The drug may then be transferred to an IV bag or bottle. If the dose is to be dispensed in the syringe, the plunger should be drawn back to clear fluid from the needle and hub. The needle should be replaced with a locking cap, and the syringe should be surface decontaminated and labeled.

- Use double-gloving procedures, as appropriate; the inner gloves should be placed under the gown cuff and the outer gloves should cover the gown cuff. Use non-powdered gloves.
- Use CSTDs, glove bags, and needleless systems during compounding, if available and appropriate.
- Keep hazardous waste trash separate from other wastes.
- Use venting devices containing 0.2-μm filters or 5-μm filter needles, as appropriate.
- Minimize exposure to a patient and caregiver by presenting the final preparation in a ready-to-use form, if possible.
- Return excess drug to the drug vial or discard into a closed container (empty sterile vial), as appropriate.

Decontamination, Deactivation, and Cleaning

Contaminated equipment includes administration devices that have been used for administering hazardous drugs; contaminated wastes resulting from any step in the dispensing, compounding, or administration process; and unused hazardous drugs that remain in vials, bags, or cassettes or that are outdated.

Decontamination may be defined as cleaning or deactivating. Deactivating a hazardous substance is preferred, but no single process has been found to deactivate all currently available hazardous drugs. The use of alcohol for disinfecting the isolator will not deactivate any hazardous drugs and may result in the spread of contamination rather than any actual cleaning. Surface decontamination may be accomplished by transferring hazardous drug contamination from the surface of a nondisposable item to disposable ones (e.g., wipes, gauze, towels).

Decontamination of isolators should be conducted according to manufacturer recommendations. The MSDSs for many hazardous drugs recommend sodium hypochlorite solution as an appropriate deactivating agent. BSCs used for aseptic compounding must be disinfected at the beginning of the workday, at the beginning of each subsequent shift (if compounding takes place over an extended period of time), and routinely during compounding.

Hazardous Drug Spills and Spill Kit

Spill kits, containment bags, and disposal containers must be available in all areas where hazardous drugs are handled. Spill kits should contain materials needed to clean up spills of hazardous drugs and be readily available in all areas where hazardous drugs are routinely handled. A spill kit should accompany delivery of injectable hazardous drugs to patient-care areas even though they are transported in a sealable plastic bag or container. If hazardous drugs are being prepared or administered in a nonroutine area (e.g., home setting, unusual patient-care area), a spill kit and respirator should be available. Signs should be posted to indicate restricted access to a spill area.

The circumstances and handling of spills should be documented. Staff members and nonemployees exposed to a hazardous drug spill should also complete an incident or exposure report and notify the designated emergency service for initial evaluation. All spill materials must be disposed of as hazardous waste.

Spills should be cleaned up immediately, using proper safety precautions and personal protective equipment. If large spills occur, notify the pharmacist in charge immediately.

Spill Cleanup Procedure
- Assess the spill (size and scope).
- Spills that cannot be contained by two spill kits may require additional assistance.
- Post signs to limit access to the spill area.
- Don personal protective equipment, including inner and outer gloves and respirator.
- Once fully and properly garbed, contain the spill using the spill kit.
- Carefully remove any broken glass fragments, and place them in a puncture-resistant container.
- Absorb liquids with spill pads.
- Absorb powder with damp disposable pads or soft toweling.
- Spill cleanup should proceed progressively from areas of lesser to greater contamination.
- Completely remove all contaminated material, and place it in the disposal bags.
- Rinse the area with water and then clean with detergent, sodium hypochlorite solution, and neutralizer.
- Rinse the area several times, and place all materials used for containment and cleanup in disposal bags. Seal bags, and place them in the appropriate final container for disposal as hazardous waste.
- Carefully remove all personal protective equipment using the inner gloves. Place all disposable personal protective equipment into disposal bags. Seal bags, and place them into the appropriate final container.
- Remove inner gloves; contain in a small, sealable bag; and place into the appropriate final container for disposal as hazardous waste.
- Wash hands thoroughly with soap and water.
- Once a spill has been initially cleaned, have the area recleaned by housekeeping, janitorial, or environmental services.

Isolator Spills
- Clean up spills occurring in an isolator immediately.
- Obtain a spill kit if the volume of the spill exceeds 30 mL or the contents of one drug vial or ampul.
- Wear utility gloves (from spill kit) to remove broken glass in an isolator. Care must be taken not to damage the fixed-glove assembly in the isolator.

- Place glass fragments in the puncture-resistant hazardous drug waste container located in the isolator, or discard the fragments into the appropriate waste receptacle of the isolator.
- Thoroughly clean and decontaminate the isolator.
- If the spill results in liquid being introduced onto the HEPA filter or if powdered aerosol contaminates the clean side of the HEPA filter, suspend use of the isolator until the equipment has been decontaminated and the HEPA filter replaced.

Only trained workers with appropriate personal protective equipment and respirators should attempt to manage a hazardous drug spill. All workers who may be required to clean up a spill of hazardous drugs must receive proper training in spill management and in the use of personal protective equipment and NIOSH-certified respirators.

Closed-System Transfer Devices

Closed-system transfer devices mechanically prevent the transfer of contaminants into a system and the escape of drug or vapor out of a system. CSTDs shall be used within an International Organization for Standardization (ISO) Class 5 environment of an isolator. ADD-Vantage and Duplex devices are CSTDs currently available for injectable antibiotics. A similar system that may offer increased environmental protection for hazardous drugs is a proprietary CSTD known as PhaSeal.

Several studies have shown a reduction in environmental contamination with marker hazardous drugs during both compounding and administration when comparing standard techniques for handling hazardous drugs with the use of PhaSeal. However, PhaSeal components cannot be used to compound all hazardous drugs. The venting device does not lock onto the vial, which allows it to be transferred from one vial to another. This practice creates an opportunity for both environmental and product contamination.

Hazardous Waste

Hazardous drug waste materials include packaging materials, disposable equipment, used syringes, absorbent and cleaning materials (paper towels, gauze pads, wipes), wash and rinse water, partially filled vials, undispensed preparations, unused IV admixtures, needles and syringes, gloves, gowns, underpads, soiled materials from spill cleanups, containers containing trace amounts of hazardous drugs, weigh boats and papers, disposable spatulas, and shoe covers.

Waste vendors should ensure acceptance of all possible hazardous waste, including mixed infectious waste, if needed. Once hazardous waste has been identified, it must be collected and stored according to specific requirements of the U.S. Environmental Protection Agency and U.S. Department of Transportation. Properly labeled, leakproof, and spill-proof containers of nonreactive plastic are required for areas where hazardous waste is generated. Hazardous drug waste may be initially contained in thick, sealable plastic bags before being placed in approved accumulation containers.

All contaminated materials must be placed in leakproof, puncture-resistant containers while in the contained environment. Thereafter, these containers should be placed in larger containers outside the contained environment for disposal.

Glass fragments should be contained in small, puncture-resistant containers to be placed into larger containers approved for temporary storage. Waste contaminated with blood or other body fluids must not be mixed with hazardous waste.

Hazardous waste must be properly recorded and transported from accumulation areas by properly licensed and trained hazardous waste transporters to a licensed hazardous waste storage, treatment, or disposal facility. A licensed contractor may be hired to manage the hazardous waste program. Investigation of a contractor, including verification of possession and type of license, should be completed and documented before a contractor is engaged.

Treatment for Exposure to Hazardous Drugs

Procedures must be in place to address worker contamination and protocols for medical attention must be developed before the occurrence of an incident. Emergency kits containing isotonic eyewash supplies (or emergency eyewashes, if available) and soap must be immediately available in areas where hazardous drugs are handled. Workers who are contaminated during a spill or spill cleanup or who have direct skin or eye contact with hazardous drugs require immediate treatment.

A general procedure for immediate, emergency treatment may include the following steps:

1. Call for help, if needed.
2. Immediately remove contaminated clothing.
3. Flood affected eye with water or isotonic eyewash for at least 15 minutes.
4. Clean affected skin with soap and water; rinse thoroughly.
5. Obtain medical attention.
6. Ensure that supplies for emergency treatment (e.g., soap, eyewash, sterile saline for irrigation) are immediately located in any area where hazardous drugs are compounded or administered.
7. Document exposure in the employee's medical record and medical surveillance log.

USP Chapter <800>: Hazardous Drugs—Handling in Healthcare Settings

USP Chapter <800>, Hazardous Drugs—Handling in Healthcare Settings, is a practice standards chapter similar to *USP* Chapters <795>, Pharmacy Compounding—Nonsterile Preparations, and <797>, Pharmacy Compounding—Sterile Preparations. It establishes enforceable standards for the practice of pharmacy for handling hazardous drugs to promote patient safety, worker safety, and environmental protection. That chapter is organized into the following main sections:

1. Introduction and Scope
2. List of Hazardous Drugs
3. Types of Exposure
4. Responsibilities of Personnel Handling Hazardous Drugs
5. Facilities
6. Environmental Quality and Control
7. Personal Protective Equipment
8. Hazard Communication Program
9. Personnel Training
10. Receiving
11. Labeling, Packaging, and Transport
12. Dispensing Final Dosage Forms

13. Compounding
14. Administering
15. Deactivation/Decontamination, Cleaning, and Disinfection
16. Spill Control
17. Disposal
18. Documentation and Standard Operating Procedures
19. Medical Surveillance
Appendix A: Acronyms and Definitions
Appendix B: Examples of Design for Hazardous Drugs Compounding Areas
Appendix C: Types of Biological Safety Cabinets
Appendix D: Bibliography

Pharmacists, pharmacy students, and pharmacy technicians are encouraged to obtain a current copy of *USP* Chapter <800> for further information.

Conclusion

The protection of personnel using hazardous drugs in compounding requires careful attention to all aspects of the handling of these substances.[4] Undoubtedly, this area of compounding pharmacy will increase in importance as the number and types of hazardous drugs continue to grow.

References

1. National Institute for Occupational Safety and Health. Preventing occupational exposure to antineoplastic and other hazardous drugs in health care settings. Publication No. 2004-165. Available at: www.cdc.gov/niosh/docs/2004-165/. Accessed November 9, 2011.
2. Gebhart F. New safeguards combat chemo vial contamination. *Drug Topics.* 2005 (October 24). Available at: http://drugtopics.modernmedicine.com/drugtopics/article/articleDetail.jsp?id=187954. Accessed November 9, 2011.
3. American Society of Health-System Pharmacists. Implementation of a safety program for handling hazardous drugs in a community hospital. *Am J Health-Syst Pharm.* 2008;65(9):861–5.
4. Allen LV Jr, Okeke CC. Considerations for implementing USP <797>, Pharmaceutical Compounding—Sterile Preparations, Part 11: hazardous drugs. *Int J Pharm Compound.* 2009; 13(1):56–62.

Chapter 4

Facilities, Equipment, and Supplies

For most professions, the tools of the trade have changed over the years. Physicians now use computers, laser light, high-technology communication systems, and biotechnology-derived drug products; lawyers conduct large database searches in the courtroom; and pharmacists use computers, databases, and hand-held electronic devices in medication dispensing, patient monitoring, patient counseling, drug preparation, communication, quality control analyses, and tracking and control of drug delivery devices (pumps).

With the changes that have occurred in the delivery of medical and pharmaceutical care have come changes in the daily use of equipment and supplies. As a result, many state boards of pharmacy are revising their regulations to reflect current practice activities, particularly as those regulations apply to the preparation of drug products.

As technology advances and the pace of change quickens, new methods and techniques must be mastered, yet retaining time-honored approaches that still are useful and contribute to patient therapy is advantageous. As we are currently witnessing, computerization and robotics have important roles in compounding, dispensing, and counseling activities. Pharmacists must know what new equipment is available, how to use and maintain it, and how responsibilities and opportunities in health care are changing. But pharmacists must still be involved in the preparation, provision, and appropriate use of drugs to meet the specific needs of patients. This is especially true for new and biotechnology-derived medications and for patient-specific preparations that must be compounded.

Pharmacies that engage in compounding should have a designated area with adequate space for the orderly placement of the equipment and materials used in compounding activities. A pharmacist is also responsible for the proper maintenance, cleanliness, and use of all equipment involved in the compounding practice. This chapter provides a detailed discussion of both the physical facility and the specific equipment and supplies needed in the compounding process.

In addition, Chapter <795>, Pharmaceutical Compounding—Nonsterile Preparations, and Chapter <797>, Pharmaceutical Compounding—Sterile Preparations, of the *United States Pharmacopeia (USP)* should be consulted for comprehensive discussion of the compounding facility and equipment and the other topics covered in the following sections.

Historical Review

Historical records show that apothecaries began their ministrations by using very simple equipment and tools—mortars and pestles, knives and axes to obtain plants and plant parts, mixing vessels, and drying tables. Common dosage forms included ointments, oils, and powdered extracts from plants. Later, processes such as distillation and extraction were introduced, which resulted in more complex equipment requirements. The earliest recognized implements of pharmacy are the mortar and pestle, which became the symbol of pharmacy.

From the earliest days of pharmacy to the present, the mortar and pestle have been characteristic utensils of the profession and, since the 17th century, have been used to identify an apothecary's shop or pharmacy. Mortars and pestles are available in different sizes (from several ounces to more than 200 pounds) and shapes (e.g., bowl, V, hourglass) and are made of different materials (e.g., wood, brass, glass, porcelain). Some are plain, and some are decorated; some are functional, and some are fashionable; some are for general use, and some are for special use. Grinding (comminution and pulverization) and mixing have always been a part of pharmacy. Formerly, roots, rhizomes, dried herbs, and earth were pulverized before administration in the form of powders, poultices, or ointments. Today, mortars and pestles are used for pulverization of powders and granules and for mixing. Even pharmacists who do not compound see the mortar and pestle as a symbol of their profession.

Equipment used by pharmacists for compounding during the 1940s, 1950s, and 1960s was basic, consisting of mortars and pestles, beakers, conical graduates, prescription balances, hot plates, refrigerators, pill tiles, and spatulas. With the advent of a pharmacist's responsibility for intravenous admixtures in the 1970s, pharmacies added equipment such as laminar-airflow hoods, aseptic transfer devices and pumps, and sterile filtration units.

The resurgence of compounding in the 1980s and 1990s led to further expansion of the range of equipment used in pharmacies, depending on their scope of practice. The first contemporary compounding-only pharmacy opened in 1987. Today, there are at least 125 such pharmacies in North America.

Pharmacists have moved from traditional compounding activities—the preparation of syrups, suppositories, troches, and ointments—to aseptic compounding of total parenteral nutrition solutions with 20 or more ingredients, programming of ambulatory pumps, and other technology-based activities requiring sophisticated equipment. Often, the agencies that regulate practice have not kept up with the tremendous changes in pharmacy. Because the practice of pharmacy is now so diverse, one may doubt whether a single board-defined list of equipment will suffice for all practice settings; rather, equipment lists must be tailored to the type of practice (e.g., community, hospital, home health care, nuclear, traditional, aseptic compounding).

Compounding Facility

The compounding facility should be designed, arranged, and maintained to facilitate quality compounding. The area for compounding sterile drug preparations should be separate from the area for compounding or dispensing nonsterile drug preparations.

Traffic in the compounding area should be kept to a minimum, with only designated individuals allowed access. The area should be well lighted and have controlled heating, ventilation, and air conditioning to prevent the decomposition of chemicals and to ensure a comfortable workplace without distractions. Humidity should be monitored and controlled as appropriate. The terms *humidity* and *relative humidity* are often used interchangeably, but they are not synonymous; humidity is the amount of water in the air, and relative humidity is the ratio of the amount of water vapor in the air at a specific temperature to the maximum possible amount of water vapor in the air at that temperature. Because humidity affects drug stability and integrity, the effects of humidity are second in importance only to those of temperature in compounding and storage areas. Drugs tend to degrade in the presence of moisture. Chapter 2 of this book discusses the effects of crystal hydrates and hygroscopic, deliquescent, and efflorescent ingredients. A hygrometer should be placed on an interior wall where it will provide a representative reading of the relative humidity level in the compounding area or storage facility but will not be near an air-handling return, hot plate, or door entrance or exit.

The materials used for the floor, walls, shelving and cabinets, and ceiling should not retain dust, odors, or residues from the compounding activities. The area should be free of dust-collecting overhangs (e.g., ceiling pipes, hanging light fixtures, ledges) and of infestation by insects, rodents, and other vermin. The actual work area should be level, smooth, impervious, free of cracks and crevices, and nonshedding. The shelving and cabinets should be easy to clean.

Surfaces should be cleaned at the beginning and the end of each compounding operation. All equipment that is used should be cleaned thoroughly to avoid cross-contamination between ingredients and preparations. Cleaning should be initiated immediately after the use of any sensitizing, caustic, or dangerous substances. The entire compounding area should be cleaned daily or weekly, but not during the compounding process. Pharmacies engaged in only occasional compounding should make adequate preparations before each compounding activity.

Washing facilities should be adequate and easily accessible from the compounding area. These facilities should have satisfactory drainage and provide hot and cold water, cleansing agents, and air driers or disposable towels. There should be sufficient potable water and a source of purified water USP or other water suitable for compounding activities. Potable water should be supplied under continuous positive pressure in a plumbing system free of defects that could contribute to the contamination of the preparation. Sewage, trash, and other refuse in and from the pharmacy and immediate drug-compounding area or areas should be disposed of in a safe and sanitary manner. Trash should be collected and removed daily.

Compounding Equipment

Equipment used in the compounding of drug preparations should be appropriately designed, adequately sized, and suitably located to facilitate compounding operations. The equipment should be of a neutral and impervious composition so that ingredients, in-process materials, and drug preparations do not react with, add to, or become absorbed by it in such a way that the safety, identity, strength, quality, or purity of the drug preparation is altered beyond the desired composition.

Equipment and utensils used for compounding should be cleaned and sanitized immediately before use to prevent contamination that would alter the drug preparation. To ensure that equipment and utensils are clean, a pharmacist should inspect them immediately before compounding operations begin.

If the compounding process involves drug preparations that require special measures to prevent cross-contamination, appropriate precautions must be taken. These precautions include dedication of equipment for these operations and meticulous cleaning of the contaminated equipment.

Automatic, mechanical, or electronic equipment, or other related equipment or systems, may be used in the compounding of drug preparations. This equipment should be routinely inspected, calibrated if necessary, and checked to ensure proper performance. The maintenance of all equipment should be documented.

Equipment for Weighing and Measuring

The accurate weighing and measuring of ingredients is crucial in order to attain a compounded preparation that is safe to administer and achieves the desired therapeutic effect. For these reasons, balances and measuring equipment are discussed separately from other compounding equipment.

Balances

Compounding pharmacies use either class A torsion balances or electronic balances to weigh materials used in compounded formulations.

Electronic balances that can weigh quantities as large as 300 g and as small as 1 mg are available (Figure 4-1A). The cost of a balance is usually proportional to the lowest weight that can be accurately measured. Electronic balances weigh small quantities of materials very accurately and require a relatively low investment. These balances are easy to use, clean, and calibrate. They simplify quality control determinations, especially if a printer is attached.

Weight sets for use with prescription balances usually contain both apothecary and metric systems, but the metric system is now the only official measuring system. Brass weight sets should be used with torsion balances only.

Weigh boats (disposable plastic) and weigh papers are used so that materials to be weighed can be placed on the boat or paper and not contaminate the balance. The weigh boats (Figure 4-1B) and papers are easy to manipulate.

Spatulas (disposable plastic) are used for weighing to minimize cross-contamination of chemicals. Metal and hard rubber spatulas are also used.

Balances should be situated in areas of low humidity and placed on flat, nonvibrating surfaces away from vents, fans, and other sources of moving air. The performance of the balances should be checked and documented at least monthly.

Measuring Equipment

In addition to the customary measuring equipment consisting of graduated cylinders, pipets, calibrated syringes, and the like, micropipets are being used more commonly to accurately measure very small volumes of liquids.

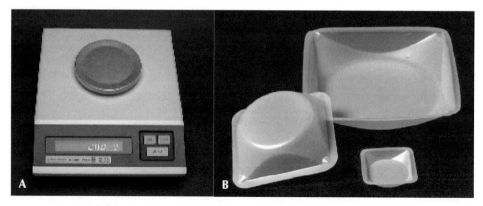

FIGURE 4-1 Weighing equipment. A: electronic balance; B: weigh boats.

Micropipets eliminate the need to prepare aliquots of drugs when only a very small quantity is required. Because various micropipets are available, the investment can be kept to a minimum. For example, one micropipet can be used for 200 μL to 1000 μL and another can be used for 5 to 200 μL. Multiple-channel micropipets can be used when simultaneous delivery of up to 12 channels (e.g., when 0.5 mL is being placed in a large number of small vials or ampuls) is necessary. Micropipets should be checked frequently to determine their accuracy for the volume of liquid delivered. This can be easily accomplished by weighing the volume of purified water USP delivered onto a tared receptacle on a balance.

Other Compounding Equipment

The equipment needs of pharmacists vary depending on the type of compounding activities performed. The basic equipment requirements for general nonsterile preparation compounding, advanced nonsterile preparation compounding, general sterile preparation compounding, and advanced sterile prep   mpounding are presented in Table 4-1. Many of these items are used for bot   le preparation compounding; the following discussion is limited   ications and uses that may be unclear or unusual.

        ding Equipment

        d protector that is convenient for picking up   e.

        erous formats. From inexpensive plastic   )- to 300-capsule machines, these devices   ing prepared. The 100-capsule units can   well with locking capsules.

        nt for storing drug preparations that   lable in glass or plastic and may have a

        y different dosage forms. Many come   s of suppositories, pill pipes, and the   ves as the primary work area. This   vith a stainless steel spatula and for

        rious compounded preparations   ved or absorbed moisture over   moisture becomes even more   re in the drug gives a greater   ed before weighing.

        . The proper pH is critical   ffered, or the pH must be   racy than can be provided

        pharmacies that com-   nacist to perform other   iting element, mixing   ossible.

        : are slowly replac-   of the dispensing   any of the metal   used with caution.

w
lik
are
mix

and fc
time. A
dangero
weight fo

pH m
for drug so
adjusted to a
by pH indicat

Stir plates
pound a large n
duties while ingr
melted ointments

Suppository, t
ing the older, heav
package. Because th
molds that were rea

TABLE 4-1 General Compounding Equipment and Supplies

Nonsterile Preparation Compounding Equipment

General Nonsterile Equipment

Balance—prescription, torsion

Balance—triple beam

Beaker hot hand

Beaker tongs

Beakers—glass/plastic/stainless steel (50, 100, 150, 250, 400, 600, 1000 mL)

Beakers—with/without handles, glass/plastic/stainless steel (1000, 2000, 3000 mL)

Capsule-filling equipment

Containers—applicators (roll on, sponge top)

Cylinders—glass/plastic (graduate 5 to 2000 mL)

Desiccant (Drier-Rite)

Desiccators—glass/plastic

Dishes—with/without handles, evaporating, porcelain

Funnels—glass/plastic (2", 3", 4", 5", 6")

Glasses—safety

Graduates—pharmaceutical/conical, glass/plastic (10, 25, 50, 100, 250, 500, 1000 mL)

Graters, hand (fine, medium, coarse, combination)

Gummy gel molds

Hot plates (various sizes and features)

Hygrometers

Molds—lollipop, rapid dissolve tablets, tablet triturates, treat, troches

Mortars/pestles—glass/porcelain (2, 4, 8 oz)

Openers—jar/bottle/tube

Ovens, drying—mechanical/convection

Pellet press

pH meters

Pill tiles—glass, frosted

Racks, drying—plastic or epoxy resin material

Refrigerator with freezer

Safety kit

Spill cleanup kit

Spatulas—plastic/stainless steel, assorted (4", 6"), regular and disposable

Stir plates—magnetic with stir bars and temperature controller

Stirring rods

Strainers (small, medium, large)

Suppository molds (rectal, vaginal, urethral, rectal-rocket)

Suppository filling rack, lighted

Thermometer clips

Thermometers—glass

Troche molds

Tubes, applicator

Weighing dishes—plastic/aluminum, disposable

Weigh papers

Weight sets, brass

TABLE 4-1 General Compounding Equipment and Supplies *(Continued)*

Advanced Nonsterile Equipment

Air compressor

Bag/tube sealer

Balance, electronic—(minimum sensitivity of 1 mg) with printer

Balance, electronic—(minimum sensitivity of 10 mg) with printer

Bath, dry—heater/incubator

Beakers, heat-resistant plastic

Beakers, insulated

Beakers, Teflon

Blender (liquefy, puree, mix; 12-mL to 4000-mL capacities; temperature-controlled, foam arrester)

Blender, hand—two-speed lab (three blades, with stand)

Blender, hand—variable speed (mixing container, stand, various blades, at least two speeds)

Boiling chips or beads

Bottles, dispensing fluid—plastic/glass

Bottles, drop dispensing—plastic/glass

Brushes, cleaning—nylon (various sizes/shapes to fit equipment)

Buckets with lids—plastic

Burets (10–50 mL)

Burners, Bunsen or similar—natural gas/propane

Carboys—with/without spigots

Carts—plastic/metal

Centrifuge

Chopper/grinder

Coffee grinder

Crimper, hand operated

Desiccator

Desiccator/micromarinader (creates vacuum; has desiccator applications)

Dispensing pumps, variable speed

Dispensing pens/syringes/canisters

Fat/oil separator (gravy separator)

Filler, piston (for thick liquids, gels, creams)

Food processor (slice, grate, chop, puree, mix, knead: various blades)

Heat gun, variable heat outputs

Homogenizers, hand operated or electric

Lead sticks, flexible

Light boxes

Magnetic stirrers

Malt shop mixer (two-speed motor, 28 oz stainless steel cup)

Microspatulas—stainless steel/Teflon coated

Mill, knife (high speed)

Mixer—orbital, single/variable speed

Mixer—Resonant Acoustic Mixer (RAM)

Mixer—professional/kitchen

Mortars/pestles (various sizes/shapes)

(continued)

TABLE 4-1 General Compounding Equipment and Supplies *(Continued)*

Ointment mill

pH meter

Pipet, motorized

Pipet bulbs

Pipet fillers, hand operated

Pipets (1–100 mL)

Pipets/micropipets (variable sizes: 5–200 mL, 200–1000 mL)

Pipets—multiple channel

Pitcher, stirring (2000-mL capacity, blades attached to handle, plastic)

Powder blender (blends powders in dust-free environment, protects operator from powder dust)

Repeating dispenser (for liquids, gels, semisolids)

Sealers, bag or suppository

Sealers, tube

Sieves, 3", 5", 7" (various mesh sizes)

Solvent dispensing/spray bottles

Spatulas—stainless steel/Teflon coated/porcelain/plastic

Sprayer bottles

Stirrer, motorized

Tablet press, single punch

Tea/spice ball

Test-tube rack, four-sided

Thermometer, digital probe

Thermometer, high-low alarm

Thermometers with alarm

Tongs, beaker/flask/tube

Tool set, cooks' heavy-gauge stainless steel (pasta fork, turner, solid spoon, ladle, server, skimmer, and hanging rack)

Tube sealer

Tubing (various sizes/types)

Tubing clamps (various sizes/types)

Ultrasonic cleaner (various capacities)

Vortex mixers

Wash bottles

Water system (high quality)

Workbench protector sheets—plastic/rubber/absorbable paper/matted

Sterile Preparation Compounding Equipment

General Sterile Equipment

Ampul openers, disposable

Anemometer, directed reading

Apparel for clean rooms (Class 10,000) (aprons, sleeves, gloves, hoods—open face/face mask, boot covers, shoe covers, frocks, coveralls, head coverings, lab coats, smocks, shirts/pants, hats/caps, face masks, beard covers)

Autoclave bags

Autoclave tape

Baggies/pouches/pouch sealers

Biohazard autoclave bags

TABLE 4-1 General Compounding Equipment and Supplies *(Continued)*

Biohazard bag holders
Cleaning materials
    Hazardous materials handling equipment
    Pickup roller—cabinet/work space
    Pickup roller—floor
    Pickup roller—wall
Filter unit—repeating syringe with three-way connector and check valve
Filter units, vacuum—disposable
Filters, sterilizing (numerous types/shapes/applications)
Forceps
Impulse or induction sealer for plastic overwraps
Laminar-airflow hood, horizontal (Class 100)
Laminar-airflow hood, vertical (Class 100)
Needle destroyer
Pumps, pressure
Pumps, vacuum, electric
Pumps, vacuum, hand operated
Refrigerator
Refrigerator with freezer
Sharps disposal unit
Stainless steel pressure filter holders (various capacities)
Tacky mats
Trash container—gowns/apparel articles
Trash container—plastic/paper articles
Wire racks/shelving

Advanced Sterile Equipment
Autoclave
Bubble point tester
Cooler/heater for medication transport in automobile (30 L)
Crimper, hand operated or electric
Decappers
Filtration, sterile—equipment
Ice replacement gel (various forms/types)
Osmometer
Particle counter
Particulate testing equipment
Pump, pressure—vacuum
Pyrogen test materials
Quality control equipment
Robotic compounding systems
Sample transporter coolant—pouch (maintains sample at about 5°C [−10°C] for 30 minutes)
Smoke sticks/devices
Spatulas and spoons, sterile (plastic for weighing and obtaining drugs)
Sterility test equipment
Ultrafreezer (capable of about −80°C)

Advanced Nonsterile Preparation Compounding Equipment

Blenders (cabinet top and hand held) are indispensable in the preparation of many formulations. Kitchen blenders are excellent for preparing solutions, suspensions, emulsions, and even gels (if used properly). They are available in the standard kitchen size of about 28 ounces and in laboratory sizes, with vessels ranging from 12 to about 4000 mL. Hand-held blenders are suitable for preparing lotions, creams, and other semisolid and liquid preparations. These appliances are available with single, dual, and variable speeds.

Carts (plastic or metal) can be used to move supplies from one area to another. They also provide working surfaces when necessary.

Choppers/grinders and *coffee grinders,* which are available in the kitchen equipment department of large stores and in gourmet shops, can be used for particle size reduction and for blending of small quantities of powders.

Crimpers (hand operated) are used to attach aluminum tamper-evident safety caps onto containers of compounded preparations. This system for packaging a preparation is very convenient when there is a need to ensure that the package has not been opened; it is similar to the seals used for injectables.

Dispensing pumps (variable speed) are invaluable when the same volume of a liquid must be repeatedly measured and dispensed. They are especially useful in packaging finished preparations into containers.

Dry baths are alternatives to hot plates, and they are replacing water baths in many facilities. A dry bath is essentially a heated chamber that can be filled with sand, salt, or aluminum blocks designed to hold various sizes of glassware. For example, a beaker can be wiggled into sand after the sand has equilibrated to the temperature required to heat a preparation. Dry baths are easy to use and clean and are virtually maintenance free.

Fat/oil separators can be used to obtain a foam-free liquid from an ingredient that has a foam on top, which makes measurement difficult. The spout originates at the bottom of the container so the liquid, not the foam, is dispensed. These items are often referred to as "gravy separators."

Food processors capable of slicing, grating, chopping, pureeing, mixing, and kneading, depending on the various blades that are available, have many applications, including the preparation of ointments and pastes.

Heat guns (variable heat) can be used in situations when heat is required and a hot plate is inconvenient. A heat gun directs the heat to the specific area where it is needed, as in sealing plastic dose containers. It can also be used to apply gentle heat to beakers of liquids and the like.

Homogenizers (hand operated) aid in the preparation of fine emulsions. They can be easily disassembled for cleaning and work with as little as 60 mL of liquid.

Homogenizers (digital) can be used for the reduction of particle size in oral suspensions and lotions of light to medium viscosity.

Lead sticks (flexible) are convenient for wrapping around beakers, flasks, and other pieces of equipment to prevent them from falling over. The sticks, which are made of soft lead with colorful plastic coatings, are available in many diameters and lengths. They can be easily shaped or formed to fit around almost any item of laboratory glassware or equipment.

Light boxes are excellent aids for determining the completeness of a solution when dissolving solids and for detecting precipitants when working with materials that may be incompatible or are near the limit of solubility. To achieve a similar outcome, one can paint a piece of Masonite half black and half white, using flat paints. When this board is hung on a wall with a fluorescent light placed immediately above it, the dark and light backgrounds help determine the presence of particles in a solution.

Mixers (professional or kitchen) can be used to beat, mix, whip, and knead with flat beaters, dough hooks, and wire whips. They aid in the compounding of preparations ranging from liquids, including emulsions, to ointments.

Orbital mixers can simultaneously mix a large number of beakers, bottles, flasks, and the like. The containers are fixed in place on a platform that moves in a circular or an orbital motion. These devices are widely used in laboratories and are especially suitable for compounding pharmacies in which a large number of containers must be mixed simultaneously.

Pipet bulbs aid in pipetting and can eliminate many of the dangers associated with pipetting by mouth. There are numerous styles of these bulbs, which may be used not only with measuring pipets but also with transfer pipets when small quantities of liquids must be moved from one vessel to another.

Powder blenders enable pharmacists to blend powders in a dust-free environment and protect the operator from powder dust. These blenders mechanically blend in enclosed plastic bags, which prevent any of the powder from escaping into the environment. V-shaped blenders and Turbo mixers provide better mixing and can be operated unattended for timed operation.

Sealers (bag or suppository) are convenient for sealing plastic bags or certain suppository molds.

Sealers (tube) are widely used for packaging large numbers of ointments, creams, or gels in plastic tubes. They are relatively simple to use and provide reproducible results with preparations that are attractively packaged.

Tablet presses (single punch) are an easy-to-use method of preparing individual tablets or pellets. A blend of the active drug and excipients can be weighed and placed in the die, the handle lowered, and a tablet produced by compression.

Tea/spice balls hold a flavoring agent while the ball is being immersed in a liquid until the desired strength is obtained.

Thermometers (with alarm) can audibly indicate when a refrigerator or an oven leaves a preset temperature range. These devices usually are used on freezers and refrigerators, especially ultrafreezers. High–low thermometers, which display the highest and lowest temperatures attained in a given period of time, will become more important as marketing requirements are implemented.

Tool sets (for cooks) contain useful implements for compounding, including a pasta fork, turner, solid spoon, ladle, server, and skimmer; often, they are complete with a hanging rack.

Ultrasonic cleaners are useful for cleaning items as well as for accelerating the dissolution of slowly dissolving drugs.

Water system (high quality) may be required if a pharmacy compounds a large quantity of preparations that require different grades of water.

Workbench protector sheets of plastic, rubber, or absorbable paper are often convenient for defining a work area for a specific project. They can be cleaned or disposed of after use.

General and Advanced Sterile Preparation Compounding Equipment
General Equipment

Many of the items listed in the categories of sterile preparation compounding and advanced sterile preparation compounding can be placed in one of four general categories. The first group includes items that are used for the compounding of sterile preparations: ampul openers, impulse sealers, vacuum pumps, sterile filtration equipment, and sterile spatulas and spoons. The second group includes items for quality control, including an anemometer, a particle counter, particulate-testing equipment, pyrogen test materials, and sterility test equipment. The third group, used for storage and delivery, includes items such as a refrigerator, a cooler and heater for use in an automobile, an ice replacement gel, and an ultrafreezer. The final group includes items used for maintenance of the clean room environment, such as apparel for personnel, cleaning materials, and high-efficiency particulate air (HEPA) filters. Also included are robotic systems.

Robotic Systems

Robotization of cancer drug preparation can reduce the risk of both accidental exposure and medication errors. Robots use a complete, double-checked prescription; are not affected by distractions; and accommodate workload increases. A robot recognizes the drugs, diluents, and containers by using a combination of barcode scanning and digital imaging. Appropriate software manages the compounding process and quality control functions as well as documentation.

Chapter 5

Records and Record Keeping

Compounding pharmacists must keep the records required by the states in which they practice, as well as those records characteristic of a well-operated compounding pharmacy. Records provide documentation of the ingredients of a preparation; facilitate a preparation recall, if necessary; and enable other compounding pharmacists to duplicate the preparation in their pharmacies. They also ensure that the compounded preparations will be consistent from one pharmacy to another, so a patient has confidence in the quality of the preparation being administered. Records and reports should be retained for the period of time required by state laws and regulations for the retention of prescription files. All records and reports should be readily available in a pharmacy for authorized inspection during the retention period. Records that should be maintained include (1) standard operating procedures (SOPs) with sign-off sheets for the procedures used; (2) formulation record, or recipe; (3) compounding record; (4) ingredient records; (5) material safety data sheets and safety data sheets; (6) certificates of analysis; and (7) hazardous drugs documentation.

Standard Operating Procedures

All significant procedures performed in the compounding area should be covered by SOPs and documentation. To ensure accountability, accuracy, quality, safety, and uniformity in a compounding practice, the practice should develop procedures for the facility; the equipment; the personnel; and the preparation, packaging, and storage of compounded preparations. More important, the implementation of SOPs establishes procedural consistency and provides a reference for the orientation and training of personnel. Documentation enables a pharmacy to systematically trace, evaluate, and replicate the steps throughout the preparation process of a compounded preparation whenever necessary.

SOPs provide assurance that (1) equipment is maintained in good working order, calibrated, and documented; (2) supplies are received, logged in, stored properly, disposed of correctly, and maintained fresh and within compendial requirements; and (3) all manipulations and procedures are performed uniformly and then documented. Because numerous forms must be completed at the end of many procedures, notebooks should be maintained to handle these forms. An important component of SOPs is keeping records of equipment maintenance. These records, which should be updated regularly, include documentation of the performance of balances, refrigerators, freezers, mixers, and all other equipment. Equipment files should be organized and updated regularly. Calibration checks should be maintained for documentation of the performance of the equipment. Refrigerator and freezer thermometers should be routinely checked and documented, and the temperatures of these pieces of equipment should be recorded on a regular basis to document their performance. Some equipment, such as laminar-airflow hoods, should be periodically certified by qualified personnel.

Figure 5-1 represents the first page of a typical SOP record. Documentation of equipment maintenance and supplies would be filed with this page. To avoid mixing or confusing records for different procedures, pharmacy personnel should mark the appropriate SOP number and, if applicable, the record's revision date on each page of the supporting documentation. Table 5-1 lists types of SOPs that might be considered for a compounding pharmacy. Appendix II provides examples of SOPs.

Standard Operating Procedure

SOP # _____

Date Effective:

Revision Number:

Person Preparing:

Person Checking:

Purpose of Procedure: [Describe]

Procedure: [Document procedure step by step so that different individuals can easily follow it and obtain the same results. Include sufficient detail and descriptive information to minimize the need for interpretation.]

1.
2.
3.
4.
5.

Documentation Forms: [The results of the SOP may need to be documented on a form and maintained in a notebook for easy retrieval. In this case, the organization of the forms notebook should parallel that of the SOP notebook. The reference point can be the SOP number, which should be placed on each page. Space should be available for a description of the procedure that was performed, date, operator's signature, and results.]

FIGURE 5-1 First page of a typical standard operating procedure record.

TABLE 5-1 Types of Compounding Pharmacy
Standard Operating Procedures

1.00	Administrative
2.00	Training
3.00	Safety
4.00	Facility—Environment and Maintenance
5.00	Facility—Cleaning
6.00	Equipment
7.00	Personnel
8.00	Compounding Procedures
9.00	Quality Assurance
10.00	Inventory Control

Formulation Record

The formulation record (Figure 5-2) provides a consistent source document for preparation of the formulation, considered the recipe, whereas the compounding record (Figure 5-3) documents the actual ingredients in the preparation and the person responsible for the compounding activity. Formulation records should be maintained in sufficient detail so that the preparations can be duplicated. Computerized records are appropriate.

Individual formulation records for compounds are obtained from a variety of sources, including journals, books, other pharmacists, organizations, and even individual development. The formulation record should include the following information:

- Name, strength, and dosage form of the preparation
- All ingredients and their quantities
- Equipment required to produce the preparation
- Pertinent calculations (see Chapter 7 of this book)
- Mixing instructions
- Quality control procedures
- Source of the recipe
- Beyond-use date
- Container used
- Storage requirements

The name, strength, and dosage form actually serve as the title of the preparation or recipe. The title should express the essence of the preparation as clearly and succinctly as possible, avoiding jargon.

Individual ingredients and their quantities should be listed. If more than one quantity of the preparation will possibly be produced in the future, a pharmacist should create a table listing the ingredients and the amounts required for various quantities. Because liquid preparations should be weighed, a notation should be made to that effect, specifying all the information regarding the quantity to be weighed or volumetrically measured. (The formulation record should also contain the specific gravity of the preparation for the conversions.)

Formulation Record

Formulation Title _____
(name, strength, dosage form)

Formula No. _____ Source _____

Quantity Prepared _____

Ingredient	Quantity	Unit	Calculation/Comments
_____	_____	_____	_____
_____	_____	_____	_____
_____	_____	_____	_____
_____	_____	_____	_____
_____	_____	_____	_____
_____	_____	_____	_____
_____	_____	_____	_____
_____	_____	_____	_____

Equipment Required _____

Compounding Instructions

1._____
2._____
3._____
4._____
5._____
6._____
7._____
8._____
9._____
10._____

Written by _____ Checked by _____

Quality Control Tests   Results

_____   _____
_____   _____
_____   _____
_____   _____

Container _____

Storage Requirements _____ Beyond-Use Date _____

FIGURE 5-2 Sample formulation record form.

Compounding Record

Formulation Title _____ Quantity _____
(name, strength, dosage form)

Formula/Rx No. _____ Prepared by _____ Checked by _____ R.Ph.

Quantity Prepared _____ Date Prepared _____ Beyond-Use Date _____

Ingredient	Quantity	Unit	Manufacturer	Lot No.	Exp. Date
_____	_____	____	_____	_____	_____
_____	_____	____	_____	_____	_____
_____	_____	____	_____	_____	_____
_____	_____	____	_____	_____	_____
_____	_____	____	_____	_____	_____
_____	_____	____	_____	_____	_____
_____	_____	____	_____	_____	_____
_____	_____	____	_____	_____	_____
_____	_____	____	_____	_____	_____
_____	_____	____	_____	_____	_____
_____	_____	____	_____	_____	_____

Compounding Instructions

1._____
2._____
3._____
4._____
5._____
6._____
7._____
8._____
9._____
10. _____

Quality Control Tests   Results

_____   _____
_____   _____
_____   _____
_____   _____

FIGURE 5-3 Sample compounding record form.

The use of different equipment yields different results. Therefore, the exact equipment used should be listed so the compounded prescriptions will be uniform in appearance and activity.

Precise mixing instructions are required in order to produce acceptable and uniform preparations. Mixing instructions include the order of mixing and any environmental or other conditions that should be monitored, such as the temperature and duration of mixing. If the mixing order is important, this order should be listed and explained in detail. Any levigating agents, solubilizing agents, and the like that are used in the preparation must also be cited and described.

Quality control procedures should be described, and a data sheet should be provided to document information such as capsule weights, as detailed in Chapter 8 of this book.

The source of the recipe should be included. If the formulation was derived from literature, a copy of the article should be appended to the formulation record. Good pharmacy practice always includes documenting the source for future reference.

The beyond-use date is assigned on the basis of the best available knowledge. Chapter 6 of this book provides some general guidelines for instances in which the beyond-use date is not known.

The container to be used should be listed on the formulation record to ensure uniformity of packaging and stability. Because much of the stability information is predicated on a certain type or composition of container, any variance from this style of container may make the beyond-use date suspect.

Storage requirements for the finished preparation should also be listed. This information should be transmitted to the patient.

Once the formulation record has been prepared and checked, it should be altered only after careful consideration is given to any changes proposed. Review by a second pharmacist of any alterations to the formulation record is always advisable.

Compounding Record

The compounding record should contain the name, strength, and dosage form as they appear in the formulation record. The compounding record is the worksheet for preparing an individual formulation. The following information should be recorded for both types of compounded formulations (individual prescriptions and preparations compounded in anticipation of orders):

- Formulation record used for the preparation
- Individual ingredients, their lot numbers, and the actual quantities measured or weighed
- Quantity of preparation prepared (i.e., weight, volume, or number of units prepared)
- Signature of the pharmacist or technician compounding the preparation
- Signature or initials of the pharmacist responsible for supervising the preparation and conducting in-process and final checks of the compounded preparation if a technician performed the compounding function
- Date of preparation
- Assigned internal identification number, if applicable
- Prescription number
- Assigned beyond-use date
- Results of the quality control procedures (e.g., the weight range of filled capsules)

In some pharmacies, the formulation record is prepared so that it can be photocopied, and space is left on it for the information required for the compounding record. This practice speeds up the record-keeping process. The compounding records are maintained for easy retrieval according to individual state requirements.

Ingredient Records

A pharmacy must maintain records of ingredients purchased, including material safety data sheets, safety data sheets, and certificates of analysis for purity of chemicals. These records should be retained as original hard copy; true copies, such as photocopies, microfilm, or microfiche; or other accurate reproduction of the original records. Computerized records are also acceptable. Employees should be instructed as to the location of the files and their format.

Material Safety Data Sheets and Safety Data Sheets

Material safety data sheets (MSDSs) should be maintained for any drug substance or bulk chemical located in the pharmacy. These data sheets are not required for commercially available finished preparations; the ingredient information on the commercial product label or package insert is sufficient. The ingredient information consists mainly of physicochemical, toxicity, and handling information. Precautions, information about potential hazards, and shipping instructions are also included. This information should be reviewed for the protection of a pharmacist as well as for that of a patient.

An MSDS is a written document that outlines information and procedures for handling and working with chemicals. The MSDS, safety data sheet (SDS), or product safety data sheet is an important component of compounding or manufacturing records. It is intended to provide workers and emergency personnel with procedures for handling or working with a specific substance in a safe manner. An MSDS includes information such as physical data (melting point, boiling point, flash point, etc.), toxicity, health effects, first aid, reactivity, storage, disposal, protective equipment, and spill-handling procedures. MSDS formats can vary from source to source within a country depending on national requirements. The sheet identifies the manufacturer of the material (name, address, phone and fax numbers) and usually includes (1) chemical identity; (2) hazardous ingredients; (3) physical and chemical properties; (4) fire and explosion data; (5) reactivity data; (6) health hazards data; (7) exposure limits data; (8) precautions for safe storage and handling; (9) need for protective gear; and (10) spill control, cleanup, and disposal procedures. MSDSs are generally not lot specific.

MSDSs can be obtained without charge from suppliers and can be easily filed in three-ring binders. They are commonly shipped with chemicals, often packaged in the same carton. They can also be obtained from the Internet or by fax from the suppliers.

Certificates of Analysis

Chapter <795>, Pharmaceutical Compounding—Nonsterile Preparations, of the *United States Pharmacopeia (USP)* states, "The compounder is responsible for compounding preparations of acceptable strength, quality, and purity with appropriate packaging and labeling in accordance with good compounding practices, official standards, and relevant scientific data and information." The compounding of quality preparations must involve the use of quality chemicals.[1]

Ingredients used in compounding official compounded preparations must meet the requirements of compendial monographs, if the substance is official. If the ingredient is not an official substance, reasonable standards can be applied for acceptance as use in compounding. If a USP or National Formulary (NF) grade is not available, or when food, cosmetics, or other substances are or must be used, the use of another high-quality source, such as analytical reagent (AR), certified American Chemical Society (ACS), or Food Chemicals

Codex (FCC) grade, is an option for professional judgment. For any substance used in compounding not purchased from a registered drug manufacturer, a pharmacist should establish purity and safety by reasonable means, which may include lot analysis, manufacturer reputation, or reliability of source.

USP Chapter <795> also states, "The bulk drug substances must be accompanied by a valid certificate of analysis."[1] For ingredients other than bulk drug substances, pharmacists should use ingredients that comply with an applicable *USP/National Formulary (NF)* monograph or *USP* Chapter <795>.

Some compounding pharmacists agree with the statement that "without the certificate of analysis, the material is valueless." The question of what tests should be conducted for evaluating ingredient quality and what tests are most important in evaluating certificates of analysis (COAs) often arise among compounding pharmacists. These tests are based on the *USP/NF*.

There are standards for active pharmaceutical ingredients (APIs) and excipients developed by the United States Pharmacopeial Convention (USP) Council of Experts, which is responsible for the content of USP's official and authorized publications. USP-NF substance and product standards are recognized widely because they are authoritative, science based, and established by a transparent and credible process. A drug or excipient monograph contains tests and acceptance criteria to comply with compendial standards for strength, quality, and purity of the substance.

A certificate of analysis is an authenticated document, issued by an appropriate authority, that certifies the quality and purity of not only pharmaceutical substances, but also animal and plant products being exported. In addition, a *certificate* is an official document attesting the truth of the facts stated. It is documentation that provides all the required information about a particular material, giving the end user confidence that the reference material is fit for its intended purposes. COAs accompanying materials are generally designed to be as clear and concise as possible, while complying with the appropriate International Organization for Standardization (ISO) guide requirements.

For official ingredients, a *monograph* in the *USP/NF* provides the article's name, definition, specifications, and other requirements related to packaging, storage, and labeling. The specification consists of tests, procedures, and acceptance criteria that help ensure the identity, strength, quality, and purity of the article. Table 5-2 provides an example of the list of specifications in monographs; not every substance will have all the specifications listed, but a list will include those that are appropriate.

A monograph may include several different tests, procedures, and acceptance criteria that reflect attributes of articles from different manufacturers. These alternatives may be presented for different polymorphic forms, impurities, hydrates, and dissolution cases.

In the *USP, manufactured product monographs* (tablets, capsules, solutions, injections, suppositories, etc.) generally include percentage strength requirements for the API, which vary depending on the drug, and so on. A product monograph also includes performance standards and specific tests for the dosage forms (e.g., disintegration and dissolution for tablets, dissolution for capsules, pH for solutions, sterility and endotoxin limits for sterile injections).

In the *USP, compounded preparation monographs* include formulas, specific directions to correctly compound the particular preparation, packaging and storage information, labeling information, pH, beyond-use dates based on stability studies, and detailed assays (majority of monographs).

Information on the name of the API or excipient and, where appropriate, its grade, batch number, and date of release should be provided on the COA. For APIs or excipients with an expiry date, the expiry date should be provided on the label and COA. For APIs or excipients with a retest date, the retest date should be indicated on the label or COA.

TABLE 5-2 Example of Monograph Specification Components for APIs or Excipients

Specification	Acceptance Criteria
Assay	Numeric value
Completeness of solution	Passes Yes/No
Congealing temperature	Numeric value
Crystallinity	Passes Yes/No
Density of solids	Numeric value
Description and solubility (Physical appearance)	Narrative
Distilling range	Numeric value
Identity	Passes Yes/No
Impurities and foreign substances	Passes Yes/No and/or Numeric values
Loss on drying	Numeric value
Loss on ignition	Numeric value
Melting range or temperature	Numeric value
Odor	Passes Yes/No
Performance tests	Varies
pH	Numeric value
Powder fineness	Passes Yes/No
Refractive index	Numeric value
Residual solvents	Passes Yes/No
Specific gravity	Numeric value
Specific surface area	Numeric value
Viscosity	Numeric value
Water	Numeric value

The COA should list each test performed in accordance with compendial or customer requirements, including the acceptance limits, and the numerical results obtained (if test results are numerical), as listed in Table 5-2. Physical descriptions and appearance are described in the *USP/NF* section, "Description and Relative Solubility of USP and NF Articles." Certificates should be dated and signed by authorized personnel of the quality unit(s) and should show the name, address, and telephone number of the original manufacturer.

The primary responsibility for preparation of the COA belongs to the manufacturer. The user of a bulk substance should always receive a certificate for the material being used. To draw on test results from a COA, the user should establish the reliability of the supplier's COA test results. Currently, few standardized requirements exist for the content or format of COAs for excipients. The certificate template generally consists of the (1) header, (2) body, (3) analysis, (4) certification and compliance statements, and (5) footer. Dates on the COA generally consist of the (1) date of manufacture, (2) expiration date and recommended reevaluation/retest dates, and (3) date retested. Other dates may be included as appropriate.

Example of a COA

If the bulk drug substance is a *USP/NF* item, then the specific tests listed in the compendia should be addressed. For example, Hydrocortisone USP includes a purity rubric ("not less than 97.0% and not more than 102.0% of $C_{21}H_{30}O_5$, calculated on the dried basis"). The individual tests may have an official *USP* chapter associated with them. If so, the method detailed should be followed unless another method has been validated to be at least as good, if not better than the method listed in the *USP*. The *USP* General Chapters associated with the tests below are provided in parentheses. Hydrocortisone USP has specific tests for which information should be provided, including the following:

- Identification (Chapters <181>, <191>, <193>, <197>, <201>, <563>)
- Specific rotation (Chapter <781>)
- Loss on drying (Chapter <731>)
- Residue on ignition (Chapter <281>)
- Chromatographic purity (Chapter <621>)
- Assay (Chapter <621>)

Therefore, the COA should address the tests and requirements listed for the specific substance or article. If a bulk drug substance is listed as "USP" or "NF," the inference is that the substance meets the standards and passes the tests required for the USP or NF designation. Some of the responses to the various tests on the COAs may be numerical and some may simply be noted "Passes," as in the following example:

Test	Requirement	Result
Specific rotation (Chapter <781S>)	Between +150° and +156°	+152°
Organic volatile impurities	Meets the requirements	Passes

If a substance is not available as a USP or NF item, then appropriate tests can be used that are similar to those required for related substances, but in all cases, tests should include a purity rubric and an assay result. An example of a *USP* monograph for Morphine Sulfate is shown in Figure 2-2, and it can be compared with the Morphine Sulfate Certificate of Analysis in Figure 2-1 in Chapter 2 of this book.

The acceptance criteria for the individual tests allow for (1) analytical error, (2) unavoidable variations in manufacturing and compounding, and (3) deterioration to an extent considered acceptable under practical conditions. The numerical standards of rounding numerical values are explained in the *USP/NF* with examples that should be followed; this approach is important for any test result on the low or high end of the range. An article that has been prepared to stricter criteria than those specified in the monograph does not constitute a basis for a claim that the article "exceeds" the compendial requirements. In some cases, an allowable range is provided, in others it may be a specification of "not less than" (or "nlt") or "not more than" (or "nmt"), "passes" or "does not pass," narrative descriptions, and so on.

COAs are lot specific and must match the current lot of bulk drug substance or excipient being used for compounding. When comparing a COA for an official ingredient, product, or preparation, one must ensure that all the specifications are within the allowable tolerances. For APIs that lack an official monograph, one can usually select a monograph of an API in a similar class to use as a guideline for individual specifications.

As previously mentioned, when manufactured drug products are used in compounding, they will be accompanied not by a COA but by a product information package insert. This information and the product's specific lot number should be maintained on file to document the specific product that was used in compounding. However, there can be difficulties in compounding with commercial products.

The USP standards for pharmaceutical compounding require the API in a compounded preparation to be present in an amount equal to 90.0% to 110.0% of the label. This requirement can pose a problem when compounding with commercially manufactured products because of the variation in allowable strengths by USP dosage form monographs or from the standards set by the U.S. Food and Drug Administration in the individual New Drug Application. To see what can occur, let's look at the following example.

Example of Variation in Allowable Strengths

A stability study was recently published.[2] The authors conducted an appropriate study, but there are some items of interest to consider. The investigators used 500-mg vials of doripenem and reconstituted them with 10 mL of 0.9% sodium chloride injection as recommended by the manufacturer. Then, the contents of one or two vials were added to either 100-mL polyvinyl chloride containers or 100-mL elastomeric infusion pumps containing either 90 mL or 80 mL of either 0.9% sodium chloride injection or 5% dextrose injection to produce solutions with doripenem concentrations of 5 mg/mL and 10 mg/mL, respectively. Six replicate bags were made for each combination of doripenem concentration, diluent, and infusion container.

An acceptable range for the 5 mg/mL concentration would be between 4.5 mg/mL and 5.5 mg/mL; for the 10 mg/mL concentration, the range would be between 9 mg/mL and 11 mg/mL. At 25°C, 4 of the 8 solutions were outside of the acceptable range; at 5°C, 3 of the 8 solutions were outside of the acceptable range; and at 25°C after being frozen and thawed, 8 solutions were outside of the acceptable range. In other words, 9 of the 24 solutions (37.5%) do not meet the standards of the USP requirement of 90.0% to 110.0%.

One can readily see that compounding with manufactured products can place a pharmacist in a situation where the final preparations are not in compliance with the USP standards. A pharmacist has no way of knowing the actual analyzed strength of the API in the commercial product. It may be anywhere in the range of 90.0% to 110.0%, or it may vary between 80.0% and 120.0% or even a broader or different range. If a pharmacist does not know the strength of the API in the commercial product, then the compounded preparation possibly will be outside the allowable USP standards that have been adopted by most states in their laws and regulations. Obviously, in many clinical situations, this variation will not be significant. It does become significant, however, when samples are selected and analyzed by regulatory agencies and found to be outside of expected specifications. A pharmacist using bulk substances accompanied by COAs does not encounter this situation, which reinforces the importance of COAs.

Hazardous Drugs Documentation[3]

Additional material on hazardous drugs can be found in Chapter 3, "Compounding with Hazardous Drugs," of this book. The following procedures regarding hazardous drugs should be documented:

- Acquisition
- Preparation
- Dispensing
- Personnel training
- Use and maintenance of equipment and supplies

The records associated with these activities must be available for review. The National Institute for Occupational Safety and Health has developed a list of hazardous drugs, which is available at www.cdc.gov/niosh/docs/2014-138/pdfs/2014-138_v3.pdf.

Personnel records should include documentation of employees' training according to Occupational Safety and Health Administration (OSHA) standards (see OSHA Standard

1910.120, "Hazardous Waste Operations and Emergency Response") and other appropriate laws and regulations.

Appropriate SOPs for the safe handling of hazardous drugs must be in place for all situations in which such drugs are used throughout a facility. The personnel responsible for compliance must review these SOPs at least annually. Examples of SOPs include the following:

- Hazard communication program
- Occupational safety program
- Labeling of hazardous drugs
- Procurement of hazardous drugs
- Use of proper engineering controls
- Use of personal protective equipment
- Decontamination and deactivation, cleaning, and disinfection
- Transport
- Environmental monitoring
- Spill control
- Medical surveillance

A facility must have an organized approach to handling hazardous drugs, and all aspects should be appropriately documented.

Record Maintenance

Neither *USP* Chapter <795>[1] nor *USP* Chapter <797>,[4] Pharmaceutical Compounding—Sterile Preparations, designates a specific length of time for maintaining COAs. If an individual state board of pharmacy has a requirement, it should be followed. If not, pharmaceutical judgment suggests that COAs be maintained on file for a designated time after the last portion of the specific lot of the substance was used, which would include the projected time of patient administration. With regard to the recommended beyond-use dates, the maximum time is generally 6 months.

When manufactured drug products are used in compounding, they will not be accompanied by a COA but instead will be accompanied by a product information package insert. This information and the product lot number should be maintained on file to document that a specific manufactured drug product was used in compounding the formulation.

Most COAs are provided in a standard 8.5 × 11 inch format and are reasonably similar in appearance between manufacturers of bulk substances. These certificates can be alphabetically arranged and maintained in standard three-ring notebooks.

References

1. United States Pharmacopeial Convention. Chapter <795>, Pharmaceutical compounding—nonsterile preparations. In: *United States Pharmacopeia/National Formulary*. Rockville, MD: United States Pharmacopeial Convention; current edition.
2. Crandon JL, Sutherland C, Nicolau DP. Stability of doripenem in polyvinyl chloride bags and elastomeric pumps. *Am J Health-Syst Pharm.* 2010;67(18):1539–44.
3. United States Pharmacopeial Convention. Chapter <800>, Hazardous drugs—handling in healthcare settings. In: *United States Pharmacopeia/National Formulary*. Rockville, MD: United States Pharmacopeial Convention; current edition.
4. United States Pharmacopeial Convention. Chapter <797>, Pharmaceutical compounding—sterile preparations. In: *United States Pharmacopeia/National Formulary*. Rockville, MD: United States Pharmacopeial Convention; current edition.

Chapter 6

Stability of Compounded Preparations

Stability is the extent to which a product retains, within specified limits and throughout its period of storage and use, the same properties and characteristics that it possessed at the time of its manufacture. The current edition of the *United States Pharmacopeia/National Formulary (USP/NF)*[1] provides definitions for five general types of stability:

- *Chemical:* Each active ingredient retains its chemical integrity and labeled potency, within the specified limits.
- *Physical:* The original physical properties, including appearance, palatability, uniformity, dissolution, and suspendability, are retained.
- *Microbiological:* Sterility or resistance to microbial growth is retained according to the specified requirements. Antimicrobial agents that are present retain effectiveness within the specified limits.
- *Therapeutic:* The therapeutic effect remains unchanged.
- *Toxicological:* No significant increase in toxicity occurs.

Instability describes chemical reactions that are "incessant, irreversible, and result in distinctly different chemical entities (degradation products) that can be both therapeutically inactive and possibly exhibit greater toxicity."[2] Incompatibility is different from instability but must be considered in the overall stability evaluation of a preparation. *Incompatibility* generally refers to visually evident and "physicochemical phenomena such as concentration-dependent precipitation and acid–base reactions, with the products of reaction manifested as a change in physical state, including protonation–deprotonation equilibria."[2]

A compounding pharmacist must avoid formulation ingredients and conditions that could result in a subpotent preparation that leads to poor clinical results. Knowledge of the chemical reactions by which drugs degrade can enable a pharmacist to establish conditions that minimize the rate of degradation. At all steps in the compounding, dispensing, and storage processes, a pharmacist should observe the compounded drug preparation for signs of instability. A discard-after or beyond-use date is the date after which a compounded preparation should be discarded. This period should be based on available stability information and reasonable patient needs with respect to the intended drug therapy.

All compounded preparations should be observed periodically for signs of physical instability, including evidence of microbiological and fungal contamination of any preparations with formulas that lack preservatives. If large quantities of a preparation have been legitimately prepared, conducting potency and stability assays to ensure the preparation's potency lasts up to the assigned beyond-use date may be advisable.[1]

Factors That Affect Stability

Numerous factors can affect the stability of a drug and dosage form, including pH, temperature, solvent, light, air (oxygen), carbon dioxide, moisture or humidity, and particle size.

pH is one of the most important factors affecting the stability of a product. A pharmacist can use published pH and stability profiles to determine the pH that will ensure the maximum stability of the product. After determining the pH range, a pharmacist can prepare buffers to maintain the pH for the expected shelf life of the product.

Temperature affects the stability of a drug by increasing the rate of reaction speed about two to three times with each 10°C rise in temperature. This temperature effect was first suggested by Arrhenius as follows:

$$k = Ae^{-Ea/RT}$$

or

$$\log k = \log A - \frac{Ea}{2.303} \times \frac{1}{T}$$

where k is the specific reaction rate, A is the frequency factor, Ea is the energy of activation, R is the gas constant (1.987 cal/deg mole), and T is the absolute temperature. As is evident from these relationships, an increase in temperature will result in an increase in the specific reaction rate, or the degradation rate of the drug. Temperature effects can be minimized by selecting the proper storage temperature: room, refrigerated, or freezing.

A *solvent* affects the stability of a product if the preparation is a liquid. The solvent can affect the pH, solubility, and solubility parameter (δ) of the active ingredient. The stability of a product may be compromised if solvents are changed indiscriminately.

Light may provide the activation energy required for a degradation reaction to occur. Many light-activated reactions are zero-order, or constant, reactions. The effects of light can be minimized by packaging products in light-resistant containers; products that are light sensitive can be covered during administration with aluminum foil or an amber-colored plastic overwrap.

Air (oxygen) can induce degradation via oxidation. Degradation can be minimized by filling the container as full as possible, thereby decreasing the headspace, or by replacing the headspace with nitrogen. Another option is to add an antioxidant to the formulation (Table 6-1).

Carbon dioxide can cause insoluble carbonates to form in the solid dosage form, which decreases the disintegration and dissolution properties of the product. Packaging in tight containers and filling the containers as full as possible minimize this condition.

Humidity, or *moisture,* can result in hydrolysis reactions and degradation of the drug product. Working in a dry environment and inserting a desiccant packet in the packaging of the product can lessen the effects of humidity.

TABLE 6-1 Suggested Antioxidants for Use in Pharmacy Compounding

Antioxidant	Mechanism	Solubility			Usual Concentration Range/Comments
		Water	Alcohol	Oil	
Acetone sodium bisulfite	Reducing	Yes	No	No	0.2%–0.4%
Acetylcysteine	True	Yes	Yes	No	0.1%–0.5%
α-Lipoic acid (sodium salt)	—	Yes	—	Yes	
α-Tocopherol (synthetic)	True	No	Yes	Yes	
α-Tocopherol acetate	True	No	Yes	Yes	≤0.001%
D-α-Tocopherol (natural)	True	No	Yes	Yes	0.05%–0.075%
DL-α-Tocopherol (synthetic)	True	No	Yes	Yes	0.01%–0.5%
Ascorbic acid	Reducing/ Synergy	Yes	Yes	No	Soluble in glycerin/ propylene glycol
Ascorbyl palmitate	True	Yes	Yes	Yes	
Butylated hydroxyanisole	True	No	Yes	Yes	0.005%–0.02%/Soluble in propylene glycol
Butylated hydroxytoluene	True	No	Yes	Yes	0.005%–0.02%/Soluble in mineral oil
Calcium ascorbate	Reducing	Yes	Yes	—	
Calcium bisulfite	Reducing	Yes	—	—	
Calcium sulfite	Reducing	Yes	Yes	—	
Cysteine	True	Yes	Yes	No	0.1%–0.5%
Cysteine HCl	True/Synergy	Yes	Yes	No	0.1%–0.5%/Bad odor
Dilauryl thiodipropionate	True	No	Yes	Yes	
Dithiothreitol	True	Yes	Yes	No	0.01%–0.1%
Dodecyl gallate	True	No	Yes	Yes	
Ethoxyquin	True	—	—	Yes	
Ethyl gallate	True	SlS	Yes	No	
Gallic acid	—	Yes	Yes	Yes	
Glutathione	True	Yes	—	—	
Gossypol	True	No	Yes	Yes	
Hydroquinone	Reducing	Yes	Yes	Yes	
4-Hydroxymethyl-2,6-di-*tert*-butylphenol	—	Yes	Yes	Yes	
Hypophosphorous acid	—	Yes	—	—	
Isoascorbic acid	Reducing	Yes	—	—	
Lecithin	True	Yes	Yes	Yes	
Monothioglycerol	Reducing	Yes	Yes	—	0.1%–1.0%/Slight odor
β-Naphthol	True	Yes	Yes	Yes	

(continued)

TABLE 6-1 Suggested Antioxidants for Use in Pharmacy Compounding *(Continued)*

| Antioxidant | Mechanism | Solubility | | | Usual Concentration Range/Comments |
		Water	Alcohol	Oil	
Nordihydroguaiaretic acid	True	No	Yes	Yes	0.001%–0.01%
Octyl gallate	True	No	Yes	Yes	
Potassium metabisulfite	Reducing	Yes	No	No	
Propyl gallate	True	SlS	Yes	SlS	0.001%–0.15% (≤2.5 mg/kg body weight)
Sesamol	—	—	—	—	
Sodium ascorbate	Reducing	Yes	Yes	No	
Sodium bisulfite	Reducing	Yes	SlS	No	0.05%–1.0%
Sodium formaldehyde sulfoxylate	Reducing	Yes	SlS	—	0.005%–0.15%
Sodium metabisulfite	Reducing	Yes	SlS	—	0.01%–1.0%/Soluble in glycerin
Sodium sulfite	Reducing	Yes	No	No	0.01%–0.2%
Sodium thiosulfate	Reducing	Yes	No	—	
Sulfur dioxide	Reducing	Yes	Yes	Yes	
Tannic acid	Reducing	Yes	—	—	
Thioglycerol	Reducing	Yes	Yes	—	
tert-Butyl-hydroquinone	True	—	—	—	
Thioglycolic acid	Reducing	Yes	Yes	Yes	
Thiolactic acid	Reducing	Yes	Yes	Yes	
Thiosorbitol	Reducing	Yes	Yes	Yes	
Thiourea	Reducing	Yes	Yes	No	0.005%
Tocopherols	True	—	—	Yes	0.05%–0.5%

— = Not available.

Particle size can have an important effect on the stability of a product. The smaller the particle size, the greater is the reactivity of the product. When working with drugs that are less stable in solid dosage forms, such as powders and capsules, using a larger particle size, as appropriate, may be advisable.

Other factors that can affect drug stability are *ionic strength* and *dielectric constant*.

Paths of Instability

Physical instability can adversely affect drug products. Some paths through which physical instability can occur include the formation of polymorphs, crystallization, vaporization, and adsorption.

Polymorphs are substances that can crystallize in different forms of the same chemical compound. Their crystallized forms differ in energy and may exhibit variations in such properties as solubility, compressibility, and melting point. Knowledge of the causative factors of polymorphs can enable a pharmacist to take steps to prevent them. For example, polymorphs can form if heat and shock cooling are used.

Crystallization of particles in suspension can alter the size distribution of the particles. Temperature fluctuations often cause such crystallization to occur, because increasing temperatures result in greater solubility (which means that smaller particles may dissolve faster) and decreasing temperatures result in some crystallization of the drug on particles that are already present. Such fluctuation cycles will cause a decrease in the proportion of smaller particles and an increase in the proportion of larger crystals present.

Vaporization increases at higher temperatures and will result in loss of solvent. When solvent or liquid is lost, the product's concentration increases. This may lead to overdosage when the product is administered. A loss of solvent could also cause precipitation of the drug if the solubility of the drug in the remaining vehicle is exceeded.

Adsorption of the drug or excipients is a common occurrence and may lessen the amount of the drug available for treatment. Drugs may adsorb to filters, the container, tubing, syringes, or other materials. This is particularly troublesome in the case of low-dose drugs. Sorption can often be minimized by pretreating equipment and containers with silain or silicone; in some instances, adding albumin or a similar material to the vehicle before adding the drug can have the same result.

Containers

In selecting a container or package for the finished compounded preparation, one must realize that although a drug may be stable when stored in one type of container (glass), it may not be stable in a plastic (polyvinyl chloride) container or an infusion device made of an elastomer. Glass is generally considered to be the most inert and stable container material, but plastic has gained wide acceptability and usefulness. The compatibility of the plastic with the drug formulation must be checked and confirmed because some plastic syringes may adversely affect the drug concentration during storage, either short or long term.

Observations of Instability

Pharmacists can often detect evidence of instability in dosage forms through observation. Table 6-2 lists physical evidence of instability that may occur in various dosage forms.

Oxidation and Antioxidants

Antioxidants are added to minimize or retard oxidative processes that occur with some drugs or excipients on exposure to oxygen or in the presence of free radicals. These processes can often be catalyzed by light, temperature, hydrogen ion concentration, presence of trace metals, or peroxides. Oxidation of a product may be manifested as an unpleasant odor or taste, discoloration or other change in appearance, precipitation, or even a slight loss of activity.

Ways to prevent or minimize oxidation are listed in Table 6-3. Removing oxygen from the ingredients before formulation and minimizing the entrapment of air during formulation are important. To minimize air entrapment, care should be taken not to foam, whip, mix too vigorously, or form a vortex during mixing. Mixing ingredients at lower-than-normal speed in sealed containers works well. For emulsions, a hand homogenizer (producing strong shear forces in a closed space) works well if the product is collected carefully and protected from air.

The most common approach to minimizing oxidation is to add an antioxidant to the system. The selection of an appropriate antioxidant depends on several factors, including solubility; location of the agent in the formulation (emulsions); chemical and physical stability over a wide pH range; compatibility; odor; discoloration; toxicity; irritation; potency;

TABLE 6-2 Physical Changes Indicating Instability

Dosage Form	Changes
Capsules	A change in the physical appearance or consistency of the capsule or its contents, including hardening or softening of the shell; also, any discoloration, expansion, or distortion of the gelatin capsule
Powders	Caking or discoloration instead of free flowing; release of pressure on opening of container, indicative of bacterial or other degradation
Solutions/elixirs, syrups	Precipitation, discoloration, haziness, gas formation resulting from microbial growth
Emulsions	Breaking, creaming
Suspensions	Caking, difficulty in resuspending; crystal growth
Ointments	Change in consistency and separation of liquid, if contained, and formation of granules or grittiness; drying
Creams	Emulsion breakage, crystal growth, shrinkage caused by evaporation of water; gross microbial contamination
Suppositories	Excessive softening, drying, hardening, shriveling; evidence of oil stains on packaging
Gels	Shrinkage, separation of liquid from the gel, discoloration, microbial contamination
Troches	Softening or hardening, crystallization, microbial contamination, discoloration
Sterile products	Discoloration, haziness, precipitation

TABLE 6-3 Ways to Minimize Oxidation in Pharmaceutical Preparations

1. Use de-aerated water. Boil the purified water for 5 minutes and immediately cover it to avoid contact with air, which may redissolve in it.

2. Incorporate the antioxidants in the preparation as early in the process as possible. If a polyphasic system is used, such as an emulsion, place an antioxidant in each phase as early in the process as possible. If this is not done, oxidation may occur and much of the added antioxidant will be consumed in neutralizing the already-present oxidation products.

3. Do not use a mixing method or device that incorporates air into the system.

4. Use a mixing container that has minimal headspace, preferably replacing the air in the headspace with nitrogen.

5. Add a buffer system to maintain a desired pH.

6. Use ingredients with low heavy metal content.

7. Decrease temperature during preparation, if possible.

8. Assay for actives and antioxidants and even excipients if compounding a preparation routinely to determine the effectiveness of the antioxidants.

9. Increase concentration of antioxidants if necessary.

effectiveness in low concentrations; and freedom from toxicity, carcinogenicity, and sensitizing effects.

The actual selection of an antioxidant depends on the (1) type of product; (2) route, dose, and frequency of administration; (3) physical and chemical properties of the preservative used; (4) presence of other components; and (5) properties of the closure and container. The effectiveness of antioxidants may actually be decreased in complex systems such as suspensions and emulsions. This decrease may be due to sorption of the antioxidant onto suspended particles or to partitioning of the antioxidant between the phases of an emulsion. Also, antioxidants may sorb to containers and closures.

In general, antioxidants are used in relatively low concentrations, usually ranging from 0.001% to 0.2%. The lowest effective concentration should be used. When formulating a product, pharmacists should remember to incorporate the antioxidant early in the preparation process to minimize the extent of oxidation, rather than at the end of preparation when much of the antioxidant will be needlessly used up in counteracting the oxidation that has already occurred. In addition, using a chelating agent together with an antioxidant to chelate trace metals that may catalyze an oxidative process is advisable. Commonly used chelating agents are shown in Table 6-4.

The formulation of an antioxidant system is accomplished primarily through trial and error. With some experimentation and patience, a suitable, stable system with the required antioxidant properties can be developed.

TABLE 6-4 Solubility of Chelating Agents and Synergists

Added Substance	Solubility			Usual Concentration Range/Comments
	Water	Alcohol	Oil	
Alkyl gallates	Yes	Yes	Yes	
Ascorbic acid	Yes	Yes	No	0.02%–0.1%
Boric acid	Yes	Yes	No	
Citric acid	Yes	Yes	—	0.005%–0.01% (incompatible with potassium tartrate, alkali, acetates, and sulfites)
Citraconic acid	Yes	Yes	No	0.03%–0.45%
Cysteine	Yes	Yes	No	
Ethylenediaminetetraacetic acid and salts (incompatible with polyvalent metal ions)	Yes	Yes	No	0.02%–0.1%
Gluconic acid	Yes	Yes	No	
Glycine	Yes	Yes	—	
Hydroxyquinoline sulfate	Yes	Yes	—	0.005%–0.01%
Maleic acid	Yes	Yes	No	
Phosphoric acid	Yes	Yes	—	0.005%–0.01%
Polysorbates	Yes	Yes	No	
Saccharic acid	Yes	Yes	No	
Tartaric acid	Yes	Yes	—	0.01%–0.02%
Tryptophan	—	Yes	No	

— = Not available.

Q_{10} Method of Predicting Shelf Life

Compounding pharmacists can use the Q_{10} method of shelf-life estimation to quickly calculate a beyond-use date for a drug preparation that is going to be stored or used under conditions that differ from the labeling requirements. The expression Q_{10} is a ratio of two different reaction rate constants, defined as follows:

$$Q_{10} = \frac{K_{(T+10)}}{K_T}$$

where K_T is the reaction rate constant at a specific temperature T, and $K_{(T + 10)}$ is the reaction rate constant at a temperature 10°C higher. The commonly used Q values of 2, 3, and 4 are related to Ea values of 12.2, 19.4, and 24.5 kcal/mol, respectively. For practical purposes, if the Ea is not known, a median value of 3 has been used as a reasonable estimate.

The actual equation used for estimating shelf life is as follows:

$$t_{90}(T2) = \frac{t_{90}(T1)}{Q_{10}^{(\Delta T/10)}}$$

where $t_{90}(T2)$ is the estimated shelf life, $t_{90}(T1)$ is the given shelf life at a given temperature $T1$, and ΔT is the temperature difference between $T1$ and $T2$.

The equation illustrates that increasing the expression $(\Delta T/10)$ will decrease the shelf life and decreasing the expression will increase the shelf life of the drug. For example, if a preparation that is normally stored at room temperature (25°C) with an expiration date of 1 week is stored in the refrigerator (5°C), what will be the approximate increase in the shelf life of the preparation?

$$t_{90}(T2) = \frac{t_{90}(T1)}{Q_{10}^{(\Delta T/10)}} = \frac{1}{3^{(-20/10)}} = \frac{1}{3^{-2}} = 9 \text{ weeks}$$

because there is a 20° decrease in temperature, from 25°C down to 5°C. Thus, the increase in shelf life will be about 9 times or, in this case, 9 weeks, when there is a 20° decrease in the storage temperature. This calculation assumes an Ea of about 19.4 kcal/mol.

Conversely, if a preparation that is normally stored at refrigeration temperature (5°C) with a shelf life of 9 weeks is stored at room temperature (25°C), what will be the approximate decrease in the shelf life of the preparation?

$$t_{90}(T2) = \frac{t_{90}(T1)}{Q_{10}^{(\Delta T/10)}} = \frac{9}{3^{(20/10)}} = 1 \text{ week}$$

because there is a 20° temperature increase, from 5°C up to 25°C. This also assumes an Ea of about 19.4 kcal/mol.

This method is applicable to preparations for which a specific shelf life has been determined and only the storage temperature, not the formulation, varies.

Beyond-Use Dating

The assignment of a beyond-use date is the responsibility of a pharmacist or compounder.

There is a difference between an expiration date and a beyond-use date. An *expiration date* is a projection of the length of time the product can be expected, on the basis of accelerated stability studies, to retain its purity and potency. Expiration dates are used for commercial products. A *beyond-use date* is an estimate of the time interval that the compounded preparation can be expected to retain its purity and potency on the basis of general guidelines, literature references, or actual real-time stability studies using prescribed conditions. In general, a maximum beyond-use date of 6 months is used because it more nearly fits into the guidelines of a compounded prescription involving a patient, physician, and pharmacist.

Unless published data are available to the contrary, the following are the maximum recommended beyond-use dates for *nonsterile* compounded drug preparations that are packaged in tight, light-resistant containers and stored at a controlled room temperature or as otherwise indicated and for sterile preparations for which a program of sterility testing is in place.[3] Drugs or chemicals known to be labile to decomposition will require shorter beyond-use dates.

- *Nonaqueous formulations:* The beyond-use date is not later than the time remaining until the earliest expiration date of any active pharmaceutical ingredient or 6 months, whichever is earlier.
- *Water-containing oral formulations:* The beyond-use date is not later than 14 days for formulations stored at controlled cold temperature.
- *Water-containing topical/dermal and mucosal liquid and semisolid formulations:* The beyond-use date is not later than 30 days.

For nonsterile compounding, numerous sources of information can be used to determine an appropriate beyond-use date, including chemical company information, manufacturers' literature, Trissel's *Stability of Compounded Formulations* (Washington, DC: American Pharmacists Association; 2012), www.CompoundingToday.com, the monographs in the latest edition of *AHFS Drug Information, International Journal of Pharmaceutical Compounding, American Journal of Health-System Pharmacy, Hospital Pharmacy,* other journals, and related books. Most pharmacists prepare or dispense small quantities of compounded preparations, recommend storage at room or cold temperatures, and use a conservative beyond-use date.

For *sterile* compounded drug preparations, check the current edition of *USP* Chapter <797>, Pharmaceutical Compounding—Sterile Preparations, for the beyond-use date.[4] When evaluating the applicability of stability studies in the literature, a pharmacist must be certain that the preparations studied are similar to the preparation under consideration in drug concentration range, pH, excipients, vehicle, water content, and the like.

Sources of drug stability and compatibility information for parenteral products (admixtures) include current editions of the *Handbook on Injectable Drugs* (G. K. McEvoy, ed., American Society of Health-System Pharmacists, Bethesda, MD), *King Guide to Parenteral Admixtures* (King Guide Publications, Napa, CA), *International Journal of Pharmaceutical Compounding,* and www.CompoundingToday.com.

Other Considerations

In the home-care setting, admixed medications typically require longer expiration dates, patients' homes are often located a considerable distance from the infusion pharmacy, and many doses are delivered at one time to eliminate the expense of additional deliveries. The stability of these medications requires additional research, and many studies are needed to generate the necessary information.

References

1. United States Pharmacopeial Convention. Chapter <1191>, Stability considerations in dispensing practice. In: *United States Pharmacopeia/National Formulary*. Rockville, MD: United States Pharmacopeial Convention; current edition.
2. McEvoy GK, ed. *Handbook on Injectable Drugs*. 18th ed. Bethesda, MD: American Society of Health-System Pharmacists; 2015.
3. United States Pharmacopeial Convention. Chapter <795>, Pharmaceutical compounding—nonsterile preparations. In: *United States Pharmacopeia/National Formulary*. Rockville, MD: United States Pharmacopeial Convention; current edition.
4. United States Pharmacopeial Convention. <797>, Pharmaceutical compounding—sterile preparations. In: *United States Pharmacopeia/National Formulary*. Rockville, MD: United States Pharmacopeial Convention; current edition.

Chapter 7

Pharmaceutical Compounding Calculations

The preparation, packaging, and dispensing of most compounded prescriptions involve a number of pharmacy calculations. These calculations present one of the greatest potential sources of error in compounding. Even though most of the mathematical processes are relatively simple, misplacing a decimal point or using an estimated value for a medication can have serious consequences, including death. When a unit of measure must be converted to an equivalent value in a different measuring system, exact equivalent values must be used. For example, the correct metric equivalent value for 1 fl oz is 29.57 mL, not 30 mL or even 29.6 mL. Any rounding of values should be saved for the final answer. Being extremely well grounded in the practice of pharmaceutical calculations is particularly important for pharmacists, because zero tolerance is allowed for errors in these vital operations. Each topic is covered in more detail in pharmaceutical calculations texts, which should be referred to during training. This chapter is simply an overview of the different calculations that are used in compounding.

Measurement Systems

The metric system is the official system of measurement used in the practice of pharmacy and medicine. Table 7-1 lists the units of measure commonly used in compounding calculations. Also listed for each unit of measure is its denomination (e.g., liter, meter) abbreviation and its equivalent value to the definitive value (i.e., largest denomination for that type of measure). Table 7-2 lists the major denominations and equivalent values for the following measurement systems used in the United States: avoirdupois weights, troy weights, and apothecary weights and measures. Table 7-3 lists equivalent values for selected units of weight and liquid measures, and Table 7-4 lists equivalent apothecary and metric values for household approximate measures. All four tables are useful references for pharmaceutical calculations.

TABLE 7-1 Metric Measures

Unit of Measure	Denomination Abbreviation	Equivalent Value to Largest Denomination
Metric Weights		
1 microgram	μg	0.000001 gram
1 milligram	mg	0.001 gram
1 centigram	cg	0.01 gram
1 decigram	dg	0.1 gram
1 gram	g	1 gram
1 dekagram	dag	10 grams
1 hectogram	hg	100 grams
1 kilogram	kg	1000 grams
Metric Liquid Measures		
1 microliter	μL	0.000001 liter
1 milliliter	mL	0.001 liter
1 centiliter	cL	0.01 liter
1 deciliter	dL	0.1 liter
1 liter	L	1 liter
1 dekaliter	daL	10 liters
1 hectoliter	hL	100 liters
1 kiloliter	kL	1000 liters
Metric Linear Measures		
1 nanometer	nm	0.000000001 meter
1 micron	μm	0.000001 meter
1 millimeter	mm	0.001 meter
1 centimeter	cm	0.01 meter
1 decimeter	dm	0.1 meter
1 meter	M	1 meter
1 dekameter	dam	10 meters
1 hectometer	hm	100 meters
1 kilometer	km	1000 meters

General Calculations

Weighing, measuring, and diluting ingredients are common preparation steps that entail calculations. The calculations may include weighing an ingredient on a balance, measuring a liquid ingredient in a graduated cylinder, or using specific gravity values (Appendix III) to convert the volume of a liquid to a weight or vice versa. Other common calculations include using the processes of dilution or aliquots to obtain an accurate quantity of material that cannot be directly weighed or measured.

Weighing or measuring ingredients is one of the first steps in preparing any prescription. One cannot expect to have a properly prepared prescription that complies with United States Pharmacopeial Convention (USP) allowable tolerances unless each

TABLE 7-2 Equivalent Values for Other Measurement Systems

Avoirdupois Weights

Pound		Ounces		Grains
1	=	16	=	7000
		1	=	437.5

Troy Weights

Pound		Ounces		Pennyweights		Grains
1	=	12	=	240	=	5760
		1	=	20	=	480
				1	=	24

Apothecary Weights

Pound		Ounces		Drams		Scruples		Grains
1	=	12	=	96	=	288	=	5760
		1	=	8	=	24	=	480
				1	=	3	=	60
						1	=	20

Apothecary Measures

Gallon		Pints		Fluidounces		Fluidrams		Minims
1	=	8	=	128	=	1024	=	61,440
		1	=	16	=	128	=	7680
				1	=	8	=	480
						1	=	60

TABLE 7-3 Equivalent Values for Selected Units of Measure

Unit of Measure	Equivalent Value
Weight Measures	
1 kilogram	2.2 pounds avoirdupois
1 pound	454 grams
1 ounce avoirdupois	28.35 grams
1 ounce apothecary	31.1 grams
1 pound apothecary	373 grams
1 gram	15.432 grains
1 grain	64.8 milligrams
Liquid Measures	
1 milliliter	16.23 minims
1 fluidounce	29.57 milliliters
1 pint	473 milliliters
1 gallon	3785 milliliters

TABLE 7-4 Equivalent Values for Household Approximate Measures

Unit of Measure	Equivalent Value	
	Apothecary	Metric
1 tumblerful	8 fluidounces	240 milliliters
1 teacupful	4 fluidounces	120 milliliters
1 wineglass	2 fluidounces	60 milliliters
2 tablespoonfuls	1 fluidounce	30 milliliters
1 tablespoonful	½ fluidounce	15 milliliters
1 dessert spoonful	2 fluidrams	8–10 milliliters
1 teaspoonful	1 fluidram	5 milliliters
½ teaspoonful	½ fluidram	2.5 milliliters

ingredient is accurately weighed or measured using properly calibrated equipment. The importance of obtaining accurate weights and measures cannot be overemphasized. In fact, good practice involves using a balance that has a printer, so that each weight reading can be printed and kept as a permanent record.

Least Measurable Quantity of Weight

A pharmacy's torsion balance has a sensitivity reading of 5 mg. What is the smallest quantity that can be accurately weighed with a maximum error of 5%?

The formula for calculating this value is expressed as

$$100\% \times \frac{\text{Maximum potential error (sensitivity reading)}}{\text{Permissible error (in percent)}} = \text{Least measurable quantity}$$

$$x = 100\% \times \frac{5 \text{ mg}}{5\%}$$

$$x = 100 \text{ mg}$$

The answer, 100 mg, illustrates the general principle of least measurable quantities with torsion balances: the value of the least measurable quantity is usually 20 times the sensitivity reading of the balance.

The pharmacy's electronic (digital) balance has a sensitivity reading of 0.1 mg. What is the least quantity that can be reasonably weighed on this balance?

A digital balance does not change its readout until a unit of material that equals or exceeds the sensitivity reading is placed on the balance pan. If, in an attempt to weigh 0.1 mg of a drug, 0.14 mg is placed on the pan, the readout will be only 0.1 mg. Therefore, use the same general principle as with torsion balances and do not weigh quantities that are less than 20 times the sensitivity reading of the balance (i.e., 20×0.1 mg = 2 mg).

Quantities of Ingredients

What quantity of each ingredient is required for the following prescription?

℞ **Clotrimazole 1% Cream**

Clotrimazole powder	1%
Dermabase	qs 30 g

Step 1. Determine the quantity of clotrimazole powder by multiplying its concentration (1% = 0.01) by the total weight of the product:

$x = 30 \text{ g} \times 0.01 = 0.3 \text{ g of clotrimazole, } answer$

Step 2. Determine the quantity of Dermabase by subtracting the quantity of clotrimazole powder from the total weight of the product:

$x = 30 \text{ g} - 0.3 \text{ g} = 29.7 \text{ g of Dermabase, } answer$

Density Factors in Weighing/Measuring

A pharmacist receives a prescription for 120 mL of a 3% (weight per volume, or w/v) hydrochloric acid (HCl) solution. The density of concentrated hydrochloric acid (37% weight per weight, or w/w) is 1.18 g/mL. How many milliliters of the concentrated acid would be required for the prescription?

Step 1. Calculate the weight of the required quantity of the 3% HCl solution:

3% (w/v) = 0.03 g/mL

0.03 g/mL × 120 mL = 3.6 g

Step 2. Calculate the volume of the required quantity of the 3% HCl solution:

$$\frac{3.6 \text{ g}}{1.18 \text{ g/mL}} = 3.05 \text{ mL}$$

Step 3. Calculate the volume of the 37% HCl required for the prescription:

37% = 0.37

$$\frac{3.05 \text{ mL}}{0.37} = 8.24 \text{ mL of 37\% HCl, } answer$$

Dilution Aliquots

A pharmacist needs 0.015 mL of a flavoring oil to prepare an oral liquid. With alcohol as a solvent and a pipet accurate to 0.01 mL, how can this volume of flavoring oil be obtained?

Step 1. Select a multiple of the desired quantity that can be accurately measured with the pipet. For this example, use 10 as the multiple and measure 0.1 mL of flavoring oil (10 × 0.01 mL). Place the oil in a suitable graduated cylinder.

Step 2. Dilute the quantity of flavoring oil calculated in step 1 with alcohol to a quantity of solution that is divisible by the selected multiple. For this example, add sufficient alcohol to make 50 mL of solution, and mix well.

Step 3. Calculate the aliquot of the solution that contains the desired quantity of flavoring oil (0.015 mL) as follows:

$$\frac{0.1 \text{ mL}}{50 \text{ mL}} = \frac{0.015 \text{ mL}}{x}$$

$x = 7.5 \text{ mL aliquot, } answer$

Step 4. Remove 7.5 mL of the solution that contains the required 0.015 mL of the flavoring oil.

Doses

Calculations concerning doses must also be performed accurately because they have a direct effect on the quantity of a medication that will be administered to a patient. Some of these calculations may involve determining the quantity of medication to be administered (e.g., teaspoonful, milliliter, tablet). Others involve converting the dose of a drug to the quantity of the final dosage form that should be administered. Appendix IV illustrates conversions to account for water of hydration and different chemical forms of a drug (base, salts, and esters).

Calibrating Droppers

A prescription for an anticholinergic liquid has been presented for a toddler at a dose of 0.25 mL. The dropper dispensed with the medication delivers 56 drops of the liquid per 2 mL. How many drops should the parents be instructed to give the toddler?

Step 1. Calculate the number of drops delivered per 1 mL:

$$\frac{56 \text{ drops}}{2 \text{ mL}} = 28 \text{ drops/mL}$$

Step 2. Calculate the number of drops delivered per 0.25 mL:

$$\frac{0.25 \text{ mL}}{1 \text{ mL}} = \frac{x}{28 \text{ drops}}$$

$x = 7$ drops, *answer*

Nasal Aerosol Doses

Qnasl nasal aerosol is available in an 8.7-g container, and each actuation delivers 100 mcg of beclomethasone dipropionate in 59 mg of solution from the valve and delivers 80 mcg of beclomethasone dipropionate from the nasal actuator. How many doses of the solution are contained in the 8.7 g container?

8.7 g × 1000 mg/g × 1 dose/59 mg = 147.46 doses = 147 full doses

How much of the drug is lost between the valve and nasal actuator?
80 mcg from actuator/100 mcg from valve = 80% delivered.
80% delivered = 20% lost between valve and actuator.

Calculating the Number of Dosage Forms/Volume to Dispense

A pharmacist receives a prescription for Wormaway 1 mg/mL for a family of five. The medication is to be given the day the prescription is filled and then repeated in 7 days. What total volume of the medication is required if the dose for each person is 0.3 mg/kg of body weight?

Step 1. Convert each person's body weight to kilograms (1 kg = 2.2 lb); multiply those values by 0.3 mg to calculate the number of milligrams per dose for each person; add the values in the last column to calculate the total number of milligrams required for one dose.

Adult 1 $\dfrac{175 \text{ lb}}{2.2} = 79.55$ kg × 0.3 mg/kg = 23.87 mg

Adult 2 $\dfrac{125 \text{ lb}}{2.2} = 56.82$ kg × 0.3 mg/kg = 17.05 mg

Child 1 $\dfrac{95 \text{ lb}}{2.2} = 43.18$ kg × 0.3 mg/kg = 12.95 mg

Child 2 $\dfrac{75 \text{ lb}}{2.2}$ = 34.09 kg × 0.3 mg/kg = 10.23 mg

Child 3 $\dfrac{60 \text{ lb}}{2.2}$ = 27.27 kg × 0.3 mg/kg = 8.18 mg

Total milligrams required for one dose = 72.28 mg

Step 2. Calculate the quantity required for two doses:

72.28 mg × 2 = 144.56 mg

Step 3. Divide the quantity for two doses by the concentration of the medication to determine the total volume required:

$\dfrac{144.56 \text{ mg}}{1 \text{ mg/mL}}$ = 144.56 mL of Wormaway 1 mg/mL, *answer*

Solutions

Solubility ratios in the literature and in the current edition of the *United States Pharmacopeia/ National Formulary* are given as "x:y" and "x in y" (e.g., 1:4 and 1 in 4). These expressions are stated as one part of *solute* plus four parts of *solvent*. The resulting product is described as a 1:5 solution; that is, the product contains one part of *solute* in five parts of *solution*. A *solubility ratio* involves the quantity of solute that will dissolve in a quantity of solvent. This ratio is usually expressed as the number of grams of solute that will dissolve in a certain number of milliliters of solvent. In contrast, a *solution concentration* involves the quantity of solute in a given quantity of solution. This concentration is usually expressed as the number of grams of solute in a certain number of milliliters of solution. Another example: a substance with a solubility of 1:3 contains 1 g of solute *plus* 3 mL of solvent. The resulting product, a 1:4 solution, contains one part of solute in four parts of solution. In contrast, a 1:3 *solution* contains 1 g of solute in 3 mL of solution (i.e., sufficient solvent is added to make 3 mL of solution).

In pharmaceutical calculations, the concentration of a solution is often expressed as "parts per *x*." Table 7-5 lists common "parts per *x*" measurements and their equivalent values in metric measures, percentage concentration, and ratio concentration.

Determining W/W and W/V of Solutions

One gram of boric acid is soluble in 18 mL of water and makes a saturated solution. What is the percentage w/w and w/v of a saturated solution of boric acid?

Step 1. Calculate the total weight of the solution:

1 mL of water weighs 1 g

1 g + 18 g = 19 g

TABLE 7-5 "Parts per *x*" Measurements and Their Equivalent Values

Parts per *x*	Metric Equivalent	Percentage Concentration	Ratio Concentration
1 pp1 (1 part per 1)	1 g/mL	100%	1:1
1 ppt (1 part per thousand)	1 mg/mL	0.1%	1:1000
1 ppm (1 part per million)	1 µg/mL, or 1 g/1,000,000 mL	0.0001%	1:1,000,000
1 ppb (1 part per billion)	1 ng/mL	0.0000001%	1:1,000,000,000

Step 2. Calculate the percentage w/w of the solution by setting up a proportion between the weights and the percentages of saturation:

$$\frac{19 \text{ g}}{1 \text{ g}} = \frac{100\%}{x \text{ (\% w/w of solution)}}$$

$x = 5.26\%$ w/w, *answer*

Step 3. Because the volume of the solution is between 18 mL and 19 mL, we know the w/v concentration is greater than 5.26%. Assume the volume is 18.2 mL, and calculate the w/v concentration:

$$\frac{1 \text{ g}}{18.2 \text{ ml}} = \frac{x(\% \text{ w/v})}{100\%}$$

$x = 5.5\%$ w/v, *answer*

Determining Quantity of Active Drug

What quantity of mannitol is required to prepare 120 mL of a 1:10 solution?

Step 1. Set up a proportion between the ratio concentrations and the quantity of the ingredients:

$$\frac{1 \text{ part}}{10 \text{ parts}} = \frac{x}{120 \text{ mL}}$$

$x = 12$ g of mannitol, *answer*

Step 2. Place 12 g of mannitol in a graduated cylinder, and add sufficient solvent to make 120 mL of solution.

A pharmacist receives a prescription for 8 oz of an oral rinse to contain 10 ppm fluoride ion (F^-) in orange flower water. How much sodium fluoride (NaF) would be required to prepare this compound?

Step 1. Convert ounces to milliliters (1 oz = 29.57 mL), and calculate the total volume of the solution:

8×29.57 mL = 237 mL

Step 2. Convert parts per million to a ratio concentration and set up the following proportion to calculate the quantity of fluoride ion required for the prescription:

$$\frac{10 \text{ g}}{1,000,000 \text{ mL}} = \frac{x}{237 \text{ mL}}$$

$x = 0.0024$ g = 2.4 mg of F^-, *answer*

Step 3. Given that 1 mg $F^- = 2.2$ mg NaF, calculate the quantity of NaF required:

$$\frac{1 \text{ mg F}^-}{2.2 \text{ mg NaF}} = \frac{2.4 \text{ mg F}^-}{x \text{ (mg NaF)}}$$

$x = 5.3$ mg NaF

Determining Quantity of Preservatives

How much 95% ethanol would be required to preserve the following prescription?

Active drug #1 (powder)	120 mg
Active drug #2 (aqueous solution)	20 mL
Water	10 mL
Syrup	qs 120 mL

As this prescription is written, the sucrose concentration and preservative properties will decrease because 10 mL of water and 20 mL of aqueous solution are diluting the syrup. To compensate for this decrease, adding 95% alcohol is the simplest solution. The quantity of alcohol required can be calculated as follows:

Step 1. Determine the quantity of syrup required for the prescription:

$$120 \text{ mL} - (10 \text{ mL} + 20 \text{ mL}) = 90 \text{ mL}$$

Step 2. Determine the quantity of sucrose present in 90 mL of syrup (w/v of sucrose = 85%):

$$85\% \times 90 \text{ mL} = 76.5 \text{ g}$$

Step 3. Given that 1 g of sucrose preserves 0.53 mL of water, determine the quantity of water that 76.5 g of sucrose will preserve:

$$76.5 \text{ g} \times 0.53 \text{ mL} = 40.5 \text{ mL}$$

Step 4. Given that 1 g of sucrose occupies a volume of 0.647 mL, determine the volume occupied by 76.5 g of sucrose:

$$76.5 \text{ g} \times 0.647 \text{ mL} = 49.5 \text{ mL}$$

Step 5. Determine the volume of solution preserved by the sucrose:

$$40.5 \text{ mL} + 49.5 \text{ mL} = 90 \text{ mL}$$

Step 6. Determine the volume of solution that is not preserved:

$$120 \text{ mL} - 90 \text{ mL} = 30 \text{ mL}$$

Step 7. Determine the quantity of absolute (18%) alcohol required to preserve the unpreserved solution:

$$18\% \times 30 \text{ mL} = 5.4 \text{ mL}$$

Step 8. Determine the quantity of 95% alcohol required to preserve the unpreserved solution:

$$\frac{5.4 \text{ mL}}{0.95} = 5.7 \text{ mL of 95\% alcohol, } answer$$

Reducing and Enlarging Formulas

The actual quantity of a formula to be prepared is often not the same quantity that is described in a formulation record. Consequently, in many cases, the quantity must be increased or decreased to achieve the required quantity of product. To ensure that the relative quantities of the ingredients remain consistent, the quantities of all ingredients must be increased or decreased by the same factor.

Semisolids

A formula for compounding 100 mL of an ibuprofen gel requires 2 g of ibuprofen powder. What quantity of the ibuprofen powder would be required for 240 mL of the product?

Set up a proportion to express the quantities of ingredients per total quantities of product, and solve for *x:*

$$\frac{2 \text{ g}}{100 \text{ mL}} = \frac{x}{240 \text{ mL}}$$

x = 4.8 g of ibuprofen, *answer*

A formula for heparin 335 units/g gel cream is as follows:

Heparin sodium	186 mg
Polyethylene glycol 400	15 g
Mineral oil	10 g
Pluronic F-127	23 g
Purified water	qs 100 g

A pharmacist needs to prepare sufficient mixture to fill twelve 30-g ointment tubes. How much of each ingredient would be required?

Step 1. 12 tubes × 30 g/tube = 360 g of mixture

Step 2. Formula conversion factor: 360 g/100 g = 3.6

Step 3.
Heparin sodium	186 mg × 3.6 = 669.6 mg
Polyethylene glycol 400	15 g × 3.6 = 54 g
Mineral oil	10 g × 3.6 = 36 g
Pluronic F-127	23 g × 3.6 = 82.8 g
Purified water	360 g − (0.67 + 54 + 36 + 82.8) = 186.53 g

Partial Dosage Units

How would a pharmacist determine the quantity of indomethacin required for the following prescription if indomethacin 25 mg capsules are used?

℞ **Indomethacin 5 mg/5 mL Suspension**

Indomethacin	5 mg/5 mL
Ora-Plus	60 mL
Ora-Sweet	qs 120 mL

Step 1. Determine the total quantity of indomethacin required for the prescription:

5 mg/5 mL = 1 mg/mL

1 mg/mL × 120 mL = 120 mg

Step 2. Calculate the number of capsules required to supply 120 mg of indomethacin:

$$\frac{120 \text{ mg}}{25 \text{ mg/capsule}} = 4.8 \text{ capsules}$$

Step 3. Empty the contents of 5 capsules onto a tared weighing paper, and weigh the contents. Given that the weight is 1.6 g, calculate the quantity of mixture to remove to use in the prescription:

$$\frac{x}{1.6 \text{ g}} = \frac{4.8 \text{ capsules}}{5 \text{ capsules}}$$

$x = 1.536$ g of mixture, *answer*

Hydrated and Anhydrous Crystals

How much magnesium sulfate heptahydrate ($MgSO_4 \cdot 7H_2O$) must be weighed to obtain 5 g of magnesium sulfate? (Formula weights: Mg = 24 g; S = 32 g; O = 16 g; H = 1 g)

Step 1. Using the given formula weights of the elements, calculate the weight of $MgSO_4$:

Weight Mg: 1×24 g $= 24$ g
Weight S: 1×32 g $= 32$ g
Weight O: 4×16 g $= 64$ g
Weight $MgSO_4 = 24$ g $+ 32$ g $+ 64$ g $= 120$ g

Step 2. Calculate the weight of $MgSO_4 \cdot 7H_2O$:

Weight $MgSO_4$: 1×120 g $= 120$ g
Weight H: 14×1 g $= 14$ g
Weight O: 7×16 g $= 112$ g
Weight $MgSO_4 \cdot 7H_2O = 120$ g $+ 14$ g $+ 112$ g $= 246$ g

Step 3. Calculate the quantity of $MgSO_4 \cdot 7H_2O$ that contains 5 g of $MgSO_4$:

$$\frac{120 \text{ g}}{246 \text{ g}} = \frac{5 \text{ g}}{x}$$

$x = 10.25$ g of $MgSO_4 \cdot 7H_2O$, *answer*

Stock Solutions

A pharmacist is preparing an ophthalmic decongestant solution in batch form. Each of three bottles will contain 15 mL of the ophthalmic solution. The formula requires 0.01% (w/v) benzalkonium chloride (BAK) as a preservative. The pharmacist has a stock solution containing 17% (w/v) BAK. How much of the BAK stock solution would be required for the three bottles of batch solution?

Step 1. Calculate the total weight of the ophthalmic batch solution:

15 mL $\times 3 = 45$ mL

Step 2. Calculate the weight of the BAK solution required for the batch solution:

$0.01\% = 0.0001$

45 mL $\times 0.0001 = 0.0045$ g

Step 3. Calculate the quantity of the 17% BAK solution required for the batch solution:

$$\frac{0.0045 \text{ g}}{x} = \frac{17 \text{ g}}{100 \text{ mL}}$$

$x = 0.026$ mL of 17% BAK solution, *answer*

Potency of Salt Forms

Polymyxin B sulfate has a potency of 6000 units/mg. How much polymyxin B sulfate, in milligrams, is required to prepare 10 mL of an ophthalmic solution containing 10,000 units/mL?

Step 1. Calculate the number of units of polymyxin B sulfate required for 10 mL of the solution:

10,000 units/mL $\times 10$ mL $= 100,000$ units

Step 2. Calculate the milligrams of polymyxin B sulfate required for the prescription:

$$\frac{6000 \text{ units}}{1 \text{ mg}} = \frac{100,000 \text{ units}}{x}$$

$x = 16.67$ mg of polymyxin B sulfate, *answer*

Mixing Products of Different Strengths

A pharmacist receives an order for 120 g of a 0.1% corticosteroid ointment. Three concentrations of corticosteroid ointment (30 g of 0.1%, 15 g of 0.15%, and 75 g of 0.005%), all in the same ointment base, are on hand. If these three ointments are mixed together, how much additional corticosteroid powder should be added to prepare the prescription? Assume the quantity of corticosteroid powder added will be negligible compared with the total weight of 120 g.

Step 1. Calculate the total milligrams of corticosteroid required for the prescription:

0.1% = 0.001; 0.15% = 0.0015; 0.005% = 0.00005

120 g × 0.001 = 0.12 g = 120 mg

Step 2. Calculate the total milligrams of corticosteroid contained in the three ointments on hand:

x (mg of corticosteroid in 0.1% ointment) = 30 g × 0.001 = 0.03 g = 30 mg

y (mg of corticosteroid in 0.15% ointment) = 15 g × 0.0015 = 0.0225 g = 22.5 mg

z (mg of corticosteroid in 0.005% ointment) = 75 g × 0.00005 = 0.00375 g = 3.8 mg

Total mg of corticosteroid in ointments = $x + y + z$ = 56.3 mg

Step 3. Calculate the amount of additional corticosteroid powder required for the prescription:

120 mg − 56.3 mg = 63.7 mg of corticosteroid power, *answer*

What quantities of a 50% dextrose in water solution ($D_{50}W$) and a 5% dextrose in water solution (D_5W) should be mixed to obtain 900 mL of a 15% dextrose in water solution?

Step 1. Determine the number of parts of $D_{50}W$ and D_5W required for the solution, using the following diagram:

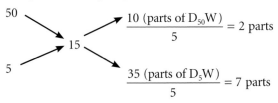

Total = 9 parts

This step can also be calculated using the following equations:

Number of parts of $D_{50}W$ = Desired strength (15%) − Strength of weaker component (5%) = 10 parts

Number of parts of D_5W = Strength of stronger component (50%) − Desired strength (15%) = 35 parts

Reduce the number of parts to lowest multiple, and calculate the total number of parts:

$$\text{Parts } D_{50}W = \frac{10 \text{ parts}}{5} = 2 \text{ parts}$$

$$\text{Parts } D_5W = \frac{35 \text{ parts}}{5} = 7 \text{ parts}$$

Total = 9 parts

Step 2. Calculate the volumes of $D_{50}W$ and D_5W required for the solution:

$$\frac{2 \text{ parts}}{9 \text{ parts}} = \frac{x \text{ (mL of } D_{50}W)}{900 \text{ mL}}$$

$x = 200$ mL of $D_{50}W$, *answer*

$$\frac{7 \text{ parts}}{9 \text{ parts}} = \frac{y \text{ (mL of } D_5W)}{900 \text{ mL}}$$

$y = 700$ mL of D_5W, *answer*

Reconstituting Powders

For reconstitution of a 1.5-g vial of Zerbaxa (1 g of ceftolozane and 0.5 g of tazobactam), 10 mL of 0.9% sodium chloride should be added. The resulting final volume is 11.4 mL. What is the actual concentration of each drug in the reconstituted solution?

Step 1. Calculate the concentration of ceftolozane:

1 g/11.4 mL × 1000 mg/g = 87.72 mg/mL

Step 2. Calculate the concentration of tazobactam:

0.5 g/11.4 mL × 1000 mg/g = 43.86 mg/mL

The directions to constitute 150 mL of an amoxicillin suspension 250 mg/5 mL call for 111 mL of purified water. The physician has requested the product be constituted at a concentration of 500 mg/5 mL. How much purified water is required for the higher concentration?

Step 1. Calculate the volume of the 250 mg/5 mL solution occupied by the amoxicillin powder:

150 mL − 111 mL = 39 mL

Step 2. Calculate the quantity of amoxicillin present in 1 mL of solution:

$$\frac{250 \text{ mg}}{5 \text{ mL}} = \frac{x}{150 \text{ mL}}$$

$x = 50$ mg/mL × 150 mL = 7500 mg

Step 3. Calculate the total volume of the requested concentration (500 mg/5 mL) of the solution:

$$\frac{500 \text{ mg}}{5 \text{ mL}} = \frac{7500 \text{ mg}}{x} = 75 \text{ mL}$$

Step 4. Calculate the quantity of purified water to add:

75 mL − 39 mL = 36 mL of purified water, *answer*

Ingredient- and Product-Specific Calculations

Some ingredients are prescribed in units of measure other than weight or volume. For example, electrolytes are prescribed in milliequivalents, and certain elements are prescribed in millimoles. Other units of measure are used for products in which activity or potency is of concern. These units of measure can be converted to a metric quantity so that the ingredient can be measured; however, specific calculations and a knowledge of how to use degrees of ionization, potency expressions, and the like are required to convert the units of measure accurately. Further, effervescent mixtures involve the use of stoichiometric ratios to determine the quantities of acids and bases that will react together. Finally, hydrophile–lipophile balance values can be used to determine the proper blending of surfactants for emulsions.

Milliequivalents

A prescription calls for 25 mEq of sodium chloride (NaCl). What quantity of sodium chloride, in milligrams, is required for the prescription? (1 equivalent NaCl = 58.5 g; 1 mEq NaCl = 58.5 mg)

Step 1. Given that 1 mEq of NaCl weighs 58.5 mg, calculate the weight of 25 mEq of NaCl:

$25 \text{ mEq} \times 58.5 \text{ mg/mEq} = 1463 \text{ mg of NaCl}$, *answer*

A pharmacist receives an order for 10 mEq of calcium ion (Ca^{++}). How much of a standard 10% calcium chloride ($CaCl_2$) solution should be used for this order? (Formula weight: Ca^{++} = 40 g; Cl^- = 35.5 g)

Step 1. Calculate the equivalent weight of Ca^{++}. Ca^{++} combines with two Cl^-; therefore, the formula weight of Ca^{++} is divided by 2 to obtain the equivalent weight:

$$\frac{40 \text{ g}}{2} = 20 \text{ g}$$

Step 2. Calculate the milliequivalent weight of Ca^{++}:

$$\frac{20 \text{ g}}{1000} = 0.02 \text{ g} = 20 \text{ mg}$$

Step 3. Calculate the quantity of Ca^{++}, in milligrams, required for the prescription:

$$\frac{1 \text{ mEq}}{10 \text{ mEq}} = \frac{20 \text{ mg}}{x}$$

$x = 200 \text{ mg}$

Step 4. Calculate the quantity of $CaCl_2$ required to supply 200 mg of Ca^{++}:

$$\frac{40 \text{ g}}{111 \text{ g}} = \frac{200 \text{ mg}}{x}$$

$x = 555 \text{ mg} = 0.555 \text{ g}$

Step 5. Calculate the quantity of the 10% $CaCl_2$ solution required to supply 555 mg of $CaCl_2$:

$10\% = 10 \text{ g}/100 \text{ mL}$

$$\frac{10 \text{ g}}{100 \text{ mL}} = \frac{0.555 \text{ g}}{x}$$

$x = 5.55 \text{ mL of 10\% } CaCl_2 \text{ solution}$, *answer*

A prescription calls for 240 mL of a solution that contains 15 mEq of potassium ion (K$^+$) as potassium chloride (KCl) and 10 mEq of sodium ion (Na$^+$) as sodium chloride (NaCl) per tablespoonful of solution. The compound is to be prepared in a suitable vehicle that contains no potassium or sodium ions. How much potassium chloride and sodium chloride would be required for this prescription? (Formula weights: K$^+$ = 39 g; Cl$^-$ = 35.5 g; Na$^+$ = 23 g; KCl = 74.5 g; NaCl = 58.5 g)

Step 1. Given that 1 mEq of KCl weighs 74.5 mg, calculate the weight of 15 mEq of KCl:

$$74.5 \text{ mg} \times 15 \text{ mEq} = 1118 \text{ mg} = 1.118 \text{ g}$$

Step 2. Calculate the quantity of KCl required for the prescription:

1 tablespoon = 15 mL

$$\frac{15 \text{ mL}}{240 \text{ mL}} = \frac{1.118 \text{ g}}{x}$$

x = 17.89 g of KCl, *answer*

Step 3. Given that 1 mEq of NaCl weighs 58.5 mg, calculate the weight of 10 mEq of NaCl:

$$58.5 \text{ mg} \times 10 \text{ mEq} = 585 \text{ mg} = 0.585 \text{ g}$$

Step 4. Calculate the quantity of NaCl required for the prescription:

$$\frac{15 \text{ mL}}{240 \text{ mL}} = \frac{0.585 \text{ g}}{x}$$

x = 9.36 g of NaCl, *answer*

Millimoles

How many millimoles of sodium chloride (NaCl) are contained in 1 liter of a 0.9% solution? (Formula weights: Na$^+$ = 23 g; Cl$^-$ = 35.5 g; NaCl = 58.5 g)

Step 1. Calculate the quantity of NaCl in the solution:

$$0.009 \times 1000 \text{ mL} = 9 \text{ g}$$

Step 2. Calculate the millimoles of NaCl contained in the solution:

1 equivalent weight NaCl = 1 mole of NaCl; therefore 1 mole of NaCl weighs 58.5 g

$$\frac{1 \text{ mole}}{58.5 \text{ g}} = \frac{x}{9 \text{ g}}$$

x = 0.154 mole = 154 millimoles of NaCl, *answer*

Osmolarity

What is the osmolarity (number of milliosmoles) of 1 L of 0.9% sodium chloride (NaCl) solution? Assume complete dissociation of the ions (NaCl → Na$^+$ + Cl$^-$). (Formula weights: Na$^+$ = 23 g; Cl$^-$ = 35.5 g; NaCl = 58.5 g)

Step 1. Calculate the number of millimoles of NaCl in the solution:

Millimoles/L of NaCl = 154 (see previous problem)

Step 2. Calculate the osmolarity of the solution by multiplying the answer in step 1 by the number of species:

NaCl → Na$^+$ + Cl$^-$ = 2 species

154 millimoles/L × 2 = 308 mOsm/L, *answer*

What is the osmolarity of 1 L of a 10% calcium chloride ($CaCl_2$) solution? Assume complete dissociation of the ions ($CaCl_2 \rightarrow Ca^{++} + 2Cl^-$). (Formula weights: $Ca^{++} = 40$ g; $Cl^- = 35.5$ g; $CaCl_2 = 111$ g)

Step 1. Calculate the number of millimoles of $CaCl_2$ in the solution:

10% = 100 g/1000 mL

$$\frac{100 \text{ g}}{111 \text{ g}} = \frac{x}{1 \text{ mole}}$$

$x = 0.9$ moles = 900 millimoles

Step 2. Calculate the osmolarity of the solution:

$CaCl_2 \rightarrow Ca^{++} + 2Cl^- = 3$ species

900 millimoles/L $\times$ 3 = 2700 mOsm/L, *answer*

Units-to-Weight Conversions

A prescription calls for 150,000 units of nystatin per gram of ointment with 60 g to be dispensed. What quantity of nystatin 4400 units/mg USP should be weighed for the prescription?

Step 1. Calculate the number of units of nystatin required:

150,000 units/g $\times$ 60 g = 9,000,000 units

Step 2. Calculate the weight of the required units of nystatin:

$$\frac{9,000,000 \text{ units}}{4400 \text{ units/mg}} = 2045 \text{ mg} = 2.045 \text{ g of nystatin, } answer$$

Shelf-Life Estimates

The shelf life of a compound can be estimated by using the equation

$$t_{90} \text{ New} = \frac{t_{90} \text{Original}}{Q^{\Delta T/10}}$$

where t_{90} equals the period of time over which a product retains 90% of its potency, ΔT equals change in temperature, and 3 is a reasonable estimate for the "Q" value, based on energies of activation (Ea) from the Arrhenius equation. (See Chapter 6 of this book for a discussion of this equation.)

An antibiotic solution has a shelf life of 96 hours when refrigerated (5°C). If a patient needed to use the solution in an ambulatory pump at approximate body temperature (30°C) for 6 hours, would the compound still retain at least 90% of its original potency during the entire period of administration?

Step 1. Calculate the change in temperature the solution will undergo:

$\Delta T = 30°C - 5°C = 25°$

Step 2. Calculate the shelf life of the solution at the new temperature:

$$t_{90} = \frac{96 \text{ hours}}{3^{25/10}} = \frac{96 \text{ hours}}{3^{2.5}} = 6.16 \text{ hours}$$

Step 3. Compare the new shelf life with the period of administration:

$t_{90} = 6.16$ hours; period of administration = 6 hours; *therefore, the answer is yes.*

A prescription is received for an ophthalmic solution with a shelf life of 4 hours at room temperature (25°C). The preparation is to be administered in a physician's office at 12:00 noon the next day. Can the solution be prepared the evening before at about 8:00 pm and still retain at least 90% of its shelf life if stored in a refrigerator?

Step 1. Calculate the change in temperature the solution will undergo:

$$\Delta T = 5°C - 25°C = -20°$$

Step 2. Calculate the shelf life at the new temperature:

$$t_{90} = \frac{4 \text{ hours}}{3^{-20/10}} = \frac{4 \text{ hours}}{3^{-2}} = 4 \text{ hours} \times 9 = 36 \text{ hours}$$

Step 3. Compare the new shelf life with the period of refrigeration:

$t_{90} = 36$ hours; period of refrigeration = 16 hours; *therefore, the answer is yes.*

A reconstituted antibiotic has a shelf life at room temperature of 3 days. How long would the preparation be stable if refrigerated (i.e., a reasonable estimate based on t_{90})?

Step 1. Calculate the change in temperature:

$$\Delta T = 5°C - 25°C = -20°$$

Step 2. Calculate the shelf life at the new temperature:

$$t_{90} = \frac{3 \text{ days}}{3^{-20/10}} = \frac{3 \text{ days}}{3^{-2}} = 3 \text{ days} \times 9 = 27 \text{ days, } answer$$

Effervescent Mixtures

A prescription calls for an effervescent mixture of citric acid/tartaric acid (1:2) molar ratio with sodium bicarbonate to mask the taste of the active drug, potassium chloride (KCl). How much active drug, citric acid ($C_6H_8O_7 \cdot H_2O$), tartaric acid ($C_4H_6O_6$), and sodium bicarbonate ($NaHCO_3$) would be required for the prescription? (Formula weights: KCl = 74.5 g; $C_6H_8O_7 \cdot H_2O = 210$ g; $C_4H_6O_6 = 150$ g; $NaHCO_3 = 84$ g)

℞ **Potassium Chloride 1 mEq/5 g tsp Effervescent Mixture**

Potassium chloride	1 mEq/5 g tsp
Citric acid	
Tartaric acid	
Sodium bicarbonate	
Lime flavor crystals	qs
Dispense 100 g.	

Step 1. Assuming the powder in final form will weigh 5 g per teaspoonful, calculate the number of doses in the prescription:

$$\frac{100 \text{ g}}{5 \text{ g/dose}} = 20 \text{ doses}$$

Step 2. Using the formula weight of each ingredient and assuming the lime flavor crystals contribute negligible weight, calculate the quantity of KCl and the acids required for this prescription:

x (g of KCl required) = 20 doses × 74.5 mg/dose = 1.49 g of KCl, *answer*

y (g of acids required) = 100 g − 1.49 g = 98.51 g of acids, *answer*

Step 3. Given the ratio of 1 part citric acid to 2 parts tartaric acid, calculate the quantity of sodium bicarbonate that will react with citric acid:

$$3NaHCO_3 \quad + \quad C_6H_8O_7 \cdot H_2O \rightarrow 4H_2O + 3CO_2 + Na_3C_6H_5O_7$$
$$(3 \times 84 \text{ g}) \qquad\qquad (210 \text{ g})$$

$$\frac{1 \text{ part}}{210 \text{ g}} = \frac{x}{3 \times 84 \text{ g}}$$

$$x = 1.2 \text{ g (parts)}$$

Step 4. Calculate the quantity of sodium bicarbonate that will react with tartaric acid:

$$2NaHCO_3 \quad + \quad C_4H_6O_6 \rightarrow 2H_2O + 2CO_2 + Na_2C_4H_4O_6$$
$$(2 \times 84 \text{ g}) \qquad\qquad (150 \text{ g})$$

$$\frac{2 \text{ parts}}{150 \text{ g}} = \frac{x}{2 \times 84 \text{ g}}$$

$$x = 2.24 \text{ g (parts)}$$

Step 5. Calculate the total quantity of sodium bicarbonate required to react with the acids:

$$1.2 \text{ g} + 2.24 \text{ g} = 3.44 \text{ g (parts)}$$

Step 6. Knowing that the prescription requires 98.51 g of the effervescent mixture, calculate the required weight of each ingredient:

Total parts of ingredients = 1 part citric acid + 2 parts tartaric acid + 3.4 parts sodium bicarbonate = 6.4 parts

$$\text{Quantity of citric acid} = \frac{1 \text{ part}}{6.4 \text{ parts}} \times 98.51 \text{ g} = 15.39 \text{ g, } answer$$

$$\text{Quantity of tartaric acid} = \frac{2 \text{ parts}}{6.4 \text{ parts}} \times 98.51 \text{ g} = 30.78 \text{ g, } answer$$

$$\text{Quantity of sodium bicarbonate} = \frac{3.4 \text{ parts}}{6.4 \text{ parts}} \times 98.51 \text{ g} = 52.34 \text{ g, } answer$$

Step 7. Prepare the prescription by accurately weighing the following quantities of the ingredients:

℞

Potassium chloride	1.49 g
Citric acid	15.39 g
Tartaric acid	30.78 g
Sodium bicarbonate	52.34 g
Total weight	100 g

Surfactant Blending

A prescription calls for preparation of 120 g of a cream using 3% Tween 80 and 1% Span 40. What is the hydrophile–lipophile balance (HLB) value of this mixture? (HLBs: Tween 80 = 15.0; Span 40 = 6.7)

Step 1. Calculate the required weight of each ingredient:

Weight of Tween 80 = 120 g × 0.03 = 3.6 g

Weight of Span 40 = 120 × 0.01 = 1.2 g

Step 2. Calculate the contribution of each ingredient to the total HLB of the mixture:

$$\text{HLB contribution of Tween 80} = \frac{3.6 \text{ g}}{4.8 \text{ g}} \times 15 = 11.25$$

$$\text{HLB contribution of Span 40} = \frac{1.2 \text{ g}}{4.8 \text{ g}} \times 6.7 = 1.68$$

Step 3. Calculate the HLB of the mixture:

HLB of mixture = 11.25 + 1.68 = 12.9, *answer*

Dosage Form–Specific Calculations

Solutions

Certain dosage forms (ophthalmic, nasal, and parenteral) must be prepared to be isotonic with body fluids to increase the patient's comfort during administration of the medication and to minimize the damage that can be done when a hypotonic or hypertonic product is administered. The sodium chloride equivalent method can usually be used in calculations dealing with isotonicity. Appendix V, which lists sodium chloride equivalents for many agents, is a useful resource for this type of calculation.

In addition, some preparations must be buffered within a certain pH range to enhance the stability of the active drug(s). Appendix VI provides tabular data for preparing various types of buffers at specific pH values. Use of this information can speed up calculations dealing with buffer solutions.

For sterile preparations, particularly in high-risk compounding from bulk substances, calculation of the endotoxin load is also necessary. The steps in this calculation and a sample worksheet are provided in chapter 25 of this book. Pharmacists performing this calculation need access to a current *USP/NF* or an endotoxin limit table (Appendix VII) and a calculator.

Sodium Chloride Equivalents for Nasal and Ophthalmic Solutions

How much sodium chloride (NaCl) is required to render the following prescription isotonic?

℞ **Lidocaine Hydrochloride 1% Solution**

Lidocaine hydrochloride	1%	(NaCl equiv. = 0.22)
Cocaine hydrochloride	1%	(NaCl equiv. = 0.16)
Epinephrine bitartrate	0.1%	(NaCl equiv. = 0.18)
Sterile water	qs 50 mL	
Sodium chloride	qs	

Step 1. Using the NaCl equivalents provided, calculate the tonicic equivalents of the ingredients required for the prescription:

x (g of lidocaine HCl) = (50 mL × 0.01 g/mL) × 0.22 = 0.5 g × 0.22 = 0.110 g

y (g of cocaine HCl) = (50 mL × 0.01 g/mL) × 0.16 = 0.5 g × 0.16 = 0.080 g

z (g of epinephrine) = (50 mL × 0.001 g/mL) × 0.18 = 0.05 g × 0.18 = 0.009 g

Step 2. Calculate the total NaCl equivalents represented by the ingredients:

Total NaCl equivalents = $x + y + z$ = 0.110 g + 0.080 g + 0.009 g = 0.199 g

Step 3. Calculate the quantity of NaCl required to make 50 mL of water isotonic (NaCl equivalent of isotonic sodium chloride solution = 0.009 g/mL):

50 mL × 0.009 g/mL = 0.45 g

Step 4. Calculate the quantity of NaCl required to make this solution isotonic:

0.45 g – 0.199 g = 0.251 g of NaCl, *answer*

Buffer Solutions and pH

A prescription for optimycin 1% calls for a phosphate buffer with a pH of 6.5. Sorensen's modified phosphate buffer will be used to prepare this buffer solution. Sorensen's modified phosphate buffer is prepared by mixing the appropriate quantities of a 1/15 M stock acid solution and a 1/15 M stock alkaline solution. What quantities of these two solutions are required to make the phosphate buffer for this prescription?

℞ Optimycin 1% Solution

Optimycin	1%
Sodium chloride	qs
Phosphate buffer (pH 6.5)	qs 100 mL

Step 1. Use the Preparation of Sorensen's Modified Phosphate Buffer with Specific pH, in Appendix VI, to determine the quantity of sodium biphosphate solution and sodium phosphate solution needed to prepare 100 mL of a phosphate buffer with a pH of 6.5:

Required mL of 1/15 M sodium biphosphate solution = 70 mL, *answer*

Required mL of 1/15 M sodium phosphate solution = 30 mL, *answer*

Calibrating a Dropper/Sprayer for Nasal Solutions

The dose for a nasal solution is 250 µg. A 0.5% solution was prepared and placed in a nasal spray bottle. The patient squeezed the bottle 10 times into a plastic bag; the squeezed-out product weighed 500 mg. Assuming the weight of the solution is 1 g/mL (i.e., 500 mg = 0.5 mL), how many squeezes are required to administer the 250-µg dose?

Step 1. Convert percentage concentration of the solution to a "parts per x" concentration:

0.5% = 0.5 g/100 mL

Step 2. Calculate the quantity of the solution expelled in 10 squeezes:

$$\frac{0.5 \text{ g}}{100 \text{ mL}} = \frac{x}{0.5 \text{ mL}}$$

x = 0.0025 g/0.5 mL = 2.5 mg/0.5 mL = 2500 µg/0.5 mL

Step 3. Calculate the number of squeezes required to administer the 250-µg dose:

$$\frac{10 \text{ squeezes}}{2500 \text{ µg}} = \frac{x}{250 \text{ µg}}$$

x = 1 squeeze, *answer*

Displacement Factors

In the preparation of many dosage forms, the volume occupied by the various ingredients must be determined. Some examples are fixed-volume dosage forms such as capsules, molded suppositories, molded troches and lozenges, and molded tablets. Because of the differences in densities of the ingredients, different substances will occupy different volumes in the dosage form. When the actual densities of the ingredients are not known, ratios can be used instead to determine the volumes they occupy. The following problems illustrate both methods of calculating the volume occupied by ingredients.

Powder-Filled Capsules

A pharmacist receives a prescription for forty-eight 15 mg piroxicam capsules. A #1 capsule filled with piroxicam weighs 245 mg; a capsule filled with lactose weighs 180 mg. What quantities of piroxicam and lactose are required for the prescription? Prepare sufficient powder for 50 capsules (2 extra).

Step 1. Calculate the quantity of piroxicam required for 50 capsules:

50 capsules × 15 mg = 750 mg of piroxicam, *answer*

Step 2. Calculate the volume equivalent of lactose that is occupied by the piroxicam in a #1 capsule:

$$\frac{15 \text{ mg}}{245 \text{ mg}} = \frac{x}{180 \text{ mg}}$$

$x = 11$ mg

Step 3. Knowing that 15 mg of piroxicam occupies a similar volume as that of 11 mg of lactose, calculate the quantity of lactose required for the prescription:

Quantity of lactose per capsule = 180 mg − 11 mg = 169 mg

Required quantity of lactose = 169 mg × 50 capsules = 8450 mg = 8.45 g, *answer*

Molded Tablets

A pharmacist receives a prescription for 30 molded tablets. Each tablet is to contain 5 mg of the active drug. The average weight of a tablet containing only base is 65 mg. This value was determined by preparing 30 tablets that contained only the base, weighing the entire batch, and dividing the weight by 30. Because the active drug weighs more than a few milligrams, its density factor should be determined. This factor is equal to the average weight of a tablet containing only active drug, which is 85 mg for this prescription. This value was determined by the same method described for obtaining the average weight of base per tablet.

Determine the quantity of base required for each tablet. Also, determine the total weight per tablet. This value can be used in quality control checks of the finished product.

Step 1. Determine the percentage of the tablet occupied by the active drug by dividing the quantity of drug per tablet by the average weight of the pure drug tablet:

$$\frac{5 \text{ mg}}{85 \text{ mg}} \times 100 = 5.9\%$$

Step 2. Determine the percentage of the tablet occupied by the base:

100% − 5.9% = 94.1%

Step 3. Determine the weight of the base per tablet:

94.1% × 65 mg = 61.2 mg

Step 4. Knowing that each tablet will contain the following quantity of each ingredient, determine the total weight per tablet:

Active drug   5 mg
Base   61.2 mg

Total weight per tablet = 5 mg + 61.2 mg = 66.2 mg, *answer*

Molded Suppositories, Troches, and Lozenges

A prescription for 300 mg zinc oxide suppositories calls for cocoa butter to be used as the vehicle. The density factors for cocoa butter and zinc oxide are 0.9 and 4.0, respectively. Given that the suppository mold holds 2.0 g of cocoa butter, what quantities of zinc oxide and cocoa butter would be required to prepare 12 suppositories?

R_x **Zinc Oxide 300 mg Suppositories**

Zinc oxide	300 mg
Cocoa butter	qs

Step 1. Calculate the total weight of 12 suppositories that contain only cocoa butter:

$12 \times 2.0 \text{ g} = 24 \text{ g}$

Step 2. Calculate the density ratio of zinc oxide to cocoa butter:

$$\frac{4}{0.9} = 4.44$$

Step 3. Calculate the weight of zinc oxide required for the prescription:

300 mg $\times$ 12 supp. = 3600 mg = 3.6 g of zinc oxide, *answer*

Step 4. Calculate the amount of cocoa butter displaced by the active drug:

$$\frac{3.6 \text{ g}}{4.44} = 0.81 \text{ g}$$

Step 5. Calculate the weight of cocoa butter required for the prescription:

24 g − 0.81 g = 23.19 g of cocoa butter, *answer*

Determination of Density Factor: Paddock Method

The Paddock method is a more accurate, but also more time-consuming, method for calculating the replacement value (occupied volume) of the suppository base and ultimately the quantity of active drug required for a prescription. Before these values can be calculated, the density factor, *df*, must be determined, using the following equation:

$$df = \frac{B}{A - C + B}$$

where *A* equals the average weight of a blank, *B* equals the weight of active drug per suppository, and *C* equals the average weight of a medicated suppository.

Each step in this method will be described first, and then a sample calculation for which the values of *A*, *B*, and *C* are given will be explained through each step.

Step 1. Determine the average blank weight (i.e., weight of a suppository containing only the base), *A*, per mold using the suppository base of interest.

Step 2. Weigh the quantity of suppository base required for 10 suppositories.

Step 3. Weigh 1 g of the active drug.

The weight of active drug per suppository, *B*, is then equal to

$$\frac{1 \text{ g}}{10 \text{ supp.}} = 0.1 \text{ g/supp.}$$

Step 4. Melt the suppository base, and incorporate the active drug. Mix the ingredients, pour into molds, cool, trim, and remove from the molds.

Step 5. Weigh the 10 suppositories, and determine the average weight, *C*.

Step 6. Using the equation provided, determine the density factor, *df.*

Step 7. To find the replacement value of the suppository base, divide the weight of the medication required for each suppository by the density factor of the medication.

Step 8. Subtract the value in step 7 from the value for the average weight of a blank suppository, calculated in step 1.

Step 9. Multiply the value in step 8 by the number of required suppositories to obtain the quantity of suppository base required for the prescription.

Step 10. Multiply the weight of drug per suppository by the required number of suppositories to obtain the quantity of active drug required for the prescription.

A prescription calls for 12 acetaminophen 300 mg (B) suppositories using cocoa butter as the vehicle. The average weight of the cocoa butter blank (A) is 2.0 g, and the average weight of the medicated suppository (C) is 1.8 g. What quantities of cocoa butter and acetaminophen are required for the prescription?

Step 1. Determine the average weight of a blank suppository, *A:*

$$A = 2.0 \text{ g}$$

Step 2. Determine the quantity of cocoa butter required for 12 blank suppositories:

$$12 \times 2.0 \text{ g} = 24 \text{ g}$$

Step 3. Determine the weight of acetaminophen per suppository, *B:*

$$B = 0.3 \text{ g}$$

Step 4. Melt the cocoa butter and incorporate the acetaminophen. Mix the ingredients, pour into molds, cool, trim, and remove from molds.

Step 5. Weigh the 12 suppositories, and determine the average weight of a medicated suppository, *C.*

$$C = 1.8 \text{ g}$$

Step 6. Determine the density factor:

$$df = \frac{0.3 \text{ g}}{2.0 \text{ g} - 1.8 \text{ g} + 0.3 \text{ g}} = 0.6$$

Step 7. Determine the replacement value of the cocoa butter:

$$\frac{0.3 \text{ g}}{0.6} = 0.5 \text{ g}$$

Step 8. Subtract the replacement value of cocoa butter from the average blank weight:

$$2.0 \text{ g} - 0.5 \text{ g} = 1.5 \text{ g}$$

Step 9. Determine the quantity of cocoa butter required for the prescription:

$$12 \times 1.5 \text{ g} = 18 \text{ g of cocoa butter, } answer$$

Step 10. Determine the quantity of acetaminophen required for the prescription:

$$12 \times 0.3 \text{ g} = 3.6 \text{ g of acetaminophen, } answer$$

Dosage Replacement Factor Method

The Dosage Replacement Factor method is another method of calculating the quantity of base that will be occupied by the active drug. The dosage replacement factor is determined by the following equation:

$$f = \frac{100(E - G)}{(G)(x)} + 1$$

where *f* equals the dosage replacement factor, *E* equals the weight of a pure base suppository, and *G* equals the weight of a suppository containing *x*% of the active ingredient.

Table 15-5 in Chapter 15 of this book lists dosage replacement factors for selected active drugs. When this factor is not known, the equation above can be used to calculate it. As illustrated in the following problem, the equation can also be used to calculate the total weight of a prepared suppository or other dosage form.

Prepare a suppository containing 100 mg of phenobarbital (f = 0.81) using cocoa butter as the base. The weight of the pure cocoa butter suppository (E) is 2.0 g. Because 100 mg of phenobarbital is to be contained in an approximately 2.0 g suppository, the phenobarbital will occupy 5% (x) of the total weight. What will be the total weight of each suppository?

Step 1. Use the dosage replacement factor equation to solve for the total weight of each suppository, *G*.

$$0.81 = \frac{100(2.0 - G)}{(G)(5)} + 1$$

$G = 2.019$ g, *answer*

Primary Emulsions Calculation
If a ratio of 4:2:1 is used for the oil:water:acacia (i.e., the Continental method) called for in the following prescription, what quantity of acacia is required? (See Chapter 19 of this book for a discussion of the Continental method.)

℞ Acacia Emulsion

Mineral oil	30%
Acacia	
Flavor	qs
Purified water	qs 120 mL

Step 1. Calculate the volume of mineral oil required for the prescription:

0.3×120 mL $= 36$ mL

Step 2. Using the given ratio, calculate the quantity of acacia required for the prescription:

$$\frac{36 \text{ mL}}{4 \text{ parts}} = \frac{x}{1 \text{ part}}$$

$x = 9$ g of acacia, *answer*

Patch Calculations
One strength of Daytrana patch contains 41.3 mg of methylphenidate and delivers 15 mg of drug over a 9-hour period. The surface area of the patch is 18.75 cm². What percentage of the drug is remaining in the patch when it is removed?

41.3 mg − 15 mg = 26.3 mg remaining

26.3 mg remaining/41.3 mg total × 100 = 63.68% remaining

What is the release rate from the patch in mcg/cm²/hr?

15 mg/18.75 cm²/9 hr × 1000 mcg/mg = 88.89 mcg/cm²/hr

Chapter 8

Quality Control

A quality program is an essential feature of any compounding activity. An effective quality program must ensure that a preparation is compounded properly and is stable for the expected duration of its use. Although most pharmacies do not have fully equipped quality control laboratories, establishing an adequate quality control program is possible. Setting up such a program begins with the proper facility, equipment, and supplies. All personnel involved in compounding, including technicians, must be properly trained. Appropriate standard operating procedures (SOPs) should be implemented to ensure that equipment is working satisfactorily and that preparations are compounded properly. Procedures must be in place for monitoring room air temperature and humidity and maintaining air quality in the pharmacy compounding laboratory. At a minimum, SOPs should be in place for the use of electronic balances, pH meters, and pipets; for air quality monitoring; and for personnel training.

This chapter discusses quality control, quality assurance, and continuous quality improvement and describes the components of an in-house quality program and the role of outside analytical laboratories.

Quality Control

Written procedures for the compounding of drugs should be available and followed to ensure the identity, strength, quality, and purity of the finished preparation. Such procedures should include a listing of the ingredients, quantities, order of mixing or preparation, and detailed description of the compounding process. The equipment and utensils used should be listed, as well as the container and closure packaging system. Information concerning stability and compatibility should be included, together with any documentation related to the preparation.

A compounding pharmacy should confirm that ingredients have been accurately weighed, measured, or subdivided as indicated. A compounding pharmacist should check and recheck these operations at each step in the compounding process to ensure that weights or measures are correct.

SOPs that describe the tests or examinations to be conducted on the finished preparation should be prepared and followed. These tests could include physical examination and measurements of pH, weight, and volume. Such procedures are established to monitor the output of the compounding pharmacy and to validate the performance of compounding processes that may cause variability in the completed drug preparation.

A pharmacist should review all compounding records for accuracy and conduct in-process and final checks to ensure that errors have not occurred in the compounding process.

Quality Assurance

A quality assurance program is a system of steps and actions taken to ensure the maintenance of proper standards in compounded preparations, including good documentation of the compounding activities. A good documentation system does not guarantee a good quality system, but it can help in minimizing errors and provide a record of changes that may affect a preparation. A good quality assurance program involves all individuals in the organization. The purpose of the system is to ensure that adequate controls are in place throughout the compounding and dispensing process so that medication is compounded correctly. The heart of any quality system is the written and approved documentation that is followed in the day-to-day operation, that is, the SOPs. These documents are prepared in order to link people with operational responsibilities. Consequently, all personnel involved in compounding must be well trained and well versed in the SOPs as they apply to each individual's functions.

Failures in quality tend to occur when individuals (1) do not know their responsibilities, (2) have not received the education and training needed, (3) are not well versed in the SOPs, (4) have not received the necessary resources (financial or time), or (5) do not take their responsibilities seriously.

Continuous Quality Improvement

Before dispensing a prescription to a patient, a pharmacist should ensure the accuracy and completeness of the compounded preparation by reviewing each step in the preparatory, compounding, final-check, and sign-off phases. In the preparatory review, a pharmacist checks that all preparations for the compounding process were handled appropriately. Aspects to be reviewed include the following:

- Appropriate ingredients, adjuvants, and equipment were selected for the specific preparation.
- Calculations are correct.
- Measurements were performed accurately with properly functioning equipment.
- The formulation is appropriate for the intended use and stability limits of the preparation.

A pharmacist then reviews the compounding steps to ensure that the procedures and techniques used to prepare the formulation were faithfully followed and appropriately documented. This review also ensures that the formulation is reasonably aesthetic and uniform in content.

A pharmacist's review of the final-check phase should be comprehensive. It is intended to verify the following:

- The calculated yield is consistent with the actual yield.
- The tolerance for weight variation of individual doses has been met by a sampling technique when appropriate (e.g., capsule weight).
- The physical characteristics (clarity, color, odor) of the preparation are consistent with those predicted for the preparation.
- Physical tests have been performed when appropriate, and the preparation meets the test limits.
- The preparation is suitably labeled, and the contents have been verified with the prescription order. All legal requirements have been imprinted on the label and in the compounding record.
- The preparation is suitably packaged for patient use, and the container that is selected will protect the preparation from undue environmental exposure until at least the discard-after or beyond-use date.
- Documentation is appropriate, as listed in Chapter 5 of this book.
- The patient or caregiver has been adequately informed about ways to identify obvious evidence of instability in the compounded preparation.
- The preparation is labeled with explicit storage and administration instructions.

A pharmacist may also decide to submit samples of the compounded preparation to an analytical testing laboratory registered with the U.S. Food and Drug Administration (FDA) for complex testing or to test it within the pharmacy using simple tests. Such analytical testing could include active drug concentrations of compounded medications and sterility and endotoxin testing. Additional tests, assays, or visual observations of samples of the preparation may be performed to ensure the content, stability, pH, particles, preservative effectiveness, and so on.

Quality Control Records and Procedures

A compounder should have established, written procedures that describe the tests or examinations to be conducted on the preparation compounded (e.g., the degree of weight variation among capsules) to ensure uniformity and integrity of compounded drug products. A reasonable quality assurance program consists of at least five separate, but integrated, components: (1) SOPs, (2) documentation, (3) verification, (4) data collection forms, and (5) testing.

Standard Operating Procedures

Pharmacy compounding requires the development and maintenance of SOPs to ensure quality and to minimize errors. SOPs should be followed in the day-to-day operation of the pharmacy. A good document system strongly supports a good quality assurance system.

SOPs are documents that describe how to perform routine tasks in the environment of formulation development, purchasing, compounding, testing, maintenance, materials handling and storage, quality assurance, labeling of beyond-use dates, cleaning, safety, and dispensing. They are basically step-by-step instructions on how to perform tasks reliably and consistently; they describe how a task will be performed, who will do it, why it is done, what limits apply to work performed, and what action to take when unacceptable deviations or discrepancies occur. An SOP should be specific to each device and process used in compounding. Master Formula records should be written to provide adequate instruction and documentation of the compounding operation.

SOPs must be reviewed regularly and updated as necessary. Auditing and verifying compliance with established SOPs should be performed periodically. Properly maintained and implemented SOPs should result in quality preparations and fewer compounding errors. SOPs are ongoing, never complete, and the best defense if anything goes wrong.

Documentation

Documentation is the act of furnishing or authenticating with documents. It is a record of the activities involved and performed. Documentation can be accomplished electronically or by use of paper and pencil. It can be as simple as initialing and dating a form, filling in data, or completing a narrative. Many SOPs require data collection forms, or documents, which should be prepared specifically to match certain SOPs; they should also be cross-referenced. These data collection forms are completed while personnel are performing the routine tasks directed by the SOPs. The purpose of the documentation is to provide a permanent record of all aspects of each compounding operation.

Verification

Verification of a compounding procedure involves checking to ensure that calculations, weighing and measuring, order of mixing, and compounding techniques were appropriate and accurately performed and recorded. It involves assurance and documentation that a process, procedure, or piece of equipment is functioning as it should and producing the expected results. Verification may require that an outside laboratory conduct tests to confirm the accuracy of the results. Process verification may include activities such as weighing, measuring, blending, filling, sterilization, and so on. Procedure verification may include cleaning and other activities. For the purposes of compounding, these processes are usually simply verified qualitatively. Equipment verification methods are sometimes available from manufacturers of the specific equipment or can be developed in house. Compounding personnel are responsible for ensuring that equipment performance is verified, but contractors may perform the verification.

Data Collection Forms

Data collection forms, or documents, are required for many SOPs and should be prepared specifically to match particular SOPs, In addition, they should be cross-referenced. Personnel complete these forms while performing the routine tasks directed by the SOPs. The forms contain fill-in-the-blank spaces for the collection of data and can include logbook entries, data printouts, and reports. Thus, the documentation supplies a permanent record of all details of each compounding operation.

Testing

Analytical and microbiological testing is like pharmaceutical compounding; only those who are trained and experienced and who can demonstrate validated performance of their operations should perform it. A quality assurance program should include some level of testing of finished compounded preparations. A compounder must have a basic understanding of pharmaceutical analysis to ensure that valid results are obtained when tests are conducted, whether they are done in house or outsourced. A pharmacist must know (1) when to test, (2) what to test, (3) what method(s) to use, (4) how to interpret the results, and (5) what limits apply to the test. In addition, a pharmacist must appreciate the importance of analytical testing in the overall quality program in the pharmacy. Although one need not be a pharmaceutical or chemical analyst or a microbiologist, one should have a basic understanding of testing methods that are used and the sample handling requirements that will ensure valid results.

The goal in testing is to produce results as accurately, efficiently, and quickly as possible. Any method used should have accuracy, speed, reproducibility, and specificity. No single method is ideally suited for all drugs; each method has its own strengths and weaknesses, and a number of factors determine the validity and reliability of results.

In-House or Outsourced Testing

Compounding pharmacies have two options when analytical or microbiological testing is required. Some methods can easily be used in house (in the pharmacy) or within an institution (hospital laboratory), but some testing needs to be outsourced to a contract laboratory. The use of an outside laboratory is particularly helpful when large quantities of a preparation are compounded. A pharmacist can periodically send samples for assay and, as appropriate, content uniformity testing; the results can serve as documentation of the performance of the compounding pharmacy. Once a good relationship has been established with a laboratory, a pharmacy can initiate a program to ensure preparation stability. Any preparation compounded in accordance with a *United States Pharmacopeia* (*USP*) monograph must meet the requirements set forth in that monograph. These requirements are designed to be within the capabilities of the compounding pharmacist.

Relatively simple tests that can be conducted in house with a moderate investment in equipment include measurements of weight and volume, pH, density and specific gravity, and refractive index, and, in some cases, sterility testing and endotoxin testing. Testing that can be outsourced to a contract laboratory includes high-performance liquid chromatography (HPLC), gas chromatography (GC), mass spectroscopy (MS), hyphenated methods (HPLC-MS and GC-MS), ultraviolet and visible spectroscopy, and other sophisticated methods. Some pharmacies perform HPLC testing, and their number is likely to grow as requirements for quality control testing increase.

Any in-house testing should be initially and periodically validated by sending a sample to a contract laboratory for comparison with in-house results. This is best done by splitting a sample, having one portion analyzed (blindly) by the in-house analyst, and sending the other portion to the outside laboratory. Personnel must be appropriately trained and evaluated if in-house testing is done. If testing is outsourced, one needs to be assured of the proper training of the personnel in the contract laboratory. Laboratory personnel need to participate in continuing competency activities. An FDA-registered laboratory is preferable, and a laboratory that works with pharmaceutical companies may be advantageous.

Chemical and Analytical Testing

Equipment Calibration and Maintenance

A compounding pharmacy must have access to an accurate, well-maintained prescription balance (preferably an electronic balance) and a set of calibration weights for assessing the performance of the balance. The balance must be placed in an area free of drafts and vibrations and should not be moved around. It should not be placed near an exhaust source or air-handling vent, which could alter its accuracy.

A compounding pharmacy should have access to an accurate pH meter and accompanying pH standard solutions for checking the pH of liquid preparations. The pH meter should be calibrated before each use.

Pharmacies should have manual (and in some cases automatic) pipets for measuring small volumes accurately, as well as a method of ensuring that the pipets are calibrated for delivering the required volumes.

Selection of an Analytical Method

The overall picture of pharmaceutical analysis includes not only the selection of a method, but also administrative and economic factors, the need to obtain a representative sample, storage or shipping of the sample, preparation of the sample for analysis, actual analysis, data acquisition, and data treatment and interpretation. A pharmacist must also consider the requirements for handling, preparation, and purification of the sample; the type of data needed; and the necessary levels of specificity and accuracy.

The needed information may be quantitative (e.g., potency or concentration), semi-quantitative (involving a cutoff level, as in endotoxin testing), or qualitative (involving a yes or no result, such as sterility testing or substance identification). Another consideration in selecting a method is the analyte's physical and chemical characteristics, including its solubility, partition coefficient, dissociation constant (pK_a), volatility, and binding, and the quantity of analyte present.

The degree of accuracy, reproducibility, and precision must be considered. Usually, the higher these requirements, the more sophisticated (and often more expensive) are the analytical methods that must be used. A related consideration is the types of instrumentation that are on hand or available from outside sources.

Sample Selection and Requirements

The choice of analytical method is influenced by factors related to the sample, such as the number of samples needed, the difficulty of obtaining a representative sample, the physical state of the sample (solid, liquid, or gas), and the type of container required for sample collection and storage. Sample analysis can be affected if analytes sorb to the walls or cap liner of the container or if leaching of the container material into a liquid sample occurs. In the case of sorption, siliconization of the sample vials may help.

Requirements for storage after the sample is collected must also be considered. What are the effects of air (e.g., carbon dioxide reacting to form insoluble carbonates, pH, free versus bound drug)? Should the sample be stored at a certain temperature (refrigerated, frozen, or room temperature) before and during shipment? What would happen if the sample were accidentally frozen or underwent a freeze–thaw cycle?

Factors that could affect chemical stability during the sample's storage, extraction, and preparation must be considered. What are the effects of water? Should the sample be maintained in a dry environment, and is a desiccant needed? Could the sample be affected by enzymatic breakdown, pH, temperature, solvents, or bacterial growth? Are volatile solvents used? If so, and if some of the solvent is allowed to evaporate, the concentration of the sample will increase.

What are the sample matrix effects? Will testing be affected by sample viscosity (pipetting, aspiration), ionic strength (immunoassays, dialysis), buffers (ionized/unionized ratio can alter the extraction efficiency of an analyte before analysis), or vapor pressure (drug can be lost)? If any pretreatment of samples is required before shipment or in-house testing, inaccuracies that may result from pipetting—one of the most common sources of analytical errors when sample volumes are small—must be considered.

What physical methods of separation and purification are used? Most analytical methods require some degree of pretreatment to prepare samples for analysis. This may include crystallization from solution, distillation, sublimation, solvent extraction, solid-phase extraction, chromatography, or centrifugation. The proper technique for separation and purification depends on the physical and chemical properties of the sample (both active drug and excipients), such as solubility, volatility, and binding, and on the quantity present.

The effect of any interfering substances in the formulation that may alter the results must be known beforehand. When sending a preparation to a contract laboratory, providing the complete formulation is wise so the laboratory can quickly determine if any interfering substance is present or, if the results are unexpected, it can determine whether the variation may be due to another ingredient.

Transportation requirements or limitations on the sample must be accommodated if it is a controlled drug substance, a dangerous or hazardous chemical, a flammable, or a caustic or if it requires refrigeration or freezing.

Data Interpretation Requirements

How are the raw data collected? What descriptive statistics are used to analyze the data and the operating parameters of the analytical instruments? Are reference values available and provided with the analytical results? What analytical controls are used by the laboratory? What reference standards are used to establish the standard curves? Is rounding of the data done in accordance with *USP/National Formulary* (*NF*) General Notices? Are cumulative data results for specific tests available or maintained at the laboratory or on-site in the pharmacy to detect any trends?

Reference values, if available, should be provided with the analytical results. A description of the analytical controls used by the laboratory is important for documentation, as is the source of reference standards used to establish standard curves.

Types of Analytical Methods

Table 8-1 lists different physical quality control tests that can be used for various compounded formulations. Table 8-2 categorizes the types of methods used in pharmaceutical analysis, including physical testing, methods involving electromagnetic radiation, conductometric techniques, immunoassays, and separation techniques. Within these categories, testing procedures may be nonspecific (melting, freezing, and boiling points; density; refractive index; polarimetry; ultraviolet or visible spectroscopy; and pH) or somewhat more specific if

TABLE 8-1 Physical Quality Control Tests for Compounded Formulations

Dosage Form	Individual Dosage Unit	Weight Average Individual Dosage Unit	Total Preparation	pH	Physical Observation[a]
Bulk powder			√		√
Powder papers	√	√	√		√
Capsules	√	√	√		√
Tablets	√	√	√		√
Troches	√	√	√		√
Liquids			√	√	√
Ointments			√		√
Suppositories	√	√	√		√
Gels			√	√	√

[a]Appearance, odor, taste, texture.

TABLE 8-2 Classification of Analytical Methods

Physical Testing Procedures
Melting point
Freezing point
Boiling point
Density
Refractive index
Optical rotation (polarimetry)
Thermal analysis

Interaction of Electromagnetic Radiation with Matter
Ultraviolet/visible spectroscopy
Infrared spectroscopy
Fluorescence/phosphorescence spectroscopy
Mass spectroscopy
Raman spectroscopy
X-ray spectroscopy
Flame emission and atomic absorption spectroscopy
Polarimetry
Refractometry
Interferometry

Conductometric Methods
pH
Ion-selective electrodes
Polarography

Immunoassay
Radioimmunoassay
Enzyme-multiplied immunoassay technique (EMIT)
Enzyme-linked immunosorbent assay (ELISA)
Fluorescent immunoassay (FIA)

Separation Techniques
High-performance liquid chromatography (HPLC)
Gas chromatography (GC)
Thin-layer chromatography (TLC)
Paper chromatography (PC)
Column chromatography (CC)

Gravimetric
Balance

Other
Osmolality

proper standards are used (infrared spectroscopy, mass spectroscopy, ion-selective electrodes, immunoassay methods, HPLC, and GC). Suggested analytical methods for different dosage forms are shown in Table 8-3.

Methods that can be routinely used for testing incoming bulk materials, whether active ingredients or excipients, include melting, freezing, and boiling points; density; refractive index; ultraviolet or visible spectroscopy; infrared spectroscopy; polarimetry; pH; and the separation methods. Final preparations usually require a method such as HPLC or GC.

Analytical testing will no doubt become a more important part of pharmaceutical compounding as the public and regulatory agencies demand increasing documentation of the quality of compounded preparations. Compounding pharmacists must decide what types of testing and what amount of testing to include in their quality control programs and whether testing should be done in house or outsourced. Like pharmaceutical compounding, analytical testing should be performed only by those who are appropriately trained and qualified.

Pharmacists can perform physical quality control tests to ensure the uniformity and accuracy of many small-scale compounded preparations. These tests include individual dosage unit weights; average individual dosage unit weights; total preparation weight; pH; and physical observations such as appearance, taste, and smell. As previously mentioned,

TABLE 8-3 Suggested Analytical Methods for Various Dosage Forms (Depending on Active Drug)

Dosage Form	Wt	Vol	pH	Osm	RI	Sp Gr	MP	UV/Vis	HPLC	GC	IR	Steril	Endo
Bulk substances	✓		✓		✓		✓	✓	✓	✓	✓		
Powders	✓								✓	✓			
Capsules	✓								✓	✓			
Tablets	✓								✓	✓			
Lozenges	✓								✓	✓			
Suppositories	✓					✓	✓		✓	✓			
Sticks	✓					✓	✓	✓	✓	✓			
Solutions	✓	✓	✓	✓	✓	✓		✓	✓	✓			
Suspensions	✓	✓	✓			✓			✓	✓			
Emulsions	✓	✓	✓		✓	✓			✓	✓			
Semisolids	✓					✓	✓		✓	✓			
Gels	✓	✓	✓		✓	✓			✓	✓			
Ophthalmics, otics, nasals	✓	✓	✓	✓	✓	✓		✓	✓	✓		✓	
Inhalations	✓	✓	✓	✓	✓	✓		✓	✓	✓		✓	
Injections	✓	✓	✓	✓	✓	✓		✓	✓	✓		✓	✓

[a]Analytical methods are weight (Wt), volume (Vol), pH, osmolality (Osm), refractive index (RI), specific gravity (Sp Gr), melting point (MP), ultraviolet/visible spectroscopy (UV/Vis), high-performance liquid chromatography (HPLC), gas chromatography (GC), infrared spectroscopy (IR), sterility (Steril), and endotoxin (Endo).

Table 8-1 indicates which physical tests can be appropriate for the various dosage forms, and individual chapters on specific dosage forms in this book describe these quality control tests in more detail.

Microbiological Testing

When sterile preparations are involved, testing for sterility and endotoxins may be advisable. Ophthalmic and inhalational preparations should be tested for sterility. Injectable preparations should be tested for both sterility and endotoxins. One additional test that may be considered for both nonsterile and sterile preparations in multiple dose containers is the preservative effectiveness test. Also, the microbial limit test may be applicable in some situations.

Sterility Testing

Sterility tests can be conducted by using commercial kits or by developing and validating USP sterility testing protocols, which are somewhat more detailed than the commercial sterility-testing kits. Standards and procedures are explained in *USP* Chapter <71>, Sterility Tests.[1]

Endotoxin Testing

Endotoxin tests can be conducted using commercially available kits or by purchasing the components separately. Endotoxin testing endpoints can be difficult to interpret, and in-house testing should be done only after obtaining training and experience. See *USP* Chapter <85>, Bacterial Endotoxins Test.[2]

An extract of the horseshoe crab, *Limulus* amebocyte lysate, is used to test the pyrogenicity and endotoxin level of a preparation. The procedure is complicated, and care must be taken to use correct technique to attain the test's endpoint—a reading of the presence or absence of a gel clot. With practice and careful attention to technique, however, one can perform the test easily and routinely. See *USP* Chapter <85>, Bacterial Endotoxins Test.[2]

Preservative Effectiveness Testing

Preservative effectiveness testing may be conducted during preparation of a frequently compounded formulation that contains a preservative. When such a test is performed, the results shall support the beyond-use-date assigned to the compounded preparations. See *USP* Chapter <51>, Antimicrobial Effectiveness Testing.[3]

Any in-house testing should be verified initially and periodically by sending a sample to an outside contract laboratory to verify and validate the in-house results. Splitting a sample, having a portion analyzed (blindly) by the in-house analyst, and sending the remaining portion to the outside laboratory is the best approach.

Microbial Limit Testing

Microbial limit testing may be conducted to provide an estimate of the number of viable aerobic microorganisms (see *USP* Chapter <61>, Microbiological Examination of Nonsterile Products: Microbial Enumeration Tests[4]) or to demonstrate freedom from designated microbial species (see *USP* Chapter <62>, Microbiological Examination of Nonsterile Products: Tests for Specified Microorganisms[5]).

Out-of-Specification Results

Increasingly, compounding pharmacies are submitting samples for potency or strength testing. If a potency test yields unexpected results, a contract laboratory performs an investigation to determine whether this is due to a substandard compounded preparation or to flawed testing. In this inquiry, the responsibilities of investigators are established, a step-by-step method is followed, and results are documented.[6]

When a result obtained in the analytical testing of raw materials, in-process materials, drug substances, drug preparations, or drug preparations undergoing stability testing fails to meet established specifications, the result is termed *out of specification* (OOS).[6] Limits are defined by *USP* or other pharmacopeias within the monograph of each drug.[7–9] In most cases, test results are expected to meet a specification of between 90.0% and 110.0% of the stated concentration. Although the typical range is ±10%, it can be as high as ±20% for some proteins and as low as ±5% for some potent analgesics. The *USP* criterion for compounded preparations is ±10% unless otherwise indicated within a specific drug monograph.[10]

Unexpected results can be due to sample preparation, transcription errors, calculations, standards and reagents used, methods used, or instrumentation.[11] Only when a quality team of laboratory personnel and the scientific director have investigated and ruled out all of these causes is a compounded preparation suspected of being OOS. An OOS result for a compounded formulation usually originates from errors in the method of preparation. For example, some drugs tend to precipitate out of solution if the alcohol content is too low. Another common error is autoclaving samples that are heat sensitive, thereby decomposing the active ingredient and lowering its concentration.

Laboratories that meet International Organization for Standardization (ISO) 9001:2000 and FDA requirements should have SOPs that describe the protocol used in investigations. When retesting clearly identifies a laboratory error, the retest results are to be substituted for the original results, the original results retained, and an explanation recorded.[10] When an OOS sample of a compounded preparation is retested and OOS values are found on the retest, the investigation should try to isolate the source of the error. The goal is to identify the problem and implement a permanent solution.[11]

Reasons for OOS potency results include the following:[12]

- *Mixtures that are not homogeneous:* This is probably the biggest issue for compounding pharmacies. Whether one mixes powders to make capsules or incorporates ingredients of a cream, proper mixing to homogeneity is necessary for accurate potency results. Possible remedies for lack of homogeneity include the use of new equipment (e.g., V-shaped blenders), longer mixing time, proper aliquot technique (smaller dilutions), and training courses and hands-on instruction for technicians.

- *Solubility issues:* Testing laboratories deal with this issue frequently. Many of the drugs currently compounded have little or no solubility in water and need alcohol to dissolve. For example, budesonide will dissolve readily in alcohol but will precipitate out if the alcohol content is diluted below a certain percentage. This will cause potency results to fall below the acceptable range. Possible remedies include determining solubility limits through a literature search, understanding the difference between a solution and a suspension, and testing to ensure proper concentration.

- *Sterilization methods:* Sterilization can affect potency when filtration is used improperly or when autoclaving is used on heat-sensitive drugs. Filtration should be used only for solutions, not for suspensions. Special attention should be paid to the heat-sensitive nature of drugs when autoclaving is used. For example, betamethasone acetate/betamethasone sodium phosphate will degrade if autoclaved, and potency results will be lower than expected. Possible remedies include filtering only solutions and understanding the thermal sensitivity of drug molecules.

Errors that lead to OOS results can be minimized through the use of the following:

- Proper equipment
- Personnel training (experienced technicians, compounding techniques courses, proficiency tests)
- Step-by-step instructions or SOPs
- Adequate facilities
- Thorough documentation and record keeping
- Research into each drug's physicochemical characteristics (salt form, hydration, pH, solubility)
- End-preparation testing (potency testing by a quality control laboratory)

OOS investigations can benefit the compounding community by providing greater understanding of each compound and permanent solutions to common problems. OOS results will occur. Analytical laboratories and pharmacists will continue to be allies in solving compounding issues.

Costs

Analytical testing costs money. Testing every preparation compounded by a pharmacy is not feasible. However, SOPs should be in place for a quality control program requiring some routine testing. Starting slowly and carefully with testing, and using contract laboratories if necessary, is best. When large quantities of selected items are being compounded, initiating in-house testing may be reasonable.

The price of analytical instruments varies from a few hundred dollars to tens of thousands or even hundreds of thousands of dollars, depending on the type of method and the sophistication of the instruments. New, reconditioned, or used instruments can be purchased. Internet auctions can be a good source of instruments if the buyer purchases wisely. Nonetheless, any instrument must be calibrated and validated before being placed in operation. In some instances, purchasing a used instrument and having it serviced by the instrument manufacturer is financially feasible.

References

1. United States Pharmacopeial Convention. Chapter <71>, Sterility testing. In: *United States Pharmacopeia/National Formulary*. Rockville, MD: United States Pharmacopeial Convention; current edition.
2. United States Pharmacopeial Convention. Chapter <85>, Bacterial endotoxins test. In: *United States Pharmacopeia/National Formulary*. Rockville, MD: United States Pharmacopeial Convention; current edition.
3. United States Pharmacopeial Convention. Chapter <51>, Antimicrobial effectiveness testing. In: *United States Pharmacopeia/National Formulary*. Rockville, MD: United States Pharmacopeial Convention; current edition.
4. United States Pharmacopeial Convention. Chapter <61>, Microbiological examination of non-sterile products: microbial enumeration tests. In: *United States Pharmacopeia/National Formulary*. Rockville, MD: United States Pharmacopeial Convention; current edition.
5. United States Pharmacopeial Convention. Chapter <62>, Microbiological examination of non-sterile products: tests for specified microorganisms. In: *United States Pharmacopeia/National Formulary*. Rockville, MD: United States Pharmacopeial Convention; current edition.

6. U.S. Food and Drug Administration. Guidance for industry: investigating out-of-specification (OOS) test results for pharmaceutical production. October 2006. Available at: www.fda.gov/downloads /Drugs/GuidanceComplianceRegulatoryInformation/Guidances/ucm070287.pdf. Accessed November 11, 2011.

7. Hoinowski AM, Motola S, Davis RJ, McArdle JV. Investigation of out-of-specification results. *Pharm Technol.* 2002;26(1):40–50.

8. Lanier L, Kemp J. Quality control analytical methods: common concerns about out-of-specification results. *Int J Pharm Compound.* 2006;10(1):41–2.

9. Odegard RD. Quality-control analytical methods: minimizing the probability of out-of-specification preparations: results that make you say . . . Hmmm! *Int J Pharm Compound.* 2008;12(3):130–5.

10. United States Pharmacopeial Convention. Chapter <795>, Pharmaceutical compounding—nonsterile preparations. *U.S. Pharmacopeia/National Formulary.* Rockville, MD: United States Pharmacopeial Convention, current edition.

11. Lanese J. Handling out-of-specification results: a current FDA view. *J cGMP Compliance* (Special Edition—Laboratory Compliance) [Institute of Validation Technology]. 2000:57–61.

12. Allen L, Kupiec T. Major issues affecting pharmacy compounders. Presented at: American College of Apothecaries 2005 Annual Conference, September 29, 2005, Coeur d'Alene, ID.

Chapter 9

Flavors, Sweeteners, and Colors

When medication is administered orally, flavoring, sweetening, and coloring are vital to patient compliance. Many drugs have disagreeable tastes, and the stronger the taste, the more difficulty patients have in adhering to their medication regimens. Pharmacists cannot simply add a flavor to a dosage form containing a bad-tasting drug and expect it to taste good. A related challenge is to minimize the taste and optimize the texture of dosage forms that remain in the mouth for an extended time, such as troches, lollipops, and gummy gels. For patient acceptance, these dosage forms must have a smooth surface texture but not be disagreeably sticky.

A pharmacist willing to spend the time can usually convert a bad-tasting medication into an acceptable preparation by choosing one or more of the following:[1]

- Select the proper flavor or flavor blends, not necessarily relying on what is traditionally used.
- Replace or adjust a vehicle if it is inadequate.
- Select a nonoffending preservative.
- Use artificial sweeteners in the proper amount and balance.
- Use desensitizing agents or flavor enhancers.
- Obtain the proper mouth feel, such as smoothness that results with increased viscosity.
- Complement any bitterness with an acceptable bitter flavor, such as coffee, chocolate, or maple.
- Mask objectionable tastes by using the cooling effect of mint and the anesthetizing effect of spices.
- Use acids, such as tartaric, citric, and maleic, to enhance fruit flavors.

Flavor and Taste

The flavor experience is very complex and is a combination of the sensations of taste, smell, touch (texture), sight, and even sound. In general, individuals are more sensitive to odors than to tastes. However, the sense of smell declines with age, and older people may be able to detect odors only when they are several times as strong as would be noticeable to younger people. Females tend to have a greater sensitivity to odors than do males. Furthermore, disease can alter taste and smell, as is evident when one has a cold or the flu. Infants and children tend to prefer sweet tastes and do not respond well to bitter substances; they like flavors such as butterscotch, citrus, berry, and vanilla. Adults accept reasonable levels of bitterness in drug products; thus, wine, spice, chocolate, or anise combinations can be used. For those who fall between the pediatric and geriatric populations, almost any flavor can be used. Patients who must take a preparation for an extended time may require milder flavors, which are less likely to cause flavor fatigue.

Basics of Taste

The four primary tastes are sweet, sour, salty, and bitter. Table 9-1 lists solutions that exemplify these four primary tastes. The chemical structure of a drug can indicate the drug's possible taste. Table 9-2 lists some correlations between chemical properties and taste and odor. For example, inorganic salts in solution will result in anions, cations, or both in solution, which will produce a salty taste. Many drugs are organic compounds that have high molecular weights; these compounds have a bitter taste that is difficult to mask. The presence of unsaturated double bonds results in a sharp, biting taste. Sugars, sorbitol, glycerin, and other polyhydroxyl compounds have a sweet taste, as do alpha-amino acids.

TABLE 9-1 Solutions Illustrating the Four Primary Tastes

Solution Strength	Sweet (% sucrose)	Sour (% citric acid)	Salty (% NaCl)	Bitter (% caffeine)
Slight	5	0.05	0.4	0.05
Moderate	10	0.10	0.7	0.10
Strong	15	0.20	1.0	0.20

Source: Reference 1.

TABLE 9-2 Correlations between Chemical Properties and Taste and Odor

	Chemical Property
Taste	
Sour	H^+
Salty	Simultaneous presence of anions and cations
Bitter	High molecular weight salts
Sweet	Polyhydroxyl compounds, polyhydrogenated compounds, alpha-amino acids
Sharp, biting	Unsaturation
Odor	
Fruity	Esters, lactones
Pleasant	Ketones
Camphoraceous	Tertiary carbon atom

Source: Reference 3.

Other factors to consider in deriving good-tasting products are as follows: (1) a hot taste is due to a mild counterirritant effect, (2) an astringent taste is due to tannins and acids, (3) coarseness or grittiness is due to texture, and (4) coolness is due to a negative heat of solution. Preservatives also have characteristic flavors, odors, and sensations. Alcohol has a biting taste. Methylparaben has a floral aroma similar to that of gauze pads. Propylparaben and butylparaben produce numbness in the mouth; thus, using the lowest concentration possible of these preservatives is best.

Flavoring Techniques

Flavoring is both a challenge and an opportunity. It is a challenge because no single correct method exists for solving an ill-defined problem; it is an opportunity because it enables a pharmacist to compound a preparation that a patient is willing to take. By following the basic principles presented in this chapter, pharmacists should be able to handle successfully many of the flavoring problems that occur in compounding preparations, particularly for pediatric patients.

An acceptable flavor for a patient involves such aspects as (1) immediate flavor identity, (2) rapid full flavor development, (3) acceptable mouth feel, (4) short aftertaste, and (5) no undesirable sensations.[2]

Many approaches can be used to compound an acceptable preparation that minimizes the bad taste of drugs. These approaches include blending, overshadowing, physical methods, chemical methods, and physiological methods.[3]

Blending is the use of a flavor that blends with the drug taste. Drugs with an acidic taste can be blended with citrus fruit flavors. For example, orange might be used to blend with ascorbic acid. Salty, sweet, and sour tastes can be used to blend with a bitter taste. The addition of a slightly salty taste may decrease sourness and increase sweetness. Bitter tastes can also be partially overcome by adding a sour flavor.

Overshadowing, or overpowering, involves the use of a flavor with greater intensity and longer residence time in the mouth than the original preparation. Examples are wintergreen oil and *Glycyrrhiza*.

Physical methods include (1) formulation of insoluble compounds as a suspension (a drug cannot be tasted if it is not in solution); (2) emulsification of oils (i.e., placing the bad-tasting drug in the internal phase of an emulsion and flavoring or sweetening the external phase that will come in contact with the oral cavity); (3) use of effervescent additives, a good approach for salty-tasting drugs; and (4) use of high-viscosity fluids, such as syrups, which tend to keep the flavor in the mouth longer.

Chemical methods of overcoming bad tastes include adsorbing or complexing the drug with an ingredient that eliminates the undesirable taste.

Physiological techniques involve the cooling sensation produced by mannitol, which is caused by its negative heat of solution, or the anesthetic action of products such as menthol, peppermint, and spearmint. These products serve as desensitizers; they reduce the sensitivity of the taste buds to bitterness. Some spices, such as clove and cinnamon, can achieve the same end because they introduce heat and numbness, creating a mild pain reaction.

Flavor intensifiers, such as monosodium glutamate, can serve as flavor enhancers. Citrus enhancers include citric, maleic, and tartaric acids. Enhancing flavor by adding small amounts of vanilla to the basic flavor is a technique long used in the flavor industry. Vanilla seems to intensify and stimulate other flavors for a quicker taste response without altering their basic taste or adding its own taste.

A flavor or sweetener can provide more than one sensation in the mouth. Saccharin may create a rapid bitter sensation followed by a sweet flavor sensation. Sucrose gives a fast sweet sensation that intensifies the full-bodied taste of other flavors. This reaction may be related to the high viscosity of the product. Many natural flavors have a prominent ingredient. For example, the primary active constituent in cherry is benzaldehyde; in banana, isoamyl acetate; in spearmint, L-carvone; and in orange, lemonene. Table 9-3 lists some flavors that mask basic tastes.

Lozenges and gummy gels present a challenge because of their long residence time in the mouth. The quantity of flavoring for these medications is recommended to be about 5 to 10 times that used in candy products.

If flavoring oils are to be added to aqueous-based products, the oils can be dissolved in a small quantity of glycerin or sorbitol and then incorporated into the preparation. This technique can also be used to incorporate an oily drug into a lozenge, lollipop, or gummy gel. The solvent technique often uses a ratio of 1 part of solvent, such as glycerin, for 3 to 5 parts of the drug.

Examples of flavors for various classes of drugs are provided in Table 9-4.[4] Table 9-5 lists some general techniques for selecting flavors.

Flavoring Agents

Definitions and Properties

Some terms used to describe flavors and their definitions are as follows.

- *Natural flavor:* Essential oil, oleoresin, essence or extractive, protein hydrolysate, distillate, or any product of roasting, heating, or enzymolysis, which contains flavoring constituents derived from a spice, fruit or fruit juice, vegetable or vegetable juice, edible yeast, herb, bark, bud, root, leaf or similar plant material, meat, seafood, poultry, eggs, dairy products, or fermentation products thereof whose significant function in food is flavoring rather than nutritional.[5] (The exact composition of "all natural" flavors is unknown.)
- *Artificial flavor:* Any substance used to impart flavor that is not derived from a spice, fruit or fruit juice, vegetable or vegetable juice, edible yeast, herb, bark, bud, root, leaf or similar plant material, meat, fish, poultry, eggs, dairy products, or fermentation products thereof.[5]
- *Spice:* Any aromatic vegetable substance in whole, broken, or ground form, except those substances that have been traditionally regarded as foods, such as onions, garlic, and celery; that has a significant function in food as seasoning rather than nutrition; that is true to name; and that has had no portion of any volatile oil or other flavoring principle removed.[5]

TABLE 9-3 Flavors Used to Mask Basic Tastes

Taste	Flavor
Sweet	Berry, bubblegum, fruit, grape, vanilla
Acid/sour	Acacia, cherry, grapefruit, lemon, lime, orange, raspberry
Salty	Butter, butterscotch, maple, nut, spice
Bitter	Cherry, chocolate, coffee, grapefruit, lemon, licorice (anise), lime, mint, orange, peach, raspberry
Oily	Anise, peppermint, wintergreen
Metallic	Berry, grape, marshmallow, mint

Source: References 2 and 3.

TABLE 9-4 Suggested Flavors by Drug Class or Population

Drug Class or Population	Flavors
Antibiotics	Banana-pineapple, banana-vanilla, cherry, cherry-custard, coconut-custard, fruit-cinnamon, lemon-custard, maple, orange, pineapple, raspberry, strawberry-vanilla
Antihistamines	Apricot, black currant, cherry, cinnamon, custard, grape, honey, lime, loganberry, peach-orange, peach-rum, raspberry, root beer, wild cherry
Barbiturates	Banana-pineapple, banana-vanilla, black currant, cinnamon-peppermint, grenadine-strawberry, lime, orange, peach-orange, root beer
Decongestants and expectorants	Anise, apricot, black-currant, butterscotch, cherry, coconut-custard, coriander, custard-mint-strawberry, gooseberry, grenadine-peach, lemon, loganberry, maple, orange, orange-lemon, orange-peach, pineapple, raspberry, strawberry, tangerine
Electrolytes	Cherry, grape, lemon-lime, raspberry, wild cherry syrup
Patients of advanced age	Black currant, grenadine-strawberry, lime, root beer, wild strawberry

Source: Reference 4.

TABLE 9-5 Techniques for Selecting Flavors

Type of Flavoring	Test Medium	Preparation
Water-Soluble Flavors		
Generally begin at 0.2% for artificial flavors and 1%–2% for natural flavors	Sweetened water containing 8%–10% sugar	Add sugar to water, then add flavoring. Add 0.2%–0.3% citric acid if a fruit flavor.
	Sugar syrup, high-fructose corn syrup, or corn syrup	Add flavor to choice of sweetener. Heat mixture in a microwave for 10–20 seconds. Cool before tasting.
Oil-Soluble Flavors		
Generally begin at 0.1% in finished product for artificial flavors and 0.2% for natural flavors	Powdered sugar and melted shortening in 1:1 ratio	Mix sugar and melted shortening. Add flavor, and taste.
	Vegetable oil (especially good for butter and nutty tastes)	Mix oil and flavoring, and taste.
Powdered Flavors		
Generally begin at 0.1% in finished product for artificial flavors and 0.75% for natural flavors	Fruit flavors: sugar 98% and citric acid 2%	Mix sugar, citric acid, and flavoring. Add about 75 g/L of water to mixture.
	Other flavors: sugar	Mix sugar and flavoring. Add about 75 g/L of water to mixture.

Flavors can be obtained as oil- or water-soluble liquids and as dry powders; most are diluted in carriers. Oil-soluble carriers include soybean and other edible oils. Water-soluble carriers include water, ethanol, propylene glycol, glycerin, and emulsifiers. Dry carriers include maltodextrins, corn syrup solids, modified starches, gum arabic, salt, sugars, and whey protein.

Flavors can degrade as a result of exposure to light, temperature, headspace oxygen, water, enzymes, contaminants, and other product components.

Flavors are regulated as follows: the Food and Drug Administration, food and pharmaceutical products; the U.S. Department of Agriculture, meat products; and the Bureau of Alcohol, Tobacco, Firearms, and Explosives, alcoholic products.

Commercial Flavor Designations

Some commonly used commercial designations and their components can be found in Table 9-6.

Effect on Drug Stability

Not all drugs are stable in the presence of flavoring materials. Flavors are complex mixtures that are composed of many chemicals. For example, natural cherry flavor contains more than 70 components, and artificial cherry flavor has more than 20; natural banana flavor has more than 150 components, and artificial banana has more than 17; and natural grape flavor has about 225 components, and artificial grape flavor has more than 18. Because each component is a chemical, it may potentially affect the stability of the drug(s) in the formulation. Many natural flavors have a prominent ingredient, for example, benzaldehyde in cherry, isoamyl acetate in banana, L-carvone in spearmint, and lemonene in orange.

Another factor to consider is whether the flavors adsorb to containers during compounding of the drug preparation or during storage. Flavors can also sorb to suspended materials or be partitioned into the internal phase of emulsions. Any flavor loss should be investigated and corrected.

TABLE 9-6 Selected Commercial Flavor Designations and Their Components

Flavor Designation	Components
Natural ABCD[a] flavor	All components are derived from ABCD.
ABCD flavor: natural and artificial	At least one component is derived from ABCD.
	No definition exists of natural-to-artificial ratio.
ABCD flavor: with other natural flavors (WONF)	All components are natural.
	At least one component is derived from ABCD.
Natural flavor: ABCD type	All components are natural.
	No components are derived from ABCD.
ABCD flavor: artificial flavor	All components are artificial.
Conceptual flavors	Product may contain artificial flavors.
	No reference point is given.
	Flavors may have to be declared only in ingredient declaration.

[a]ABCD represents the flavor name, such as cherry.

Flavor-Enhancing Agents

Flavor is a key determinant of the palatability of pharmaceutical products administered in oral liquid and oral semisolid dosage forms. Enhancers are useful for covering or masking off-notes and tastes.

Excessive bitterness of active compounds in oral medications is a major problem for the pharmaceutical industry. Certain ions, such as sodium, suppress bitterness well and serve to enhance certain flavors. Sodium chloride is also used to enhance sweetness. Sweet-tasting spices, including anise, cinnamon, cloves, ginger, and nutmeg, can also enhance flavor.

Flavor enhancers are used in relatively low concentrations. They can produce a primary, rapid release of flavor that a patient experiences before the drug taste. Alternatively, they can provide a lingering flavor in cases in which the disagreeable drug taste tends to persist.

Commonly used flavor enhancers include citric acid USP (United States Pharmacopeia), ethyl maltol, ethyl vanillin NF (National Formulary), fructose USP, fumaric acid NF, malic acid NF, maltol, menthol USP, monosodium glutamate NF, sodium chloride USP, stevia, tartaric acid NF, and vanillin NF. Table 9-7 lists properties of some flavor enhancers.

Sweeteners

Sucrose, dextrose, corn syrup, sorbitol, mannitol, and other sugars are commonly used as sweeteners. Sugars often are used in relatively high concentrations, and their effect on viscosity may retard the rate of dissolution of some drugs. Therefore, dissolving the active drugs and other excipients in the aqueous vehicle before adding the sugar(s) may be advisable.

Noncaloric sweeteners include saccharin (sodium) and aspartame. Saccharin is about 250 to 500 times as sweet as sucrose, but its bitter aftertaste must be addressed. Aspartame is approximately 200 times sweeter than sucrose and is very widely used. It does not have a prominent aftertaste, but it does have a stability profile that is pH and temperature dependent. For example, aspartame is most stable between pH 3.4 and 5 at refrigerated temperatures. Because it is often used in products that are heated (e.g., syrups, troches), compounders must be aware of its potential degradation at elevated temperatures. During the compounding of most pharmaceutical preparations, the ingredients do not remain at an elevated temperature for long, and hence the aspartame should be stable.

A wide variety of sweeteners is available for liquid, semisolid, and solid dosage forms. The *United States Pharmacopeia/National Formulary* does not list all commonly used sweeteners, but it contains 22 monographs in the category of Sweetening Agents: Acesulfame Potassium, Aspartame, Aspartame Acesulfame, Dextrates, Dextrose, Dextrose Excipient, Fructose, Galactose, Maltitol, Maltose, Mannitol, Saccharin, Saccharin Calcium, Saccharin Sodium, Sorbitol, Sorbitol Solution, Sucralose, Sucrose, Compressible Sugar, Confectioner's Sugar, Syrup, and Tagatose. Table 9-8 lists properties of some of the sweetening agents.

Acesulfame potassium, an intense sweetening agent that is also a flavor enhancer, can be effectively used to mask some unpleasant tastes. It is quite stable in the solid state, in solution, and at elevated temperatures. Synergism with other sweeteners, especially aspartame or sodium cyclamate, has been effectively used.[1]

Aspartame has an intensely sweet taste. It is stable when dry but can hydrolyze in the presence of moisture. It degrades during prolonged heating, but the use of higher temperatures for short time periods followed by rapid cooling can minimize this problem. Aspartame can be used synergistically with cyclamate, glucose, saccharin, and sucrose, and its taste can be enhanced with sodium bicarbonate, gluconate salts, and lactose. It does not have the

TABLE 9-7 Physicochemical Properties of Commonly Used Flavor Enhancers

Substance	Usual Concentration (%)	pH (% w/v)	Melting Range (°C)	Solubility				
				Water	Alcohol	Glycerin	Propylene Glycol	Packaging
Citric acid	0.2–2.0	2.2 (1%)	153	FS	FS	—	—	T
Ethyl maltol	0.005	—	89–93	1:55	1:10	1:500	1:17	—
Ethyl vanillin	0.01	—	76–78	1:250	1:2	Sol	Sol	T, LR
Fructose	—	5.35 (9%)	102–105	1:0.3	1:15	—	—	W
Fumaric acid	—	2.45 (ss)	287	1:200	1:17	—	1:33	W
Malic acid	—	2.35 (15)	131–132	1:1.5–2.0	1:2.6	—	1:1.9	W
Maltol	—	5.3 (0.5%)	162–164	1:83	1:21	1:80	1:28	W
Menthol	0.003–0.015	—	41–44	SlS	VS	—	—	T
Monosodium glutamate	—	—	—	FS	SpS	—	—	T
Sodium chloride	—	6.7–7.3 (ss)	801	1:2.8	1:250	1:10	—	W
Stevia	0.1–0.75	—	198	1:800	SlS	—	—	T
Tartaric acid	—	2.2 (1.5%)	168–170	1:0.75	1:2.5	Sol	—	W
Vanillin	0.01–0.02	—	81–83	1:100	1:2	1:20	—	T, LR

— = Not available; ss = saturated solution.

TABLE 9-8 Usual Concentrations and Solubilities of Selected Sweetening Agents

Sweetener	Usual Concentration (%)	Sweetness[a]	Solubility[b] (mL solvent/1 g sweetener)		
			Water	Alcohol	Other
Acesulfame potassium	—	180–200	3.7	1000	100 (50% alcohol)
Aspartame	—	180–200	SpS	SIS	
Cyclamate calcium	0.17	30	FS	PrIn	
Cyclamate sodium	0.17	30	5	250	Propylene glycol (25)
Dextrates	—	0.5	1	PrIn	
Dextrose	—	0.65	1	60	Sol in glycerin
Fructose	—	1.17	0.3	15	
Liquid glucose	20–60	—	Misc	PartMisc	
Glycerin	≤20	—	Misc	Misc	
Maltitol solution	—	0.75	Misc	Misc (<55% ethanol)	
Mannitol	—	0.5	5.5	83 (18)	Glycerin
Saccharin	0.02–0.5 w/w	500	290	31 (50)	Glycerin
Saccharin calcium	0.075–0.6	300	2.6	4.7	
Saccharin sodium	0.075–0.6	300	1.2	50	Propylene glycol (3.5)
Sorbitol	20–70	0.5–0.6	0.5	25	
Stevia powder	<0.3	30	Sol		
Stevioside	<0.03	300	Sol		
Sucrose	≤85 w/v	1	0.5	170	
Sugar, compressible	10–60	0.98	0.5 (sucrose)	170 (sucrose)	
Sugar, confectioner's	10–50	0.95	0.5 (sucrose)	170 (sucrose)	
Syrup	—	0.85	Misc	Misc	
Xylitol	—	1.0	1.6	80	Propylene glycol (15)

— = Not available.
[a]Sweetness relative to sucrose, with sucrose being 1.0.
[b]Solubility at 20°C unless otherwise specified.

aftertaste associated with saccharin, but it does have a pH- and temperature-dependent stability profile. It is most stable between pH 3.4 and 5 at refrigerated temperatures.

Dextrates is a purified mixture of saccharides from the controlled enzymatic hydrolysis of starch. Dextrates may be heated to 50°C without any appreciable darkening in color.

Dextrose is widely used as a sweetening and tonicity-adjusting agent and as a tablet diluent and binder. It is a stable material and should be stored in a cool, dry place. One gram of anhydrous dextrose is approximately equivalent to 1.1 g of dextrose monohydrate.

Fructose is used as a flavor enhancer, sweetening agent for syrups and solutions, and tablet diluent. Fructose is sweeter than mannitol and sorbitol and is effective at masking unpleasant flavors in tablet formulations; its sweetness profile is experienced more rapidly in the mouth than that of sucrose and dextrose. Also, its greater solubility in alcohol is sometimes an advantage.

Liquid glucose can be used to provide body and sweetness to liquid formulations. It contains dextrose and smaller amounts of dextrins and maltose, being prepared by the partial hydrolysis of starch with acid. Although not a pure, specific chemical entity, it is reasonably uniform from batch to batch.

Glycerin is about two-thirds as sweet as sucrose. It is a hygroscopic liquid and should be stored in airtight containers in a cool place. It is not prone to oxidation but will decompose on heating. When glycerin is mixed with water, ethanol, and propylene glycol, the mixtures are chemically stable.

Maltitol solution is an aqueous solution of a hydrogenated, partially hydrolyzed starch that is used as a sweetening and suspending agent. It is noncrystallizing and prevents cap locking in syrups and elixirs. It is a colorless, odorless, clear viscous liquid that is sweet tasting.

Mannitol is a hexahydric alcohol related to mannose and is isomeric with sorbitol. It imparts a cooling sensation in the mouth, which is due to its negative heat of solution. It is used as a sweetening agent, tablet and capsule diluent, tonicity agent, and bulking agent and is especially useful for chewable tablet formulations.

Saccharin is odorless or has a faint aromatic odor, and its solutions are acid to litmus. Its relative sweetening power is increased by dilution.

Saccharin calcium is odorless or has a faint aromatic odor. Saccharin sodium is an intense sweetening agent. It is a white, odorless or faintly aromatic, efflorescent, crystalline powder with an intensely sweet taste and a metallic or bitter aftertaste. It decomposes on heating to a high temperature (125°C) at a low pH (about pH 2).

Cyclamate sodium can be used to enhance flavor systems and to mask some unpleasant taste characteristics. It is often used in combination with saccharin.

Sorbitol occurs as a white, hygroscopic powder, granules, or flakes with a sweet taste. It is also commercially available as a 70% solution.

Stevia (honey leaf, yerba dulce) powder is a relatively new sweetening agent. It is the extract from the leaves of the *Stevia rebaudiana* Bertoni plant. Its sweet taste is attributed to sweet glycosides such as the steviosides, rebaudiosides, and a dulcoside. It is natural, nontoxic, and safe and occurs as a white, crystalline, hygroscopic powder. It can be used in both hot and cold preparations. The source of stevia is important, because some countries (e.g., Paraguay) produce a sweeter and higher-quality product than that obtained from other countries.

Sucrose has a long history of use and is available in highly purified form at a reasonable cost. It is obtained from sugar cane, sugar beet, or other sources. When finely divided, it is hygroscopic and can absorb up to 1% water. Sucrose is stable at room temperature. When heated, it caramelizes at temperatures greater than 160°C. Its dilute solutions support microbial growth and can be sterilized by filtration or autoclaving. When sucrose is used in candy-based preparations, at temperatures rising from 110°C to 145°C, some inversion of sucrose to dextrose and fructose occurs; one potential problem is that fructose may cause stickiness, but it will inhibit cloudiness and graininess. This inversion process is enhanced in the presence of acids and at temperatures greater than 130°C. The tendency of sucrose to crystallize as seen in cap locking (i.e., sucrose crystallizes on the threads of the bottle cap and makes cap removal difficult) can be minimized if sucrose is used in conjunction with sorbitol, glycerin, or other polyols.

Syrup NF is a solution of 85% weight per volume sucrose in purified water. It may be prepared by the use of boiling water or, preferably, by the percolation method, which requires no heat. Unless used when freshly prepared, it should contain a preservative; it has a specific gravity of not less than 1.30.

Xylitol is a noncariogenic sweetening agent used in tablets, syrups, and coatings. It has a sweet taste and imparts a cooling sensation in the mouth. It is heat stable but can caramelize if heated for several minutes near its boiling point (215°C–217°C).

The cooling sensation of some sugars is due to their negative heats of solution; for example, the following comparisons are given in joules per gram (J/g): mannitol (−120.9), sorbitol (−111.3), sucrose (−18.0), and xylitol (−153.1).

Coloring Agents

Coloring a preparation is not always necessary. If a coloring agent is used, however, it should be selected to match the flavor (i.e., green for mint, red for cherry). Better results are generally obtained by using minimal quantities of dyes, which will produce light-to-moderate color densities.

References

1. *The PFC Index—A Guide to Flavor and Fragrance Elegance.* Camden, NJ: The Pharmaceutical Flavor Clinic, Division of Foote & Jenks; 1986;10, 16–17.
2. Reiland TL. Physical methods of taste-masking. Presented at the 1990 Annual Meeting of the American Association of Pharmaceutical Scientists, Las Vegas, November 4–8, 1990.
3. Allen LV Jr., Ansel HC. *Ansel's Pharmaceutical Dosage Forms and Drug Delivery Systems,* 10th ed. Philadelphia PA: Wolters Kluwer; 2014:156–8.
4. Neuroth MI. Liquid medications. In: Martin EW. *Dispensing of Medication.* 7th ed. Easton, PA: Mack Publishing Co.; 1971:859.
5. Code of Federal Regulations. April 1, 2015; 21 CFR 101.22(a). Available at: https://www.accessdata.fda.gov/scripts/cdrh/cfdocs/cfcfr/cfrsearch.cfm?fr=101.22. Accessed November 28, 2015.

Chapter 10

Preservation, Sterilization, and Depyrogenation

Many pharmaceutical products are injected into the body or applied to compromised areas. If a product containing microorganisms is introduced into or applied to the body, severe infections may result. Such infections could result in the loss of an organ (e.g., an eye) or a limb, or even death. Consequently, certain pharmaceutical preparations must be sterile and contain preservatives to maintain their sterility. Parenteral medications must also be free of pyrogens and have endotoxin levels within allowable limits.

Preservation

Preservation is the prevention or inhibition of microbial growth. In pharmacy, preservatives are typically added to a product either to minimize microbial growth, as is the case with oral liquids, topical preparations, and the like, or to prevent microbial growth, as is necessary for sterile preparations such as parenteral medications, ophthalmic preparations, and oral inhalation solutions.

Methods of Preservation
Preservation involves the addition of a substance to a product; the choice of preservative to be added depends on the characteristics of the product and its acceptability to the patient. Table 10-1 lists preservatives that can be used in various types of preparations.

Selection Factors
Factors that must be considered in selecting a preservative include concentration, pH, taste, odor, and solubility. Some preparations, such as syrups (discussed in Chapter 17 of this book), are inherently preserved by their high concentration of sugar, which acts as an osmotic preservative. For most preparations, however, a suitable preservative is necessary. In choosing a preservative, a pharmacist must ensure that the compounded preparation is stable. A preservative must be nontoxic, stable, compatible, and inexpensive and have an acceptable taste, odor, and color. It should also be effective against a wide variety of bacteria, fungi, and yeasts.

TABLE 10-1 Concentrations of Preservatives Used in Pharmaceutical Products

Preservative	Concentration (%)				
	Liquids	**Emulsions**	**Ointments/ Creams**	**Parenteral Preparations**	**Ophthalmic/ Nasal/Otic Products**
Alcohol/ethanol	15–20	15–20	—	—	—
Benzalkonium chloride	0.004–0.02	0.002–0.1	0.01	0.013	—
Benzethonium chloride	0.004–0.02	0.005–0.02	0.01	0.01	—
Benzoic acid and salts[a]	0.1–0.3	0.1–0.3	—	—	—
Sodium benzoate	0.1–0.3	0.1–0.3	—	—	—
Benzyl alcohol	1.0–3.0	1.0–4.0	1	2	—
Boric acid and salts	0.5–1	—	—	—	—
Cetylpyridinium chloride	0.01–0.02	0.01–0.02	—	—	—
Cetyltrimethyl ammonium bromide	—	0.01–0.02	—	—	—
Chlorobutanol[b]	0.3–0.5	0.5	—	0.25–0.5	—
Chlorocresol	0.05–0.1	—	—	0.1–0.3	—
Cresol	0.3–0.5	0.3–0.5	0.3–0.5	—	—
Imidazolidinyl urea	—	0.05–0.5	—	—	—
Metacresol	—	—	0.1–0.3	—	—
Myristyl gamma picolinium chloride	0.17	—	—	—	—
Nitromersol	0.001–0.1	—	—	—	—
Parabens[c]	0.001–0.2	0.001–0.2	0.001–0.2	0.02–0.2	0.1
Benzyl	—	—	—	—	—
Butyl	—	—	—	0.015	—
Methyl	—	—	—	0.1–0.2	—
Propyl	—	—	—	0.02–0.2	—
Phenol[d]	0.2–0.5	0.2–0.5	0.2–0.5	—	—
o-Phenyl phenol	0.005–0.01	—	—	—	—
β-phenylethyl alcohol	0.2–1	—	—	—	—
Phenylmercuric acetate/nitrate	0.002–0.005	0.002–0.005	0.002	0.004	—
Sorbic acid and salts	0.05–0.2	0.05–0.2	—	—	—
Thimerosal	0.001–0.1	0.005–0.02	0.01	0.01	—

— = Not available.

[a]Benzoic acid/sodium benzoate are most effective at pH 4 or below.

[b]The anhydrous form of chlorobutanol should be used if a clear solution is desired in liquid petrolatum. Chlorobutanol needs a pH <5; also, it will sorb to plastic.

[c]Parabens are usually used in pairs. They have low water solubility and poor taste. They may degrade at a pH >8; they are best used at a range of pH 4 to 8. The parabens may interact with certain macromolecular compounds and bind, resulting in a loss of some effectiveness.

[d]Phenol forms a eutectic mixture with a number of compounds and may soften cocoa butter in suppository mixtures. Phenol may precipitate albumin, gelatin, and collodion. A green color may be produced in the presence of alum or borax.

Dosage Form Considerations

The following dosage forms should be considered during selection of a preservative.

Emulsions. Preservatives may partition into the oil phase of an emulsion and lose their effectiveness. The preservative should be concentrated in the aqueous phase, because bacterial growth usually occurs then. In addition, because the unionized form of the preservative is more effective against bacteria, most of the preservative should be present in the nonionized state. To be effective, the preservative must be neither bound nor adsorbed to any agent in the emulsion or the container. In summary, only preservative in the aqueous phase in the free, unbound, unadsorbed, unionized state will be effective in emulsions. The parabens (methylparaben, propylparaben, butylparaben) are among the most satisfactory preservatives for emulsions.

Gels. When added to an aqueous system, 0.1% methylparaben or propylparaben is an acceptable preservative and does not affect the efficiency of the polymer to maintain viscosity.

Oral Inhalations. Any preparation that is not in unit dose containers should contain a preservative, especially with the latest requirement of sterility for this class of dosage forms. The minimum amount of preservative that is effective should be used. If too high a concentration is used, it may initiate a cough reflex in the patient. Also, too high a concentration of certain preservatives that are also surfactants may cause foaming that can interfere with the delivery of the complete dose.

Lozenges and Troches. The flavors and effects of preservatives included in these preparations are varied. A 0.08% solution of methylparaben has an odor described as "floral," "gauze pad," or "face powder" sweet. A 0.015% solution of propylparaben has minimal aroma and a tongue-numbing effect, producing a slight sting. A 0.125% butylparaben solution has the least aroma of all. Preservatives may have a tendency to partition into flavors, because preservatives are not always water soluble and most flavors are oily in nature.

Preservative Selection

Preservation involves the addition of a substance to a preparation; the choice of preservative to be added depends on the characteristics of the preparation and its acceptability to the patient. Table 10-1 lists preservatives that can be used in various types of preparations. Factors that must be considered in selecting a preservative include concentration, pH, taste, odor, and solubility. Some preparations, such as syrups, are inherently preserved by their high concentration of sugar, which acts as an osmotic preservative. For most preparations, however, a suitable preservative is necessary. In choosing a preservative, a pharmacist must ensure that the compounded preparation is stable. A preservative must be nontoxic, stable, compatible, and inexpensive and have an acceptable taste, odor, and color. It should also be effective against a wide variety of bacteria, fungi, and yeasts.

When personal experience or shelf storage experiments indicate that a preservative is required in a pharmaceutical preparation, its selection is based on many considerations, including some of the following:

- The preservative prevents the growth of the type of microorganisms considered the most likely contaminants of the preparation.
- The preservative is sufficiently soluble in water to achieve adequate concentrations in the aqueous phase of a system with two or more phases.
- The proportion of preservative remaining undissociated at the pH of the preparation makes it capable of penetrating the microorganism and destroying its integrity.
- The required concentration of the preservative does not affect the safety or comfort of a patient when the pharmaceutical preparation is administered by the usual or intended route; that is, it is nonirritating, nonsensitizing, and nontoxic.

- The preservative has adequate stability and will not be reduced in concentration by chemical decomposition or volatilization during the desired shelf life of the preparation.
- The preservative is completely compatible with all other formulative ingredients and does not interfere with them, nor do they interfere with the effectiveness of the preservative agent.
- The preservative does not adversely affect the preparation's container or closure.

Mode of Action
Preservatives interfere with microbial growth, multiplication, and metabolism through one or more of the following mechanisms:

- Modification of cell membrane permeability and leakage of cell constituents (partial lysis)
- Lysis and cytoplasmic leakage
- Irreversible coagulation of cytoplasmic constituents (e.g., protein precipitation)
- Inhibition of cellular metabolism, such as by interfering with enzyme systems or inhibiting cell wall synthesis
- Oxidation of cellular constituents
- Hydrolysis

Physicochemical Considerations for Common Preservatives
Preservatives have unique characteristics that must be taken into account during the selection process. For example, the anhydrous form of chlorobutanol should be used if a clear solution is desired in liquid petrolatum. Ethylenediamine may irritate the skin and mucous membranes and thus should be used with caution, sodium benzoate is most effective at a pH of 4 or below, and a green color may be produced in the presence of alum or borax. The parabens may interact with certain macromolecular compounds, binding and thereby losing some of their effectiveness (Table 10-2). Phenol forms a eutectic mixture with a number of compounds and may soften cocoa butter in suppository mixtures. Also, phenol may precipitate albumin, gelatin, and collodion.

Quaternary Ammonium Compounds
Benzalkonium chloride is an antimicrobial agent commonly used as a preservative. It acts by emulsification of the bacterial cell walls, probably the cell membrane lipids. Ethylenediaminetetraacetic acid (EDTA) is often added in concentrations ranging from 0.01% to

TABLE 10-2 Binding Percentages of Parabens with Macromolecular Compounds

Compound	% of Methylparaben Bound	% of Propylparaben Bound
Gelatin	8	11
Methylcellulose	9	13
Polyethylene glycol 4000	16	19
Polyvinylpyrrolidone	22	36
Polyoxyethylene monostearate	45	84
Polyoxyethylene sorbitan monolaurate	57	86
Polyoxyethylene sorbitan monooleate	57	90

0.1% to enhance the activity of benzalkonium chloride against *Pseudomonas aeruginosa.* Listed incompatibilities include aluminum, anionic materials, citrates, cotton, fluorescein, hydrogen peroxide, hydroxypropyl methylcellulose, iodides, kaolin, lanolin, nitrates, high concentrations of nonionic surfactants, permanganates, protein, salicylates, silver salts, soaps, sulfonamides, tartrates, zinc oxide, and zinc sulfate.

Benzethonium chloride is a detergent antiseptic with the same limitations and behavior characteristics as benzalkonium chloride. It is incompatible with soaps. One advantage of benzethonium chloride is that its germicidal activity increases with an increase in pH. For example, at pH 10 it is several times more active against selected bacteria than at pH 4.

Chlorobutanol

Chlorobutanol is both antibacterial and antifungal. Its antibacterial effectiveness is reduced above pH 5.5. Aqueous solutions of chlorobutanol will degrade in the presence of hydroxide ions. Chlorobutanol aqueous solutions have good stability at pH 3, but stability decreases with an increase in pH. Chlorobutanol may diffuse through polyethylene or other porous containers, resulting in a decreased concentration and effectiveness. Incompatibilities include plastic vials, rubber stoppers, bentonite, magnesium trisilicate, polyethylene, and poly-hydroxyethylmethacrylate (in some soft contact lenses). Some antimicrobial activity is lost on contact with carboxymethylcellulose or polysorbate 80 because of sorption or complex formation. Greater antimicrobial effectiveness can be obtained by combining 0.5% chlorobutanol with 0.5% phenylethanol. The anhydrous form of chlorobutanol should be used if a clear solution is desired in a liquid petrolatum vehicle.

Parabens

Methylparaben is most effective in solution between pH 4 and 8; its efficacy decreases at higher pH levels. It can be autoclaved in aqueous solution, and it is stable in aqueous solution in the range of pH 3 to 6 for up to 4 years at room temperature. Methylparaben is incompatible with nonionic surfactants (its antimicrobial activity is reduced) and with atropine, bentonite, essential oils, magnesium trisilicate, talc, tragacanth, sodium alginate, and sorbitol. It may sorb to some plastics and is discolored in the presence of iron.

Propylparaben is also most effective in solution between pH 4 and 8; its efficacy decreases at higher pH levels. It can be autoclaved in aqueous solutions of pH 3 to 6 without decomposition; aqueous solutions within this pH range are stable for up to 4 years. Propylparaben is incompatible with nonionic surfactants (reduced effectiveness); in addition, sorption has been reported to magnesium aluminum silicate, magnesium trisilicate, ultramarine blue, and yellow iron oxide. Discoloration in the presence of iron and hydrolysis by weak alkalis and strong acids can also occur. Some plastics will adsorb propylparaben. Sodium propylparaben is a more water-soluble form that may be used in place of propylparaben, but the pH of the formulation may be increased.

Phenylmercuric Acetate/Nitrate

Phenylmercuric acetate should be protected from light. It is reported to be incompatible with anionic emulsifying agents and suspending agents; disodium edetate, halides, silicates, sodium metabisulfite, sodium thiosulfate, starch, talc, and tragacanth; and some types of filter membranes used for sterilization.

Phenylmercuric nitrate is effective over a broad pH range against both bacteria and fungi. It is the preferred form in acidic solutions.

Phenylmercuric salts are used in preference to benzalkonium chloride in solutions of salicylates and nitrates, as well as in solutions of physostigmine and epinephrine that contain sodium sulfite. Its solutions can be autoclaved, but significant amounts of the salt may be lost; therefore, they are best sterilized by filtration. Incompatibilities include anionic emulsifying agents and suspending agents; disodium edetate, halides, silicates, sodium metabisulfite, sodium thiosulfate, starch, talc, and tragacanth; and some types of filter membranes used for sterilization.

Thimerosal
Thimerosal is an antibacterial agent with weak bacteriostatic and mild fungistatic properties. It is affected by light.

Preservative Effectiveness Testing
Although not required, *United States Pharmacopeia (USP)* tests for the effectiveness of antimicrobial preservatives should be conducted on any formulation that is expected to be prepared in quantity and used for an extended period of time. The purpose of the tests, which can be conducted by a testing laboratory, is to demonstrate effectiveness against five different organisms (*Candida albicans, Aspergillus niger, Escherichia coli, P. aeruginosa,* and *Staphylococcus aureus*). Test results are applicable only to the specific preparation, packaged in the original, unopened containers.

Sterilization

Sterilization is the process of destroying or eliminating microorganisms that are present in or on an object or a preparation. Sterility is defined as the absence of all viable life forms. Parenteral and ophthalmic preparations have long had sterility requirements, but now a number of dosage forms, including oral inhalations, nasal solutions, implants, irrigations, metered sprays, and certain swabs, also have sterility requirements.

Methods of Sterilization
The five basic methods of sterilization are moist heat, dry heat, chemical use, filtration, and radiation. Of these, moist heat, dry heat, some forms of chemical sterilization, and filtration are appropriate for pharmacists to use. Pharmacists can, however, use contract facilities for gaseous and radiation sterilization. A pharmacy should validate all of its sterilization methods on a regular basis; the routine use of devices or kits that indicate sterility is recommended. Heat is the most reliable method of sterilization. The efficiency of heat in destroying microorganisms is dependent on temperature, time, moisture, and pressure. Both moist-heat and dry-heat sterilization processes are used.

Moist-Heat Sterilization
In moist-heat sterilization (steam under pressure), an autoclave provides a saturated steam environment, typically 121°C at 15 psi, with variation depending on the autoclave being used. After the correct temperature and pressure are reached, the sterilization process continues for an additional 20 minutes, at which time the pressure and temperature are allowed to return to ambient levels at a rate depending on the load of items in the autoclave.

The saturation of water, or steam, at high pressure is the foundation for the effectiveness of moist-heat sterilization. When steam makes contact with a cooler object, it condenses and loses latent heat to the object. Under autoclaving conditions, the amount of energy released is approximately 524 cal/g, whereas 1 cal/g of energy is released in dry-heat sterilization. The difference explains why moist heat under pressure is more effective than dry heat at the same temperature in destroying microbial life. It also helps explain why objects or preparations to be sterilized in an autoclave must contain water or permit saturated steam to penetrate and make contact with all surfaces to be sterilized. Air pockets are of great concern in the steam sterilization process because the steam must reach all sites to be effective.

Sealed containers must contain water in order to be sterilized by this method. Sealed, dry containers will reach only 121°C inside, and the heat will not be moist; thus, sterilization will likely not occur. Similarly, anhydrous and oily solutions that contain no water will reach only 121°C and the heat will be dry. To sterilize glycerin in sealed containers, about 1% sterile water for injection can be added before the autoclaving process. Moist-heat sterilization is the desired method of sterilization for any item that can withstand high temperatures, including rubber closures, high-density plastic tubing, filter assemblies, sealed-glass ampuls containing solutions that can withstand high temperatures, stainless-steel vessels, gowning materials, and various hard-surface equipment items.

Dry-Heat Sterilization

Dry-heat sterilization requires heat in excess of that produced by autoclaving and involves the use of a high-temperature oven. The following operating conditions have been established: at 160°C, 120 to 180 minutes; at 170°C, 90 to 120 minutes; and at 180°C, 45 to 60 minutes. However, pharmacists should not assume that any of the three conditions will automatically suffice for all formulations; sufficient time at the various temperatures must be determined to achieve the desired sterilization. Dry-heat sterilization is used to sterilize glass, stainless steel, and other hard-surface materials, as well as dry powders not labile to high temperatures. Injectable oily solutions also can be dry-heat sterilized if the active ingredient remains potent and stable; a time and temperature cycle that produces a validated finished sterile preparation must be used.

Chemical Sterilization

Chemical sterilization involves the use of a gas, such as ethylene oxide, or chemical solutions, such as isopropanol and ethanol. The items to be sterilized are placed in an apparatus that is specially designed to expose them to the sterilizing agent. After sterilization, the items are aerated to remove any residual chemical agent. Gaseous sterilization is employed primarily to sterilize items such as medical devices and plastic materials that cannot withstand heat or radiation sterilization. Gases commonly used include ethylene oxide, formaldehyde, methyl bromide, β-propiolactone, and propylene oxide. Approximately 75% of all single-use, disposable devices are sterilized by ethylene oxide. Two other agents that are gaining popularity are peracetic acid and vapor-phase hydrogen peroxide. Peracetic acid decomposes to nontoxic products of acetic acid and water without leaving adsorbable residues. Vapor-phase hydrogen peroxide is a powerful antimicrobial and is very effective in killing spore-forming bacteria. Contract facilities that will sterilize small lots for a fee can be found on the Internet.

Filtration Sterilization

Filtration, one of the oldest methods of sterilization, is a process whereby particulate matter from a flowing liquid is removed by the use of a filter. Filtration is not actually a terminal sterilization process, because the preparation is then aseptically packaged in the dispensing container.

Filtration, which is recommended for most compounding situations, removes but does not destroy microorganisms; particulate matter is unable to penetrate the smaller pores in the filter matrix and is retained on the filter. After filtration has been completed, the sterile solution should be removed immediately because microorganisms can eventually penetrate the pores of some filters if left on the filter surface for a prolonged period.

Also, as bacteria grow on a filter, their byproducts (pyrogenic substances) may pass into the sterile solution.

As a general rule, aqueous and organic solvent-based fluids can be filtered with polyvinylidiene fluoride and cellulosic esters; aqueous solutions at extreme pH values, with polyvinylidiene fluoride filters; and organic solvents and gases, with polyvinylidiene fluoride and polytetrafluoroethylene filters. When using filtration, a pharmacist should know whether the drug, preservative, or any other component in the solution tends to sorb to the filter material. If so, an alternative filter material should be used.

Filtration sterilization is used for drug preparations that are chemically or physically unstable if sterilized by heat, gas, or radiation sterilization. Currently, probably more than 80% of all small-volume parenteral preparations may be sterilized by filtration followed by aseptic processing.

Filters suitable for sterilization of pharmaceutical preparations have a nominal rated pore size of 0.22 µm or less. Membrane filters are available either as flat discs or as cartridges. The cartridges have much larger surface areas and should be used for filtering large volumes of solution or solutions of high viscosity. Filters of different materials are available for a wide variety of solvents and gases; filter compatibility tables should be checked before the selection of a filter for each procedure.

Radiation (Ionizing) Sterilization

Radiation, or ionizing, sterilization is a low-temperature method used in situations similar to those in which gaseous sterilization is used—for products or systems that cannot withstand high-temperature sterilization. There are two types of radiation sterilization processes: particulate and electromagnetic. Particulate radiation sterilization commonly uses cobalt-60 or cesium-137. Electromagnetic radiation includes gamma radiation and ultraviolet light. Radiation (gamma) is used for sterilizing compounded implantable pellets, dry powders, and some packaging materials.

Sterility Testing

Two common sterility tests are (1) direct inoculation of media and (2) either membrane filtration or incubation with media. Commercial kits and supplies can be purchased for conducting these tests, or samples of the compounded preparation can be forwarded to a testing laboratory. Sterility testing is commonly used to document the quality of compounded preparations. Newer, rapid sterility-testing methods are now available and in use by some contract laboratories. They can usually provide results in about 48 hours.

Validation

Whatever sterilization method is used, the equipment and processes must be validated. Appropriate biological indicators for use in validation include *Bacillus subtilis* var. *niger* spores for dry heat, *B. stearothermophilus* for moist-heat sterilizers, and *B. pumulis* spores for ionizing radiation.

Performance

Two different types of procedures are used to test the performance of an autoclave. A physical test can be performed by applying autoclave tape to the preparation containers and checking whether the temperature required to kill microorganisms was reached, as indicated by a color change on the tape. A second, microbiological method is to place ampuls of viable microorganisms with the preparations to be autoclaved. After the autoclaving process, either the ampul or a sample from the ampul can be placed on a culture plate and the plate can be checked after the appropriate time interval to determine whether any micro-organisms survived the sterilization process. The absence of any sign of microbial growth indicates that the sterilization process was successful. A more appropriate test is to place some of the actual sterilized preparation on culture plates or in tubes of broth media and, after the proper time interval, to check for signs of growth of microorganisms. Preparations that have been sterilized by filtration can be similarly tested by inoculating a sterile media plate with a sample of the preparation, incubating it, and observing it for signs of growth.

Endotoxins and Depyrogenation

Pyrogens are metabolic products produced by microorganisms. Depyrogenation is the destruction or removal of pyrogens. Endotoxins, the most pathogenic pyrogens, are pro-duced from the lipopolysaccharide constituents of microorganism cell walls, primarily of gram-negative bacteria (especially the *Pseudomonas* species and *E. coli*). The molecular weight of these endotoxins is about 20,000 daltons. When injected, these substances can cause fever, chills, pain, and malaise. Although such reactions are rarely fatal, they do cause great discomfort and can even produce shock in seriously ill patients.

An essential part of quality assurance and quality control is testing end-product inject-able drugs, medical devices, and raw materials for endotoxins. Compounding pharmacies often omit endotoxin testing because of their reliance on sterility testing. However, a sterility test does not accurately detect endotoxins.

The importance of testing for endotoxins cannot be overemphasized. Humans are par-ticularly sensitive to minute amounts of endotoxins, and mild gram-negative bacterial infec-tions can cause a pyrogenic response. The presence of endotoxin in the bloodstream can cause fever, inflammation, and (frequently) irreversible shock known as septic shock. High concentrations of endotoxins that cause irreversible shock have been observed in patients with fulminating gram-negative bacteremia.[1] Each year in the United States, approximately 300,000 cases of septic shock result in about 100,000 deaths.[1]

The steps in calculating the endotoxin load in a compounded sterile preparation are provided in Chapter 25 of this book.

Methods of Depyrogenation

Pyrogen removal can be accomplished by any of the following seven methods:

- Heat the equipment or materials at high temperatures (≥170°C for several hours).
- Use charged modified 0.2- and 0.1-μm filter cartridges in a dead-end filtration mode.
- Perform ultrafiltration by size exclusion (using cutoff filters of 10,000 to 100,000 daltons).
- Use reverse osmosis membranes.
- Use activated carbon.
- Use distillation.
- Rinse with sterile, pyrogen-free water.

The two methods most often used in a pharmacy are heating and rinsing. Equipment, containers, and stable materials can be depyrogenated by using dry heat at a high tempera-ture. At 230°C, the time of exposure is 60 to 90 minutes; at 250°C, the exposure time is 30 to 60 minutes. Rinsing involves the use of large quantities of sterile water for injection USP to rinse equipment or containers. Because sterile water for injection USP is pyrogen free, using it as a rinse removes pyrogens, which are water soluble, from equipment or supplies.

Endotoxin and Pyrogen Testing

Originally, pyrogen testing was performed by injecting a group of rabbits with the injectable product and monitoring them for an increase in body temperature. The rabbit pyrogen test is detailed in *USP* Chapter <151>.[2]

In vitro tests developed more recently have a higher level of sensitivity than that of the rabbit test. These tests use *Limulus* amebocyte lysate (LAL), which is an aqueous blood cell extract from the horseshoe crab. Three types of LAL endotoxin testing methods (the gel-clot method, the chromogenic method, and the turbidimetric method) have been approved by USP for the evaluation of end-product injectable drugs, medical devices, and raw materials. Each of these three methods has advantages and disadvantages, but all can be used to accurately and effectively determine the presence of endotoxins in various products. Many scientists believe that the gel-clot method is the most accurate for determining endotoxin content; with this method, fewer interactions that can inhibit the reaction occur, but the long preparation process can delay results. The turbidimetric method can be performed with an automated system; although it is easy to perform, many individuals believe that it often yields false-positive results. The chromogenic method is user friendly and can be performed with an automated system; however, many compounds can interact when this method is used, so its usefulness is limited. Errors by technicians and misinterpretation of results are common among these three methods. Laboratories and pharmacies should ensure that their technicians are well trained and educated in the endotoxin testing method of choice.

The LAL kits used in pyrogen testing usually are complete with endotoxin standards and require only sterile water for injection USP for dilutions. All equipment, materials, and supplies used must be depyrogenated, and strict aseptic technique must be followed. Testing involves the manipulation of samples and dilutions and the capability to read a gel endpoint. Although pyrogen testing requires some experience and careful technique, compounding pharmacists can perform such testing in their facilities.

References

1. Volk WA, Gebhardt BM, Hammarskjold ML, Kadner RK, eds. *Essentials of Medical Microbiology.* 5th ed. Philadelphia: Lippincott-Raven; 1996:47, 327.
2. United States Pharmacopeial Convention. Chapter <151>, Pyrogen test. *United States Pharmacopeia/ National Formulary.* Rockville, MD: United States Pharmacopeial Convention; current edition.

Chapter 11

Powders and Granules

Definitions and Types

Powders and granules not only are dosage forms themselves but also are a beginning point for other dosage forms. Powders are the fine particles that can result from the comminution of any dry substance. They consist of particles ranging in size from about 0.1 μm to about 10,000 μm, although the most useful pharmaceutical range is approximately 0.1 to 10 μm. To describe particle size, pharmacists usually use the sieve number or mesh fraction terminology. The *United States Pharmacopeia/National Formulary (USP/ NF)* uses descriptive terms, such as very coarse, coarse, moderately coarse, fine, and very fine, in referring to sieve size (Table 11-1). Figure 11-1 shows a No. 80–mesh sieve; this number correlates with the *USP* description standard of "very fine."

As dosage forms, *powders* are thorough mixtures of dry, finely divided drugs and excipients that are intended for internal or external use. Powders are easy to administer to pediatric patients or patients of advanced age because the contents of divided powder papers (charts) or bulk powders can be mixed with foods or liquids. One factor that limits their use is the taste of the active drug. Powders are also prepared for use as douches and as tooth powders.

Granules are dosage forms that consist of particles ranging in size from about No. 4 to No. 10 mesh. The particles are formed when blended powders are moistened and passed through a screen or a special granulator. These moist granules are dried in the air or in an oven. Effervescent granules are especially suitable for products with a salty or bitter taste. Mixtures of citric acid or tartaric acid, or both, combined with sodium biphosphate or sodium carbonate, or both provide the effervescence. When the mixture is placed in water, it effervesces with the production of carbon dioxide.

Calculations for sample preparations that contain effervescent granules are explained in Chapter 7 of this book. Readers who are uncertain about how to determine the required quantities of these granules for a formulation should review that chapter.

TABLE 11-1 Sieve Numbers, Openings, and Descriptions

Sieve No.	Sieve Opening mm	Sieve Opening μm	Descriptive Standard (USP)	General Applications
2	9.52	9520	Very coarse	Sieve Nos. 2 through 40 are used to sift granulated effervescent salts and granulations for compressed tablets.
3.5	5.66	5660		
4	4.76	4760		
8	2.38	2380		
10	2	2000		
20	0.84	840	Coarse	
30	0.59	590		
40	0.42	420	Moderately coarse	
50	0.297	297		Sieve Nos. 50 through 120 are used to sift powdered effervescent salts and divided powders.
60	0.25	250	Fine	
70	0.21	210		
80	0.177	177	Very fine	
100	0.149	149		
120	0.125	125		
200	0.074	74		Sieve Nos. 200 through 400 are used to sift divided powders for dusting, adsorbents, inhalants, and others.
230	0.063	63		
270	0.053	53		
325	0.044	44		
400	0.037	37		

Historical Use

Originally, powders were found to be a convenient mode of administering drugs derived from hard vegetables such as roots (e.g., rhubarb), barks (e.g., cinchona), and woods (e.g., charcoal). As synthetic drugs were introduced, powders were used to administer insoluble drugs such as calomel, bismuth salts, mercury, and chalk.

Powders as a solid dosage form have been used historically as internal and external medications. For internal use, they can be taken orally, administered through the nose as snuffs, or blown into a body cavity as an insufflation. For external use, solid powders can be applied to compromised areas of the body. Powders have also been used to make solutions for topical and oral use and for use as douches. Such traditional applications and modes of administration of the dosage form continue today. Additional applications have also been developed; for example, powders containing a bioadhesive material can be applied to a specific body area so that the medication will adhere for a prolonged drug effect.

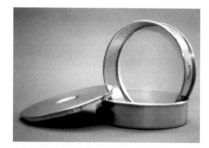

FIGURE 11-1 Brass sieve (No. 80 mesh).

Applications

Powders have qualities that make them an attractive dosage form for certain situations. Unlike a standardized capsule or tablet, powders enable a primary care provider to easily alter the quantity of medication for each dose. Powders can also aid in clinical studies of drug preparations because the dose can be so readily adjusted. Doses can be individually weighed and placed in folded powder papers, envelopes, or small vials or bottles (e.g., in powder-in-a-bottle research studies). In another example, infants and young children who cannot swallow tablets or capsules will accept powders that can be mixed with a formula or sprinkled in applesauce or some other appropriate food. Also, if a drug is too bulky to be prepared as a capsule or tablet, it may be suitable for a powder dosage form. Powders provide a rapid onset of action because they are readily dispersed; have a large surface area; and usually require only dissolution, not disintegration, before absorption.

Composition

Properly prepared, powders have a uniform, small particle size that has an elegant appearance. In general, powders are more stable than liquid dosage forms and are rapidly soluble, enabling the drug to be absorbed quickly.

The properties of powders are related to the size and surface area of the particles. For example, large particles that are more dense tend to settle more rapidly than small particles; particles that are more bulky will settle more slowly. This characteristic must be considered in the mixing or the storing and shipping of powders, when powders of different particle size may become segregated. Another concern is that powder dosage forms have a large surface area that is exposed to atmospheric conditions. Thus, powders should be dispensed in tight containers. Further, because powders of small particle size present a greater surface area to the atmosphere, they are more reactive in nature and can adsorb larger quantities of gases, such as carbon dioxide. However, a powder with a smaller particle size can dissolve at a more rapid rate, unless adsorbed gases prevent the water from surrounding the individual particles and wetting them, thereby decreasing their wetting properties. This increase in surface free energy can increase the absolute solubility of the drug and have a positive effect on its bioequivalence.

This dosage form should not ordinarily be used for drugs with a disagreeable taste or caustic nature. If taste is not a consideration, a powder can simply be prepared as powder papers and packaged in paper, glassine paper, waxed paper, or small plastic bags, depending on the characteristics of the powder.

Bulk oral powders require a patient to measure the desired quantity of each dose, and thus a measuring device must be provided to ensure accurate measurement. Divided oral powder papers (charts), however, are prepackaged individual doses; a patient simply removes the dose and takes its contents at the appointed time.

Topical powders should have a uniform, small particle size that will not irritate the skin when applied. They should be impalpable and free flowing, easily adhere to the skin, and be passed through at least a No. 100–mesh sieve to minimize skin irritation. The powder should be prepared so that it adheres to the skin.

Highly sorptive powders should not be used for topical powders that are to be applied to oozing wounds, because a hard crust may form. A more hydrophobic, water-repellent powder will prevent loss of water from the skin and will not cake on the oozing surfaces. Talc, or any other naturally derived product that is to be used on open wounds, should first be sterilized to avoid an infection in the area.

Topical powders usually consist of a base or vehicle, such as cornstarch or talc; an adherent, such as magnesium stearate, calcium stearate, or zinc stearate; and possibly an active ingredient, together with an aromatic material. The powder should provide a large surface area, flow easily, and spread uniformly. The large surface area will aid in absorbing perspiration and give a cooling sensation to the skin.

Insufflated powders are finely divided powders that are intended for application in a body cavity, such as the ears, nose, vagina, tooth socket, or throat. When using an insufflator, or puffer unit, a patient simply puffs the desired quantity of powder onto the affected area or into the cavity. This device is particularly appropriate for anti-infective preparations. Also, a moisture-activated adherent, such as Polyox, can be incorporated into the powder. Polyox is an ethylene oxide polymer with a high molecular weight that forms a viscous, mucoadhesive gel when in contact with moisture. The gel serves to provide a depot for long-term drug delivery spanning several hours.

Preparation

Particle Size Reduction

The first step in preparing powders is to generally ensure that all the ingredients are in the same range of particle size. This task is accomplished through particle size reduction, or comminution. Comminution includes both manual (trituration, levigation, pulverization by intervention) and mechanical methods (ball mills, grinders, coffee mills). The method of particle size reduction chosen depends on the characteristics of the drug. For example, gummy-type materials are best comminuted using pulverization by intervention; insoluble materials for ointments and suspensions by levigation; tough, fibrous materials by coffee grinders or mills with blades; and hard, fracturable powders by trituration. Potent materials and dyestuffs should be comminuted in nonporous mortars, such as glass, so that none of the drug remains in the pores of the mortar to decrease the dose for the current patient or to contaminate the next formulation to be prepared. For most other purposes, a standard Wedgwood or porcelain mortar and pestle will suffice. Figure 11-2 shows the types of mortars and pestles available from commercial equipment suppliers.

The type of powder that is the starting point and the type of powder that is the desired product will dictate which technique should be used. For example, if one wants to produce a light, fluffy powder but is starting with a dense powder, then light trituration with periodic fluffing using a spatula works well. Conversely, if one starts with a fluffy powder and desires to produce a more dense powder, then heavy and prolonged trituration with a mortar and

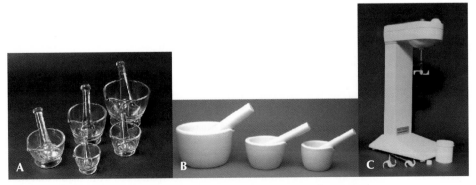

FIGURE 11-2 Mortars and pestles. A: glass; B: ceramic; C: electric.

pestle is the preferred approach. In any case, all ingredients should be approximately the same particle size for best mixing.

If topical powders are being prepared, the powders are usually passed through a sieve after comminution. In general, passing powders for liquid suspensions through a sieve is not necessary.

Particle Characteristics
When two or more powdered substances are to be combined to form a uniform mixture, one must be aware of the following characteristics of powders that affect blending.

Particle Size
Generally, particles of uniform size are blended more easily. One can visualize a mixture of large and small marbles and the difficulty involved in blending because the smaller marbles in this case tend to sink, pushing the larger marbles to the surface. This is visually evident when baking if one shakes back and forth a substance such as flour and the larger particles rise to the surface.

Particle Shape
Spherical particles tend to mix more readily because they are transported more easily from areas of high concentration to lower concentrations. Needle-shape particles and cube-shaped particles do not slide over each other as easily and tend to clog or stick together.

Particle Density
Higher density, or heavier, particles tend to sink, and less dense, or lighter, particles tend to rise. Consequently, when blending particles of different densities, one must be careful to ensure uniformity of mixing.

Electrostatic Charge
Static electricity tends to hamper blending and needs to be addressed. This can often be overcome by humidification of the work area or the inclusion (if appropriate) of a small quantity of sodium lauryl sulfate or similar material to neutralize the charges.

Adhering or Repelling Properties
By their nature, some particles may tend to either adhere or repel each other. Hence, the faster they are individually diluted with an inert substance or nonreactive material in the formulation, the easier they can be blended.

Other Characteristics
Some substances, such as camphor, are slightly gummy in nature and need to be reduced in particle size (pulverization by intervention) and immediately mixed with an inert material in the formulation to aid in the overall blending process.

Mixing Methods
Powders are generally blended for compounding by manual mixing (spatulation, trituration, sifting) or by mechanical mixing (tumbling, resonant mixing, etc.).

Manual
Pharmaceutical mixing uses a process called geometric dilution; that is, one starts with the ingredient in the smallest quantity, then adds other ingredients in order of quantity required

---

BOX 11-1 Hints for Compounding Powders

Suggestions to aid in the compounding of powders are as follows:

- A coffee grinder will aid in particle size reduction for small amounts of powder. It can be cleaned with a camel's hair brush, and some grinders can be washed with soap and water.
- Mixing powders with similar particle size and density characteristics in a plastic bag using a spatula will lessen the amount of powder floating around the compounding area.
- Dust masks can be used if a powder is excessively light and escapes into the work area.
- Powder that is too fluffy can be compacted slightly by the addition of a few drops of alcohol, water, or mineral oil.
- Magnesium stearate—less than 1% of the total weight of the mix—can be used to enhance the lubrication and flow characteristics of powders.
- Sodium lauryl sulfate—up to 1%—can be added to powders to neutralize electrostatic forces for powders that tend to float away or are difficult to handle.
- After mixing the powders, pass them through a fine sieve to remove any clumps and produce a fine, textured well-mixed powder.

---

by approximately doubling the portion being mixed with each addition. Mixing can be done in a mortar with a pestle; pill tile with spatula; or a bottle, sieve, sifter, or other suitable device. See Box 11-1 for suggestions on compounding powders.

Mechanical
Mechanical methods of mixing in compounding can include the use of a V-blender, Turbula mixer, and the ResonantAcoustic mixing technology.

V-Blender. This method involves tumbling the powders in a rotating chamber designed to enhance the mixing process. Mixing by this process is thorough but can be time consuming; however, it can be done while performing other duties. The speed of the rotating chamber causes the powders to tumble over and over and not simply slide down the side of the chamber. This type of blender is very widely used in the pharmaceutical industry on a large scale.

Triple V-Type Blender. This V-blender consists of three individual chambers attached to the blender power unit. It allows up to three different blending processes to be conducted simultaneously.

Turbula Mixer. This blender is used to obtain a homogeneous mixing of powders with different specific weights and particle sizes. The powders can be mixed in their own closed container. The efficiency of this shaker-mixer is derived from the use of rotation, translation, and inversion, according to the Schatz geometric theory. The mixing container is subjected to a three-dimensional movement that exposes the product to continuously changing, rhythmically pulsing motion.

ResonantAcoustic Mixing Technology. This technology uses low frequency, high-intensity acoustic energy to establish a uniform shear field throughout the entire mixing container, resulting in rapid fluidization (movement) and dispersion of the material. An oscillating mechanical driver generates motion in the mechanical system that is then acoustically transferred to the material to be mixed. The system operates at resonance, and in this mode, a nearly complete exchange of energy occurs between the mass elements and the spring elements in the mechanical system.

In summary, tumbling devices have numerous advantages. They are relatively easy to use, and the containers can, in some cases, be the ultimate dispensing container. These units revolve at about 40 rpm, which is about half the critical speed wherein the centrifugal force on the particles exceeds the pull of gravity, so there are no complex controls to adjust and so on. They do occupy approximately 4 to 9 sq ft of space on a workbench, but the benefits are many. The technology continues to evolve to produce uniform, homogeneous mixtures of powders for dispensing or for additional processing.

Physicochemical Considerations

Eutectics

Some powders may become sticky or pasty or they may liquefy when mixed together, such as those listed in Table 11-2. To keep the powders dry, one can mix them with a bulky powder adsorbent such as light magnesium oxide or magnesium carbonate. Also, these powders should be triturated very lightly on a pill tile (Figure 11-3) by using a spatula for mixing rather than a mortar and pestle. The latter will cause compression and magnify the problem. Double wrapping the papers may also be advisable. Mixing these powders with the bulky powders first and then performing a light blending can minimize the problem.

Another approach is to make the eutectic first and then adsorb the paste or liquid that results onto a bulky powder. One also has the option of dispensing the ingredients separately. After preparation, the charts can be dispensed in a plastic bag.

Hygroscopic and Deliquescent Powders

Hygroscopic powders will absorb moisture from the air. Deliquescent powders will absorb moisture from the air to the extent that they will partially or wholly liquefy. These problems must be overcome for a powder to be acceptable to a patient and usable. The best approach is to dispense the ingredients in tight containers and incorporate a desiccant packet or capsule when necessary. A patient should be instructed to store the powder in a dry place in a tightly closed container. To lessen the extent of the problem, a compounding pharmacist can in some situations dilute the powder with an inert drying powder to reduce the amount of surface area exposed to moisture. Common hygroscopic and deliquescent powders are listed in Table 11-3.

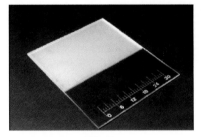

FIGURE 11-3 Pill tile.

TABLE 11-2 Common Substances That Soften or Liquefy When Mixed Together

Acetanilid	Benzocaine	Menthol	Resorcinol
Acetophenetidin	β-naphthol	Phenacetin	Salicylic acid
Aminopyrine	Camphor	Phenol	Thymol
Antipyrine	Chloral hydrate	Phenyl salicylate	
Aspirin	Lidocaine	Prilocaine	

TABLE 11-3 Common Hygroscopic and Deliquescent Powders

Ammonium bromide	Hyoscyamine hydrobromide	Physostigmine sulfate
Ammonium chloride	Hyoscyamine sulfate	Pilocarpine alkaloid
Ammonium iodide	Iron and ammonium citrate	Potassium acetate
Calcium bromide	Lithium bromide	Potassium citrate
Calcium chloride	Pepsin	Sodium bromide
Ephedrine sulfate	Phenobarbital sodium	Sodium iodide
Hydrastine hydrochloride	Physostigmine hydrobromide	Sodium nitrate
Hydrastine sulfate	Physostigmine hydrochloride	Zinc chloride

Efflorescent Powders

An *efflorescent powder* (Table 11-4) is a crystalline powder that contains water of hydration or crystallization. This water can be liberated either during manipulations or on exposure to a low-humidity environment. If this occurs, the powder will become sticky and pasty or it may even liquefy. One approach is to use an anhydrous salt form of the drug, keeping in mind the potency differential between its anhydrous form and its hydrated form. Another method is to include a drying bulky powder and to use a light, noncompacting method of mixing the powders.

Effervescent Salts

Effervescent salts are usually mixtures of effloresced citric acid or tartaric acid, or both, combined with sodium biphosphate or sodium carbonate, or both. These salts can also be prepared by using uneffloresced citric acid and tartaric acid. After the powders are blended, they are placed in an oven at 95°C to 105°C until a pasty mass is formed. The powders liberate their water of crystallization or hydration, forming a moist powder. The mass is then passed through a No. 10–mesh sieve onto a drying tray, where it is dried, broken apart into granules, and packaged. One disadvantage of effervescent powders is their large exposed surface area, which provides for greater reactivity (effervescence) and creates potential stability problems. Granules offer the ability to control the rate of effervescence that occurs when the preparation is added to water. A powder will rapidly effervesce when added to water and may overflow the container. Because granules expose less surface area, they will hydrate and dissolve more slowly, resulting in a slower, more controlled effervescence.

TABLE 11-4 Common Efflorescent Powders

Alums	Codeine phosphate	Scopolamine hydrobromide
Atropine sulfate	Codeine sulfate	Sodium acetate
Caffeine	Ferrous sulfate	Sodium carbonate (decahydrate)
Calcium lactate	Morphine acetate	Sodium phosphate
Citric acid	Quinine bisulfate	Strychnine sulfate
Cocaine	Quinine hydrobromide	Terpin hydrate
Codeine	Quinine hydrochloride	

Explosive Mixtures

Some combinations of powders (Table 11-5) may react violently when mixed together. Special precautions must be taken if one must prepare a formulation containing these mixtures.

Incorporation of Liquids

A liquid that is to be incorporated into a dry powder can be adsorbed onto an inert material (carrier) such as lactose and then geometrically introduced into the bulk of the powder. Pasty material can be added to dry powder by mixing it with increasing quantities of the powder, which will dry out the paste. Adding some materials is best done by preparing an alcoholic solution and spraying it evenly on the powder, which has been spread out on a pill tile.

TABLE 11-5 Common Oxidizing and Reducing Agents That May React Violently When Mixed

Oxidizing Agents	*Reducing Agents*
Bromine	Alcohol
Chlorates	Bisulfites
Chloric acid	Bromides
Chlorine	Charcoal
Chromates	Glycerin
Dichromates	Hydriodic acid
Ethyl nitrite spirit	Hypophosphites
Hydrogen peroxide	Hypophosphorous acid
Hypochlorites	Iodides
Hypochlorous acid	Lactose
Iodine	Nitrites (in some situations)
Nitrates	Organic substances in general
Nitric acid	Phosphorus
Nitrites	Sugar
Nitrohydrochloric acid	Sulfides
Nitrous acid	Sulfites
Perborates	Sulfur
Permanganates	Sulfurous acid
Permanganic acid	Tannic acid
Peroxides	Tannins
Potassium chlorate	Thiosulfates
Potassium dichromate	Volatile oils
Potassium nitrate	
Potassium permanganate	
Sodium peroxide	
Silver nitrate	
Silver oxide	
Silver salts	
Trinitrophenol	

The alcohol, or another suitable solvent, should then be allowed to evaporate, leaving the ingredient uniformly dispersed. This method may be especially suitable for high-potency drugs or flavoring agents because it minimizes the possibility that clumps of active drug will develop in the powder blend.

Quality Control

Bulk Powders

A pharmacist should compare the final weight of the preparation with the theoretical weight. The powder should be examined for uniformity of color, particle size, flowability, and freedom from caking.

Divided Powders

For divided powders, a pharmacist should individually weigh the divided papers and then compare that weight with the theoretical weight. The packets should be checked to confirm uniformity.

Packaging and Dispensing

The powder mixture is packaged according to its use. Bulk oral powders can be packaged in glass, plastic, metal, or other containers that have a wide mouth to allow use of the powder measure. Divided powders, or powder papers, can be individually folded. Topical powders can be poured into sifter-top containers or powder shakers (Figure 11-4), and insufflations can be filled into plastic puffer units.

Techniques for Preparing Charts

Preparing charts requires placing a specific quantity of powder into individual papers. A number of methods can be used to determine the correct quantity, including weighing each powder quantity, blocking and dividing, or using a miniature powder measure. The most accurate method is to weigh each powder quantity, a technique that should be used for potent drugs. Blocking and dividing consists of placing a powder in a smooth, even-depth rectangular pile and using a spatula to cut or divide the pile into the desired number of portions. These portions are then placed on the powder paper for folding and dispensing. A miniature powder measure, when full, will contain the correct quantity of drug required for each dose. One approach to making a miniature powder measure is to glue a handle to a base from the appropriate size capsule that, when full, contains the desired quantity of powder. This device can then be used to measure the doses for a chart. After the dose is placed on the paper, the paper is folded and placed in the dispensing package. In the preparation of powder papers, preparing sufficient powder for one extra paper is common practice, because some of the powder will be lost during the manipulations.

Methods of dispensing divided powder dosage forms have included such traditional approaches as (1) placing the weighed powder onto powder papers, which are then folded and boxed; (2) placing the weighed powder into small zipper storage bags; (3) using a continuous tube of plastic that is then

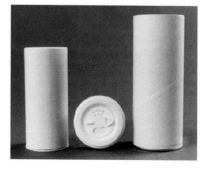

FIGURE 11-4 Powder shaker.

heat sealed to form the bottom of the pouch, after which the weighed powder is introduced and the pouch sealed; and (4) placing self-contained powder papers into a zipper storage bag.

Charts or powder papers can be fashioned from white bond paper, glassine paper, vegetable parchment, waxed paper, or other suitable material. The paper of choice for hygroscopic or deliquescent materials is waxed paper because it is waterproof and its edges can be heat sealed. If limited water resistance is desired, glassine or parchment paper may be satisfactory. Although bond paper has no moisture resistance capability, it has a neat, aesthetic, and pleasing appearance.

A common practice is to double-wrap hygroscopic powders by using glassine, parchment, or waxed paper as the inner wrap and bond paper as the final or outer wrap. Powders containing volatile ingredients should also be double-wrapped to prevent ingredient loss. Double wrapping provides ingredient protection and a uniform, pleasing appearance to the final dosage form. After the papers are folded, they are usually packaged in slide-type boxes or shouldered boxes with either hinged or removable lids. The label directions are placed on or, preferably, inside the lid.

Techniques for Folding Powder Papers

The two common methods of preparing folded papers for compounded powder dosage forms are shown in Figures 11-5 and 11-6.[1,2] The directions and diagrams are provided to aid the novice in visualizing the final folded preparation. These techniques are used to package compounded, individualized powder dosage forms. By following the steps, a pharmacist can, with practice, make a neatly folded preparation.

Storage and Labeling

Powder and granule dosage forms should be stored in dry places. They may also require protection from light, depending on the active drug they contain.

Stability

Because powders are dry, they generally provide a stable dosage form as long as they are protected from moisture and heat. According to *USP* Chapter <795>,[3] powders prepared from a manufactured product should have the beyond-use date of 25% of the time remaining on the product's expiration date or 6 months, whichever is earlier. If the preparation is prepared from USP or NF grade substances, a beyond-use date of 6 months is appropriate, unless evidence is available to support other dating.

Patient Counseling

If bulk oral powders are prescribed, explaining to a patient the exact technique for measuring the dose to be administered and the proper mode of administration is critical. Should the powder be mixed with a liquid? If so, what liquid? Can it be premixed and stored for a day? A week? What happens if some water drops into the package containing the powder? Can the powder be mixed with food(s)? If so, which foods? Hot or cold?

If bulk topical powders are prescribed, a patient should be counseled about the quantity of powder to apply and whether or not rubbing or patting the powder is recommended. What happens if much of the powder falls off the skin? Can a patient safely apply the powder in areas where children will be playing? Does the skin need to be dry? What happens if the skin is sweaty?

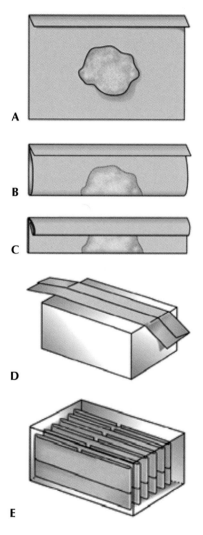

A

B

C

D

E

Fold down the long edge of the paper about ½ inch. Several papers may be folded at one time to save time and promote uniformity. A note of caution: Do not try to fold too many papers at one time because the fold on the top piece of paper will be larger than the fold on the bottom piece of paper. The reason is that the paper will not stretch around corners (Figure 11-5A).

1. Place the papers on the counter in a convenient arrangement, out of the way of wind or drafts, with the folded tops away from but facing the pharmacist.
2. Place the weighed individual doses on the center of each paper (Figure 11-5A).
3. Bring up the lower edge of the paper and insert it completely into the top fold of the powder paper (Figure 11-5B).
4. Fold down the top fold toward the pharmacist until the paper fits exactly to the top of the powder box. This can be approximated by folding the paper until the remainder of the paper is divided approximately in half (Figure 11-5C).
5. Center the folded paper lengthwise over an open powder box of the size intended to be used. (Note: The center of the box, as well as the paper, should be marked with a pencil on its edge to remove any guesswork associated with this measurement.) Fold the equal overhanging ends down while pressing in on the sides of the box. Fold cautiously because pressing too hard may bend the box; however, adequate pressure must be applied to allow the powder paper to fit snugly, without bending, when placed into the box (Figure 11-5D).
6. Fold back the ends of the powder paper completely, and sharply crease the end folds with a clean spatula to make a permanent fold. All of the ends of the powder papers should lie on a straight line.
7. Place the filled powder papers into the box, with the folds away from the pharmacist (Figure 11-5E). Usually, all top folds are up. However, on occasion, they may be alternately up and down. The appearance may not be as neat with this latter procedure, but more folded papers can be placed into the box and there is less tendency for several papers to pop out when a single powder is removed.

FIGURE 11-5 Folding technique for a traditional powder paper.

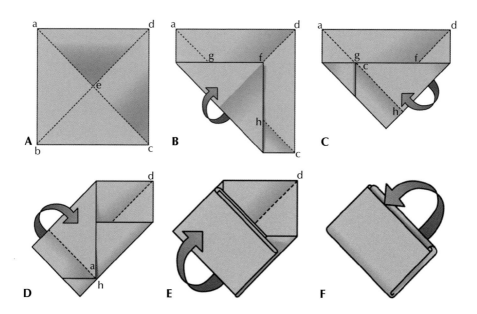

1. Use a square piece of powder paper. (Note: If the powder is to be double-wrapped, then both papers must be folded together.) Fold the paper diagonally from point a to point c and then again from point b to point d. When the paper is unfolded, the two diagonal lines will meet at point e. Take point d and fold in to point e to give point f. Unfold the paper to the open position (Figure 11-6A).
2. Bring point b to point f and crease, using a spatula. The fold intersects the ac diagonal line at point g (Figure 11-6B).
3. Bring point c to point g and crease, using a spatula. The fold intersects the ac diagonal line at point h (Figure 11-6C).
4. Bring point a to point h and crease, using a spatula. This fold forms an elongated envelope (Figure 11-6D).
5. Bring the bottom of the envelope up so that it divides it into thirds and leaves the flap to be tucked into the envelope after filling (Figure 11-6E).
6. Place the weighed powder dose into the envelope.
7. Tuck point d into the opening at the bottom, which was previously brought up to form the envelope. This secures the powder packet, which can then be placed into a zipper storage bag and labeled appropriately with the physician's directions (Figure 11-6F).

FIGURE 11-6 Folding technique for a self-contained powder paper.

Sample Formulations

℞ Bulk Oral Powder

Dextrose	25 g	Active
Sodium chloride	2.5 g	Active
Potassium citrate	4.5 g	Active

For electrolyte and rehydration solution

1. Calculate the quantity of each ingredient required for the prescription.
2. Accurately weigh each ingredient.
3. Mix the powders together.
4. Place in container.
5. Label product to be diluted to 1000 mL for drinking.

℞ Bulk Topical Powder

Menthol	0.1 g	Active
Camphor	0.2 g	Active
Zinc stearate	0.8 g	Adherent
Zinc oxide	8 g	Adherent/Astringent
Talc	31 g	Vehicle/Protectant

Make dusting powder.

1. Calculate the quantity of each ingredient required for the prescription.
2. Accurately weigh each ingredient.
3. Mix the menthol and camphor together to form a liquid (eutectic).
4. Mix the zinc stearate, zinc oxide, and talc by geometric dilution.
5. Incorporate the powders into the liquid geometrically, and mix well.
6. Package and label the product.

℞ Divided Oral Powder

Scopolamine hydrobromide	5 mg	Active
Lactose	2.495 g	Vehicle

Prepare 10 powder papers.

1. Calculate the quantity of each ingredient required for the prescription.
2. Accurately weigh each ingredient. (Note: Depending on the total quantity to be prepared, preparing a dilution of the scopolamine hydrobromide to accurately obtain the 5 mg may be necessary.)
3. Geometrically incorporate the lactose into the scopolamine hydrobromide.
4. Place 250 mg of the mixture onto each of 10 powder papers.
5. Package and label the product.

℞ Powdered Dentifrice

Triclosan	1 g	Active
Precipitated calcium carbonate	98 g	Active
Sodium lauryl sulfate	0.4 g	Active/Surfactant
Saccharin sodium	0.2 g	Sweetener
Peppermint oil	0.4 mL	Flavor
Cinnamon oil	0.2 mL	Flavor
Wintergreen oil	0.8 mL	Flavor

Prepare tooth powder.

1. Calculate the quantity of each ingredient required for the prescription.
2. Accurately weigh each ingredient.
3. Mix the triclosan, sodium lauryl sulfate, and saccharin sodium together.
4. Geometrically incorporate the mixture into the precipitated calcium carbonate.
5. Mix the oils together.
6. Incorporate the powder into the oil geometrically, and mix until uniform.
7. Package and label the product.

℞ Powdered Douche

Boric acid	80 g	Active
Ammonium aluminum sulfate	15 g	Active
Tannic acid	0.5 g	Active
Sodium lauryl sulfate	0.5 g	Surfactant
Thymol	0.3 g	Active/Aromatic
Phenol	0.2 g	Active/Aromatic
Menthol	0.5 g	Active/Aromatic

Prepare douche powder.

1. Calculate the quantity of each ingredient required for the prescription.
2. Accurately weigh each ingredient.
3. Mix the boric acid, ammonium aluminum sulfate, tannic acid, and sodium lauryl sulfate together. (Note: Boric acid powder should be used.)
4. Mix the thymol, phenol, and menthol together to form a liquid.
5. Geometrically incorporate the powder mixture from step 3 into the liquid, and mix thoroughly.
6. Package and label the product.

℞ Misoprostol 0.0027% Mucoadhesive Powder

Misoprostol	400 µg	Active
Polyethylene oxide (Polyox 301)	200 mg	Vehicle/Adherent
Hydroxypropyl methylcellulose (Methocel E4M)	qs 15 g	Vehicle

1. Calculate the quantity of each ingredient required for the prescription.
2. Obtain two misoprostol 200 µg tablets.
3. Accurately weigh each of the other ingredients.
4. Pulverize the misoprostol tablets to a very fine powder.
5. Add the polyethylene oxide (Polyox 301) followed by the hydroxypropyl methylcellulose (Methocel E4M), and mix well. (Note: Using only materials of approximately the same particle size is important.)
6. Package and label the product.

℞ Adhesive Hydrating Powder

Carboxymethylcellulose sodium	35 g	Vehicle/Carrier
Polyox WSR-301	15 g	Adherent
Calcium phosphate	50 g	Vehicle/Carrier

1. Calculate the quantity of each ingredient required for the prescription.
2. Accurately weigh each of the ingredients.
3. Geometrically, add the carboxymethylcellulose sodium to the Polyox WSR-301 powder using a pill tile and spatula or a mortar and pestle.
4. Incorporate the calcium phosphate geometrically, and mix well.
5. Package and label the product.

References

1. Dittert LW. *Sprowl's American Pharmacy.* 7th ed. Philadelphia: Lippincott; 1974:316–7.
2. Hendrickson R, ed. *Remington: The Science and Practice of Pharmacy.* 21st ed. Baltimore: Lippincott Williams & Wilkins; 2006:718–9.
3. United States Pharmacopeial Convention. Chapter <795>, Pharmaceutical compounding—nonsterile preparations. In: *United States Pharmacopeia/National Formulary.* Rockville, MD: United States Pharmacopeial Convention; current edition.

Chapter 12

Capsules

The most versatile of all dosage forms is probably the capsule. Capsules have been used for more than a century and have an important role in drug delivery. In addition to being relatively easy to manufacture, they are amenable to small-scale compounding by a pharmacist, who is able to prepare specific formulations for individual patient needs. The process of designing and developing preparations is aided by new excipients that not only can improve bioavailability and ensure site-specific release of the preparation, but also can enhance the elegance of this popular dosage form. When a primary care provider prescribes a tablet, the choice is usually, but not always, limited to commercially available products. However, a capsule can be prepared extemporaneously, which provides dosing flexibility for a primary care provider and pharmacist. Capsules can be prepared to be elegant, convenient, and easily identifiable; they are available in many different sizes, shapes, and colors.

Definitions and Types

Dosage forms in which unit doses of powder, semisolid, or liquid drugs are enclosed in either a hard or a soft envelope, or shell, are called capsules. Usually, the shells are composed of gelatin. Capsules are generally of the hard-gelatin or soft-gelatin type. Hard-gelatin capsules can be prepared to release the drug rapidly or over a predetermined time, whereas soft-gelatin capsules usually provide standard release.

Hard-gelatin capsules consist of two parts: the base or body, which is longer and has a smaller diameter, and the cap, which is shorter and has a slightly larger diameter. The cap is designed to slide over the base portion and form a snug seal.

This dosage form is intended to be swallowed whole. Only with the concurrence of a pharmacist should capsules be opened and the contents administered in food or liquids.

Historical Use

Mothes, a French pharmacist, invented the soft-gelatin capsule in 1833; Dublanc made improvements to this invention. Patents were issued to both inventors in 1834. Lehuby developed the hard-gelatin capsule, for which a patent was issued in 1846, and in 1848 Murdock created a two-piece hard-gelatin capsule, which was patented in 1865. Initially, the rate of usage and acceptance of capsules was low. During the 1900s, however, a growing number of drugs became available in solid powder form in dosages that could be easily administered orally, leading to a phenomenal increase in the capsule's popularity. This dosage form was included for the first time in the 12th revision of the *United States Pharmacopeia (USP)*.

Because they can be prepared in many colors, capsules are considered elegant and make an agreeable presentation for administration to a patient. They are popular also because they conceal taste. Their portability, light weight, and rapid drug release have contributed to their increased use.

Applications

In recent years, pharmacists have been preparing ever-greater numbers of capsules extemporaneously. This growth may be due to several marketplace factors. First, low volume has forced some manufacturers to take certain drug products off the market. A pharmacist, who has access to the pure drug chemical or another dosage form of the drug, can easily prepare the required formulation to serve the needs of an individual primary care provider and patient. Second, some patients cannot swallow a tablet but can swallow a capsule. To aid these individuals, a pharmacist can convert many tablets into a capsule dosage form. Third, capsules enable a primary care provider and pharmacist to combine several drug products into one dosage form to minimize the number of prescription medications to be taken by a patient. With only one dosage form instead of several, patients are more likely to adhere to their regimens and thus have more positive therapeutic outcomes. Finally, the proper formulation of a capsule can affect the release of a drug preparation; that is, it can slow down or speed up the release.

The primary application of capsules is the oral administration of drugs. The capsule incorporates drugs that might have an unpleasant odor or taste within a practically tasteless shell that dissolves or digests in the stomach after about 10 to 20 minutes.

Capsules can be administered rectally or vaginally if the capsule is pierced with a pin or needle to allow aqueous body fluids to penetrate the capsule and dissolve its contents more easily. In these instances, excipients that are highly water soluble should be used, because hydrophobic materials may release a smaller quantity of the drug than is desired.

Capsules are not suitable for drugs that are very soluble, such as salts (e.g., potassium chloride, potassium bromide, ammonium chloride). With such drugs, the fluid penetrating the capsule rapidly dissolves the salt and creates a highly concentrated solution that may cause nausea and vomiting when it comes in contact with the gastric mucosa.

Capsules are also not appropriate for strongly efflorescent or deliquescent materials. An efflorescent material may cause the capsule to soften when water is lost, whereas a strongly deliquescent powder may make the shell of the capsule brittle when the powder extracts its moisture.

Composition

Hard-gelatin capsules are actually cartridges, shells, or envelopes that are designed to serve as a carrier for a drug preparation. Their primary ingredients are gelatin, sugar, and water, but they may contain a dye or an opacifying agent, or both. Hard-gelatin capsules may also contain about 0.15% sulfur dioxide to prevent decomposition. Soft-gelatin, or elastic, capsules are prepared from gelatin, glycerin, and water and can be filled with a liquid, suspension, or powder. The hard- and soft-gelatin capsules protect the ingredients from direct exposure to the atmosphere before administration and provide a barrier so that a patient will not taste the enclosed contents. After reaching the gastrointestinal tract, capsules may release their contents at different rates based on the physicochemical properties of the active drug and the excipients.

Colored capsules are available in almost any form and combination: solid colors (base and cap are the same color) or mixed colors (base and cap are different colors). Special orders of almost any color can be prepared. In addition, a pharmacist can add an approved dye to the powdered material and place the colored powder inside a clear capsule if colored capsules are not available. Double-blind (DB) capsules are available for research purposes. These capsules are opaque and slightly larger in diameter than routine capsules. They are often used in studies in which small tablets or capsules are placed inside the DB capsule, which is then closed and locked.

Preparation

Source of Equipment and Materials

Materials for the extemporaneous preparation of capsules can be obtained from a variety of sources. Equipment for preparing up to 300 capsules at a time is available at a reasonable cost. Some of the equipment already on hand in a pharmacy can be used for preparing capsules and for carrying out related quality control procedures.

Sources of drugs for capsules include the pure powder, tablets, capsules, and even liquids. Pure powders, which are generally used in their original state, present the fewest complications. Tablets usually must be finely comminuted before they can be incorporated into the capsule powder mix. Obviously, only immediate-release tablets should be used, not altered- or controlled-release tablets. Capsules can be a source of the drug if one opens the capsule shell and uses the contents. Closed capsules, which have gelatin bands, seals, or locking mechanisms, provide a greater challenge. They should be cut into two pieces with a clean razor blade to remove the powder. Some pharmacists, however, break up the capsules in a mortar and then separate the powder from the shell fragments by passing it through a sieve. Liquids can be evaporated to dryness by using appropriate means, or they can be soaked up with an adsorbent before their incorporation into the capsule powder mix. Injectable preparations can be reconstituted and used, but they may be somewhat more expensive as a source of the active ingredient.

Preparation of the Powder

To prepare the powder, one must first weigh or measure the individual ingredients. Preparation of a sufficient quantity to produce an extra capsule or an additional 5% to 10% of the formulation is best, because it will allow for any loss of powder during manipulations. However, preparing excess quantity does not apply to controlled drug substances. The particle sizes of solid ingredients should be reduced by comminution to approximately the same size range. The powders should then be passed through a sieve (Nos. 60 to 100 mesh, depending on the powders). Then the preparation should be mixed by geometric dilution to ensure that the active drugs are distributed uniformly throughout the mix. If the powders are light and fluffy and difficult to manage, a few drops of alcohol, water, or mineral oil can be added to improve workability. The choice of material to add depends on the powders involved; usually, one or two drops of liquid are sufficient. Personal safety may dictate that a mask or other protective gear be worn. Whichever method is used, the primary goal in mixing ingredients is homogeneity.

Capsule Size Selection

For human consumption, eight sizes of gelatin capsules are in general use, ranging from the smallest, No. 5, through the largest, No. 000 (Table 12-1). The numerical designations are arbitrary and do not indicate a capsule's capacity. The capacity of a capsule depends on the density and characteristics of the powders it contains. The capsule size offers only a relative volume designation. Examples of the weights of materials that can be held by capsules are shown in Table 12-2. Selected physicochemical properties of some capsule diluents are shown in Table 12-3.

Veterinary compounding has increased dramatically in recent years. Capsules for veterinary use are available in sizes designated as No. 10, No. 11, and No. 12, with capacities of 1 oz, 1/2 oz, and 1/4 oz, respectively.

In general, capsules can be used to encapsulate between 65 and 1000 mg of powdered material. Capsule selection is usually a simple matter. Some patients may have difficulty swallowing larger capsules (No. 00, No. 000), but others, especially patients of advanced age, may find smaller capsules (No. 5, No. 4) difficult to handle. The capsule size selected should be slightly larger than is needed to hold the powder; additional powder will be added to produce a full capsule. Compounding pharmacists have ways of compensating for problems with swallowing or handling capsules. If the active drug powder bulk is large, the total amount can be divided into two smaller capsules that are easier to swallow. If the powder bulk is small, more diluent can be added to increase the size of a capsule for handling convenience.

TABLE 12-1 Approximate Capacities of Capsules (in milliliters)

Size	Capacity (mL)
Human	
5	0.12
4	0.21
3	0.30
2	0.37
1	0.50
0	0.67
00	0.95
000	1.36
Veterinary	
10	30
11	15
12	7.5

TABLE 12-2 Weights of Powder Material by Capsule Size[a]

Powder Material	Weight (mg) by Capsule Size							
	5	4	3	2	1	0	00	000
Acetaminophen	130	180	240	310	420	540	750	1100
Aluminum hydroxide	180	270	360	470	640	820	1140	1710
Ascorbic acid	130	220	310	400	520	700	980	1420
Aspirin	65	130	195	260	325	490	650	975
Bismuth subnitrate	120	250	400	550	650	800	1200	1750
Calcium carbonate	120	200	280	350	460	600	790	1140
Calcium lactate	110	160	210	260	330	460	570	800
Cornstarch	130	200	270	340	440	580	800	1150
Lactose	140	210	280	350	460	600	850	1250
Quinine sulfate	65	97	130	195	227	325	390	650
Sodium bicarbonate	130	260	325	390	510	715	975	1430

[a]Depending on the actual powder density.

TABLE 12-3 Physicochemical Characteristics of Selected Capsule and Tablet Diluents

Diluent[a]	Density (g/mL)	Bulk Density (g/mL)	Tapped Density (g/mL)	Melting Point (°C)	pH (concentration)	Hygroscopic?
Calcium carbonate	2.70	0.80	1.2	825[b]	—	—
Calcium phosphate, dibasic						
Anhydrous	2.89	0.78	0.82	—	7.3 (20%)	No
Hydrate	2.39	0.92	1.17	—	7.4 (20%)	No
Calcium phosphate, tribasic	3.14	0.80	0.95	1670	6.8 (20%)	—
Calcium sulfate						
Anhydrous	2.96	0.70	1.28	1450	10.4 (10%)	Yes
Dihydrate	2.32	0.67	1.12	—	7.3 (10%)	No
Cellulose, microcrystalline	1.59	0.34	0.48	260–270 (chars)	5–7	Yes
Cellulose, powdered	1.50	0.14–0.39	0.21–0.48	—	4–7.5 (10%)	Little
Dextrates	1.54	0.68	0.72	141	3.8–5.8 (20%)	—
Dextrin	1.50–1.59	0.80	0.91	178[b]	—	—
Dextrose excipient	1.54	0.83	1.00	83	3.5–5.5 (20%)	No
Fructose	1.58	—	—	102–105	5.35 (9%)	Yes
Kaolin	2.60	—	—	—	—	—
Lactitol	1.54	—	—	—	4.5–7 (10%)	No
Lactose	1.55	0.62	0.94	202	—	No
Mannitol	1.51	0.43	0.73	166–168	—	No
Sorbitol	1.50	0.45	0.40	110–112	4.5–7 (10%)	Yes
Starch	1.48	0.46	0.66	—	5.5–6.5 (2%)	Yes
Starch, pregelatinized	1.52	0.59	0.88	—	4.5–7.0 (10%)	Yes
Sucrose	1.6	0.60	0.82	160–186[b]	—	Yes
Sugar, compressible	—	0.49	0.60	—	—	Yes
Sugar, confectioner's	—	0.47	0.83	—	—	Yes

— = Not available.
[a]All are stable. Lactose and sorbitol require a tightly closed container; all others require a well-closed container.
[b]Ingredient melts with some decomposition.

The Rule of Sixes is a method for the extemporaneous filling of conventional hard-gelatin capsules. The steps are as follows:

1. Set up six "6s."	6	6	6	6	6	6
2. List the capsule size.	0	1	2	3	4	5

3. Subtract values in step 2 from those in step 1 to determine the average fill weight in grains.

	6	5	4	3	2	1

4. Convert fill weight to grams (1 grain = 0.065 g).

	0.390	0.325	0.260	0.195	0.130	0.065

5. Determine fill volume in milliliters (see Table 12-4).

	0.67	0.50	0.37	0.30	0.21	0.12

6. Calculate and list average capsule fill density (divide weight values in step 4 by volume values in step 5).

	0.58	0.65	0.70	0.65	0.62	0.54

As can be seen, the average fill density of the capsules is about 0.62 g/mL.

Table 12-4 gives the bulk densities of typical active drugs and excipients. The bulk densities of most of these materials are within the range of 0.4 and 0.8 g/mL, for an average 0.6 g/mL, which is close to the fill density of empty, two-piece, hard-gelatin capsules; therefore, the fill density forms the basis for the Rule of Sixes.

The bulk density of a powder is determined by adding a known weight of powder mix to a 100-mL graduated cylinder and measuring the volume. For example, if 75 g of powder is added to a 100-mL graduated cylinder and occupies 100 mL volume, the powder's bulk density is 75 g/100 mL, or 0.75 g/mL. However, if the cylinder is gently tapped on a padded counter surface 100 to 200 times, the powder will settle and occupy less volume. If the weight is divided by this new volume, a new measurement, known as the *tapped density* or *packed bulk density,* is obtained. If the new volume is now 85 mL, then the tapped density is 75 g/85 mL, or 0.88 g/mL. Figure 12-1 illustrates the effect of tapping on the bulk density of a powder. The difference between the bulk density and the tapped density is used to determine the approximate compressibility of the powder mix in percentages.

The percentage of compressibility is determined by subtracting the ratio of the bulk density divided by the tapped bulk density from 1 and multiplying by 100, as shown here using the values in the previous example: $1 - (0.75/0.88) \times 100 = 14.8\%$ compressibility. This information can be used to estimate the quantity of powder that can be placed into the overfill capacity of empty, two-piece, hard-gelatin capsules. As the percentage of compressibility increases, more powder mix can be placed inside the empty capsule. This information should aid in calculating the size of capsules to be used for various powder mixes.[1]

Another general rule that can be used in selecting capsule size is the Rule of Seven. This rule has several easy steps: (1) convert the weight of the powder per capsule to grains, (2) subtract the number of grains from 7, and (3) match the result with the following listing:

If the resulting number is	Then choose capsule size
−3	000
−2	00
−1 or 0	0
+1	1
+2	2
+3	3
+4	4
+5	5

TABLE 12-4 Bulk Densities of Typical Active Drugs and Excipients

Material	Bulk Density (g/mL)
Activated charcoal	0.32
Aluminum magnesium silicate	0.34
Ascorbic acid	0.51, 0.72
Barium sulfate	0.96
Bentonite	0.8, 0.96
Cab-O-Sil	0.03
Calcium carbonate	0.7
Calcium phosphate	0.77
Calcium sulfate	0.72
Cellulose derivatives	0.41, 0.43, 0.45, 0.72
Citric acid	0.77
Cornstarch	0.64, 0.67, 0.69
Dextrose	0.58, 0.62
FDC dye mixes	0.62
Kaolin	0.80
Magnesium carbonate	0.19
Magnesium oxide	1.04
Magnesium stearate	0.33
Maltodextrin	0.48
Mannitol	0.61
Meprobamate	0.56
Pentaerythritol	0.7
Sodium bicarbonate	0.80, 0.99
Sodium chloride	1.28
Sodium phosphate	1.28
Sodium sulfate	1.36
Sucrose	0.56, 0.85
Talc	0.56
Thiamine hydrochloride	0.75
Titanium dioxide	0.77
Urea	0.62
Vitamin mixes	0.56, 0.67, 0.70
Zinc oxide	0.88

Source: *Dry Materials Feeding Handbook.* Whitewater, WI: AccuRate Bulk Solids Metering.

If, for example, the weight of powder per capsule is 325 mg (5 grains), then $7 - 5 = 2$. The capsule size is 2.

This method does not work if the resulting number is higher than 5 or lower than 3. Nevertheless, because it is quick and easy, it serves as a good beginning point for the preparation of hard-gelatin capsules.[2]

In selecting the size of a capsule, one should be aware that the required quantity of powder is to be held in the base of the capsule, with the cap simply ensuring powder retention.

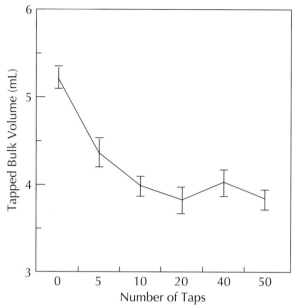

FIGURE 12-1 Tapped bulk volume decreases with number of taps used. Observations are mean ± standard error.

After the cap is in place, the capsule can be tapped to spread the contents throughout the entire capsule if a clear capsule is used.

Once the proper capsule size has been selected, the entire quantity of capsules required for the specific prescription should be removed from bulk stock. The container should then be closed to reduce any risk of contamination.

Encapsulation Process

Two general methods of encapsulation of powders are commonly used today: individual hand filling and capsule-machine filling. These approaches for encapsulating powders and methods for encapsulating semisolids and liquids are described in the following sections.

Filling Capsules Individually by Hand

When hand filling, a pharmacist should arrange the powder on a suitable surface using a spatula so that the thickness of the pile is about one-third the length of the capsule body. A pharmacist's hands should not touch the powder while punching the capsules. Wearing gloves or finger cots will minimize contact with the powder and prevent fingerprints from appearing on the capsules. Another option is to slip the cap from a second capsule over the base of the capsule to be filled (the filling capsule). The second cap thus acts as a holder. Using this technique, the compounding pharmacist does not touch the capsules directly.

As the capsule is pressed into the powder on the working surface, the pharmacist should rotate it slightly to pack the powder in the capsule. When the capsule is full, the pharmacist will feel a slight resistance as the capsule is pressed through the powder. After a few capsules have been filled and weighed, the pharmacist will usually develop a feel for how much resistance is required for the capsule to be full.

After the capsule has been filled according to this method, the pharmacist should check its weight and then add or remove powder to obtain the weight desired. Weighing should be performed on a pharmaceutical or electronic laboratory balance by using an empty gelatin capsule of the same size as a tare.

An alternative method involves blocking and dividing the powder into individual portions for each capsule. This approach results in an approximation, which is not always accurate and thus is not recommended.

Some powders will not stick in the capsules when they are punched out. One way to solve this problem is to place the capsule base on its side and use a spatula to guide or fill the powder. Care must be taken to ensure that the capsule is not scraped or scratched.

Granular materials are particularly difficult to punch into capsules because they are not adequately cohesive. Reducing the particle size to the point at which the powders become more cohesive may alleviate the problem.

Filling Capsules by Machine

A number of manually operated capsule-filling devices are commercially available for filling up to 50, 100, or 300 capsules at a time (Figure 12-2). These machines can be used for preparing smaller quantities by blocking off unused holes with an index card or self-sticking note.

Using these machines requires a careful determination of the capsule formulation. The powder is blended as previously discussed. Empty gelatin capsules are placed into the device so that the cap is on top. The machine is worked to separate the base from the cap, and the portion of the machine holding the caps is removed and set aside. The capsule bases are allowed to drop into place so that the top of the base is flush with the working surface.

The powder mix is then spread over the working surface. A plastic scraper can be used to spread the powder evenly into the capsule bases. The plastic scraper should be held perpendicular to the plate to allow the powder to simply fall into the empty capsule shells by gravity. The plastic scraper should not be used to push the powder into the capsule shell; if this occurs, varying quantities of powder will be forced into the shells. A special tamper is designed for the purpose of compressing the powder in the shell. Before using a tamper, a pharmacist moves the excess powder by scraping it to one side of the capsule plate; the tamper is then used in the cleaned area. The excess powder is moved over the tamped shells, and the remaining shells are tamped. The plastic scraper is then used to move the excess powder over the shells, allowing them to again fill by gravity. The tamping process is repeated as required until all

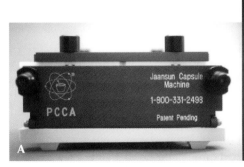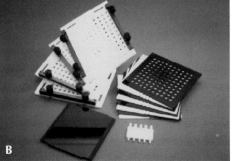

FIGURE 12-2 A: Jaansun capsule machine; B: Base unit for capsule sizes Nos. 00, 0, 1, and 3.

the powder is filled into the capsules. If any excess powder is built up on some of the capsules before tamping, those capsules may receive more powder than others; therefore, the process just described should result in less variation in capsule fill.

Alternatively, a capsule vibrator machine can be used to help compress the powder in the capsules. The entire capsule plate is set on the machine, and the rate of vibration is slowly increased to allow the powder to settle in the capsule shells. This can be repeated until the desired quantity of powder is filled into the shells.

After filling, the portion of the machine holding the capsule caps is fitted over the machine and fixed in place. The filled capsules are capped, removed, dusted with a clean cloth, and packaged.

Filling Capsules with a Semisolid Mass

Producing a capsule containing a semisolid material requires a different approach. Two methods are used to place semisolid materials into hard-gelatin capsules: forming a pipe or pouring a melt.

Material that is sufficiently plastic can be rolled to form a pipe with a diameter slightly less than that of the inner diameter of the capsule in which it will be enclosed. The quantity of material desired is cut with a spatula or knife, with the length removed determining the weight of the material to be enclosed in the capsule shell. The pieces can be dusted with cornstarch and then inserted individually into the capsules.

If a material is too fluid, cornstarch or a similar material can be added to achieve a firmer consistency. The quantity to add can be determined empirically.

If the material is too firm to roll into a pipe but its melting point is in a satisfactory temperature range, it can be melted until it is fluid and then poured into the bases of the gelatin capsules. After the capsules have cooled, the caps are replaced. When this technique is used, using a stand to hold the capsule bodies is helpful. The stand can be made by drilling holes slightly larger than the diameter of the caps into a block of wood or plastic. Caps are inserted into the holes and glued in place to prevent any scratching of the capsule bodies. The bases and caps of the required quantity of capsules are separated. The capsule bases are then inserted into the stationary caps, and the melt is poured into the bases and allowed to cool. The separated caps are placed on the bases, and the completed capsules are removed from the holder.

This method can also be used to enhance the bioavailability of drugs that are poorly soluble and exhibit bioavailability problems. In these cases, the drug is added to a melt of a material such as polyethylene glycol (PEG). The mixture is heated and stirred until the powder is either melted or thoroughly mixed in the PEG. After the melt is cooled to just above the melting point of the PEG, it is poured into the capsule shells as described. When this method is used, the desired quantities can be measured using a pipet, syringe, or calibrated dropper to deliver the volume to the individual capsules. Excipients useful in formulating these preparations are shown in Table 12-5.

Filling Capsules with Liquids

Occasionally, pharmacists must prepare hard-gelatin capsules containing liquid materials. This task can be accomplished easily as long as the liquid material does not dissolve the gelatin. The method should work with alcoholic solutions, fixed oils, or volatile oils because gelatin is not soluble in these materials. A partially hydrogenated cottonseed oil can be used as a vehicle because it has a low melting point, oil-soluble drugs are soluble in it, and it is a solid at room temperature. Experimentation may be required, however, to determine the solubility of the gelatin in the liquid.

This approach calls for the liquid to be measured accurately with a pipet (micropipet) or a calibrated dropper and then dropped into the capsule base, with care not to touch the

TABLE 12-5 Excipients Used as Matrices for Semisolid Capsules

Vegetable Oils	*Animal Fats*	*Esters*
Cottonseed	Beeswax	Ethyl oleate
Maize	Lanolin	Glycol stearates
Nut	Spermaceti	Isopropyl myristate
Olive	*Hydrocarbons*	*Mixed Esters*
Soya	Paraffin	Liquid
Hydrogenated Vegetable Oils	*Fatty Alcohols*	Labrafil
Castor	Cetyl	Miglyol 812
Coconut	Lauryl	Solid
Cottonseed	Stearyl	Suppocire
Palm	*Fatty Acids*	Witepsol
Soya	Lauryl	
Vegetable Fats	Myristic	
Carnauba wax	Palmitic	
Cocoa butter	Stearic	

opening. To soften the gelatin at the opening of the caps, one can either touch the gelatin cap, open end down, to a moist towel or dip a cotton swab in warm water and then rub it around the edge of the cap. The cap is placed over the base containing the liquid with a slight twist, enabling the softened edge of the cap to form a seal with the base to prevent leakage. Before the capsules are packaged, they should be placed on a clean, dry sheet of paper to check for leakage. Sealing can also be accomplished by painting a warm gelatin solution around the capsule, as well as along the inside of the cap, before placing the cap on the base.

Cleaning Capsules

A compounding pharmacist must take every precaution to minimize traces of moisture or body oils on capsules because moisture causes powders to stick to the surface, creating an unsightly appearance and a disagreeable taste. Cleaning the capsules is difficult if they become moist or sticky. The use of gloves ensures that the working environment is hygienic and helps preserve the capsule's dry, shiny appearance.

If gloves are not available, a pharmacist should (1) wash and dry hands thoroughly, (2) keep the fingers dry by stripping a towel through tightly clenched fingers until friction develops and a clearly perceptible heat is generated, and (3) prepare four or five capsules before repeating the hand-cleaning procedure.

If the capsules have been kept dry, clinging surface powder can be removed by rolling the capsules between the folds of a cloth or shaking them in a cloth that has been formed into a bag or hammock. Another method of cleaning capsules is to place them in a container filled with sodium bicarbonate, sugar, or salt and then gently roll the container. The contents are next poured into a No. 10–mesh sieve, which allows the cleaning salt to pass through but retains the capsules.

These cleaning methods are effective only if the capsules have been kept clean and dry. Once capsules have become soiled and dull, they cannot be effectively cleaned.

See Box 12-1 for additional tips for preparing capsules.

BOX 12-1 Hints for Compounding Capsules

Recommendations for compounding capsules are as follows:

- Sodium lauryl sulfate, up to 1%, can be added to powders to neutralize electrostatic forces.
- Capsules may be colored by adding a dye to the powder before it is placed in a clear capsule. This helps distinguish various strengths of powders and capsules. Also, mixing bases and caps of different-colored capsules customizes the colors. Using two capsule machines for this process is best.
- Liquids can be incorporated into capsules by mixing with melted polyethylene glycol 6000 or 8000 or a related concentration of this substance. The mixture can be poured into capsules, where it will solidify. The capsules can then be closed and dispensed.
- Liquids can be dispensed in capsules by using a syringe to drop the liquid into the capsule base. Oils can be mixed with a fat or fatty acid, such as cocoa butter, and slightly heated. The mixture can then be poured into capsules.
- The locking-type capsules available today minimize the loss of their contents, whether powder, liquid, or semisolid; they also work well with hand-operated capsule-filling machines.

Physicochemical Considerations

Physical and chemical interactions between active drugs, between active drugs and excipients, and between active drugs and excipients and the gelatin shell must be considered. For example, hard-gelatin capsules normally contain about 10% to 15% moisture, yet gelatin can absorb up to 10 times its weight in water. Capsules stored in high humidity absorb moisture and can become misshapen. If stored in low humidity, they become dry and brittle and can crack. A relative humidity range of 30% to 45% is best for good encapsulation. If the drug to be encapsulated requires a drier environment, such an environment should be provided.

Various agents can be added to improve the characteristics of the material used in the preparation or administration of a capsule. Magnesium stearate is sometimes used to enhance the flowability of particles, which allows capsules to be filled more easily. Although it is usually present at concentrations less than 1%, it is hydrophobic and can affect the bioavailability of a drug. Thus, up to 1% of sodium lauryl sulfate can be incorporated to enhance the bioavailability of drugs contained within capsules.

Deliquescent powders can be prepared by adding a finely powdered bulking material such as starch or magnesium oxide. This practice lessens the tendency of the powders to absorb moisture.

Eutectic mixtures can be incorporated into capsules by keeping the problematic ingredients separate, adding an inert powder, and mixing lightly before encapsulating the ingredients. Also, using the next-larger size capsule will decrease the contact of the powder particles with each other and hence minimize their tendency to liquefy. Materials that help to prevent or correct eutectics are included in Table 12-6, together with other excipients that are useful in capsule preparation. An alternative technique is first to form the eutectic and subsequently absorb the liquid into a powder, which is then encapsulated.

TABLE 12-6 Useful Excipients in Capsule Preparation

Excipients That Enhance Compatibility of Eutectic Mixtures	Excipients Used as Diluents for Other Purposes in Capsules
Effective	Bentonite
Magnesium carbonate	Calcium carbonate
Kaolin	Lactose
Light magnesium oxide	Mannitol
Less effective	Magnesium carbonate
Heavy magnesium oxide	Magnesium oxide
Tribasic calcium phosphate	Silica gel
Silica gel	Starch
Relatively ineffective	Talc
Talc	Tapioca powder
Lactose	
Starch	

Capsules within Capsules

If one ingredient must be separated from the others in a formulation, a pharmacist may have to fill a small capsule, such as a size No. 5, with one powder and then place that capsule, together with the remaining ingredients, within a larger capsule. For elegance, the inside capsule should not be visible through the larger capsule.

Tablets within Capsules

If a small tablet containing a necessary ingredient is commercially available, it can be placed inside the capsule. A small quantity of the additional powder should be deposited in the base before and after adding the tablet. The inside tablet should not be visible through the filled capsule.

Altered-Release Capsules

The rate of release of a capsule's contents will vary according to the nature of the drug and the capsule's excipients. If the drug is water soluble and a fast release is desired, the excipients should be hydrophilic and neutral. If a slow release of a water-soluble drug is desired, the excipients should be hydrophobic to delay the rate at which the drug dissolves. If the drug is insoluble in water and a fast release is desired, hydrophilic excipients should be used. Release of a drug may be slowed by adding hydrophobic and neutral excipients or gel-forming excipients.

Rapid-Release Capsules

A more rapid or immediate release of the capsule contents can be accomplished by piercing holes in the capsule to allow faster penetration of fluids in the gastrointestinal tract or by adding a small quantity of sodium bicarbonate and citric acid to help open the capsule through the production of carbon dioxide. Adding 0.1% to 1% of sodium lauryl sulfate can allow water to penetrate the capsule more quickly and speed dissolution.

Slow-Release Capsules

If a slower release of the active drug is desired, the active drug powder can be mixed with various excipients, such as cellulose polymers (methylcellulose, hypromellose [Methocel E4M]) or sodium alginate. In general, the rate of release is delayed as the proportion of polymer or alginate is increased relative to water-soluble ingredients, such as lactose. Because predicting the exact release profile for a drug and obtaining consistent results from batch to batch is difficult, attempts to alter release rates to this extent should be used only in special circumstances.

Delayed-Release Capsules

Capsules can be coated to delay the release of the active drug until it reaches a selected portion of the gastrointestinal tract. Materials that have been found to be suitable include stearic acid, shellac, casein, cellulose acetate phthalate, and natural and synthetic waxes; they are suitable because they have acid insolubility but are soluble in alkaline environments. Many of the newer coating materials depend on time erosion rather than acid–base factors; that is, rather than being pH dependent, their coating erodes over timed exposure to gastrointestinal contents. A number of newer materials have predictable pH solubility profiles. A dispensing pharmacist should avoid coatings applied to modify the release of a drug but can add a coating to conceal taste, which can enhance patient compliance.

The application of a coating requires skill and additional equipment. A general coating can be applied, but it should be used only for medications that are not critical in nature. In many cases, a pharmacist must develop experience in preparing specific formulations, depending on the requests of primary care providers and the needs of individual patients.

Three methods are commonly used to coat compounded capsules: beaker-flask coating, dipping, and spraying.

- *Beaker-flask coating:* Place a small quantity of the coating material in the flask and gently heat until it has melted. Add a few capsules, remove from the heat, and rotate the flask to start applying the coating. Periodically add a few more drops of melted coating while continuing to rotate the flask. The addition of small quantities of coating material keeps the capsules from sticking together and clumping.
- *Dipping:* Heat the coating material in a beaker at the lowest feasible temperature. Dip the individual capsules, using tweezers. Allow the coating to cool, and repeat the process until a sufficient layer has been applied to the capsule.
- *Spraying:* Prepare an alcoholic or ethereal solution of the coating material. Place solution in a small sprayer. (A model airplane paint sprayer works well). Place the capsules on a screen in a well-ventilated area. Apply the solution of the coating material in thin coats, allowing sufficient time for drying between coats. (A hair dryer may be used for this step if care is taken.) Repeat the process until a sufficient layer has been developed.

Quality Control

Because a pharmacist is responsible for the quality of the capsules prepared, keeping the work area clean and neat and conducting quality control checks to ensure that the preparations contain the correct material in the right quantity are important. One check is to routinely read the label on the bottle at least three times and record the necessary information (e.g., source, lot number) on the compounding formulation record.

The only reliable method of filling capsules accurately is to weigh each capsule. Because such an approach is generally not feasible, a pharmacist can instead weigh representative samples. A good practice is to weigh some capsules individually and weigh others in groups of 10. The two methods together provide data that document the accuracy of the capsule fill, which can be included in the formulation record. Weighing groups of at least 10 capsules at a time is advised because empty gelatin capsules can vary in weight by as much as 15%. Although this variation seems large, the capsule shell is light and represents little of the total weight of a filled capsule. Composite weighings will average out any small variations in the weight of the empty capsules.

Packaging and Storage

Empty gelatin capsules should be stored at room temperature at constant humidity. High humidity can cause the capsules to soften, and low humidity can cause them to dry and crack. Storing capsules in glass containers is best, because they protect against both extreme humidity and dust.

Storage of filled capsules depends on the characteristics of the drug they contain. For example, hard-gelatin capsules filled with semisolids should be stored away from excessive heat, which can cause the contents to soften or melt.

Stability

Capsules are dry or, if they are filled with liquids or semisolids, they contain nonaqueous liquids. For this reason, they generally provide a stable dosage form as long as they are protected from moisture and heat. According to *USP* Chapter <795>,[3] powders prepared from a manufactured product should have a beyond-use date of 25% of the time remaining on the product's expiration date or 6 months, whichever is earlier. If the preparation is compounded from USP or NF grade substances, a beyond-use date of 6 months is appropriate unless evidence is available to support other dating.

Patient Counseling

Capsule sizes Nos. 5 through 0 are not too difficult to swallow in most cases; however, many patients can have difficulty swallowing No. 00 and No. 000 capsules. In such a case, a patient may be advised to place the capsule on the back of the tongue before drinking a liquid or to place the capsule in warm water for a few seconds before taking it, which makes it slide over the mucous membranes more easily. Also, a teaspoonful of a flavored candy gel can be placed in the mouth and swished around; the capsule is then placed into the mouth and easily swallowed. A pharmacist can also suggest alternatives such as smaller capsules or even a liquid preparation.

Sample Formulations

Capsules with Dry Powder Fill

℞ Morphine Sulfate 10 mg and Dextromethorphan Hydrobromide 30 mg Capsules (#100)

Morphine sulfate	1 g	Active
Dextromethorphan hydrobromide	3 g	Active
Lactose	35.5 g	Diluent

1. Calculate the quantity of each ingredient required for the prescription.
2. Accurately weigh the morphine sulfate, dextromethorphan hydrobromide, and lactose.
3. Reduce the particle size, if necessary, and mix well.
4. Fill 100 No. 1 capsules with 395 mg of the powder mix. (Note: Altering the quantity of lactose per capsule may be necessary, depending on the bulk density of the lactose being used.)
5. Check the weights of the capsules.
6. Package and label the product.

Capsules with Semisolid Fill

℞ Estradiol 0.25 mg and Estrone 0.25 mg Capsules (#100)

Estradiol	25 mg	Active
Estrone	25 mg	Active
Polyethylene glycol 1450	20 g	Diluent
Polyethylene glycol 3350	20 g	Diluent

1. Calculate the quantity of each ingredient required for the prescription.
2. Accurately weigh each ingredient.
3. Using geometric dilution, mix the estrogen powders.
4. Using low heat (to about 65°C), melt the polyethylene glycols.
5. Sprinkle on the estrogen powders, and thoroughly mix.
6. Load a capsule machine, if available, with 100 No. 1 capsules, and remove the caps.
7. To determine the volume of mixture to place in each capsule, perform the following steps:
   - Using a micropipet, place 330 µL of the estrogen–polyethylene glycol melt into each of three capsule bases.
   - Weigh the three capsules, and obtain the average weight for each.
   - Adjust the volume delivered, if necessary, to obtain capsules with a tared weight of 403 mg.
8. Place the required volume in each of the capsules, according to step 7.
9. Allow the mixture to harden, and replace the caps on the capsules.
10. Check the weights of about 10 capsules for uniformity and accuracy.
11. Package and label the product.

℞ Progesterone 100 mg Semisolid-Fill, Hard-Gelatin Capsules (#100)

Progesterone	10 g	Active
Polyethylene glycol 1450	20 g	Diluent
Polyethylene glycol 3350	20 g	Diluent

1. Calculate the quantity of each ingredient required for the prescription.
2. Accurately weigh or measure each ingredient.
3. Using low heat (60°C–65°C), melt the polyethylene glycols (PEGs).
4. Sprinkle on the progesterone powder, and thoroughly mix.
5. Load a capsule machine with 100 capsules (No. 1), and remove the caps.
6. Using a micropipet, place 330 µL of the progesterone–PEG melt into each of three capsule bases. Weigh the three capsules, and obtain the average weight for each. Adjust the volume delivered, if necessary, to obtain capsules that weigh 500 mg each.
7. Fill all the capsules with the progesterone–PEG melt mixture.
8. Allow the mixture to harden, and replace the caps on the capsules.
9. Check the weights of 10 capsules for uniformity and accuracy.
10. Package and label the product.

Capsules with Liquid Fill

℞ Progesterone 100 mg in Peanut Oil Capsules (#100)

Micronized progesterone	10 g	Active
Peanut oil	qs 30 mL	Diluent

1. Calculate the quantity of each ingredient required for the prescription.
2. Accurately weigh the progesterone.
3. Mix the progesterone with about 20 mL of peanut oil, in small portions.
4. Add sufficient peanut oil to make 30 mL, and mix well.
5. Load a capsule machine with 100 No. 1 capsules.
6. Using a micropipet, add 300 µL of the mixture to each of the 100 capsules.
7. Remove the filled capsules from the capsule machine.
8. Package and label the product.

References

1. Nash RA. The "Rule of Sixes" for filling hard-shell gelatin capsules. *Int J Pharm Compound.* 1997;1(1):40–1.
2. Al-Achi A, Greenwood RB. The "Rule of Seven" for determining capsule size. *Int J Pharm Compound.* 1997;1(3):191.
3. United States Pharmacopeial Convention. Chapter <795>, Pharmaceutical compounding—nonsterile preparations. In: *United States Pharmacopeia/National Formulary.* Rockville, MD: United States Pharmacopeial Convention; current edition.

Chapter 13

Tablets

The tablet is the most frequently prescribed commercial dosage form. It is stable, elegant, and effective. It provides a patient with a convenient product for handling, identification, and administration. Commercially available tablets can be made at a rate of thousands per minute, but they are available in only fixed dosage strengths and combinations. In many instances, the available products do not match the requirements of specific patients. Until recently, tablets were beyond the scope of a compounding pharmacist. Today, however, some pharmacists extemporaneously prepare molded and compressed tablets for their patients. Pellet presses and single-punch tableting machines now make compounding tablets feasible. In some cases, pre-blended powders are available that allow for easier incorporation of small quantities of active drugs into a tablet preparation, provided the tablet's hardness, friability, and disintegration rates are considered.

Definitions and Types

Sublingual molded tablets are placed under the tongue. They dissolve rapidly, releasing the medication for absorption sublingually, or they can be swallowed. Usually, sublingual tablets contain lactose and other ingredients that are quite water soluble and dissolve quickly.

Buccal molded tablets are administered in the cheek pouch. They dissolve rather quickly, and the released medication can be absorbed or swallowed. The excipients can be manipulated between hydrophilicity and hydrophobicity according to the desired release rate.

Rapid-dissolving tablets (compressed, molded, or sintered tablets [if prepared using heat]) are prepared for rapid disintegration and even dissolution in the mouth. They generally contain the active drug, a diluent, and, if sintered, a meltable binder such as polyethylene glycol (PEG) 3350.

Rapid-dissolving lyophilized tablets are prepared for quick dissolution in the mouth, releasing the active drug either for absorption in the oral cavity or for swallowing.

Compressed tablets are designed to be swallowed. Although they are generally prepared by using large, expensive tableting machines, they can be extemporaneously prepared by using pellet punches or single-punch tableting machines. They can also be used to prepare fast-dissolving tablets depending on the selection of excipients and the compression pressures used during the tableting process.

Chewable tablets must be chewed and swallowed. Formulated to be pleasant tasting, they should not leave a bitter or unpleasant aftertaste. Chewable tablets are typically prepared by compression and usually contain sugars (mannitol, sorbitol, or sucrose) and flavoring agents.

Soluble effervescent tablets are prepared by compression and contain mixtures of acids and sodium bicarbonate, which release carbon dioxide when dissolved in water. Citric acid or tartaric acid may be used. These tablets are intended to be dispersed in water before they are administered and should not be swallowed whole.

Lyophilized tablets are characterized by a very high porosity that allows water or saliva to rapidly penetrate into the tablet, resulting in very rapid disintegration. Pharmacists prepare them by using a suspension or solution of drug with other excipients together with a mold or blister pack to form tablet-shaped units. The tablets are then frozen and lyophilized in the pack or mold, which often becomes the dispensing package.

Implants or pellets are small, sterile, solid masses containing a drug with or without excipients. They can be prepared by compression or molding. Implants are intended for implantation in the body, usually subcutaneously, and provide continuous release of the drug over time. These preparations must be sterile and free of pyrogens and prepared in a clean environment. They can be implanted by means of a special injector or by a superficial incision. Testosterone and estradiol are two agents that have been prepared as implants or pellets.

Historical Use

The tablet originated in England in the 1800s as a compressed pill. In 1878, Burroughs Wellcome and Company applied the term *tablet* to this dosage form. John Wyeth and his brother introduced compressed tablets into the United States in 1882 in the form of compressed hypodermic tablets and compressed tablet triturates. In 1892, a British manufacturer was granted use of the term *tablet* for biconvex discs. Today, tablets make up most of the drug dosage forms on the market because of their economy, ease of preparation, accuracy of dosage, and simplicity of administration.

Applications

With the exception of molded tablets, few tableted dosage forms have been compounded in recent years. This situation may soon change as new methods and techniques are developed and new equipment becomes available. Tablets are likely to be compounded in greater numbers in the future by using single-punch tableting machines and preblended excipients. Compounding pharmacists would simply weigh the required ingredients, mix the powders, punch out the tablets, check them for hardness and disintegration, and dispense them to a patient.

Composition

Tablets are generally composed of the active drug, diluents, binders, disintegrants, lubricants, coloring agents, and flavoring agents. Diluents include lactose, sucrose, mannitol, and starch. (See Table 12-3 in Chapter 12 of this book.) Binders are adhesive materials used to hold the powders together and include water, alcohol, starch paste, sucrose syrup, gelatin solutions,

TABLE 13-1 Characteristics of Capsule and Tablet Disintegrating Agents

Agent	Solubility Water	Solubility Alcohol	pH of Aqueous Dispersion (concentration)	Container Specifications
Alginic acid	IS	—	1.5–3.5 (3%)	W
Microcrystalline cellulose	IS	—	5.0–7.0 (supernatant)	T
Croscarmellose sodium	PartSol	—	5.0–7.0 (1%)	T
Crospovidone	IS	—	5.0–8.0 (1%)	T
Polacrilin potassium	IS	—	—	W
Sodium starch glycolate	—	—	3.0–5.0 (3.3%)	W
Starch, potato	IS	IS	4.5–7.0 (20%)	W
			5.0–8.0 (20%)	
Starch, pregelatinized	SlS	IS	4.5–7.0 (10%)	W

— = Not available.

acacia mucilage, glucose solutions, and polymer solutions (PEG, polyvinylpyrolidone) in water, alcohol, or hydroalcoholic mixtures. Disintegrants include cellulose derivatives, starch, and some commercially available superdisintegrants (Table 13-1). Lubricants are commonly used for high-speed tableting machines, but they can be used for extemporaneously preparing tablets if a punch and die system is available to minimize tablet sticking. Lubricants include PEG, starch, calcium stearate, magnesium stearate, zinc stearate, talc, and numerous other waxes or waxlike materials (Table 13-2). The actual composition of a tablet depends on the method of preparation and the characteristics desired. Different excipients that may be included are shown in Table 13-3.

TABLE 13-2 Characteristics of Capsule and Tablet Lubricants

Lubricant	True Density (g/mL)	Bulk Density (g/mL)	Tapped Density (g/mL)	Melting Point (°C)	Container Specifications
Calcium stearate	1.064–1.096	0.16–0.38	0.20–0.48	149–160	W
Glyceryl behenate	—	—	—	70	T
Glyceryl palmitostearate	—	—	—	52–55	T
Magnesium stearate	1.092	0.159	0.286	117–159	T
Mineral oil, light	0.818–0.880	—	—	—	T
Polyethylene glycol	1.15–1.21	—	—	Varies	W
Sodium stearyl fumarate	1.107	0.2–0.35	0.3–0.5	224–245	W
Stearic acid	0.980	0.537	0.571	≥54	W
Stearic acid, purified	0.847 (70°C)	—	—	66–69	W
Talc	2.7–2.8	—	—	—	W
Vegetable oil, hydrogenated, type I	—	—	0.57	61–66	W
Zinc stearate	1.09	—	0.26	120–122	W

— = Not available.

TABLE 13-3 Categories of Tablet and Capsule Excipients

Anticaking agents	Diluents	Lubricants
Antioxidants	Disintegrants	Preservatives
Binders	Dissolution retardants	Solubilizers
Coating agents	Flavorings	Sweeteners
Colorants	Glidants	Wetting agents

Preparation

Tablets that can be compounded include those that are molded, sintered, and even compressed. A compounding pharmacist can prepare compressed tablets, but generally in unique situations only.

Molded Tablets

Molded tablets are generally prepared by mixing the active drug with lactose, dextrose, sucrose, mannitol, or some other appropriate diluent that can serve as the base. This base must be readily soluble and should not degrade during the tablet's preparation. Lactose is the preferred base, but mannitol adds a pleasant, cooling sensation and additional sweetness in the mouth. Combinations of sugars can also be used.

Tablet triturate molds can be made from plastic or metal, with the latter more commonly used today (Figure 13-1). A formula must be developed to determine the capacity of the mold based on the respective tablet base. Because different bases have different densities, the capacity must be determined for each base. This determination is made by preparing tablets that consist of the base alone, weighing the entire batch, and then dividing the weight by the number of tablets to obtain the average weight per tablet for that base.

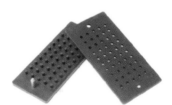

FIGURE 13-1 Tablet triturate molds.

The preparation of molded tablets involves forcing a dampened mass into the cavities of a tablet mold. Generally, these molds are made from plastic or metal and are designed as two plates, one containing pegs and the other containing matching holes or cavities. The mass is moistened and pressed into the plate containing the holes. While the mass remains moist, the cavity plate is situated on the peg plate with the pegs or pins aligned. The cavity plate is then allowed to drop, causing the pegs to push out the moist tablets. The tablets are left undisturbed as they dry, after which they are removed and packaged.

If the active drug used weighs more than a few milligrams, the drug's density factor should be determined. This determination involves moistening a portion of the active drug with 50% ethanol in water, filling some of the mold cavities, drying the tablets, and then weighing them. Dividing the total weight by the number of tablets prepared will give the average weight of the tablet consisting of the active drug. The quantity of drug that will be required in the prescription per tablet can then be divided by the weight of the pure drug tablet to obtain a percentage of the tablet cavity that will be occupied by the active drug. This percentage subtracted from 100 will give the percentage of the tablet cavity that will be occupied by the tablet base. Multiplying this percentage by the weight of the pure base tablet will give the quantity of base that is required per tablet. (See Chapter 7 of this book for a sample calculation and step-by-step instructions for its solution.)

Rapid-Dissolving Sintered Tablets

Sintered tablets are modified molded tablets. They are prepared by blending the active drug and a diluent, which together make up approximately 65% of the tablet weight. The remaining 35% consists of PEG 3350 or a mixture of PEGs with various molecular weights. The powder mixture is pressed firmly into the cavity portion of a tablet triturate mold, which rests on a flat surface. The mold should be lubricated with a vegetable oil spray before use. The cavity portion of the mold containing the tableting materials is placed on a sieve or similar device and set in an oven at about 90°C for about 10 to 12 minutes. The mold is removed from the oven and allowed to cool. The cavity mold is then placed on top of the matching peg mold so that the individual tablets can be worked free.

Alternatively, a small quantity of 50% ethanol in water can be used to form a mass to aid in filling the cavities. The cavity portion of the mold is placed on the peg portion and allowed to slide down, exposing the individual tablets. The entire unit is placed inside an oven at around 90°C for about 12 minutes. After the unit is removed and allowed to cool, the tablets can be removed and packaged. In general, rapid-dissolving tablets prepared by sintering are more robust than other molded tablets and can better withstand handling.

Chewable Tablets

Chewable tablets can be prepared with a single-punch press or a single-punch tableting machine. The matrix consists largely of mannitol, a sugar that has a sweet, cooling taste and is easy to manipulate. Other ingredients can include binders, lubricants, colors, and flavors. The mixture is prepared and the required quantity weighed. The powder is then placed into the cavity of a press, where the tablet is compressed. If a tableting machine is used to punch out the tablets, the powder blend is placed in the hopper and the tablet size and hardness are adjusted before the operation begins.

Effervescent Tablets

Effervescent tablets can be prepared by compressing mixtures of sodium bicarbonate with either citric acid or tartaric acid. A formulation is as follows:

℞ Effervescent Tablets

Active drug	**g	Active
Effervescent mixture	qs	Effervescent Vehicle
Citric acid	15.6%	Acidifier
Tartaric acid	31.3%	Acidifier
Sodium bicarbonate	53.1%	Alkalizer

These tablets must be packaged in tight containers to prevent moisture from causing premature effervescence. They are prepared with either a single-punch press or a single-punch tableting machine.

Compressed Tablets

If the need occurs, small quantities of compressed tablets can be prepared with a pellet press (Figure 13-2). If the quantity of tablets is large enough to justify the expense, a small tableting machine can be used. Usually, the active drug is mixed with a diluent (e.g., lactose), a disintegrant (e.g., starch), and a lubricant (about 1% magnesium stearate) to form a powder blend. Ingredients can be modified on the basis of the desired qualities of the tablets.

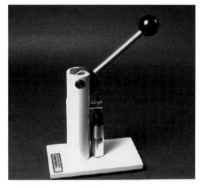

FIGURE 13-2 Pellet press.

Quality Control

Routine quality control tests for tablets should address tablet weight, weight variation, appearance, and disintegration. To test for disintegration, a pharmacist can drop tablets (except chewable tablets) into a beaker containing a No. 10–mesh screen situated about 2 inches from the bottom of the beaker. The screen should be supported by hooks attached to the top of the beaker. A stir bar is placed in the bottom of the beaker, and the entire apparatus is set on a magnetic stirrer. A total of 1 L of water is placed in the beaker, and the stirrer is turned on at a moderate speed. The pharmacist should note and record the time taken for the tablet to break apart. Although the disintegration time depends on the preparation, it generally should be within 15 to 30 minutes. Although dissolution is the determining test, most compounding pharmacies lack the analytical instruments needed to determine the actual quantity of drug that has gone into solution.

Storage and Labeling

Tablets should be stored at room temperature unless directions indicate otherwise. Tablets should be labeled as to the proper mode of administration, that is, swallowable, sublingual, buccal, or chewable.

Stability

Because tablets are dry, they generally constitute a stable dosage form as long as they are protected from moisture and heat. According to *United States Pharmacopeia (USP)* Chapter <795>,[1] tablets prepared from a manufactured product should have a beyond-use date of 25% of the time remaining on the product's expiration date or 6 months, whichever is earlier. If the preparation is compounded from USP or NF (National Formulary) grade substances, a beyond-use date of 6 months is appropriate unless evidence is available to support other dating.

Patient Counseling

A patient should be counseled about the proper mode of administration. If chewable, the tablet should be thoroughly chewed before it is swallowed. Sublingual tablets should be placed under the tongue, whereas buccal tablets should be placed in the cheek pouch between the cheek and gum. After these types of tablets dissolve, the medication should still be held in the mouth for a brief time to allow absorption. Patients should be informed that the buccal and sublingual routes of administration are used when rapid action is desired or when the prescribed drugs might degrade in the stomach if swallowed. Instructions about proper storage in a cool, dry place and away from children should be included.

Sample Formulations

℞ **Sodium Fluoride 2.2 mg Tablet Triturates (#100, using a 60-mg mold)**

Sodium fluoride	220 mg	Active
Sucrose, powdered	1.150 g	Diluent
Lactose, hydrous	4.630 g	Diluent

1. Calculate the quantity of each ingredient required for the prescription.
2. Accurately weigh or measure each ingredient.
3. Mix the powders together geometrically, starting with the sodium fluoride and the sucrose, then the lactose, until thoroughly mixed.
4. Prepare about 10 mL of a solution containing 7.5 mL ethanol (95%) in water.
5. Add the alcohol solution to the powder a drop at a time, and mix well until the mixture attains the consistency of a playing dough or modeling clay.
6. Fill the holes of a tablet triturate mold plate with the mixture until all holes are uniformly filled.
7. Place this portion of the mold plate onto the portion containing the pegs, and gently push down until the tablets are sitting on top of the pegs.
8. Allow tablets to air dry.
9. Gently remove the tablets.
10. Package and label the product.

℞ **Ibuprofen 200 mg Compressed Tablets (#100)**

Ibuprofen	20 g	Active
Caffeine	10 g	Active
Avicel PH 101	14 g	Diluent
Stearic acid	200 mg	Lubricant

1. Calculate the quantity of each ingredient required for the prescription.
2. Accurately weigh or measure each ingredient.
3. Using geometric dilution, mix the powders, starting with the ibuprofen and caffeine. Then incorporate the Avicel PH 101 and, finally, the stearic acid. (Note: The stearic acid is used as a lubricant to prevent the powder from sticking to the tablet press; therefore, it should be added last so that it is distributed uniformly on the other powders.)
4. Weigh 442 mg of the mixture, place it in a tablet press, and then prepare the tablet, ensuring that the amount of pressure used is consistent and that the tablet will disintegrate within 10 minutes when placed in water.
5. Package and label the product.

℞ **Rapid-Dissolving and Fast-Dissolving Tablet Composition**

Ingredient	Use
Active pharmaceutical ingredient (API)	API
Sucrose	Base
Mannitol	Base
Citric acid, anhydrous	Saliva stimulant
Sodium bicarbonate	Saliva stimulant
Polyethylene glycol 3350	Base/Binder
Stevia	Sweetener
Flavors	Flavor for compliance

Reference

1. United States Pharmacopeial Convention. Chapter <795>, Pharmaceutical compounding—nonsterile preparations. In: *United States Pharmacopeia/National Formulary.* Rockville, MD: United States Pharmacopeial Convention; current edition.

Chapter 14

Lozenges, Troches, and Films

Dosage forms that dissolve slowly in the mouth or that can be chewed and swallowed easily are gaining in popularity, especially for pediatric patients. Hard (compressed or molded) preparations of this dosage form are called lozenges, troches, or drops. Soft (molded) lozenges or troches are often called pastilles, and chewable, gelatin-based lozenges or troches are often called gummy, novelty-shaped products. The term *lozenge* will be used in this chapter to refer to all variations of the dosage form.

Definitions and Types

Lozenges are various-shaped solid dosage forms, usually containing a medicinal agent and a flavoring substance, that are intended to be dissolved slowly in the oral cavity for localized or systemic effects. Molded lozenges have a softer texture because they contain a high percentage of sugar or a combination of a gelatin and sugar.

Hard lozenges have hard candy bases made of sugar and syrup and often incorporate an adhesive substance such as acacia. Commercial lozenges are made on a tableting machine using high compression pressures. Ingredients should be heat stable if they are to be incorporated into compounded lozenges.

Recently, soft lozenges and chewable lozenges have been reintroduced into pharmacy and are enjoying increased popularity. *Soft lozenges* generally have a polyethylene glycol (PEG) base, whereas *chewable lozenges* have a glycerinated gelatin base. These dosage forms, usually chewed, are a means of delivering the product to the gastrointestinal tract for systemic absorption.

Films are thin sheets placed in the oral cavity for dissolution and absorption of the active drug. They contain one or more layers and may be indicated for application to different areas of the oral cavity: sublingual, buccal, or even on the tongue surface. Films must be sufficiently strong to maintain their integrity during preparation, packaging, and handling. They should generally provide rapid dissolution, pleasant taste, and satisfactory mouthfeel.[1]

Historical Use

Lozenges have long been used to deliver topical anesthetics and antibacterials for the relief of minor sore throat pain and irritation. Today, they are used for analgesics, anesthetics, antimicrobials, antiseptics, antitussives, aromatics, astringents, corticosteroids, decongestants, demulcents, and other classes and combinations of drugs.

Soft lozenges are similar to a historical form of medication that is now making a comeback—the *confection.* Confections are heavily saccharinated, soft masses containing medicinal agents. Their growing popularity is largely due to the use of polymers (PEGs) as the matrix for the dosage form. Confections are easy to use, convenient to carry, easy to store (i.e., at room temperature), and generally pleasant tasting. PEG-based lozenges have a tendency to be hygroscopic and may soften if exposed to high temperatures; storage in a cool, dry place is recommended.

Currently, a popular lozenge for pediatric use is the chewable lozenge, or gummy-type candy product. The gelatin base for these chewable lozenges is similar to traditional glycerin suppositories or glycerinated gelatin suppositories that consisted of 70% glycerin, 20% gelatin, and 10% purified water. Some of the earlier soft lozenges consisted of a gelatin or a glycerogelatin base. These lozenges were prepared either by pouring the melt into molds or by pouring it out to form a sheet of uniform thickness. The dosage forms were then punched out using various-shaped punches. The last step often included dusting the preparation with cornstarch or powdered sugar to decrease tackiness.

Films are gaining popularity along with rapid-dissolving tablets (RDTs). Similar to RDTs, films are designed to dissolve on contact with a wet surface, such as the tongue, within a few seconds, meaning a patient can take them without the need for additional liquid. This convenience can aid increased patient compliance and, when the drug is directly absorbed into systemic circulation, decrease its degradation in the gastrointestinal tract and avoid the first-pass effect. These factors make this formulation popular and acceptable among pediatric and geriatric patients and patients who fear choking. Examples of commercial thin-film products include Benadryl, Chloraseptic, Gas-X, Klonopin wafers, Listerine, Orajel, Sudafed-PE, Suppress, Theraflu, and Triaminic.

Applications

Lozenges are regaining popularity as a means of delivering drugs, especially for patients who cannot swallow solid oral dosage forms. Lozenges are also used for medications designed for slow release. This dosage form maintains a constant level of the drug in the oral cavity or bathes the throat tissues in a solution of the drug. Medicated lozenges are usually intended for local treatment of infections of the mouth or throat; however, they may contain active medications that produce a systemic effect.

The lozenge dosage form has a number of advantages. It is easy to administer to both pediatric patients and patients of advanced age, it has a pleasant taste, and it extends the time that a quantity of drug remains in the oral cavity to elicit a therapeutic effect. Also, pharmacists can prepare lozenges extemporaneously with minimal equipment and time.

One disadvantage of the lozenge is that children can mistake it for candy. Parents should be cautioned both not to refer to medications as candy and to keep the product out of the reach of children.

Films can be used for local or systemic administration of drugs. Locally, they can include anesthetics, antibacterials, and others; systemically, they can include analgesics and many other drugs where a rapid release of a drug for systemic effect is required. The dissolution rate of the film can be controlled to facilitate the incorporation of the medication into saliva or the absorption by the proximal mucosa.

Composition

Hard Lozenges

Hard candy lozenges are mixtures of sugar and other carbohydrates in an amorphous (non-crystalline) or glassy condition. These lozenges can be considered solid syrups of sugars and usually have a moisture content of 0.5% to 1.5%. Hard lozenges should not disintegrate but instead should provide a slow, uniform dissolution or erosion over 5 to 10 minutes. They should have a smooth surface texture and a pleasant flavor that masks the drug taste. Their primary disadvantage is the high temperature required for preparation. Hard candy lozenges generally weigh between 1.5 and 4.5 g.

Excipients such as sorbitol and sugar have demulcent effects, which relieve the discomfort of abraded tissue caused by coughs and sore throat. A portion of the active drug product may actually be absorbed through the buccal mucosa, thereby escaping the first-pass metabolism that occurs when a drug is swallowed and absorbed through the gastrointestinal tract.

Soft Lozenges

Soft lozenges have become popular because of the ease with which they can be extemporaneously prepared and their applicability to a wide variety of drugs. The bases usually consist of a mixture of various PEGs, acacia, or similar materials. An alternative and older form of soft lozenges is the pastille, which is usually transparent and consists of a medication in a gelatin, a glycerogelatin, or an acacia:sucrose base. These lozenges may be colored and flavored, and they can be either slowly dissolved in the mouth or chewed, depending on the intended effect of the incorporated drug.

Chewable Lozenges (Gummy, Novelty-Shaped Preparations)

Chewable lozenges have been on the market for a number of years. They are highly flavored and frequently have a slightly acidic taste. Because their fruit flavor often masks the drug taste, they are an excellent way of administering drugs. These lozenges are relatively easy to prepare extemporaneously. The most difficult task involves preparing the gelatin base. Chewable lozenges are especially useful for pediatric patients and are an effective means of administering medications for gastrointestinal absorption and systemic use.

Films

Films are typically formed by casting or extrusion. They are generally formulated with edible polymers such as pullulan or with water-soluble polymers such as modified cellulose, edible gums, and copolymers. Rapid-dissolving films often dissolve within 1 minute, are 2 to 8 cm^2 in size, and can incorporate up to about 30 mg of active drug. Typical components of a film are listed as follows:

Ingredients	Amounts (w/w)	Use
Active pharmaceutical ingredient (API)	5%–30%	API
Water-soluble polymer	45%	Vehicle
Plasticizer	0%–20%	Pliability
Saliva stimulation	2%–6%	Dissolution Increaser
Surfactant	qs	Wettability Enhancer
Sweetener	3%–6%	Taste Masker
Flavors, colors, fillers	qs	Compliance Enhancer

Preparation

Lozenges are prepared by molding a mixture of carbohydrates to form hard candies, by molding a matrix to form a soft lozenge, or by molding a gelatin base into a chewable mass. Each approach is described below.

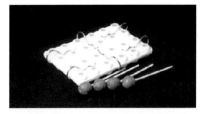

FIGURE 14-1 Lollipop mold.

Hard lozenges are usually prepared by heating sugar and other components to a proper temperature and either pouring the mixture into a mold or pulling the mass out into a ribbon while it cools and then cutting the ribbon to the desired lengths. A commercial method is to compress the materials into a very hard tablet. The mold shown in Figure 14-1 can be used to make lollipops.

Both soft lozenges and chewable lozenges are usually prepared by pouring a melted mass into molds (Figure 14-2). Another method, which depends on the ingredients, involves pouring the

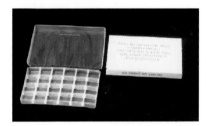

FIGURE 14-2 Troche mold.

mass out to form a sheet of uniform thickness and then punching out the lozenges by using a punch of the desired shape and size.

If molds are unavailable, the plastic snap cap from a plastic vial can be used as a mold. A vegetable spray can be applied to the cap, if needed, and the preparation can be poured into the cap. After solidification, the cap can be peeled away from the lozenge. Alternatively, the melt can be dropped onto a heavy sheet of aluminum foil that is sitting on a bed of ice cubes. The drops will immediately solidify, usually in a circular form, on contact with the cold foil.

Molds used in the preparation of lozenges must be calibrated to determine the weight of the lozenge, using the applicable base. The calibration can be done as follows:

1. Prepare the lozenge mold, and confirm that the cavities are clean and dry.
2. Obtain and melt sufficient lozenge base to fill 6 to 12 molds.
3. Pour the molds, cool the blank lozenges, and trim if necessary.
4. Remove the blank lozenges, and weigh them.
5. Divide the total weight by the number of blank lozenges to obtain the average weight of each lozenge for this particular base. Use this weight as the calibrated value for that specific mold when using that specific lot of lozenge base.

The powders contained in the lozenges may also occupy a specific volume, and an adjustment may be required in the quantity of the base used. These dosage replacement calculations are analogous to those used with suppositories. (See Chapter 7 of this book for sample calculations.)

In general, the quantity of flavoring agent added to medicated lozenges is about 5 to 10 times that used in candy lozenges, which compensates for the flavor of the medication. If the flavoring agent (an oil) is immiscible with the base, it can be dissolved in glycerin; the glycerin solution is then incorporated into the preparation. The same technique can be used to incorporate an oily drug into a lozenge. The solvent technique often uses a ratio of 1 part solvent to 3 to 5 parts drug.

An oral film generally is composed of a water-soluble polymer for the support, a plasticizer for pliability, and sweeteners and flavors. In addition, a saliva stimulant can be included to enhance dissolution, a surfactant to facilitate spreading of the dissolved drug and enhance wettability, colors, fillers, and other ingredients as required. Films are generally made by (1) preparing a fluid mixture of the ingredients and casting them onto a plate where they are allowed to cool, harden, and then be divided into dosage units and packaged or (2) preparing a plastic mass, extruding the mass and dividing it into appropriate dosage units, and then packaging the units.

Lozenges and Troches

Physicochemical Considerations

A binder is used in most lozenges. *Binders* are substances added to tablet or lozenge formulations to add cohesiveness to powders, providing the necessary bonding that contributes to the maintenance of the integrity of the final dosage form. Binders are usually selected on the basis of previous experience of the formulator, particular preparation needs, literature or vendor information, and individual preferences. Binders can be added at any of several steps in the process, depending on the specific procedure being used and the speed at which the lozenge should disintegrate. Table 14-1 lists the official binding agents and their physicochemical characteristics.

Dosage forms are removed from the mouth at various rates. Generally, the rate of removal, from the fastest to the slowest, is as follows: tablets and capsules, solutions, suspensions, chewable tablets, and lozenges. According to salivary kinetics, about 1.07 mL of saliva resides in the mouth before swallowing and about 0.71 mL after swallowing. The baseline flow rate for saliva of about 0.3 mL/minute may be increased to about 10.6 mL/minute when stimulated. The frequency of swallowing is about 0.6 to 2.3 times per minute. Given these calculations, a lozenge can increase the residence time of a drug in the oral cavity.

If flavors and preservatives are included in the preparation formulation, their characteristics should be considered. For example, the odor of a 0.08% solution of methylparaben has been described as "floral," "gauze pad," or "face powder" sweet. A 0.015% solution of propylparaben has a tongue-numbing effect, producing a slight sting and minimal aroma. A 0.125% butylparaben solution has the least aroma of all. Preservatives have a tendency to partition into flavors, because they are not always water soluble and most flavors are oily in nature.

The type of medication prepared as a lozenge is limited only by flavor, dose restrictions, or chemical compatibility, or a combination of these factors. Some materials are so unpalatable or irritating that they are unsuitable for this type of administration. The following are examples of active ingredients used in lozenges:

- *Benzocaine:* The usual dose of benzocaine is in the range of 5 to 10 mg per lozenge. Benzocaine is extremely reactive with the aldehydic components of candy base and flavor components. As much as 90% to 95% of available benzocaine may be lost when added to a candy base, but a PEG base is compatible.
- *Hexylresorcinol:* The dose of hexylresorcinol is about 2.4 mg per lozenge. Hexylresorcinol is somewhat susceptible to reaction with aldehydic components. No flavoring or mouthfeel problems are associated with this material because of its low dose and lack of appreciable flavor.
- *Dextromethorphan:* The dose of dextromethorphan hydrobromide is about 7.5 mg per lozenge. Dextromethorphan is easy to incorporate into a candy base because of its melting point (122°C–124°C) and solubility (1.5 g/1000 mL of purified water). It is compatible with most flavors and stable over a wide pH range. Conversely, it does have a bitter taste, an anesthetic mouthfeel, and an unpleasant aftertaste. Masking doses greater than about 2 mg per lozenge requires special considerations.

TABLE 14-1 Characteristics of Binding Agents

Agent	Usual Concentration (%)	Solubility		pH of Aqueous Dispersion (concentration)	Container Specifications
		Water	Alcohol		
Acacia NF	2–5	FS		4.5–5.0 (5%)	T
Alginic acid NF	2–5	IS		1.5–3.5 (3%)	W
Carboxymethyl-cellulose sodium USP	1–5		IS	6.5–8.5 (1%)	T
Cellulose, microcrystalline NF	1–90	IS		5.0–7.0 (12.5%)	T
Dextrin NF		VS			W
Ethylcellulose NF	1–5	IS	FS	5.0–7.5 (2%)	W
Gelatin NF					
Type A	1–5	Sol	IS	3.8–6.0 (1%)	W
Type B	1–5	Sol	IS	5.0–7.4 (1%)	W
Glucose, liquid NF	—	Misc	SpS	—	T
Guar gum NF	1–10	Disp	—	5.0–7.0 (1%)	W
Hydroxypropyl methylcellulose USP	1–5	Swells	IS	5.5–8.0 (1%)	W
Methylcellulose USP	1–5	Swells	IS	5.5–8.0 (1%)	W
Polyethylene glycol NF	5–50	FS	Sol	4.5–7.5 (5%)	T
Polyethylene oxide NF	—	Sol	—	—	T, LR
Povidone USP	2–5	FS	FS	3.0–7.0 (5%)	T
Starch, pregelatinized NF	—	SlS	IS	4.5–7.0 (10%)	
Syrup NF	2–25	Misc	Misc	—	T

— = Not available.

Quality Control
The weight and uniformity of individual lozenges can be easily determined. Appearance, odor, and hardness can be observed and recorded.

Storage and Labeling
Lozenges (hard, soft, and chewable) should be stored either at room temperature or in a refrigerator, depending on the active drug incorporated and the type of vehicle used. These preparations should be kept in tight containers to prevent drying; this is especially important for chewable lozenges, which can dry out and become difficult to chew. If a disposable mold with a cardboard sleeve is used, slipping this unit into a properly labeled, sealable plastic bag is best.

Stability

The completed preparations are dry and thus generally provide a stable dosage form as long as they are protected from moisture and heat. According to Chapter <795> of the *United States Pharmacopeia (USP)*, lozenges prepared from a manufactured product should have a beyond-use date of 25% of the time remaining on the product's expiration date or 6 months, whichever is earlier. If the preparation is compounded from USP or NF (National Formulary) grade substances and is anhydrous, a beyond-use date of 6 months is appropriate, unless evidence is available to support other dating. Other considerations are described below.

Hard candies are hygroscopic and are usually prone to absorption of atmospheric moisture. Therefore, considerations must include the hygroscopic nature of the candy base, storage conditions of the lozenges, length of time they will be stored, and potential for drug interactions.

Lozenges should be stored away from heat and out of the reach of children. They should be protected from extremes of humidity. Depending on the storage requirement of both the drug and the base, either room temperature or refrigerated temperature is usually indicated.

Because lozenges are solid dosage forms, preservatives are generally not needed. However, hard candy lozenges are hygroscopic; therefore, their water content may increase, and bacterial growth can occur if they are not packaged properly. Nevertheless, any water present would dissolve some sucrose; the resulting highly concentrated sucrose solution would be bacteriostatic and would not support bacterial growth. The paraben preservatives were discussed earlier in this chapter.

All hard candy lozenges eventually become grainy, but the speed at which this occurs depends on the ingredients. When the concentration of corn syrup solids is greater than 50%, the graining tendencies decrease but moisture absorption tendencies can increase. Increased moisture absorption increases product stickiness and causes the medications to interact. Sucrose solids in concentrations greater than 70% tend to increase graining tendencies and the speed of crystallization. Formulations that contain between 55% and 65% sucrose or between 35% and 45% corn syrup solids generally offer the best compromise in terms of graining, moisture absorption, and preparation time.

Acidulents, such as citric, tartaric, fumaric, and malic acids, can be added to a candy base to strengthen the flavor characteristics of the finished preparation and to control pH to preserve the stability of the incorporated medication. Regular hard candy has a pH of about 5 to 6, but it may be as low as 2.5 to 3 when acidulents are added. Sodium bicarbonate, calcium carbonate, and magnesium trisilicate can be added to increase the lozenge pH to as high as 7.5 to 8.5.

Patient Counseling

A patient should be counseled about the purpose of a hard lozenge, which is to provide a slow, continuous release of the drug over a prolonged period of time. Hard lozenges should not be chewed. Soft and chewable lozenges are to be taken only as directed and should not be considered candy. They should be kept out of the reach of children.

Because hard lozenges are designed to provide a slow, uniform release of the medication directly onto the affected mucous membrane, a compounding pharmacist is faced with a challenge: developing flavor blends that mask any unpleasant taste produced by the medication while maintaining a smooth surface texture as the lozenge slowly dissolves. If a medication has no significant taste, flavoring will not be a problem. If it has a strong, disagreeable taste, however, that taste should be minimized to enhance patient compliance.

Films

Thin-film drug delivery technology has emerged as an advanced alternative to traditional tablets, capsules, and liquids. Similar in size, shape, and thickness to a postage stamp, thin-film strips are typically designed for oral administration, with the user placing the strip on or under the tongue (sublingual) or along the inside of the cheek (buccal).

Formulation of fast-dissolving buccal film involves material such as film-forming polymers, plasticizers, active pharmaceutical ingredient, sweetening agents, saliva-stimulating agent, flavoring agents, coloring agents, stabilizing and thickening agents, permeation enhancers, and superdisintegrants. All the excipients used in the formulation of fast-dissolving film should be approved for use in oral pharmaceutical dosage forms in accordance with regulatory perspectives.

Active Pharmaceutical Ingredient

Because the size of the dosage form has limitations, high-dose drugs are difficult to incorporate into oral films. Generally, 5% weight per weight (w/w) to 30% w/w of active pharmaceutical ingredients can be incorporated.

Film-Forming Polymers

The polymer employed should be nontoxic and nonirritant, and it should have good wetting and spreadability qualities. It should also exhibit sufficient peel, shear, and tensile strengths. The obtained film should be strong enough to not be damaged during handling or transportation. A combination of microcrystalline cellulose and maltodextrin has been used to formulate oral strips of piroxicam made by the hot melt extrusion technique. Pullulan has been the most widely used film-forming polymer (used in Benadryl, Listerine PocketPak, etc.). Also, carboxymethylcellulose, ethylcellulose, gelatin, hydroxypropylcellulose, hydroxypropyl methylcellulose, maltodextrins, methylcellulose, pectin, polyvinyl alcohol, polyvinylpyrrollidone, sodium alginate, starch, and others are used.

Plasticizers

A plasticizer is a vital ingredient in the film formulation. It helps improve flexibility and reduce the brittleness of the strip. Some of the commonly used plasticizer excipients include castor oil; glycerol; low molecular weight polyethylene glycols; propylene glycol; citrate derivatives such as acetyl, triacetin, tributyl, and triethyl citrate; and phthalate derivatives such as dibutyl, diethyl, and dimethyl phthalate.

Sweetening, Flavoring, and Coloring Agents

An important aspect of thin-film drug technology is the taste and color. The sweet taste of the formulation is especially important in pediatrics. Natural and artificial sweeteners are used to improve the flavor of the mouth-dissolving formulations; the flavors can be tailored specifically for individuals. Examples include saccharin, cyclamate, and aspartame. Pigments, such as titanium dioxide, are incorporated for coloring.

Saliva-Stimulating Agents

Salivary stimulation can aid in dissolving the thin film together with the active drug, which is necessary for absorption. Common saliva-stimulating agents include ascorbic acid, citric acid, lactic acid, and malic acid.

Stabilizing and Thickening Agents

Stabilizing and thickening agents are used to improve the viscosity and consistency of dispersion or solution of the strip preparation solution or suspension before casting. Drug content uniformity is a requirement for all dosage forms, particularly those containing low-dose highly potent drugs. Surfactants, including benzalkonium chloride, polysorbates, sodium lauryl sulfate, and others, have been used to stabilize the film and improve its uniformity; they also serve as penetration enhancers.

Preparation

Extemporaneously prepared oral thin films can be made from a standard casting solution in which different active pharmaceutical ingredients are dissolved or suspended. The desired composition and characteristics of a standard casting solution should be defined in relation to the properties of the final product. Different methods can be used for the preparation of oral thin films, including solvent casting (most common), hot-melt extrusion, semisolid casting, solid dispersion extrusion, and rolling. Only the solvent casting method is presented here.

In the solvent casting method, the water-soluble polymers are dissolved in rapidly stirred water that is heated to about 60°C. All the other excipients, such as colors, flavoring agent, and sweetening agent, are dissolved separately. Then both solutions are combined and mixed thoroughly with rapid stirring. The active drug, previously dissolved in a suitable solvent, is added and thoroughly mixed. Next, the entrapped air is removed by vacuum, and the resulting solution is cast as a film and allowed to dry. Thereafter, it is cut into pieces of the desired size.

Sample Formulations

Lozenge Vehicles

For the following vehicles, the gelatin is dissolved in a hot mixture of the glycerin, water, and sorbitol solution in which the parabens have been previously dissolved. Use of a tared vessel to determine water loss during heating is advisable, so that an appropriate amount can be replaced. The amount of flavor oil can be determined by trial-and-error taste tests; one can start at about 0.1% and make adjustments as needed.[2]

Ingredients	Vehicle						
	A	B	C	D	E	F	G
Sodium saccharin	0.1 g	—	0.1 g	0.05 g	0.05 g	0.05 g	0.05 g
Gelatin	20 g	20 g	20 g	30 g	30 g	30 g	20 g
Glycerin	70 mL	20 mL	40 mL	30 mL	30 mL	30 mL	40 mL
Sorbitol 70% solution	—	50 mL	30 mL	30 mL	25 mL	26 mL	26 mL
Polyethylene glycol 6000	—	—	—	—	5 g	4 g	4 g
Methylparaben	0.15 g	0.15 g	0.15 g	0.15 g	0.15 g	0.15 g	0.15 g
Propylparaben	0.05 g	0.05 g	0.05 g	0.05 g	0.05 g	0.05 g	0.05 g
Flavor oil	qs mL	qs mL	qs mL	qs mL	qs mL	qs mL	qs mL
Purified water USP qs	100 mL	100 mL	100 mL	100 mL	100 mL	100 mL	100 mL

Ingredient-Specific Formulations

Sample formulations are presented to illustrate the differences in the types of lozenges and their applications. These formulas can be adjusted according to the quantity of active drug to be used.

Hard Lozenges

℞ Hard Sugar Lozenges

Powdered sugar	42 g	Base/Vehicle
Light corn syrup	16 mL	Base/Vehicle
Purified water	24 mL	Base/Vehicle
Active drug, example	1.0 g	Active
Mint extract	12 mL	Flavor
Food coloring, green	qs	Color

1. Calculate the quantity of each ingredient required for the prescription.
2. Accurately weigh or measure each ingredient.
3. Combine the sugar, corn syrup, and water in a beaker, and stir until well mixed.
4. Cover the mixture, and heat on a hot plate at a high setting until the mixture boils; continue boiling for 2 minutes.
5. Uncover and remove the mixture from heat at 61°C. Do not stir the mixture until the temperature drops to 55°C.
6. Quickly add the active drug, mint extract, and food coloring, and stir until well mixed.
7. Coat the mold to be used with a vegetable spray.
8. Pour the melt into the mold.
9. Cool, package, and label the product.

℞ Anti-Gag Lollipops (36 lollipops)

Sodium chloride	46.56 g	Active
Potassium chloride	3 g	Active
Calcium lactate	6.12 g	Active
Magnesium citrate	2.04 g	Active
Sodium bicarbonate	22.44 g	Active
Sodium phosphate monobasic	3.84 g	Active
Silica gel	3.60 g	Thickener
Polyethylene glycol 1450	qs	Base

1. Calculate the quantity of each ingredient required for the prescription.
2. Calibrate the lollipop mold for the formula.
3. Accurately weigh or measure each ingredient.
4. Triturate all the powders together to obtain a small, uniform particle size.
5. Melt the polyethylene glycol 1450 at a temperature in the range of 50°C to 55°C in a suitable beaker or other container.
6. Slowly add the powders with thorough mixing.
7. Cool the mixture to approximately 45°C.
8. Pour the mixture into a mold that has been previously sprayed with a vegetable-based oil, wiping off the excess.
9. Cool the mixture for approximately 90 minutes, and remove from the mold.
10. Package and label the product.

℞ Pediatric Chocolate Troche Base

Chocolate (good quality)	60 g	Base
Vegetable oil (bland)	40 g	Base

1. Calculate the quantity of each ingredient required for the prescription.
2. Accurately weigh or measure each ingredient.
3. Heat the vegetable oil by using low heat or a double boiler/water bath.
4. Add the chocolate, stir until melted, and then cool.
5. Package the product, and use for compounding.

℞ Sildenafil Citrate 25 mg Sublingual Troches (#24)

Sildenafil citrate	600 mg	Active
Aspartame	500 mg	Sweetener
Silica gel	480 mg	Suspending Agent
Acacia	360 mg	Demulcent/Smooth Texture
Flavor	qs	Flavor
Polyethylene glycol 1450	22 g	Base

(Note: Amount of polyethylene glycol 1450 will vary depending on mold and size of tablet used as the source of the drug.)

1. Calculate the quantity of each ingredient required for the prescription.
2. Accurately weigh or measure each ingredient, and obtain the required number of sildenafil citrate tablets (24 of the 25 mg, 12 of the 50 mg, or 6 of the 100 mg tablets).
3. In a mortar, triturate the sildenafil citrate tablets to a very fine powder.
4. Add the aspartame, silica gel, and acacia, and triturate further to a fine powder.
5. Melt the polyethylene glycol 1450 to about 55°C to 60°C.
6. Add the powders from step 4, and mix well.
7. Cool the mixture a few degrees, add the flavor(s), and pour into troche molds.
8. Allow the mixture to solidify.
9. Package and label the product.

Soft Lozenges

℞ Steroid Linguets *** mg

Fattibase/cocoa butter	76 g	Base
Steroid powder	** g	Active
Acacia	3 g	Demulcent/Smooth Texture
Cinnamon oil	5 drops	Flavor
Artificial sweetener	14 drops	Sweetener

1. Calculate the quantity of each ingredient required for the prescription.
2. Accurately weigh or measure each ingredient.
3. Melt the Fattibase/cocoa butter at about 35°C to 40°C.
4. Add the acacia powder followed by the steroid, and mix well.
5. Add the cinnamon oil and the artificial sweetener, and mix well.
6. Pour the mixture into 1-g molds, and place in a refrigerator to cool and harden.
7. Package and label the product, and store in a refrigerator.

℞ Polyethylene Glycol Troches

Polyethylene glycol 1000	10 g	Base
Active drug, example	1 g	Active
Aspartame sweetener	20 packets	Sweetener
Mint extract	1 mL	Flavor
Food color	2 drops	Color

1. Calculate the quantity of each ingredient required for the prescription.
2. Accurately weigh or measure each ingredient.
3. Melt the polyethylene glycol 1000 on a hot plate to about 70°C, and gradually add the active drug powder and the aspartame sweetener by stirring.
4. Add the coloring and flavoring, and pour the mixture into troche molds.
5. Allow the mixture to cool at room temperature.
6. Package and label the product.

℞ Polyethylene Glycol Troches with Suspending Agent

Polyethylene glycol 1000	34.5 g	Base
Active drug, example	4.8 g	Active
Silica gel	0.37 g	Suspending Agent
Acacia	0.61 g	Demulcent/Smooth Texture
Flavor	5 drops	Flavor

1. Calculate the quantity of each ingredient required for the prescription.
2. Accurately weigh or measure each ingredient.
3. Blend the powders together until uniformly mixed.
4. Heat the polyethylene glycol 1000 until melted at approximately 70°C.
5. Add the powder mix to the melted base, and blend thoroughly.
6. Cool the mixture to less than 55°C, add the flavor, and mix well.
7. Pour the mixture into troche or cough drop molds.
8. Cool, package, and label the product.

(Note: This formulation is based on a mold that weighs approximately 1.8 g. The formula can be adjusted to other mold weights.)

℞ Powdered Sugar Troches

Powdered sugar	10 g	Base
Active drug, example	1 g	Active
Acacia	0.7 g	Demulcent/Smooth Texture
Purified water	qs	Base

1. Calculate the quantity of each ingredient required for the prescription.
2. Accurately weigh or measure each ingredient.
3. Mix the acacia and purified water together in a mortar to form a mucilage.
4. Sift the powdered sugar and active drug together, and gradually add sufficient mucilage to make a mass of the proper consistency.
5. Roll the mass into the shape of a cylinder, cut into 10 even sections (approximately twice the length of the diameter), and allow to air dry.
6. Package and label the product.

Chewable Lozenges

℞ Gelatin Base

Glycerin	155 mL	Base
Gelatin	3.4 g	Base
Purified water	21.6 mL	Base
Methylparaben	0.44 g	Preservative

1. Calculate the quantity of each ingredient required for the prescription.
2. Accurately weigh or measure each ingredient.
3. Heat a water bath to boiling.
4. In a beaker, add the purified water, glycerin, and methylparaben; stir and heat for 5 minutes.
5. Over a 3-minute period, add the gelatin very slowly while stirring until it is thoroughly dispersed and free of lumps.
6. Continue to heat the mixture for 45 minutes.
7. Remove the mixture from heat, cool, and refrigerate until used.

℞ Drug Preparation in Gelatin Base

Gelatin base	43 g	Base
Bentonite	800 mg	Suspending Agent
Aspartame	900 mg	Sweetener
Acacia powder	720 mg	Demulcent/Smooth Texture
Citric acid monohydrate	1.08 g	Acidifier
Flavor	14–18 drops	Flavor
Active ingredient	—	Active

1. Calculate the quantity of each ingredient required for the prescription.
2. Accurately weigh or measure each ingredient.
3. Calibrate the particular mold to be used for this preparation.
4. Melt the gelatin base using a water bath.
5. Triturate the powders together, and add to the gelatin base melt; thoroughly mix until evenly dispersed.
6. Add the desired flavor, and mix.
7. Continuously mix the melt, pour into the pediatric chewable lozenge molds, and allow to cool. If the mixture congeals during pouring, one may need to reheat and then continue pouring.
8. Package and label the product.

℞ Morphine 10 mg Troches (#24)

Morphine sulfate	240 mg	Active
Aspartame	250 mg	Sweetener
Flavor	qs	Flavor
Polybase	24 g	Base

1. Calculate the quantity of each ingredient required for the prescription.
2. Accurately weigh or measure each ingredient.
3. Melt the Polybase using gentle heat to about 60°C.
4. Add the morphine sulfate and the aspartame powders, and mix well.
5. Cool the mixture a few minutes, and add flavor while the mixture is still fluid.
6. Mix thoroughly, and pour the mixture into 1-g molds.
7. Cool, package, and label the product.

℞ Fentanyl 50 µg Chewable Gummy Gels (24 chewable gels)

Fentanyl citrate	1.884 mg	Active
Chewable gummy gel base	23.35 g	Base
Bentonite	0.5 g	Suspending Agent
Aspartame	0.5 g	Sweetener
Acacia powder	0.5 g	Demulcent/Smooth Texture
Citric acid monohydrate	0.65 g	Acidifier
Flavor concentrate	10–12 drops	Flavor

1. Calculate the quantity of each ingredient required for the prescription.
2. Accurately weigh or measure each ingredient.
3. Blend the fentanyl citrate, bentonite, aspartame, acacia powder, and citric acid monohydrate together.
4. Heat the chewable gummy gel base on a water bath until fluid.
5. Incorporate the dry powder from step 3 into the base, and stir until evenly dispersed.
6. Add the flavor concentrate, and mix well.
7. Pour the mixture into suitable molds, and allow to cool.
8. Package and label the product.

(Note: Because mold capacities vary, it may be necessary to calibrate the specific mold being used and to adjust the formula before actual preparation.)

Oral Thin Films

℞ Oral Thin-Film Vehicle

Hydroxypropyl methylcellulose	9 g	Vehicle
Glycerin 85%	1.99 g	Vehicle
Carbomer 974P	450 mg	Vehicle/Thickener
Disodium ethylenediaminetetraacetic acid	45 mg	Chelator
Tromethamine	45 mg	Alkalinizing Agent
Purified water	qs 100 g	Vehicle

1. Calculate the quantity of each ingredient required for the prescription.
2. Accurately weigh or measure each ingredient.
3. Mix the hydroxypropyl methylcellulose and carbomer 974P with the glycerin.
4. Add the disodium ethylenediaminetetraacetic acid and tromethamine in the purified water with constant high-speed stirring at room temperature with a magnetic stirring bar until a clear solution is obtained.
5. Stir the solution at room temperature overnight at 100 rpm to allow entrapped air bubbles to disappear.
6. Cast the solution onto a release liner (Primeliner 410/36, Loparex, Apeldoorn, the Netherlands) with a quadruple film applicator using a casting height of 1000 microns.
7. Apply vacuum suction to remove any air bubbles.
8. Dry the film at a set temperature and ambient relative humidity (40%RH–50%RH).
9. Carefully remove dry films from the release liner, and divide or punch into squares of 1.8 × 1.8 cm, yielding stamp-shaped orally dissolving films.
10. Seal product in plastic, and store under ambient conditions.

℞ Nicardipine Hydrochloride 20 mg Films

Nicardipine hydrochloride	2 g	Active
Pullulan	20 mg	Vehicle
Locust Bean Gum	2 mg	Vehicle
Mannitol	5 mg	Vehicle
Purified water	qs 50 mL (depending on mold size)	Vehicle

1. Calculate the quantity of each ingredient required for the prescription.
2. Accurately weigh or measure each ingredient.
3. Dissolve the nicardipine hydrochloride, pullulan, locust bean gum, and mannitol in hot purified water, and mix until clear.
4. Pour the solution into molds, and dry at 40°C over 8 hours.
5. Package in tight containers.

References

1. United States Pharmacopeial Convention. Chapter <795>, Pharmaceutical compounding—nonsterile preparations. In: *United States Pharmacopeia/National Formulary*. Rockville, MD: United States Pharmacopeial Convention; current edition.
2. Palmer HA, Semprebon M. Extemporaneous lozenge formulations. *Int J Pharm Compound.* 1998;2(1):71–2.

Chapter 15

Suppositories and Inserts

Definitions and Types

These solid dosage forms are used to administer medicine through the rectum (*suppositories*) and the vagina or urethra (*inserts*). They melt, soften, or dissolve in the body cavity.

Rectal suppositories are cylindrical or conical and are tapered or pointed at one end. They generally weigh approximately 2 g and are about 1 to 1.5 inches long. Infant rectal suppositories weigh about half as much as adult suppositories.

Vaginal inserts, formerly called pessaries, are available in ovoid, globular, and other shapes and weigh about 3 to 5 g each. Compounded vaginal inserts that use water-soluble bases, such as polyethylene glycol (PEG) or glycerinated gelatin, are the preferred form because they minimize leakage. Some vaginal inserts are actually compressed tablets.

Urethral suppositories, formerly called bougies, vary in their dimensions, depending on the sex of the patient. Suppositories for females are about 5 mm in diameter, 50 mm in length, and 2 g in weight. Suppositories for males are 5 mm in diameter, 125 mm in length, and 4 g in weight.

Historical Use

Suppositories and inserts have been used for several thousand years and were cited in the early writings of the Egyptians, Greeks, and Romans. Suppositories at that time consisted of pieces of cloth, plants, wood, or other material that were used plain or soaked in a solution of a "medication" and administered. Cocoa butter revolutionized the preparation of suppositories and has served as a suppository base for many years.

Applications

Suppositories and inserts can be used to administer drugs to infants and small children, to severely debilitated patients, to those who cannot take medications orally, and to those for whom the parenteral route might be unsuitable. The drugs contained in this dosage form have either local or systemic application. Local applications include the treatment of hemorrhoids, itching, and infections. Systemic applications involve a variety of drugs, including antinauseants, antiasthmatics, analgesics, and hormones. A detailed presentation of the applications and all aspects of suppositories has been published.[1]

Suppositories could be used more often in compounded formulations. For example, compounded suppositories that contain benztropine, dexamethasone, diphenhydramine, haloperidol, and metoclopramide can be administered prophylactically to control severe nausea and vomiting; salbutamol can be administered rectally for long-term prophylactic treatment of asthma; and a prolonged-release morphine alkaloid suppository has been introduced for chronic pain.

Types and Composition of Bases

A suppository or insert base should be stable, nonirritating, chemically and physiologically inert, compatible with a variety of drugs, stable during storage, and aesthetically acceptable. It should not melt or dissolve in rectal fluids and should not bind or otherwise interfere with the release or absorption of drug substances. Other desirable characteristics depend on the drugs to be added. For example, bases with higher melting points can be used to incorporate drugs that generally lower the melting point of the base (e.g., camphor, chloral hydrate, menthol, phenol, thymol, and volatile oils) or to formulate suppositories for use in tropical climates. Bases with lower melting points can be used when adding materials that will raise the melting point or when adding large amounts of solids. Examples of suppository bases are shown in Table 15-1.

Oil-Soluble Bases

Cocoa butter, or theobroma oil, is an oleaginous base that softens at 30°C and melts at 34°C. It is a mixture of liquid triglycerides entrapped in a network of crystalline, solid triglycerides. Palmitic and stearic acids make up about half of the saturated fatty acids in cocoa butter, and oleic acid is the one unsaturated fatty acid. Cocoa butter has four different forms—α, β, β', and γ—with melting points of 22°C, 34°C to 35°C, 28°C, and 18°C, respectively. The β form, which is the most stable, is preferable for suppositories. Cocoa butter will melt to form a nonviscous, bland oil. Because it is immiscible with body fluids, it may leak from the body orifice. Polymorphs with lower melting points will eventually convert to a more stable form over time. Chloral hydrate will decrease the melting point of cocoa butter. To avoid problems with cocoa butter suppositories sticking when released from their molds, a pharmacist must not overheat the cocoa butter and must ensure the molds are clean and dry before use.

Hydrogenated Vegetable Oil Bases

Fattibase is a preblended suppository base that offers the advantages of a cocoa butter base with few of the drawbacks. It is composed of triglycerides derived from palm, palm kernel, and coconut oils, with self-emulsifying glyceryl monostearate and polyoxyl stearate used as emulsifying and suspending agents. This base is stable, with a low irritation profile; needs no special storage conditions; is uniform in composition; and has a bland taste and controlled melting range. It exhibits excellent mold-release characteristics and does not require mold lubrication. Fattibase is a solid with a melting point of 35°C to 37°C, has a specific gravity of 0.890 at 37°C, is opaque white, and is free of suspended matter.

Wecobee bases are derived from palm kernel and coconut oils; they are rendered emulsifiable by the incorporation of glyceryl monostearate and propylene glycol monostearate. These bases also exhibit most of cocoa butter's desirable features but few of its shortcomings. They are stable and exhibit excellent mold-release characteristics.

TABLE 15-1 Suppository Bases, Primarily of U.S. Origin and Availability

Base	Composition	Melting Range/ Point (°C)
Cocoa butter	Mixed triglycerides of oleic, palmitic, stearic acids	34–35
Cotomar	Partially hydrogenated cottonseed oil	35
Dehydag	Hydrogenated fatty alcohols and esters	
Base I		33–36
Base II		37–39
Base III	Glycerides of saturated fatty acids C-12–C-16 also present	9 ranges
Fattibase	Triglycerides from palm, palm kernel, and coconut oils with self-emulsifying glyceryl monostearate and poly-oxyl stearate	35.5–37
Hexaride Base 95		33–35
Hydrokote 25	Higher melting fractions of coconut and palm kernel oil	33.6–36.3
Hydrokote 711	Same as above	39.5–44.5
Hydrokote SP	Same as above	31.1–32.3
Polybase	Homogeneous blend of polyethylene glycols and poly-sorbate 80	60–71
S-70-XX95	Rearranged hydrogenated vegetable oils	34.4–35.6
S-070-XXA	Same as above	38.2–39.3
Suppocire OSI	Eutectic mixtures of mono-, di-, triglycerides derived from natural vegetable oils, each type having slightly different properties	33–35
Suppocire OSIX	Same as above	33–35
Suppocire A	Same as above	35–36.5
Suppocire B	Same as above	36–37.5
Suppocire C	Same as above	38–40
Suppocire D	Same as above	42–45
Suppocire DM	Same as above	42–45
Suppocire H	Same as above but with the addition of polyoxyethylated glycerides	36–37.5
Suppocire L	Same composition as Suppocire H	38–40
Tegester Triglycerides	Specially prepared triglyceride bases	
TG-95		32.2–34.5
TG-MA		34.5–36
TG-57		34–36.5
Tween 61	Used alone or in combination with polyethylene glycol sorbitan monostearate	35–49
Wecobee FS	Triglycerides derived from coconut oil	39.4–40.5
Wecobee M	Same as above	33.3–36
Wecobee R	Same as above	33.9–35
Wecobee S	Same as above	38–40.5
Wecobee SS	Same as above	40–43
Wecobee W	Same as above	31.7–32.8
Witepsol (selected examples)	Triglycerides of saturated fatty acids C-12–C-18 with varied portions of the corresponding partial glycerides	
H-5		35.2
H-12		32–33
H-15		33–35
H-19		34.8
H-85		42–48

Witepsol bases number about 12 and are nearly white and almost odorless. The melting range and release characteristics of Witepsol H-15 are similar to those of cocoa butter. These bases solidify rapidly in the mold, and lubrication is not necessary because the suppositories contract nicely. Witepsol bases with a high melting point can be mixed with those with a low melting point to provide a wide array of possible melting ranges (i.e., 34°C to 44°C). Because the Witepsol bases contain emulsifiers, they will absorb limited quantities of water.

Water-Soluble Bases

When a water-soluble base is used, the drug dissolves and mixes with the aqueous body fluids. Water-soluble bases may cause some irritation, however, because they may produce slight dehydration of the rectal mucosa by taking up water and dissolving. Nevertheless, they are a widely used base for suppository formulation.

PEG suppository bases are the most popular water-soluble bases. The ratios of low to high molecular weight individual PEGs can be altered to prepare a base with a specific melting point or one that will overcome any problems that result from having to add excess powder or liquid to a suppository. Table 15-2 lists characteristics of various PEGs. PEG bases are incompatible with aminopyrine, aspirin, benzocaine, clioquinol, ichthammol, quinine, silver salts, sulfonamides, and tannic acid. Salicylic acid, sodium barbital, and camphor will crystallize out of PEG suppositories. High concentrations of salicylic acid will soften PEGs, and aspirin will complex with PEGs. PEG-based suppositories may be irritating to some patients. Suppositories prepared with PEG should not be stored or dispensed in a polystyrene prescription vial because PEG interacts adversely with polystyrene. All PEG suppositories should be dispensed in glass or cardboard containers.

Polybase is a preblended suppository base. A white solid, it consists of a homogeneous mixture of PEGs and polysorbate 80. It is a water-miscible base that is stable at room temperature, has a specific gravity of 1.177 at 25°C with an average molecular weight of 3440, and does not require mold lubrication.

Glycerinated gelatin suppositories, composed of 70% glycerin, 20% gelatin, and 10% water, should be packaged in tight containers because they are hygroscopic. They are not recommended as a rectal suppository base because they can exert an osmotic effect and a defecation reflex. A glycerin base is composed of glycerin (87%), sodium stearate (8%), and purified water (5%). These bases have occasionally been used for the preparation of vaginal inserts.

TABLE 15-2 Characteristics of Polyethylene Glycols

Average Molecular Weight	Molecular Weight Range	Melting Range (°C)	Water Solubility (approximate % by weight)
300	285–315	−15 to −8	100
400	380–420	4–8	100
600	570–630	20–25	100
1000	950–1050	37–40	80
1450	1300–1600	43–46	72
3350	3000–3700	54–58	67
4600	4400–4800	57–61	65
8000	7000–9000	60–63	63

Preparation

Three methods are used to prepare a suppository: hand molding, fusion, and compression. Compounding suppositories generally involves hand molding and fusion, but compression can be used in some instances. Powders to be incorporated into suppositories should be in an impalpable form.

Hand molding requires considerable skill, but it enables one to avoid using heat while preparing the suppository because this technique generally uses cocoa butter, which can easily be manipulated, shaped, and handled at room temperature. Hand molding involves grating the cocoa butter, adding the active ingredient, mixing the ingredients thoroughly by using either a mortar and pestle or a pill tile and spatula, pressing the mix together until it resolidifies, shaping the mixture into a long cylinder with a diameter the size of the suppository to be prepared, cutting it into the desired lengths, rounding the tips, and packaging and labeling the units. Plastic gloves can be worn when forming the suppository; working through a filter paper or using cornstarch or talc to decrease the tackiness of the cocoa butter is advisable also.

When using the fusion method, a pharmacist gently heats the base material and then mixes in the active ingredients and any excipients. The melt is then poured into molds and allowed to cool. After cooling, the suppositories are trimmed, packaged, and labeled. Disposable molds, such as the suppository strips and shells shown in Figure 15-1, can be used for molding and dispensing suppository formulations.

A straw or thin glass tube can be used as the mold for preparing urethral suppositories. A 1-mL tuberculin syringe can also be used if the lower portion of the barrel is cut off in a tapered shape (this can be done with a pencil sharpener). A large-diameter needle can be attached to a separate syringe and filled with the suppository melt for transferring the preparation into the 1-mL tuberculin syringe. The urethral suppository can be removed from the 1-mL syringe barrel by inserting the plunger and forcing out the suppository after slight warming. Also, the syringe can be used as an aid for administering the urethral suppository; pressing on the plunger will force the suppository directly into the urethra. Commercial reusable molds for urethral suppositories are also available (Figure 15-2).

Cold compression is suitable for bases that can be formed into suppositories under pressure. It is especially appropriate for ingredients that are heat labile. Cold compression can be used for such bases as a mixture of 6% hexanetriol-1,2,6 with PEG 1450 and 12% polyethylene oxide polymer 4000.

If fusion or cold compression is used, blanks must be prepared to calibrate the molds. These steps should be followed in performing this calibration:

1. Prepare the suppository molds, and confirm that the cavities are clean and dry.
2. Obtain and melt sufficient suppository base to fill 6 to 12 molds.

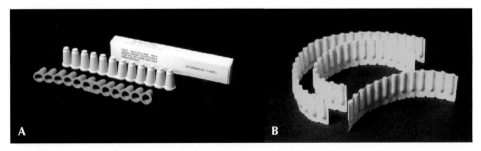

FIGURE 15-1 Disposable suppository molds. A: Shells; B: Strips.

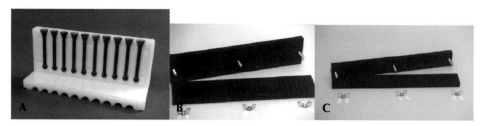

FIGURE 15-2 Urethral suppository molds. A: Ball end; B: Male; C: Female.

3. Pour the base into the molds, cool, and trim.
4. Remove the suppositories, and weigh.
5. Divide the total weight by the number of blank suppositories prepared to obtain the average weight of each suppository for this particular base.
6. Use this weight as the calibrated value for that specific mold using that specific lot of suppository base.

The following five steps are involved in the preparation of suppositories: (1) preparing the mold, (2) preparing the base, (3) preparing the active drug, (4) mixing and pouring, and (5) cooling and finishing.

Preparing the Mold

Molds should be clean and dry at the start. If prepared and heated properly, good suppository bases should require no lubricants applied to a mold; however, if a lubricant is needed, the choice depends on the properties of the base. If a water-soluble base is used, light mineral oil is a good lubricant. Glycerin and propylene glycol are good lubricants for oil-soluble bases. Only enough lubricant should be used to provide a thin layer on the walls of the mold. Excessive lubricant will pool at the tip of the mold and produce misshapen suppositories, whereas inadequate lubricant will result in difficulty in removing the suppositories. The lubricant can be applied either by spraying or by using a lubricant-treated cloth to wipe the molds. Some pharmacists have also used a commercial vegetable spray as a lubricant. The mold should be equilibrated at room temperature for the pouring procedure.

Preparing the Base

The method of preparation will determine the type of base. If hand molding is used, a pharmacist must grate the cocoa butter. The pharmacist can also grate it for the fusion method. If fusion is used, one must take care not to exceed a temperature of about 34° to 35° in order to prevent the formation of an unstable polymorph of the cocoa butter base, which would produce a suppository with a low melting point that would melt at room temperature and might stick to the mold. Cocoa butter should be melted to form a mixable, pourable liquid that is creamy but hazy in appearance; it should not be melted to a clear yellow state.

For cold compression, the desired base is obtained in grated or granular form and mixed with the active drug. The required quantity of the mix is placed in the chamber or barrel and the piston or plunger is moved into place, forcing the material into the attached mold unit. Pressure is then released, and the molded, compressed suppositories are removed.

PEG bases can be melted by using either a water bath or direct heat to a temperature of approximately 60°C. Even though PEG bases are very heat stable, they should not be heated excessively. Rather, they should be heated gently to just a few degrees above their melting range.

Preparing the Active Drug

The active drug should be comminuted to a uniform, small particle size to ensure that it is distributed evenly throughout the base and to minimize settling in the melt. The best source of ingredients for the extemporaneous compounding of suppositories is the pure drug powder. If pure powder is unavailable, commercial dosage forms such as injections, tablets, or capsules can be used. If any excipients are present in these dosage forms, however, they may affect the physicochemical properties and stability of the finished preparation. In many cases, depending on the solubility of the drug and the excipients, one may possibly first mix the dosage form with a solvent (alcohol 95%) and then filter the solution, collect the filtrate, dry it, and use the resulting active drug powder.

In general, the maximum quantity of excipient that can be incorporated is about 30% of the blank weight of the suppository. For example, for a 2-mL disposable mold, the maximum excipient would be about 600 mg.

Liquids may occupy too much volume to be easily incorporated, and the vehicles may not be compatible with selected suppository bases. Tablets and capsules may contain excessive powder, which could produce suppositories that are too brittle. Adding a large quantity of liquid to an oily suppository base may require the preparation of a water-in-oil emulsion. This preparation can be made by incorporating 10% wool fat or 2% cholesterol in up to 15% aqueous solutions in cocoa butter, or by using one of the modern triglyceride vegetable oil bases such as Fattibase, Wecobee, or Witepsol. In the case of PEG bases, a greater percentage of higher molecular weight PEGs can be used to accommodate the liquid.

Mixing and Pouring

The drug is either mixed directly into the base or wetted before incorporation. A stirring rod or a magnetic stirring setup can be used for mixing. The mixing process should be long enough to distribute the drug uniformly but not so long as to lead to drug or base deterioration. As soon as the melt is ready, it can be poured into a mold, which has been brought to room temperature and is situated with the openings on top. A cold or frozen mold should never be used because it can cause fractures and fissures throughout the suppository. The pharmacist should fill each cavity slowly and carefully, starting at one end of the mold and ensuring that no air bubbles are incorporated into the suppository. A slight excess of material may be allowed to build up on the top of the mold as the next cavity is filled, and so on. To prevent layering in the suppositories, the pouring process should not be stopped until all the molds have been filled. The pharmacist can use a 10-mL syringe, or other suitable size, filled with melt to fill the molds as long as the melt does not cool too rapidly. The mold should be at room temperature so that the melt does not solidify prematurely as it is poured down the sides of the mold cavity. Premature solidification could result in unfilled mold tips and deformed suppositories. If disposable molds are used, PEG melts should be poured at a minimum temperature; some molds may collapse at about 70°C. If the melt is poured at around 60°C, such a collapse should not occur. Other bases should be kept near their respective melting temperatures.

Cooling and Finishing

The molds should be allowed to set for 15 to 30 minutes at room temperature and then refrigerated for 30 minutes, if necessary. Any excess material can be removed from the top of the mold (the back of the suppository) with the blade of a stainless steel spatula that has first been dipped in a beaker of warm water. Removing this excess will also give the backside of the suppository an even, smooth surface. A razor blade also works well. The suppositories should then be carefully removed from the molds, packaged, and labeled. If the mold is still cool from refrigeration, the suppositories should be slightly contracted, which will

---

BOX 15-1 Hints for Compounding Suppositories

Suggestions for compounding suppositories are as follows:

- A 10% overage of materials should be calculated to allow for loss during preparation and overpouring.
- If disposable molds are not marked with lines for reproducible filling, the extent of fill should be determined from the blank.
- If plastic disposable molds are used, the temperature of the melt must be lower than the temperature that will melt or soften the mold.
- A constant-temperature dry bath filled with sand set at 37°C provides the proper temperature for softening and melting fatty acid and cocoa butter bases in a short time.
- Vegetable extracts, moistened by levigation with a small quantity of melted base, will more readily distribute the active drug throughout the base.
- A large quantity of powder, if dampened with a few drops of a bland oil, such as mineral oil, or a water-miscible liquid, such as glycerin, will be easier to incorporate into some bases.
- Liquid ingredients, if mixed with a powder such as starch, will be less fluid and easier to incorporate into a base.

---

make removal easier. Wrapping the individual suppositories with foil wrappers, although not necessary, presents an elegant preparation to a patient.

Additional suggestions for preparing suppositories are provided in Box 15-1.

Physicochemical Considerations

A number of factors affect the decisions a pharmacist must make when preparing a suppository. Questions the pharmacist should ask before formulating this dosage form include the following:

- Is the desired effect to result from systemic or local use?
- Is the route of administration rectal, vaginal, or urethral?
- Is a rapid or a slow and prolonged release of the medication desired?

The rate of drug release is an important factor in the selection of a suppository base. If a drug does not release its medication within 6 hours, the patient may not receive its full benefit, because the drug may be expelled. Thus, among the factors that must be considered in the selection of a suppository base is the drug's solubility. One way to ensure maximum release of the drug from the base is to apply the principle of opposite characteristics: water-soluble drugs should be placed in oil-soluble bases, and oil-soluble drugs should be placed in water-soluble bases. Oil-soluble bases (e.g., cocoa butter) melt quickly in the rectum to release the drug, whereas PEG bases must dissolve in mucosal fluids, a process that can take longer. If PEGs with a higher molecular weight are used, the dissolution time is extended. Moistening the suppositories with warm water immediately before insertion facilitates not only insertion, but also dissolution.

The release of the drug and the onset of drug action thus depend on the liquefaction of the suppository base, the dissolution of the active drug, and the diffusion of the drug through the mucosal layers. For example, the time for liquefaction of a suppository with a hydrogenated vegetable oil—or cocoa butter—base is approximately 3 to 7 minutes; for a glycerinated gelatin suppository, about 30 to 40 minutes; and for a PEG suppository, about 30 to 50 minutes. Table 15-3 shows the relationships among drug release rates, the drug, and the suppository base. For instance, if diazepam (very lipophilic) is incorporated into an oleaginous base, the plasma concentration of diazepam and the anticonvulsant effect decrease.[2]

Other factors that must be considered in preparing a suppository include the presence of water, hygroscopicity, viscosity, brittleness, density, volume contraction, special problems, incompatibilities, pharmacokinetics, and bioequivalence.

Presence of Water

When preparing suppositories, a pharmacist should avoid using water to incorporate an active drug. Water may accelerate the oxidation of fat, increase the degradation rate of many drugs, enhance reactions between the drug and other components in the suppository, support bacterial or fungal growth, and necessitate the addition of bacteriostatic agents. Furthermore, if the water evaporates, the dissolved substances may crystallize.

Hygroscopicity

Glycerin- and PEG-containing suppositories are hygroscopic. The rate of moisture change depends on the chain length of the molecule as well as the temperature and humidity of the environment. PEGs with molecular weights greater than 4000 have less tendency to be hygroscopic than do PEGs with lower molecular weight.

Viscosity

Viscosity considerations are also important in the preparation of suppositories and release of the drug. If the viscosity of a base is low, adding a suspending agent such as silica gel may be necessary to ensure that the drug is uniformly dispersed until solidification occurs. When preparing the suppository, a pharmacist should stir the melt constantly and keep it at the lowest possible temperature to maintain high viscosity. After the suppository has been administered, the release rate of the drug may be slowed if the viscosity of the base is very high. The increased viscosity causes the drug to diffuse more slowly through the base to reach the mucosal membrane for absorption.

To increase the viscosity of a fatty base, a pharmacist can increase the fatty acid chain length of compounds in the base. For example, increased C-16 and C-18 monoglycerides and diglycerides can be added to the base. Other approaches involve adding cetyl, stearyl, and myristyl alcohols and stearic acid in concentrations of about 5% or adding about 2% aluminum monostearate to the base.

Brittleness

Brittle suppositories can be difficult to handle, wrap, and use. Cocoa butter suppositories are usually not brittle unless the percentage of solids present is high. In general, brittleness results

TABLE 15-3 Drug Release Rates of Suppository Formulations

Drug:Base Characteristics	Approximate Drug Release Rate
Oil-soluble drug:Oily base	Slow release; poor escaping tendency
Water-soluble drug:Oily base	Rapid release
Oil-soluble drug:Water-miscible base	Moderate release
Water-miscible drug:Water-miscible base	Moderate release; based on diffusion; all water soluble

when the percentage of nonbase materials exceeds about 30%. Synthetic fat bases with high stearate concentrations or those that are highly hydrogenated are typically more brittle. *Shock cooling* occurs when the melted base is chilled too rapidly, possibly causing fat and cocoa butter suppositories to crack. This condition can be prevented by ensuring that the temperature of the mold is as close to the temperature of the melted base as possible. Suppositories should not be placed in a freezer, which also causes shock cooling. The addition of a small quantity (usually less than 2%) of castor oil, glycerin, fatty acid monoglycerides, propylene glycol, Tween 80, or Tween 85 will make these bases more pliable and less brittle.

Density

To determine the weight of the individual suppositories, a pharmacist must know the density of the incorporated materials. For example, if the density of the insoluble powders is too great, the suspended materials will have a tendency to settle and stratify in the molds, resulting in a poor appearance and possibly a brittle suppository.

One principle states that if the quantity of the active drug is less than 100 mg, the volume occupied by the powder is insignificant and need not be considered. This approach is generally based on a 2-g suppository weight. Obviously, if a suppository mold weighing less than 2 g is used, or if the quantity of the active drug to be added is greater than 100 mg, the powder volume should be considered. A pharmacist should know the density factors of various bases and drugs to determine the proper weights of the ingredients to be used.

The density factors of cocoa butter are known. For other bases, the density factor can be calculated as the ratio of the blank weight of the non-cocoa butter base to the blank weight of the cocoa butter base. Density factors for a number of ingredients are shown in Table 15-4.

Two methods of calculating the quantity of base that will be occupied by the active medication are the Dosage Replacement Factor method and the Paddock method. The following equation is used to determine the dosage replacement factor:[3]

$$f = \frac{100\,(E-G)}{(G)(x)} + 1$$

where *f* equals the dosage replacement factor, *E* equals the weight of the pure base suppository, and *G* equals the weight of a suppository with *x*% of the active ingredient.

This equation can be used both for calculating the dosage replacement factor (Table 15-5) and for calculating the weight of the prepared suppositories. A sample calculation for each method is given in Chapter 7 of this book.

Volume Contraction

Bases, excipients, and active ingredients generally occupy less space at lower temperatures than at higher temperatures. When preparing a suppository, a pharmacist pours hot melt into a mold and allows the melt to cool. During this cooling process, the melt has a tendency to contract in size. This contraction allows for easier release of the suppository from the mold, but it may also produce a cavity at the back, or open end, of the mold. Such a cavity is undesirable and can be prevented if the melt is permitted to approach its congealing temperature immediately before it is poured into the mold. Pouring a small amount of excess melt at the open end of the mold to allow for the slight contraction during cooling is advisable. Scraping with a blade or spatula dipped in warm water will remove the excess after solidification, but care must be taken not to remove the metal from the mold. The heated instrument can also be used to smooth out the back of the suppository.

TABLE 15-4 Density Factors for Cocoa Butter Suppositories

Active Drug	Density Factor	Active Drug	Density Factor
Aloin	1.3	Menthol	0.7
Alum	1.7	Morphine hydrochloride	1.6
Aminophylline	1.1	Opium	1.4
Aminopyrine	1.3	Paraffin wax	1.0
Aspirin	1.1	Pentobarbital sodium	1.2
Barbital sodium	1.2	Peruvian balsam	1.1
Belladonna extract	1.3	Phenobarbital	1.2
Benzoic acid	1.5	Phenol	0.9
Bismuth carbonate	4.5	Potassium bromide	2.2
Bismuth salicylate	4.5	Potassium iodide	4.5
Bismuth subgallate	2.7	Procaine	1.2
Bismuth subnitrate	6.0	Quinine hydrochloride	1.2
Boric acid	1.5	Resorcinol	1.4
Castor oil	1.0	Salicylic acid	1.3
Chloral hydrate	1.3	Secobarbital sodium	1.2
Cocaine hydrochloride	1.3	Sodium bromide	2.3
Codeine phosphate	1.1	Spermaceti	1.0
Digitalis leaf	1.6	Sulfathiazole	1.6
Dimenhydrinate	1.3	Tannic acid	1.6
Diphenhydramine hydrochloride	1.3	White wax	1.0
Gallic acid	2.0	Witch hazel fluid extract	1.1
Glycerin	1.6	Zinc oxide	4.0
Ichthammol	1.1	Zinc sulfate	2.8
Iodoform	4.0		

Special Problems

Some active drugs are more difficult to incorporate into a base and require additional preparation steps. Before vegetable extracts are added, they can be moistened by levigation with a small amount of melted base. This step permits easier distribution of the active drug throughout the base.

Hard, crystalline materials can be incorporated either by pulverizing them to a fine state or by dissolving them in a small quantity of solvent, which is then taken up into the base. An aqueous solvent and a PEG base are appropriate for water-soluble materials. Alternatively, if the material is water soluble and an oily base must be used, wool fat could be used to take up the solution for incorporation into the suppository base.

When liquid ingredients are mixed with an inert powder such as starch, they become less fluid, which makes them easier to handle. The suppository produced in this manner will thus hold together better.

Several methods are used to incorporate excess powder into a suppository base, depending on the base used. If the base is oil miscible, a few drops of a bland oil like sesame oil or mineral oil can be added. When excess powder is incorporated into water-soluble bases, a pharmacist can vary the ratio of low to high melting point ingredients. For example, because additional powders will make the suppository harder, using a higher percentage of a PEG having a low molecular weight would result in a suppository of the proper character.

Incompatibilities

A number of ingredients are incompatible with PEG bases. They include aspirin, benzocaine, clioquinol, ichthammol, quinine, silver salts, sulfonamides, and tannic acid. Other materials reported to have a tendency to crystallize out of PEG include salicylic acid, sodium barbital, and camphor.

Pharmacokinetics

Factors affecting absorption include anorectal or vaginal physiology, suppository vehicle, absorption site pH, drug pK_a, degree of ionization, and lipid solubility. In some instances, suppositories have been proven to have better absorption than orally administered medications.

Bioequivalence Examples

The rectal and oral routes of administration can be bioequivalent. The rectal route, however, should be considered as an alternative for some drugs, such as etodolac. Some prodrugs may degrade before they are absorbed through the gastrointestinal tract. The use of cyclodextrins to improve the pharmaceutical properties of drugs has been well documented. When a cyclodextrin is incorporated with a prodrug in a suppository dosage form, the rectal bioavailability of the prodrug may be enhanced.

Single dosing of fluconazole orally has been demonstrated to be equivalent to once-daily dosing for 3 days of terconazole (80 mg each). The terconazole was contained in a vaginal insert with a cocoa butter base. In late evaluation of the infection for which the drugs were administered, the cure rates for oral and vaginal administration were 75% and 100%, respectively.

Bioavailability of solids can be maximized by using the smallest particle size available. Also, drugs that are available as water-soluble salt forms will generally go into solution more easily in the mucosal fluids, followed by migration to the rectal wall and absorption. The addition of sodium caprate increases the bioavailability of penicillins and cephalosporins, and the addition of bile salts and fatty acids can increase the permeability of some other drugs.

TABLE 15-5 Dosage Replacement Factors for Selected Drugs[a]

Active Drug	Dosage Replacement Factor
Balsam peru	0.87
Bismuth subgallate	0.37
Bismuth subnitrate	0.33
Boric acid	0.67
Camphor	1.49
Castor oil	1.0
Chloral hydrate	1.67
Ichthammol	0.91
Phenobarbital	0.81
Phenol	0.9
Procaine hydrochloride	0.8
Quinine hydrochloride	0.83
Resorcinol	0.71
Silver protein, mild	0.61
Spermaceti	1.0
Wax, white and yellow	1.0
Zinc oxide	0.15–0.25

[a]Cocoa butter is arbitrarily assigned a value of 1 as the standard base.

Quality Control

Quality control of suppositories encompasses uniformity of weight and uniformity of texture and physical appearance. Uniformity of texture can be assessed by sectioning a suppository longitudinally and laterally and then ensuring that each section presents a smooth, uniform surface.

Patient Counseling

Patients should be instructed on how to properly store the suppository, unwrap a wrapped suppository, and resolidify a melted suppository. The proper method of disposing of unused suppositories should be discussed. Patients should also be counseled on the proper insertion of the suppository: whether to moisten it before insertion, how far to insert it, and how long to remain inactive after insertion. For rectal suppositories, a patient should lubricate the suppository with a water-soluble lubricant or a small amount of water, if needed; lie on the left side with the upper leg flexed; and gently insert the suppository into the rectum a finger's depth, at an angle toward the umbilicus so the suppository is placed against the rectal wall for absorption rather than being left in the canal or pushed into a mass of stool. After withdrawing the finger, the patient should hold the buttocks together until the urge to expel has ceased.

Packaging

Wrapping suppositories individually or dispensing them in the disposable molds in which they are prepared is best. If suppositories are not packaged properly, they may become deformed, stained, broken, or chipped. Foil suppository wrappers are available in various colors. Wrapped suppositories are usually placed in wide-mouthed containers or in sliding, folding, or partitioned boxes (Figure 15-3) for dispensing to a patient. Suppositories that are dispensed in disposable molds are often placed in cardboard sleeves or plastic bags, labeled, and dispensed.

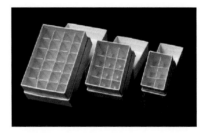

FIGURE 15-3 Suppository boxes.

Storage and Labeling

Suppositories must be protected from heat and can be stored in a refrigerator. They should not be frozen. Glycerin- and PEG-based suppositories should be protected from moisture, because they tend to be hygroscopic.

If the suppositories are wrapped, including the instruction, "Unwrap, Moisten, and Insert" or "Unwrap and Insert," on the label is a good idea.

Stability

The completed formulations are generally considered dry or nonaqueous and thus provide a stable dosage form as long as they are protected from moisture and heat. According to Chapter <795> of the *United States Pharmacopeia (USP),*[4] these preparations should have a beyond-use date of 25% of the time remaining on the expiration date if the preparation is compounded with a manufactured product or 6 months, whichever is earlier. If the preparation is compounded from USP or NF (National Formulary) grade substances, a beyond-use date of 6 months is appropriate unless evidence is available to support other dating. Most guidelines recommend storage in a refrigerator unless otherwise indicated.

According to *USP,* the major indication of instability in suppositories is excessive softening. In some cases, suppositories may dry out, harden, or shrivel. The *USP* description of stability considerations for suppositories includes observations for excessive softening and evidence of oil stains on packaging materials. A pharmacist may have to remove the wrappings of individual suppositories to check for evidence of instability.

The formation of polymorphs is evidence of cocoa butter instability during preparation. These polymorphs may be liquid at room temperature. To avoid this situation, a pharmacist may substitute an appropriate hydrogenated vegetable oil base for the cocoa butter. If necessary, fatty materials with higher melting points, such as white wax or paraffin, can be added to fatty bases or cocoa butter, with low melting points, to increase the melting point of the formulation. However, the suppository must be able to melt when administered. To check the melting point, the pharmacist can place a sample suppository in a beaker of water that has been heated to 37°C. If the suppository does not melt, the formulation should not be used for patient therapy.

If water is incorporated into an oily base with the use of an emulsifying agent (nonionic surfactant, wool fat, and the like), the preparation may become rancid. In this case, the suppository usually will not be as stable as if the same drug were added to a PEG-based suppository containing water.

Most suppository formulations do not contain preservatives or antioxidants because (1) water is usually excluded from the formulations, (2) nonoxidizing bases are generally used, and (3) the drug is generally stable in a solid dosage form.

Sample Formulations

Suppository Bases
These bases are to be prepared according to the instructions given in the subsection above, "Preparing the Base."

General Purpose #1 Base

Polyethylene glycol 8000	50%	Base
Polyethylene glycol 1540	30%	Base
Polyethylene glycol 300	20%	Base

General Purpose Soft Base

Polyethylene glycol 3350	60%	Base
Polyethylene glycol 1000	30%	Base
Polyethylene glycol 300	10%	Base

General Purpose Firm Base

Polyethylene glycol 8000	30%	Base
Polyethylene glycol 1540	70%	Base

Polyethylene Glycol Bases for Progesterone Suppositories

	Formula 1	Formula 2	
Polyethylene glycol 8000	40%	20%	Base
Polyethylene glycol 300	60%	80%	Base

Base for Water-Soluble Drugs

Polyethylene glycol 8000	60%	Base
Polyethylene glycol 1540	25%	Base
Cetyl alcohol	5%	Emulsifier
Purified water	10%	Base

Ingredient-Specific Formulations

Estradiol Suppository (#1)

Estradiol	1 mg	Active
Silica gel	20 mg	Suspending Aid
Fatty acid base	qs	Base

1. Calculate the quantity of each ingredient required for the prescription.
2. Accurately weigh or measure each ingredient.
3. Carefully heat the fatty acid base to about 35°C to 37°C, being careful not to overheat.
4. Sprinkle the estradiol powder and silica gel onto the melted base, and mix thoroughly.
5. Remove the mix from heat, and pour into mold that is at room temperature, not chilled. Once the pouring has started, do not stop. If reusable mold is used, allow a small quantity of the melt to bead up on the back of the suppository to allow for contraction.
6. Place suppository in a refrigerator to harden.
7. Remove suppository from refrigerator, and allow to set at room temperature for a few minutes.
8. Trim the suppository and package. If reusable mold is used, trim the suppository, remove from mold, wrap if desired, and package.
9. Label the product.

℞ Morphine Sulfate Slow-Release Suppository (#1)

Morphine sulfate	50 mg	Active
Alginic acid	25%	Slow-Release Agent
Fatty acid base	qs	Base

1. Calculate the quantity of each ingredient required for the prescription.
2. Accurately weigh or measure each ingredient.
3. Pass the alginic acid through a No. 200-mesh sieve.
4. Melt the fatty acid base in a glass beaker to about 50°C.
5. Sprinkle the alginic acid on the fatty acid base, and mix well.
6. Sprinkle the morphine sulfate on the mixture, and stir until well mixed.
7. Place the mixture in an ultrasonic bath for 10 minutes for thorough and complete mixing.
8. Cool the mixture slightly, and pour continuously into mold held at room temperature.
9. Cool and trim the suppository.
10. Package and label the product.

℞ Ondansetron Hydrochloride Suppository (#1)

Ondansetron hydrochloride	8 mg	Active
Micronized silica gel	25 mg	Suspending Aid
Fatty acid base	qs	Base

1. Calculate the quantity of each ingredient required for the prescription.
2. Accurately weigh or measure each ingredient.
3. Triturate the ondansetron hydrochloride with the micronized silica gel.
4. Melt the fatty acid base, and heat to approximately 50°C.
5. Sprinkle the powder on the melt, and mix thoroughly.
6. Remove the mix from heat for a few minutes.
7. Pour the mix into mold (equilibrated at room temperature).
8. Place the suppository in refrigerator to harden.
9. Trim, package, and label the product.

℞ Antiemetic Suppository (#1)

Haloperidol	5 mg	Active
Diphenhydramine hydrochloride	25 mg	Active
Lorazepam	2 mg	Active
Silicon dioxide	30 mg	Suspending Aid
Polyethylene glycol base	qs	Base

1. Calculate the quantity of each ingredient required for the prescription.
2. Accurately weigh or measure each ingredient.
3. Mix the powders together.
4. Heat the polyethylene glycol base to about 60°C.
5. Sprinkle the powders onto the melted base, and mix well.
6. Pour the melt into mold (maintained at room temperature) slowly and smoothly, and stir intermittently to ensure the powders remain well mixed.
7. Allow the suppository to solidify (refrigerate if necessary).
8. Remove the suppository from mold, and trim.
9. Package and label the product.

℞ Fluconazole 200 mg Suppository (#1)

Fluconazole	200 mg	Active
Polyethylene glycol base	qs	Base

1. Calculate the quantity of each ingredient required for the prescription.
2. Accurately weigh or measure each ingredient and/or count the required number of fluconazole tablets.
3. Pulverize the fluconazole tablets to provide the fluconazole powder.
4. Melt the polyethylene glycol base at about 60°C.
5. Sprinkle the powder onto the melted base, and stir.
6. Cool the mix slightly, and pour into mold.
7. Cool and trim the suppository.
8. Package and label the product.

℞ Nifedipine, Lidocaine, and Nitroglycerin Suppositories (#30)

Nifedipine	200 mg	Active
Lidocaine HCl	1.5 g	Active
Nitroglycerin 0.4 mg tablets	#25	Active
Polybase or fatty acid base	qs 75 g	Base

1. Calculate the quantity of each ingredient required for the prescription.
2. Calibrate the suppository mold, using the Polybase or the fatty acid base.
3. Accurately weigh or measure each ingredient, and count out the nitroglycerin tablets.
4. Mix nifedipine and lidocaine powders together.
5. Levigate the nitroglycerin tablets with a small quantity of ethyl alcohol.
6. Gently melt the selected base.
7. Add the powders and the nitroglycerin to the melted base, and mix well.
8. Pour the mix into molds, and allow to cool.
9. Cool and trim the suppositories.
10. Package and label the product.

(Note: This preparation should be prepared in a room with subdued light because of the light sensitivity of nifedipine.)

References

1. Allen LV Jr. *Suppositories.* London: Pharmaceutical Press; 2008.
2. Hidaka N, Suemaru K, Aimoto T, Araka H. Effect of simultaneous insertion of oleaginous base on the absorption and on the anticonvulsant effect of diazepam suppository. *Biol Pharm Bull.* 2006; 29(4):705–8.
3. Coben LJ, Lieberman HA. Suppositories. In: Lachman L, Lieberman HA, Kanig JL. *The Theory and Practice of Industrial Pharmacy.* 3rd ed. Philadelphia: Lea and Febiger; 1986:564–88.
4. United States Pharmacopeial Convention. Chapter <795>, Pharmaceutical compounding— nonsterile preparations. *United States Pharmacopeia/National Formulary.* Rockville, MD: United States Pharmacopeial Convention; current edition.

Sticks

Medication sticks are a convenient form for administering topical drugs; they are not limited to applications to the lips. Their development is interesting because it involves the history of cosmetics, which parallels human history. Historical uses of cosmetics and pharmacists' involvement in their development are reviewed in Chapter 31 of this book.

Although cosmetics are viewed as preparations aimed at improving a person's appearance, many cosmetic preparations also serve as either medications or drug vehicle bases. Some formulations that have been introduced and improved for cosmetic use—powders, sticks, gels, solutions, suspensions, pastes, ointments, and oils—are widely used in the pharmaceutical sciences.

The medication stick, a fairly recent preparation, is used for both cosmetic and medical purposes. Examples include styptic pencils and lip balm sticks, which became available in the early 1940s. Currently, medication sticks provide pharmacists, patients, and primary care providers with a unique, convenient, relatively stable, easy-to-prepare dosage form for the topical delivery of drugs. The use of this form will probably continue to grow.

Definitions and Types

In accordance with their characteristics, sticks can be grouped in three main categories: soft opaque, soft clear, and hard.

Soft opaque sticks can contain cocoa butter, petrolatum, and polyethylene glycol (PEG) bases. Most medication sticks are of this type.

Soft clear sticks usually contain the bases propylene glycol and sodium stearate. Water or alcohol is also added.

Hard sticks consist of crystalline powders either fused by heat or held together with a binder such as cocoa butter or petrolatum.

The same principles used in formulating lipsticks—the prototype for all cosmetic sticks—apply to the formulation of medication sticks. Lipsticks vary greatly in their physical properties. They can be quite hard, soft, greasy or sticky, brittle and crumbly, or smooth and velvety. All lipsticks, however, have a definite mechanical function, which is to provide a vehicle to facilitate easy, uniform application of color to the lips. Thus, their consistency is of vital importance. If the stick is too hard, it is difficult to apply. If it crumbles or is too sticky, it will smear, which generates consumer complaints.

The materials that give body to sticks are waxes, polymers, resins, dry solids fused into a firm mass, and fused crystals. An example of a fused stick is a styptic pencil. Resin is used in connection with epilating wax. The resin and pitch or waxes are melted and poured into molds in which they solidify in stick form.

Applications

Sticks are a convenient form for administering topical medications. They come in different sizes and shapes, are readily transportable, and can be applied directly to the affected site of the body. Sticks can be easily compounded by using different materials to produce topical or systemic effects. Medications and other ingredients that have been incorporated into sticks include local anesthetics, sunscreens, oncology drugs, antivirals, and antibiotics. Sticks containing antibiotics, antivirals, and oncology agents are usually packaged in 5-g tubes, whereas sticks containing local anesthetics are usually packaged in 1- or 2-oz tubes.

The medication in a soft stick is applied by raising the stick above the tube level and simply rubbing it onto the skin, where it softens and flows easily onto the affected area. The medication usually cannot be seen on the skin. When a hard stick is applied, the tip of the stick is moistened and then touched to the affected area. The crystalline powder used to prepare the stick can leave a white residue on the skin.

Composition

Preparing sticks requires different bases depending on the application. There are two types of bases: melting bases and moistening bases.

Melting Bases

Melting bases include the bases used to prepare soft opaque and soft clear sticks. These bases, which will soften and melt at body temperatures, include cocoa butter, PEGs, petrolatum, waxes, and the like. Active drugs can include any agent that can be applied directly to a specific skin site or over a larger area of skin to relieve such discomforts as muscle sprains and arthritis. Penetration enhancers (e.g., alcohol, glycerin, propylene glycol, and surfactants) can increase the amount of transdermal drug delivery. Using waxes, oils, or plain polymers such as PEGs alone achieves a topical effect. Melting bases can be further divided into opaque and clear. Opaque bases include waxes, oils, PEGs, and the like, whereas clear bases include sodium stearate and glycerin mixtures.

Moistening Bases

This base is used to produce solid, hard sticks that must be moistened to become activated. When the stick is moistened, a concentrated solution of the drug forms at the tip of the stick. When applied, the drug will exert its effect topically. A styptic pencil containing alum or aluminum sulfate is an example of this type of stick. Some drugs that are not stable in other forms possibly would be stable in a dry, hard crystalline stick.

Preparation

Certain characteristics are required of a good stick. It should spread easily without excessive greasiness. It should be uniform, stable, and free from mottling. It should not sweat, crumble, or crack.

Pharmacists preparing sticks need to be familiar with waxes. Some waxes such as carnauba have high melting points; others such as beeswax, cocoa butter, and paraffin have lower melting points. There are also waxy fatty acids such as stearic acid and spermaceti and waxy alcohols such as cetyl and stearyl alcohol. Table 16-1 lists the melting and congealing points of various waxes, oils, and PEGs. Clearly, no single waxy substance is appropriate for all purposes. The high-melting-point waxes must be blended with the low-melting-point waxes to produce a combination that will soften at body temperature. Adding lubricants will minimize the coherence of the waxes and make the product easier to spread. By balancing these ingredients, one can eventually develop a stick that has the desired physical properties for its application. A pharmacist's goal is to prepare a combination of waxes that will soften at body temperature and will still contain lubricants and other ingredients that promote the absorption and emollient effects.

The consistency of the stick is determined by the melting point of the waxes. To change the consistency, one must adjust the melting point by changing the percentage of the wax with the highest melting point.

A pharmacist should mold a batch of sticks all at once to ensure that the mixture does not grow cold and require reheating. All trimmings and scraps, together with any sticks rejected because of mold marks or pinholes, should be kept separate from the regular batch. This material can be remelted and will produce sticks that are as good as the others.

A pharmacist should keep in mind a number of hints when compounding a preparation. Vitamins E and A can be added to enhance emollient and skin care effects. Zinc oxide or para-aminobenzoic acid acts as a sunblock. Perfume sticks can be prepared by adding an appropriate perfume oil.

For the preparation of medication sticks, a constant-temperature dry bath filled with sand or salt at about 35°C to 40°C provides the proper temperature for softening and melting fatty acid and cocoa butter bases; the proper temperature for softening and melting PEG bases in minimal time is 55°C to 65°C.

Physicochemical Considerations

The ingredients used to formulate sticks have unique properties. A list of ingredients and their advantages and disadvantages follows.

Oils

Vegetable oils, such as olive oil and sesame oil, have a tendency to become rancid.

Mineral oils resist rancidity, but their ability to dissolve certain ingredients is limited. They also tend to make the product smear and run off. They can be used in small proportions to enhance gloss.

Castor oil is a unique vegetable oil that has a high viscosity. High viscosity helps delay the settling of ingredients from the molten stick mass and lessens the tendency of the applied stick to smear and run off.

Butyl stearate has been widely used in the preparation of sticks. A pure grade has no disagreeable odor and does not turn rancid. Fatty esters of lower alcohols are generally similar in properties to butyl stearate.

TABLE 16-1 Melting and Congealing Point Ranges of Waxes, Oils, and PEGs

Item	Melting Range or Point (°C)	Congealing Range or Point (°C)
Wax		
Carnauba wax	81–86	
Cetostearyl alcohol	48–55	
Cetyl alcohol	45–50	
Cetyl esters wax	43–47	
Cholesterol	147–150	
Cocoa butter	30–35	
Emulsifying wax	48–52	
Glyceryl monostearate	≥55	
Hard fat	27–44	
Microcrystalline wax	54–102	
Paraffin		47–65
Polyoxyl 40 stearate		37–47
Propylene glycol monostearate		≥45
Purified stearic acid		66–69
Stearic acid		≥54
Stearyl alcohol	55–60	
White wax	62–65	
Yellow wax	62–65	
Oil		
Castor oil		−10 to −18
Corn oil	−18 to −10	
Cottonseed oil		0 to −5
Hydrogenated castor oil	85–88	
Hydrogenated vegetable oil	61–66	
Oleic acid		−10
Peanut oil		−5
Polyoxyl 40 hydrogenated castor oil	20–30	
Soybean oil		−10 to −16
Polyethylene glycol (PEG)		
PEG 300		4 to 8
PEG 1500	44–48	
PEG 3350	54–58	
PEG 6000	58–63	

Cocoa butter is widely used because it melts on application at about body temperature. However, it tends to bloom, or come to the surface in an irregular fashion, which could produce unsightly craters or excrescences, a characteristic that can be overcome by the use of commercially available fatty acid bases (Fattibase).

Petrolatum is quite stable and produces good gloss, and thus, it is useful in preparing sticks.

Lanolin and absorption bases enhance the incorporation of water-containing ingredients and are useful in preparing sticks.

Lecithin improves smoothness, emollience, and ease of application.

Waxes

Carnauba wax is one of the harder waxes, so a small percentage raises the melting point and the strength.

Candelilla wax has a lower melting point than carnauba and must be used in larger proportions to obtain equal effects.

Beeswax is the traditional stiffening agent for sticks and is still used extensively. If used as the only wax, it produces a rather dull stick that does not apply easily. Hard waxes yield a better gloss.

Paraffins are too weak and brittle to be of much value in sticks, although small amounts can improve gloss. Immiscibility with castor oil can limit their use in some applications. Hydrogenated castor oil is a brittle white wax that yields a high gloss but little strength.

Synthetic waxes of many types are available. Each must be judged on its own merits.

Water-Soluble Bases

PEGs and their ethers are available in great variety. They are quite water soluble and are easy to remove from the skin.

Propylene glycol monoesters have relatively good solvent power and are found in some sticks. Sodium stearate–propylene glycol combinations are widely used for deodorant sticks and are good for the application of topical drugs. This type of base melts at body temperature, is colorless, and rubs in nicely.

A pleasant fragrance is one factor in determining consumer acceptance of some sticks. When selecting flavoring oils, one must ensure that those to be applied near or on the lips are free from irritating effects (burning) and disagreeable tastes.

Quality Control

Quality control procedures for preparing medication sticks should address weight variation, melting point, and physical observations. Preparing extra medication sticks and placing them in storage over the expected use or life of the prescription is advisable. If adverse changes are observed in the dosage form during storage, a patient can be contacted and the remaining sticks recalled.

Packaging, Storage, and Labeling

Sticks should be packaged in 5-g, 25-g, or other appropriate tube sizes (Figure 16-1), depending on the application. The sticks should be kept out of the reach of children and out of heat and direct sunlight. They are best stored at either 5°C or 25°C, depending on the composition of the stick. Appropriate labeling of these preparations includes "For External Use Only," "Do Not Take Internally," "Keep Out of Reach of Children," and "Protect from Heat."

Stability

Medication sticks are generally considered dry and thus provide a stable dosage form as long as they

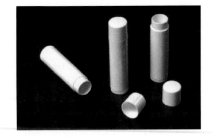

FIGURE 16-1 Applicator tube.

are protected from moisture and heat. According to Chapter <795> of the *United States Pharmacopeia (USP),*[1] sticks prepared from a manufactured product have a beyond-use date of 25% of the time remaining on the product's expiration date or 6 months, whichever is earlier. If the formulation is prepared from USP or NF (National Formulary) grade substances, a beyond-use date of 6 months is appropriate unless evidence is available to support other dating. Because many of these preparations do not contain water, the active drug should remain stable. However, using heat in the preparation could result in drug degradation. A pharmacist should estimate a reasonable beyond-use date.

Patient Counseling

When counseling a patient about the use of medications sticks, a pharmacist must consider the active drug and the method of application. In general, the patient should be instructed to apply the stick only to the involved area and not to surrounding skin. In addition, the patient should apply the medication liberally over the area but only as needed. The surface of the stick should be cleaned with a clean tissue after each use, and, to avoid transmitting infection, the product should not be shared with others.

Sample Formulations

Three categories of bases and ingredient-specific formulations for medication sticks are described in the following section: soft opaque, soft clear, and hard. Sample formulations are presented for illustrative purposes only. These sticks can be used in many ways, depending on the active ingredients incorporated into the formulation.

Soft Opaque Sticks

Several formulations for bases can be used to prepare soft opaque sticks. Nine such base formulations, followed by sample formulations for preparations containing active drugs, are presented in this section.

Sample Bases

 Stick Formulation No. 1 (general purpose, water-repellent base)

Beeswax	34 g	Base/Thickener
Cocoa butter	8 g	Base
Lanolin	6 g	Base
Petrolatum	18 g	Base
Paraffin	10 g	Base/Thickener
Talc (optional)	16 g	Base/Color
Perfume (optional)	1 g	Perfume
Active drug	qs	Active

1. Accurately weigh or measure the ingredients.
2. Triturate the active drug with the petrolatum mass until smooth.
3. Melt the beeswax, cocoa butter, lanolin, and paraffin, and add the petrolatum base; stir thoroughly, and slowly sift in the active drug and talc (optional) while mixing.
4. Add perfume to the mix, stir, and pour into molds or containers.

Stick Formulation No. 2 (softer, general purpose, water-repellent base)

Talc (optional)	19 g	Base/Color
Petrolatum	20 g	Base
Paraffin	30 g	Base/Thickener
Cocoa butter	15 g	Base
Beeswax	10 g	Base/Thickener
Perfume (optional)	1 g	Perfume
Active drug	qs	Active

1. Accurately weigh or measure the ingredients.
2. Mix the active drug and talc with the petrolatum, and triturate until smooth.
3. Melt the waxes and the cocoa butter with the petrolatum mixture, and mix thoroughly.
4. Add the perfume to the mix, and pour into molds.

 Stick Formulation No. 3 (stiff stick that will take up some water)

White beeswax	31 g	Base/Thickener
Paraffin	5 g	Base/Thickener
Cocoa butter (Fattibase)	7 g	Base
Aquabase	34.5 g	Base/Water Absorber
Castor oil, tasteless	4 g	Base
Perfume	0.9 g	Perfume
Preservative	0.1 g	Preservative
Butyl stearate	5 g	Thickener

1. Accurately weigh or measure the ingredients.
2. Mix the butyl stearate and the castor oil.
3. Melt the Aquabase using mild heat.
4. Add the butyl stearate–castor oil mixture to the Aquabase, and mix thoroughly.
5. Melt the beeswax, paraffin, and cocoa butter, and mix with the mixture prepared in step 4.
6. Mix thoroughly, and add the perfume and preservative.
7. Heat the mixture until the temperature of the mass reaches 45°C; maintain the temperature of the batch at this point while filling molds.

Stick Formulation No. 4 (hard, firm stick)

White petrolatum	70.75 g	Base
Cetyl alcohol	3 g	Emulsifier
Lanolin	10.5 g	Base/Water Absorber
White beeswax	5.25 g	Base/Thickener
Cetyl esters wax	10.5 g	Emulsifier

1. Accurately weigh or measure the ingredients.
2. Melt the cetyl alcohol, white beeswax, and cetyl esters wax together, and mix well.
3. Melt the white petrolatum and lanolin together, and mix well.
4. Mix the melt from step 2 to the melt in step 3 by stirring.
5. Cool the mix to about 45°C, and fill molds.

 ### Stick Formulation No. 5 (water-repellent stick)

Carnauba wax	10 g	Base
White beeswax	15 g	Base/Thickener
Lanolin	5 g	Base/Water Absorber
Cetyl alcohol	5 g	Emulsifier
Castor oil	65 g	Base

1. Accurately weigh or measure the ingredients.
2. Melt the carnauba wax, white beeswax, and cetyl alcohol together.
3. Add the lanolin and castor oil, and mix well.
4. Cool the mix to about 45°C, and fill molds.

 ### Stick Formulation No. 6 (smooth stick that will absorb some water)

White wax	36 g	Base/Thickener
Yellow wax	18 g	Base/Thickener
Cocoa butter	19 g	Base
Absorption base (Aquabase)	5.5 g	Base/Water Absorber
Mineral oil	9.5 g	Base
Oleyl alcohol	3 g	Base

Absorption Base:[a]

Petrolatum	94 g	Base
Cholesterol	3 g	Emulsifier
Cetyl alcohol	3 g	Emulsifier

1. Accurately weigh or measure the ingredients.
2. Melt the white wax and yellow beeswax together.
3. Melt the absorption base and cocoa butter together.
4. Add the melt from step 2 to the melt from step 3.
5. Add the mineral oil and oleyl alcohol, and mix well.
6. Cool the mix to about 45°C, and pour into molds.
7. For the absorption base, melt the cetyl alcohol and cholesterol together; add the petrolatum, mix well, and allow to cool.

[a]Alternative absorption base.

Stick Formulation No. 7 (lip balm base)

| White wax NF | 5 g | Base/Thickener |
| White petrolatum USP | 95 g | Base |

1. Accurately weigh or measure the ingredients.
2. Melt the white wax in a beaker using low heat.
3. Add the white petrolatum, and mix thoroughly with a stirring rod until uniform.
4. Cool the mix until thick, and pour into an ointment jar for storage at room temperature until used.

 Stick Formulation No. 8 (lip balm base)

White wax NF	30 g	Base/Thickener
Cetyl esters wax NF	30 g	Emulsifier
Mineral oil USP	40 g	Base

1. Accurately weigh or measure the ingredients.
2. Melt the white wax and cetyl esters wax in a beaker.
3. Stir in the mineral oil.
4. Cool the mix until thickened.
5. Pour mix into an ointment jar for storage until used.

 Stick Formulation No. 9 (lip balm base)

Glyceryl monostearate NF	20 g	Emulsifier
Span 80	2 g	Emulsifier
Oil-in-water emulsion base (Dermabase)	78 g	Base

1. Accurately weigh or measure the ingredients.
2. Melt the glyceryl monostearate at 55°C–70°C in a beaker.
3. Add the Span 80, and mix thoroughly.
4. Heat the emulsion base to about 60°C, and pour into the other melted mixture.
5. Stir the mix rapidly.
6. Cool the mix, and pour into an ointment jar until used.

Ingredient-Specific Soft Opaque Sticks

 Camphor Ice-Type Preparation (for insect stings)

Powdered camphor	20 g	Active
Light beeswax	18 g	Base/Thickener
White petrolatum	15 g	Base
Cetyl esters wax	47 g	Emulsifier

1. Calculate the quantity of each ingredient required for the prescription.
2. Accurately weigh or measure the ingredients.
3. Melt the light beeswax, white petrolatum, and cetyl esters wax.
4. Mix the ingredients. When the temperature drops to about 50°C, add the camphor and mix well.
5. Fill the molds, and allow to cool.

℞ Acyclovir Lip Balm,[a] Plain

	Formula 1	Formula 2	
Acyclovir (200 mg capsules)	#6	#6	Active
Span 80	0.5 g		Emulsifier
Glyceryl monostearate	5 g		Emulsifier
Water-in-oil emulsion base (Dermabase)	19.5 g		Base
Polyethylene glycol base (Polybase)		25 g	Base

[a]These formulas can be modified by incorporating lidocaine, para-aminobenzoic acid, or other ingredients as needed.

Formula 1
1. Calculate the quantity of each ingredient required for the prescription.
2. Accurately weigh or measure the ingredients.
3. Heat the glyceryl monostearate to about 55°C to 70°C, and add the Span 80, followed by the acyclovir powder, which has been previously removed from the capsules and comminuted to obtain a fine, uniform powder.
4. Heat the water-in-oil emulsion base; add the melted glyceryl monostearate mixture to the base; stir, and remove from heat.
5. Stir the mix rapidly, cool, and pour into tubes or molds.

Formula 2
1. Calculate the quantity of each ingredient required for the prescription.
2. Accurately weigh or measure the ingredients.
3. Heat the polyethylene glycol base to about 55°C.
4. Empty the acyclovir capsules into a mortar, and reduce the particle size to a fine powder.
5. Add these powders to the melted base, and mix thoroughly.
6. Cool the mix to just above the melting point of the preparation, until it starts to thicken.
7. While stirring, pour the mix into the lip balm molds or tubes.

℞ Lidocaine 30% Lip Balm[a]

Lidocaine	1.5 g	Active
Polyethylene glycol 4000	1 g	Base
Polyethylene glycol 400	2.5 g	Base

1. Calculate the quantity of each ingredient required for the prescription.
2. Accurately weigh or measure the ingredients.
3. Melt the polyethylene glycol bases together at about 55°C.
4. Add the powder to the melted base, and mix until evenly dispersed.
5. Cool the mix to just above the melting point of the preparation, until it starts to thicken.
6. While stirring, pour the mix into the lip balm molds or tubes.

[a]Alternative formulation: Replace polyethylene glycol bases with 3.5 g of Polybase.

℞ Camphor–Phenol–Menthol (CPM) Lip Balm

Camphor	1%	Active
Phenol	0.5%	Active
Menthol	1%	Active
Lip balm base	qs	Base

1. Calculate the quantity of each ingredient required for the prescription.
2. Accurately weigh or measure the ingredients.
3. Mix the camphor, phenol, and menthol until a eutectic liquid forms.
4. Melt the lip balm base in a beaker using gentle heat.
5. Remove the melted base from heat, add the eutectic mixture to the base while it is still fluid, and mix thoroughly with a stirring rod.
6. Pour the mix into lip balm molds or tubes, and allow to cool.

℞ Analgesic Medication Stick

Methyl salicylate	35 g	Active
Menthol	15 g	Active
Sodium stearate	13 g	Base/Emulsifier
Purified water	12 mL	Base
Propylene glycol	25 g	Base/Humectant

1. Calculate the quantity of each ingredient required for the prescription.
2. Accurately weigh or measure the ingredients.
3. Gently heat and melt the sodium stearate.
4. Mix the purified water with the propylene glycol, and add to the melted sodium stearate.
5. Mix the base thoroughly, remove from heat, and allow to cool slightly.
6. Dissolve the menthol in the methyl salicylate; add this solution to the base, and mix thoroughly.
7. As the preparation begins to thicken, continue to mix and pour into either 5-g or 20-g stick containers.
8. Allow sticks to harden at room temperature.

Soft Clear Sticks

℞ Clear Stick Base

Sodium stearate	7 g	Base
Alcohol	65 g	Base
Propylene glycol	25 g	Base
Cyclomethicone	3 g	Active

1. Calculate the quantity of each ingredient required for the prescription.
2. Accurately weigh or measure the ingredients.
3. Melt the sodium stearate.
4. Mix the alcohol, propylene glycol, and cyclomethicone, and add to the melted sodium stearate.
5. Mix well, cool the mix slightly, and pour into stick molds.

Hard Sticks

Hard sticks, or styptic pencils, are used to stop the flow of blood from cuts. There are two types of styptic pencils: those with a hard crystalline structure and those with a wax base.

℞ Styptic Pencil (hard with aluminum sulfate)

Ammonium chloride	7 g	Active
Aluminum sulfate	27 g	Active
Ferric sulfate	40 g	Active
Copper sulfate	26 g	Active

1. Calculate the quantity of each ingredient required for the prescription.
2. Accurately weigh or measure the ingredients.
3. Mix the ingredients together, and heat in a porcelain-lined vessel until they fuse.
4. While the mass is molten, pour into molds.

℞ Styptic Pencil (crayon type)

Titanium dioxide	3.7 g	Color
Alum	18 g	Active
Aluminum chloride	15 g	Active
Oxyquinoline sulfate	2.3 g	Active
Cocoa butter (Fattibase)	22 g	Base
Cetyl esters wax	19 g	Base
Petrolatum	13 g	Base
Lanolin	7 g	Base

1. Calculate the quantity of each ingredient required for the prescription.
2. Accurately weigh or measure the ingredients.
3. Triturate the titanium dioxide, alum, and aluminum chloride.
4. Add enough petrolatum to make a viscous paste.
5. Mix the rest of the petrolatum with the oxyquinoline sulfate.
6. Melt the cocoa butter, cetyl esters wax, and lanolin; stir in the titanium dioxide–petrolatum mixture, and then the oxyquinoline mixture.
7. Pour the mix into molds.

℞ Moisturizing and Cold Sore Stick

Vitamin E oil	1.1 g	Active
Lysine	1.1 g	Active
Silica gel	120 mg	Suspending Aid
Polyethylene glycol 4500	7 g	Base
Polyethylene glycol 300	14 mL	Base

1. Calculate the quantity of each ingredient required for the prescription.
2. Accurately weigh or measure each ingredient.
3. Melt the polyethylene glycol bases together at about 55°C.
4. Mix the vitamin E oil, lysine, and silica gel together, and add to the melted bases.
5. Turn off heat, and mix until uniform.
6. Pour the mix into tubes, and allow to cool.

Reference

1. United States Pharmacopeial Convention. Chapter <795>, Pharmaceutical compounding—nonsterile preparations. *United States Pharmacopeia/National Formulary.* Rockville, MD: United States Pharmacopeial Convention; current edition.

Solutions

Pharmacists are called on to compound solutions for many routes of administration, including oral, topical, rectal, vaginal, ophthalmic, and otic. The most common solution dosage form is the oral liquid, which includes solutions, syrups, elixirs, and the like. The preparation techniques for most of these liquid dosage forms are similar.

Definitions and Types

Solutions are liquid preparations containing one or more drug substances molecularly dispersed in a suitable solvent or a mixture of mutually miscible solvents. Oral liquids contain one or more substances with or without flavoring, sweetening, or coloring agents dissolved in water or cosolvent–water mixtures. They can be either formulated for direct oral administration to the patient or dispensed in a concentrated form that requires dilution before dispensing or administration.

Topical solutions usually are aqueous but may contain cosolvent systems such as various alcohols or other organic solvents with or without added active ingredients. The term *lotion* is often used for solutions or suspensions that are applied topically.

Syrups are concentrated aqueous preparations of a sugar or sugar substitute with or without flavoring agents and medicinal substances. Syrups can serve as pleasant-tasting vehicles for active drugs.

Elixirs are clear, sweetened, hydroalcoholic solutions that are usually flavored and are suitable for drugs that are insoluble in water alone but soluble in water–alcohol mixtures. Less sweet and less viscous than syrups, elixirs are generally less effective in masking taste. Elixirs can contain different solvents as cosolvent systems, such as alcohol, glycerin, polyethylene glycol 300, propylene glycol, sorbitol, and water.

Aromatic waters can be used for both internal and external purposes. They are clear, saturated aqueous solutions of volatile oils or other aromatic or volatile substances. For compounding purposes, they are usually prepared with volatile oils and water.

Historical Use

Solutions are one of the oldest dosage forms. Myrrh, laudanum, and other tinctures are mentioned in literature dating back to biblical times. For early solutions (e.g., fluid extracts, tinctures, spirits, and potions), the composition and preparation were simpler than for contemporary preparations. Solutions prepared today can be buffered, preserved, flavored, sweetened, adjusted for pH and osmolality, and protected against oxidation.

Applications

An oral liquid may be the most appropriate dosage form for a patient for a number of reasons. Some of the most common reasons for a pharmacist to compound an oral liquid dosage form are as follows:

- Many drug products are not commercially available as oral liquids.
- Infant, pediatric, and some psychiatric patients, as well as patients of advanced age, cannot swallow solid dosage forms.
- Some products are therapeutically better in liquid form.
- The bulk of some preparations makes oral liquids more feasible than other forms.
- Some patients, such as nursing home residents or persons who are incarcerated, are administered oral liquids to prevent them from placing tablets or capsules under the tongue and not swallowing them at the time of administration.
- Patients receiving enteral feedings require a liquid dosage form.
- Oral liquid dosage forms are diverse and have varying dosage strengths.
- Drugs are often more bioavailable from oral liquids than from solids.

Solubilization

The compounding of many dosage forms requires the preparation of a solution even though the final formulation may not be a solution. The proper selection of a solvent depends on the physicochemical characteristics of the solute and the solvent as well as the purpose of the solution in the formula.

The solubility of a substance represents the sum of various factors involved in the transport of a solute particle from the solid phase to the solution phase. The driving force for dissolution is the interaction of the solvent molecules with the solute molecules or solute ions. The process of dissolution involves (1) the breaking of interionic or intermolecular bonds in the solute, (2) the separation of the molecules of the solvent to provide space in the solvent for the solute, and (3) the interaction between the solvent and the solute molecule or ion. A number of forces of attraction are involved in the dissolution process, including van der Waals, dipole–dipole, and ionic forces.

A good general rule to remember is the one learned in chemistry class: "Like dissolves like." Generally, polar solutes will dissolve in polar solvents; nonpolar solutes will dissolve in nonpolar solvents. The challenge is that many solutes are of intermediate polarity.

If appropriate, official solvents should be used in pharmaceutical compounding. A number of official solvents that are listed in the *United States Pharmacopeia/National Formulary (USP/NF)* will be briefly discussed. Generally, all solvents should be preserved in tight containers, and those that are flammable should be stored away from excessive heat or sources of sparks or flame. Oils also should be stored to avoid exposure to excessive heat.

Composition

The composition of solutions can range from quite simple to very complex. The choice of active ingredient, the intended use, patient characteristics, and, potentially, the environment in which the preparation will be stored can affect its composition.

Oral liquids generally contain the active drug with or without cosolvent systems, flavorings, sweeteners, colorings, preservatives, buffering agents, antioxidants, or other ingredients. Most drugs are more susceptible to degradation in an aqueous solution. Adding buffers to adjust the pH, preservatives, and antioxidants can prevent degradation. Flavorings and sweeteners can make a drug with a disagreeable taste or odor more palatable, thereby increasing patient acceptance of the preparation and ease of administration. For physiological reasons, other additives are used to bring the solution within a suitable osmolality range.

pH

pH is important in drug formulations, especially because it affects drug solubility, activity, absorption, stability, sorption, and patient comfort. pH is related to certain physical characteristics, such as the viscosity of some polymers used as gel-forming agents and in suspensions. Tables 17-1 and 17-2 list acidifying agents and alkalizing agents, respectively, that are used to adjust pH.

pH adjustment is critical for maintaining drugs in solution. A slight increase or decrease in pH can cause some drugs to precipitate from a solution. Conversely, a slight adjustment of pH can aid in solubilizing some drugs. Drug activity can be related to pH, depending on whether the ionized or the nonionized form is desired. Drug stability, in many cases, directly depends on the pH of the environment (dosage form). pH:degradation profiles are of great value in selecting the proper pH for optimum stability of a preparation. Sorption of a drug to various excipients, packaging components, and administration devices can occur. The sorption can be pH related, depending on which species, ionized or nonionized, is sorbed to the material. Patient comfort and, ultimately, compliance can depend on the proper pH of the preparation. In some cases, a compromise must be reached between the drug requirements and patient preferences. Often, pH can be adjusted for optimum drug stability and a low buffer capacity can be used so that a patient's physiologic buffers will quickly move the pH to the physiologic range upon administration.

Vehicles

The vehicles most commonly used in oral solutions include ethanol, glycerin, syrups, water and various blends of these ingredients. A greater variety of vehicles is available for topical solutions. Most of the vehicles used for oral solutions, as well as acetone, collodion, isopropanol, the polyethylene glycols, propylene glycol, many oils, and numerous polymers, can be used in topical preparations. Another vehicle, dimethyl sulfoxide, has limited use in topical solutions. Although oral solutions are usually ready to administer, they sometimes have to be diluted or prepared before administration, particularly when a preparation is not very stable. Official solvents are listed in Table 17-3, and some oleaginous vehicles are listed in Table 17-4.

Water is the primary solvent, and the *USP/NF* lists several different waters, including pharmaceutical waters, which are clear, colorless, odorless liquids but differ in their preparation, requirements, packaging, and intended use.

Purified water (H_2O, molecular weight [MW] 18.02) is water obtained by a suitable process; distillation, deionization, reverse osmosis, and ion exchange. It is discussed thoroughly in *USP* Chapter <1231>, Water for Pharmaceutical Purposes.[1]

TABLE 17-1 Physicochemical Characteristics of Acidifying Agents

Acidifying Agent	Physical Form	% Strength	Solubility		Specific Gravity	Solution pH (%)[a]	Container Specifications
			Water	Alcohol			
Acetic acid NF	Liquid	36.5	Misc	Misc	1.04	—	T
Acetic acid, glacial USP	Liquid	100	Misc	Misc	1.05	—	T
Citric acid USP	Solid	100	VS	FS	—	2.2 (1)	T
Fumaric acid NF	Solid	100	SlS	Sol	—	2.45 (saturated)	W
Hydrochloric acid NF	Liquid	37.5	Misc	Misc	1.18	0.1 (10)	T
Hydrochloric acid, diluted NF	Liquid	10	Misc	Misc	1.06	0.1	T
Lactic acid USP	Liquid	88	Misc	Misc	1.21	—	T
Malic acid NF	Solid	100	VS	FS	—	2.35 (1)	W
Nitric acid NF	Liquid	70	Misc	Misc	1.41	—	T
Phosphoric acid NF	Liquid	87	Misc	Misc	1.71	—	T
Phosphoric acid, diluted NF	Liquid	10	Misc	Misc	1.06	—	T
Propionic acid NF	Liquid	100	Misc	Misc	0.99	—	T
Sodium phosphate monobasic USP	Solid	100	FS	PrIn	—	4.3 (5)	W
Sulfuric acid NF	Liquid	98	Misc	Misc	1.84	—	T
Tartaric acid NF	Solid	100	VS	FS	—	2.2 (1.5)	W

— = Not available.
[a]Aqueous solutions.

TABLE 17-2 Physicochemical Characteristics of Alkalizing Agents

Alkalizing Agent	Physical Form	% Strength	Solubility		Specific Gravity	Solution pH (%)[a]	Container Specifications
			Water	Alcohol			
Ammonia solution, strong NF	Liquid	29	Misc	Misc	0.90	—	T
Ammonium carbonate NF	Solid	100	FS	—	—	—	T, LR
Diethanolamine NF	Liquid	100	Misc	Misc	1.088	11 (0.1 N)	T, LR
Monoethanolamine	Liquid	100	Misc	Misc	1.012	12.1 (0.1 N)	T, LR
Potassium hydroxide NF	Solid	100	FS	FS	—	—	T
Sodium bicarbonate USP	Solid	100	Sol	IS	—	8.3 (0.1 M)	W
Sodium borate NF	Solid	100	Sol	IS	—	—	T
Sodium carbonate NF	Solid	100	FS	FS	—	—	W
Sodium hydroxide NF	Solid	100	FS		—	—	T
Sodium phosphate dibasic USP	Solid	100	FS	SlS	—	9.1 (1)	T
Trolamine NF	Liquid	100	Misc	Misc	1.12	10.5 (0.1 N)	T, LR

— = Not available; N = normal; M = molar.
[a]Aqueous solutions.

TABLE 17-3 Physicochemical Characteristics of Official Solvents

Solvent	Miscibility			General Use		Specific Gravity	Boil Point	Freeze Point	Flammable
	Water	Alcohol	Oil	External	Internal				
Acetone	Misc	Misc		Yes		0.789	56		Yes
Alcohol	Misc	Misc		Yes	Yes		78		Yes
Alcohol, diluted	Misc	Misc		Yes	Yes	0.936			
Almond oil	Immisc	SlS		Yes	Yes	0.913			
Amylene hydrate	Misc	Misc				0.805	100		
Benzyl benzoate	Immisc	Misc		Yes	Yes	1.118		18	
Butyl alcohol	Misc	Misc							
Corn oil	Immisc	SlS	Misc	Yes	Yes	0.918			
Cottonseed oil	Immisc	SlS	Misc	Yes	Yes	0.918			
Diethylene glycol monoethyl ether	Misc	Misc	PartMisc	Yes		0.991	198		Yes
Ethyl acetate	Misc	Misc	Misc	Yes		0.896			Yes
Glycerin	Misc	Misc	Immisc	Yes	Yes	1.249			No
Hexylene glycol	Misc	Misc				0.919			
Isopropyl alcohol	Misc	Misc		Yes		0.785			Yes
Methyl alcohol	Misc	Misc		Yes			65		Yes
Methylene chloride		Misc	Misc	Yes		1.320	40		Yes
Methyl isobutyl ketone	SlS	Misc		Yes					Yes
Mineral oil	Immisc	Immisc	Misc	Yes	Yes	0.870			No
Peanut oil	Immisc	VSS	Misc	Yes	Yes	0.916			No
Polyethylene glycol									
300	Misc	Misc		Yes	Yes	1.12		−11	No
400	Misc	Misc		Yes	Yes	1.12		6	No
600	Misc	Misc		Yes	Yes	1.12		20	No
Propylene glycol	Misc	Misc	Immisc	Yes	Yes	1.036			No
Sesame oil		SlS		Yes	Yes	0.918			No
Water	Misc	Misc	Immisc	Yes	Yes	1.00	100	0	No

TABLE 17-4 Physicochemical Characteristics of Oleaginous Vehicles

Vehicle	Specific Gravity	Refractive Index	Acid Value[a]	Iodine Value[b]	Saponification Value[c]	Container Specifications
Alkyl (C_{12}–C_{15}) benzoate	0.915–0.935	1.483–1.487	≤0.5		169–182	T, LR
Almond oil	0.910–0.915			95–105	190–200	T
Corn oil	0.914–0.921			102–130	187–193	T, LR
Cottonseed oil	0.915–0.921			109–120		T, LR
Ethyl oleate	0.866–0.874	1.443–1.450	≤0.5	75–85	177–188	T, LR
Isopropyl myristate	0.846–0.854	1.432–1.436	≤1.0	≤1	202–212	T, LR
Isopropyl palmitate	0.850–0.855	1.435–1.438	≤1.0	≤1	183–193	T, LR
Mineral oil	0.845–0.905					T, LR
Mineral oil, light	0.818–0.880					T, LR
Octyldodecanol			≤5.0	≤8	≤5	T
Olive oil	0.910–0.915			79–88	190–195	T
Peanut oil	0.912–0.920	1.462–1.464		84–100	185–195	T, LR
Safflower oil				135–150		T, LR
Sesame oil	0.916–0.921			103–116	188–195	T, LR
Soybean oil	0.916–0.922	1.465–1.475		120–141	180–200	T, LR
Squalane	0.807–0.810	1.451–1.452	≤0.2	≤4	≤2	T

[a]Acid value is the number of milligrams of potassium hydroxide required to neutralize the free acids in 1 g of the substance. It is a measure of the acidity of the oil.
[b]Iodine value is the number of grams of iodine absorbed, under the prescribed conditions, by 100 g of the substance. It is a measure of the unsaturation of the oil.
[c]Saponification value is the number of milligrams of potassium hydroxide required to neutralize the free acids and saponify the esters contained in 1 g of the substance.

Sterile purified water is purified water that is sterilized and suitably packaged. It contains no antimicrobial agent. (Note: It is not to be used for preparations intended for parenteral administration.)

Water for injection is water purified by distillation or by reverse osmosis. Water for injection is intended for use in preparing parenteral solutions.

Sterile water for injection is prepared from water for injection that is sterilized and suitably packaged. It contains no antimicrobial agent or other added substance.

Bacteriostatic water for injection is prepared from water for injection that is sterilized and suitably packaged; it contains one or more suitable antimicrobial agents. (Note: Bacteriostatic water for injection must be used with due regard for the compatibility of the antimicrobial agent or agents it contains with the particular drug that is to be dissolved or diluted.)

Sterile water for irrigation is prepared from water for injection that is sterilized and suitably packaged. It contains no antimicrobial agent or other added substance.

Sterile water for inhalation is prepared from water for injection that is sterilized and suitably packaged. It contains no antimicrobial agents, except when it is prepared for use in humidifiers or similar devices and is liable to contamination over a period of time, and no other added substances. (Note: Sterile water for inhalation should not be used for parenteral administration or for other sterile compendial dosage forms.)

Preparation

A variety of techniques can be used to prepare an oral liquid dosage form. The most common method is to make a simple solution by dissolving a drug in a solvent. Most materials can be dissolved simply by stirring, but others can require heat or a high degree of agitation. Methylcellulose is one material that requires a special process. Initially, it can be dispersed in an amount of hot water that is one-third to one-half of the total volume of water, with the remaining volume added as ice water or ice. To wet the methylcellulose, one should sprinkle the powder lightly on the surface of the hot water so that it can hydrate. If the powder is added too rapidly, clumps form, creating difficulty for inside particles to become wet because they are covered by the outer shell of the hydrated clump. Before water is added, an intermediate liquid, such as alcohol or glycerin, can sometimes be used to displace air entrapped in the powder, replacing it with a water-miscible liquid. Then, when water is added, it will wet the powder more easily.

Surfactants aid in solubilizing an ingredient. The surfactant can be either dispersed in the vehicle before the drug is added or mixed with the drug before addition to the vehicle.

A common technique for preparing aromatic waters is to use a solution with a dispersant. The volatile oil is mixed with small pieces of filter paper, talc, or some other appropriate dispersion medium before the water is added. The mixture is agitated and allowed to set for a time, with periodic agitation. The aromatic water is then collected by filtration. The purpose of the dispersion medium is to increase the surface area of the oil that is exposed to the water in order to increase the rate at which the solution is saturated with the oil. In working with aromatic waters, one must remember that the addition of a salt will probably salt out the volatile oils. See Box 17-1 for suggestions on other preparation techniques.

Physicochemical Considerations

To compound a successful oral liquid preparation, a pharmacist must overcome several technical difficulties. Unstable drugs are even more unstable in solution; poorly soluble drugs must be solubilized or suspended; and bad-tasting drugs must be masked to produce

BOX 17-1 Hints for Compounding Solutions

Suggestions for compounding solutions are as follows:

- A preparation should be stirred gently; shaking can entrap air, which causes foaming.
- The use of magnetic stirrers, blenders, and electric mixers can save time and produce uniform preparations.
- The dissolution step can be speeded up by immersing the beaker in an ultrasonic bath.
- A stirring rod should not be used when adding "sufficient volume" of a solvent to the graduate in which the formulation is being prepared.
- Either a stirring rod laid across the top of a beaker or an alcohol spray (ethanol for internal solutions) can aid in breaking up a foam; a silicone defoaming agent can also be used.
- Filtration of a liquid helps produce a clear preparation. During this process, one should watch the surface of the filter to determine whether the active drug is being inadvertently removed from the preparation.
- One should always know the pH and alcohol concentration of the preparations being compounded.
- The effectiveness of a preservative can be related to pH. For example, the parabens are generally used within a pH range of 4 to 8, chlorobutanol needs a pH of less than 5, and sodium benzoate is more effective at a pH of 4 or less.
- Salts should be dissolved in a small quantity of water before a viscous vehicle is added.
- When combining two liquids, one should stir the mixture constantly to lessen the occurrence of incompatibilities resulting from concentration effects.
- High-viscosity liquids should be added to low-viscosity liquids. The solution should be stirred constantly when these types of liquids are mixed.
- To obtain small quantities of active drugs or excipients (e.g., flavoring oils) when employing the dilution or aliquot method, one should use a solvent, not just a liquid.
- Hydrocolloids should be allowed to hydrate slowly before use.
- Considerations involved in selecting a vehicle include the drug concentration, solubility, pK_a, taste, and stability. Other vehicle considerations include pH, flavoring, sweetener, color, preservative, viscosity, compatibility, and, if indicated, suspending and emulsifying agents.
- In preparing elixirs, dissolving the alcohol-soluble constituents in the alcohol and the water-soluble constituents in the water is advisable. To maintain as high an alcohol concentration as possible, one should then add the aqueous solution to the alcohol solution by stirring.
- Talc can be used to remove excess flavoring oils by adding 1 to 2 g of talc per 100 mL of solution and then filtering. During the filtration process, the first portions are returned to the filter until a clear filtrate is obtained.
- Cosolvent systems (e.g., mixtures of water, alcohol, glycerin, and propylene glycol) can aid in clarifying solutions that are hazy or cloudy because of poor solubility in water.

a palatable preparation. Therefore, compounding a successful formulation requires a combination of scientific acuity and pharmaceutical art.

Physicochemical, pharmaceutical, and patient factors must be taken into account during the preparation of an oral liquid dosage form. The physicochemical and stability characteristics of the active drug determine the oral liquid dosage form that can be prepared (i.e., syrups, elixirs, suspensions). Factors to be considered in formulating an oral liquid dosage form include the following:

- Physical and chemical properties of the ingredients
- Order of mixing and adjuvants
- Pharmaceutical techniques required
- Incompatibilities in preparation and storage
- Stability and potency of the ingredients
- Proper labeling, including accessory labels

When preparing an oral liquid, a pharmacist should consider the drug's concentration, solubility, pK_a, taste, and stability. Vehicle considerations include pH, flavoring, sweetener, color, preservative, viscosity, compatibility, and, if indicated, suspending and emulsifying agents. The drug's concentration and solubility in various solvents will dictate the type of dosage form to prepare. For example, if the drug is water soluble, a syrup can be prepared; if it is soluble in water–alcohol–glycerin cosolvent systems, an elixir is appropriate. If the drug is insoluble, a suspension can be formulated; if the drug is an oil, however, an emulsion is the form of choice. The following points should be considered in solubilizing drugs:

- Small particles dissolve faster than large particles.
- Stirring increases the dissolution rate of a drug.
- The more soluble the drug, the faster is its dissolution rate.
- A viscous liquid will decrease the dissolution rate of a drug.
- An increase in temperature generally leads to an increase in the solubility and dissolution rate of a drug.
- Adding an electrolyte can increase or decrease the solubility of a nonelectrolyte drug.
- An alkaloidal base, or any nitrogenous base of relatively high molecular weight, usually is poorly soluble unless the pH of the medium is decreased (i.e., conversion to a salt occurs).
- The solubility of poorly soluble acidic substances is increased as the pH of the medium is increased (i.e., conversion to a salt occurs).

The pH of the vehicle and pK_a of the drug partially determine the drug's overall solubility. Slight adjustments in pH can greatly affect the solubility of the drug; pH should be controlled in the preparation of a solution. Buffering the solution may be necessary to maintain its solubility characteristics.

Another area affected by pH is chemical stability. Various reference sources can be consulted to determine the required pH for maximum stability for specific drugs. This information can be used to establish guidelines for selecting the best vehicle. An inexpensive pH meter (Figure 17-1) can help predict and prevent pH-related incompatibilities.

FIGURE 17-1 pH meter.

Syrups

Syrups are appropriate for water-soluble drugs. The usual pH requirement for many drugs is slightly to moderately acidic. Thus, flavored syrups can often effectively mask the disagreeable taste of certain drugs. The flavor will remain in the mouth longer because of the syrup's viscosity. Viscosity can cause the active drug to dissolve more slowly in the vehicle during preparation. The best approach is first to dissolve the active ingredient in a small quantity of water and then add a sufficient quantity of syrup to make the desired volume.

TABLE 17-5 Common Preservatives for Oral Liquid Preparations

Preservative	Concentration (%)
Alcohol	15–20
Benzoic acid	0.2
Methylparaben	≤0.2
Potassium sorbate	0.2
Propylparaben	≤0.2
Sodium benzoate	0.2
Sorbic acid	0.2

The preservative properties of a syrup depend in part on maintaining a high concentration of sucrose or sugar in the final preparation. If the sucrose concentration is decreased, adding another preservative (e.g., alcohol) to the preparation may be necessary. Table 17-5 lists preservatives that can be used in oral liquids. (See Chapter 7 of this book for an example of how to determine the required quantity of preservatives.)

Some syrup vehicles are listed in Table 17-6. As is evident from this table, most syrups have slightly acidic pH values. Commercially prepared products (e.g., Ora-Blend, Ora-Sweet, Ora-Sweet SF, PCCA Sweet-SF Sugar Free Syrup Vehicle, PCCA Syrup Vehicle, Syrpalta, and SyrSpend) generally have pH values of approximately 4.2 to 4.5. Cherry syrup, Coca-Cola syrup, orange syrup, and raspberry syrup all have a pH of less than 4. Neutral syrup vehicles include simple syrup (syrup USP) and aromatic eriodictyon syrup. Other commercial vehicles are available with alkaline pH values. Because the commercially available products contain preservative systems, additional preservatives are not normally needed unless the vehicle is significantly diluted.

In some circumstances, fruit juices, especially those that are clear and pulp free such as apple or grape, can be used and diluted with syrup to increase sweetness, if necessary. Maple syrup or ice cream sundae toppings such as butterscotch can also be adapted for use, diluted as needed with simple syrup or water. Another interesting approach is the use of soft drink concentrates or lemonade concentrates. These concentrates can be reconstituted with water to a concentrated solution or can be diluted with simple syrup instead of using the water and sucrose formulas provided on the commercial package. Still another option is diluting fruit preserves to make syrups; using a sugar-free preserve for patients with diabetes is a noteworthy option. Still other approaches involve diluting a commercial syrup with either simple syrup or methylcellulose solution; in some areas, a 1:1 mixture of simple syrup and methylcellulose solution is commonly used, flavored to the taste of a patient. One must be cognizant of the fact that when vehicles are diluted, the preservative effectiveness may also be decreased and additional preservative may need to be added.

Elixirs

Because elixirs are mixtures of water and alcohol, they dissolve both alcohol-soluble and water-soluble substances, depending on the percentage of each solvent present. Glycerin, which is also present in some elixirs, is comparable in solvent properties to alcohol, but its viscosity causes solutes to dissolve slowly. Propylene glycol is miscible with water and alcohol and is routinely substituted for glycerin.

Elixirs are usually prepared by simple solution; however, care must be taken to keep the alcohol concentration and pH within the range for maximum stability of both the drug and the dosage form. One must consider whether the salt form of the drug (more water soluble) or the free acid or base form (more alcohol soluble) should be used.

TABLE 17-6 pH and Alcohol Content of Common Oral Liquid Vehicles

Vehicle	pH	Alcohol Content (%)	Container Specifications
Official USP/NF Vehicles			
Aromatic elixir	5.5–6	21–23	T
Benzaldehyde compound elixir	6	3–5	T, LR
Peppermint water	—	0	T
Sorbitol solution	—	0	T
Suspension structured vehicle	—	0	T, LR
Suspension structured vehicle-SF	—	0	T, LR
Syrup	6.5–7	—	T
Xanthan gum solution	—	0	T, LR
Nonofficial Vehicles			
Acacia syrup	5	—	T
Aromatic eriodictyon syrup	6–8	6–8	T, LR
Cherry syrup	3.5–4	1–2	T, LR
Citric acid syrup	—	1	T
Cocoa syrup	—	—	T
Glycyrrhiza elixir	—	21–23	T
Glycyrrhiza syrup	6–6.5	5–6	T
Hydriodic acid syrup	—	—	T
Iso-alcoholic elixir, low	5	8–10	T
Iso-alcoholic elixir, high	5	73–78	T
Orange flower water	—	0	T
Orange syrup	2.5–3	2–5	T
Raspberry syrup	3	1–2	T, LR
Sarsaparilla compound syrup	5	—	T
Tolu syrup	5.5	2–4	T
Wild cherry syrup	4.5	1–2	T
Commercial Branded Vehicles			
Coca-Cola syrup	1.6–1.7	0	T
Ora-Sweet	4–4.5	0	T, LR
Ora-Sweet SF	4–4.4	0	T, LR
Syrpalta	4.5	—	T, LR

— = Not available.

The preparation of elixirs involves dissolving the alcohol-soluble components in the alcohol and the water-soluble components in the water. The aqueous phase is generally added to the alcohol solution to maintain the highest alcohol concentration possible. If the situation is reversed, the oils and drug can separate from the solution as soon as the alcohol solution contacts the water. If the preparation is cloudy, an excess of aromatic oils may have been added. In such cases, talc filtration can be used to produce a clear preparation. This technique involves adding approximately 1 to 2 g of talc per 100 mL of solution, mixing, and filtering. The liquid is then refiltered until a clear preparation is obtained.

TABLE 17-7 Elixirs for Use in Common Oral Liquids

Elixir	pH	Alcohol Content (%)
Aromatic elixir	5.5–6	21–23
Benzaldehyde compound elixir	6	3–5
Iso-alcoholic elixir (low, high)[a]	5	8–10, 73–78

[a]These two elixirs can be mixed in various ratios to obtain the required alcohol concentration.

Cosolvent systems serve to dissolve not only the active drug, but also the flavoring components, which often are volatile oils. Artificial sweeteners (e.g., saccharin) may be required for sweetening, because sucrose may not be sufficiently soluble in the alcoholic system.

Sample elixir vehicles are listed in Table 17-7. The most common elixir vehicle is aromatic elixir, which has an alcohol content of approximately 22%. Some syrups now contain alcohol, so the distinction between syrups and elixirs is sometimes vague. The two iso-alcoholic elixirs (low: 8%–10% alcohol; high: 73%–78% alcohol) can be adjusted to obtain a vehicle of the desired alcohol concentration.

Quality Control

Quality control procedures include checking the final volume, appearance, odor, clarity, and pH. Small, inexpensive pH meters are available for checking the final pH of a preparation. Preparations that do not exhibit the expected characteristics should not be dispensed; they may have to be reformulated.

Packaging

Solutions can usually be packaged in glass or plastic containers. Oral liquids and some other solutions can be packaged in squeeze bottles for application by spraying (Figure 17-2), in applicator bottles for topical application in small volumes, and in dropper bottles. Many solutions need to be in light-resistant containers.

Storage and Labeling

Oral liquids should generally be stored at room temperature or refrigerated, depending on the characteristics of the active drug. Syrups are often refrigerated to enhance their stability and palatability. If saturated solutions are stored in the refrigerator, precipitation can occur. In many cases, the precipitate will redissolve when the solution is returned to room temperature. If not, the preparation can be gently warmed to redissolve the precipitate.

Labels should contain instructions as to type of use (external or internal), proper storage conditions, and beyond-use dates. The statement "Protect from Light" should be on the label. For some solutions, the statement "Shake Well" should also be on the label.

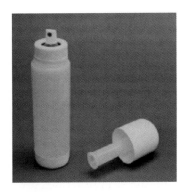

FIGURE 17-2 Pressure spray bottle.

Stability

The following physical attributes of liquid dosage forms can be observed for evidence of instability: clarity, precipitation, mold or bacterial growth, odor, and loss of volume. Solutions are particularly susceptible to chemical degradation, especially when aqueous vehicles are used. Information on chemical stability can be obtained from the literature or other appropriate sources.

Beyond-use dates for water-containing formulations stored at cold temperatures are no later than 14 days for oral preparations compounded from ingredients in solid form or 30 days for topical preparations. These dates can be extended if valid scientific information on stability supports extension, as discussed in Chapter 6 of this book.

Patient Counseling

Patients should be instructed on how to measure the dose of a liquid preparation and how to administer it. They should also be informed about shaking the preparation (if indicated), replacing and tightening the cap, and storing the preparation properly, including keeping it out of the reach of children. Patients should be taught how to check the preparation for physical stability and should be instructed to return it if signs of instability are noted. Instructions on how to dispose of preparations that have reached their beyond-use date should also be provided.

Sample Formulations

Iontophoretic Solution

℞ **Lidocaine Hydrochloride 2% Solution for Iontophoresis**

Lidocaine hydrochloride	2 g	Active
Sterile water for injection	100 mL	Vehicle

1. Calculate the quantity of each ingredient required for the prescription.
2. Accurately weigh the lidocaine hydrochloride and measure the sterile water for injection.
3. Dissolve the lidocaine hydrochloride in the sterile water for injection.
4. Package and label the product.

Oral Solutions

℞ **Methylcellulose Oral Liquid Vehicle**

Methylcellulose 1% solution	50 mL	Vehicle
Glycerin	3 mL	Cosolvent
Preserved flavored syrup	qs 100 mL	Preserved Vehicle
Sodium benzoate or potassium sorbate	200 mg	Preservative
Purified water	qs	Vehicle

1. Calculate the quantity of each ingredient required for the prescription.
2. Accurately weigh or measure each ingredient.
3. Dissolve the sodium benzoate or potassium sorbate in about 1 mL of purified water.
4. Add this solution to the methylcellulose 1% solution.
5. Add the glycerin; then add the preserved flavored syrup to 100 mL, and mix well.
6. Package and label the product.

℞ Flavored Cod Liver Oil

Spearmint oil	0.4 mL	Flavoring
Peppermint oil	0.4 mL	Flavoring
Cod liver oil	qs 100 mL	Vehicle

1. Calculate the quantity of each ingredient required for the prescription.
2. Accurately measure the two flavoring oils.
3. Mix the flavoring oils with sufficient cod liver oil to make 100 mL, and mix well.
4. Package and label the product.

Topical Solutions

℞ Dimethyl Sulfoxide 70% Topical Solution (100 g)

Dimethyl sulfoxide	70 g	Active
Alcohol 95% or purified water	30 g	Vehicle

1. Calculate the quantity of each ingredient required for the prescription.
2. Accurately weigh or measure each ingredient.
3. In a suitable container, mix the two liquids.
4. Package and label the product.

℞ Fluconazole 1.5% in Dimethyl Sulfoxide (100 mL)

Fluconazole	1.5 g	Active
Dimethyl sulfoxide	qs 100 mL	Vehicle/Penetration Enhancer

1. Calculate the quantity of each ingredient required for the prescription.
2. Accurately weigh the fluconazole powder or obtain from Diflucan tablets.
3. Dissolve the fluconazole powder in dimethyl sulfoxide, or mix the finely powdered tablets with dimethyl sulfoxide.
4. If the tablets were used, filter the preparation after the fluconazole has gone into solution.
5. Package the solution in a bottle with a glass rod applicator.

Reference

1. United States Pharmacopeial Convention. Chapter <1231>, Water for pharmaceutical purposes. In: *United States Pharmacopeia/National Formulary*. Bethesda, MD: United States Pharmacopeial Convention; current edition.

Chapter 18

Suspensions

Definitions and Types

When components of a formula are not soluble, a suspension or an emulsion (see Chapter 19 of this book) is often indicated. A *suspension* is a two-phased system consisting of a finely divided solid dispersed in a solid, liquid, or gas. Suspensions are appropriate when the drug to be incorporated is not sufficiently soluble in an ordinary solvent or cosolvent system. A good suspension ensures that the drug is uniformly dispersed throughout the vehicle. *Oral suspensions* are liquid preparations in which solid particles of the active drug are dispersed in a sweetened, flavored, and sometimes viscous vehicle. *Topical suspensions* are liquid preparations containing solid particles dispersed in a suitable liquid vehicle that are intended for application to the skin. These preparations are sometimes called lotions (e.g., calamine lotion).

Historical Use

The first suspensions may have been preparations of vegetable or earth products mixed with water. Mixing the drug with water made it easier to take orally or apply topically. This dosage form was a simple way of converting powdered leaves, bark, clays, and the like to a fluid preparation that not only would be easier to administer, but also would increase patient acceptance of the preparation.

Applications

A suitable vehicle for suspension of drugs not soluble in a solvent would have the necessary viscosity to keep the drug particles suspended separately from each other but would be sufficiently fluid to allow the preparation to be poured from the container. Suspensions can be prepared for oral use or for topical use; they can even be prepared for ophthalmic, otic, nasal, and rectal applications.

The suspension dosage form can enhance the stability of a drug that is poorly stable in solution. Using an insoluble form of the drug places more of the drug in the suspended form, not in solution, and thus the drug is not available for solution degradation.

Composition

Suspensions usually contain insoluble particles; a liquid medium; a suspending agent, surfactant, or viscosity enhancer; and a preservative. They can also contain a flavoring or perfume agent and a sweetener. The order in which these ingredients are blended is important to the stability of the preparation.

Preparation

To prepare a suspension, a pharmacist must first obtain uniform, small particles of the drug. This is accomplished through particle size reduction, which is discussed in Chapter 11 of this book. Once this step is completed, the active insoluble material should be thoroughly wetted before it is mixed with the vehicle. Hydrophilic materials are best wetted with water-miscible liquids (e.g., glycerin), whereas hydrophobic substances can be wetted with nonpolar liquids or with the use of a surfactant. See Table 18-1 for a list of commonly used wetting agents. A general guideline is to use the minimal amount of wetting agent required to produce the desired product.

After the drug and wetting agent have been combined to form a thick paste, the vehicle can be added with constant stirring. Methylcellulose preparations are best prepared by dispersing the polymer in about one-third to one-half of the total volume of hot water, and then adding the remaining water as ice water or ice. Many polymers can be sprinkled onto rapidly agitating water to improve their dispersion.

Physicochemical Considerations

Sample suspension vehicles are listed in Table 18-2. If a good suspension vehicle is unavailable, one can usually prepare a 0.5% to 5% methylcellulose dispersion. A 0.5% to 1.5% sodium carboxymethylcellulose dispersion can also be prepared. The viscosity required depends on the active drug's tendency to settle, which, in turn, is related to the powder's density and particle size. Table 18-3 provides a list of the concentrations of viscosity-increasing agents that will yield a viscosity of 800 centipoise (cP). After the suspending agent is prepared, it can be mixed 1:1 with a flavored syrup. Additional suspension agents and their characteristics are shown in Table 18-4.

Viscosity and Rheology

Viscosity plays an important role in a number of different dosage forms. It is an important factor in maintaining drugs in suspension, enhancing the stability of emulsions, altering the release rate of drugs at sites of application, and enabling easier application of drugs to various parts of the body so they do not run off. Compounding pharmacists routinely use viscosity to enhance stability of numerous preparations. As shown in Table 18-2, there are many different viscosity-increasing or suspending agents with different physical properties and, consequently, different applications and uses. Physical properties of importance include solubility in different solvents, pH range of maximum viscosity, and rheologic characterization. (See Appendix VIII for information on properties of commonly used suspending and thickening agents.)

Viscosity is an important factor in rheology, the study of flow. *Viscosity* is defined as the force required to move one plane surface past another under specified conditions when

TABLE 18-1 Some Physicochemical Characteristics of Wetting and Solubilizing Agents

Item	Physical State	Solubility Water	Solubility Alcohol	Packaging Requirements
Benzalkonium Chloride	Gel	VS	VS	TC
Benzethonium Chloride	Solid	Sol	Sol	TLR
Cetylpyridinium Chloride	Solid	VS	FS	WC
Docusate Sodium	Solid	SpS	FS	WC
Nonoxynol-9	Liquid	Sol	Sol	TC
Octoxynol-9	Liquid	Misc	Misc	TC
Poloxamer(s)	Solid	FS	FS	TC
Polyoxyl 35 Castor Oil	Liquid	VS	Sol	TC
Polyoxyl 40 Hydrogenated Castor Oil	Paste	VS	Sol	TC
Polyoxyl 10 Oleyl Ether	Semisolid/Liquid	Sol	Sol	TC
Polyoxyl 20 Cetostearyl Ether	Solid	Sol	Sol	TC
Polyoxyl 40 Stearate	Solid	Sol	Sol	TC
Polysorbate 20	Liquid	Sol	Sol	TC
Polysorbate 40	Liquid	Sol	Sol	TC
Polysorbate 60	Liquid/Gel	Sol	—	TC
Polysorbate 80	Liquid	VS	Sol	TC
Sodium Lauryl Sulfate	Solid	FS	—	WC
Sorbitan Monolaurate	Liquid	IS	—	TC
Sorbitan Monooleate	Liquid	IS	—	TC
Sorbitan Monopalmitate	Solid	IS	#	WC
Sorbitan Monostearate	Solid	##	—	WC
Tyloxapol	Liquid	Misc	—	TC

VS = Very Soluble, 1 part of solute in less than 1 part of solvent
FS = Freely Soluble, 1 part of solute in 1 to 10 parts of solvent
Sol = Soluble, 1 part of solute in 10 to 30 parts of solvent
SpS = Sparingly Soluble, 1 part of solute in 30 to 100 parts of solvent
SlS = Slightly Soluble, 1 part of solute in 100 to 1000 parts of solvent
VSS = Very Slightly Soluble, 1 part of solute in 1000 to 10,000 parts of solvent
PrIn = Practically Insoluble, IS = Insoluble; 1 part of solute in 10,000 or more parts of solvent
# = Soluble in warm absolute alcohol
= Dispersible in warm water
TC = Tight containers
TLR = Tight, light-resistant containers
WC = Well-closed containers

the space between is filled by the liquid in question. More conveniently, it can be considered as a relative property, with water as the reference material that is assigned a viscosity of 1 cP. If a liquid has a viscosity 10 times that of water, it is assigned a viscosity of 10 cP. Fluids generally fall into Newtonian or non-Newtonian flow categories.

Newtonian flow applies to a liquid whose viscosity does not change with increasing shear rate. Water is an example; regardless of how much shear is applied, its viscosity remains at 1 cP. Many pure substances, such as alcohol, glycerin, and propylene glycol, are Newtonian liquids.

Non-Newtonian flow applies to substances that fail to follow the Newton equation of flow, such as colloidal solutions, emulsions, liquid suspensions, and ointments. There are

TABLE 18-2 Suspending Agents and Vehicles for Compounding Suspensions

Suspending Agent	Final Concentration (%)	
Acacia NF	2.0–5.0	
Carbomer resins NF	0.5–5.0	
Carboxymethylcellulose sodium USP	0.5–1.5	
Colloidal silicon dioxide NF	1.5–3.5	
Methylcellulose USP	0.5–5.0	
Tragacanth NF	0.5–2.0	

Vehicle	pH	Alcohol Content (%)
Cologel[a]	4	5
Flavor Plus	Slightly acidic	0
Ora-Blend	4–4.5	0
Ora-Plus	4–4.5	0
Suspendol-S	5.3–6	0
SyrSpend SF	Slightly acidic	0
Versa-Plus	—	0

— = Not available.
[a]No longer available.

three types of non-Newtonian flow: plastic, pseudoplastic, and dilatant. *Plastic flow* is characteristic of materials (such as petrolatum) that have a certain yield value; their viscosity decreases with increasing shear rate. *Pseudoplastic* materials (such as polymer solutions) do not have a yield value, and their viscosity decreases with increasing shear rate; they are also called "shear-thinning" systems. *Dilatant* materials (such as pastes) increase in volume when sheared, and the viscosity increases with increasing shear rate; also called "shear-thickening" systems, they usually have a high percentage of solids in their formulations.

    Thixotropy is a property wherein certain gels, when stressed, become sols and then revert back to a gel state upon standing. This characteristic is desirable for increasing the

TABLE 18-3 Concentration of Viscosity-Increasing Agents for Obtaining Viscosity of 800 cP

Viscosity Agent	% Concentration Required
Acacia	35[a]
Bentonite	6.3
Carboxymethylcellulose, low	4.1
Carboxymethylcellulose, medium	1.9
Carboxymethylcellulose, high	0.7
Methylcellulose 100 cP	3.5
Methylcellulose 400 cP	2.4
Methylcellulose 1500 cP	1.7
Tragacanth	2.8
Veegum	6.0

[a]Concentration of acacia required to yield a viscosity of 600 cP.

TABLE 18-4 Properties of Commonly Used Suspending and Thickening Agents

| Substance | MW | Solubility | | | Usual Suspension Concentration | pH of Aqueous Solution | Most Effective pH Range | Recommended Preservatives |
		Water	Alcohol	Glycerin				
Acacia NF	240,000–580,000	2.7	PrIn	20	5–10	4.5–5.0 (5%)	—	Benzoic acid 0.1% Sodium benzoate 0.1% Methylparaben 0.17% with propylparaben 0.03%
Agar NF	—	Swells	IS	—	<1%	—	—	—
Alginic acid NF	20,000–200,000	Swells	PrIn	—	—	1.5–3.5 (3%)	—	Benzoic acid 0.1–0.2% Sodium benzoate 0.1–0.2% Sorbic acid 0.1–0.2% Parabens
Attapulgite, colloidal/ activated	—	PrIn	PrIn	—	—	7.5–9 (5%)	6–8.5	—
Bentonite NF	—	PrIn	PrIn	PrIn	0.5–5.0	9.5–10.5 (2%)	>6	—
Carbomer 910, 934, 934P, 940, 941, 1342 NF	—	Sol	Sol after neutralization	—	0.5–1	2.5–3.0 (1%)	6–11	Chlorocresol 0.1% Methylparaben 0.1% Thimerosal 0.1%
Carboxymethylcellulose calcium NF	—	IS	PrIn	—	0.25–5	4.5–6.0 (1%)	2–10	—
Carboxymethylcellulose sodium USP	—	Sol	PrIn	—	0.25–5	6.5–8.5 (1%)	2–10	—
Carrageenan NF	—	1:100+	—	—	—	—	—	—
Cellulose microcrystalline NF	—	PrIn	—	—	0.5–5	5–7	—	—
Microcrystalline cellulose and carboxymethylcellulose sodium NF	—	PartSol	—	—	—	6–8 (1.2%)	—	—

(continued)

TABLE 18-4 Properties of Commonly Used Suspending and Thickening Agents *(Continued)*

Substance	MW	Solubility*			Usual Suspension Concentration	pH of Aqueous Solution	Most Effective pH Range	Recommended Preservatives
		Water	Alcohol	Glycerin				
Dextrin NF	—	Sol	PrIn	—	—	—	—	—
Gelatin NF	—	Sol	PrIn	Sol	—	3.8–6 (Type A) 5.0–7.4 (Type B)	—	—
Guar gum NF	—	FS	—	—	2.5%	5.0–7.0 (1%)	4–10.5	Methylparaben 0.15% with Propylparaben 0.02%
Hydroxyethyl cellulose NF	—	Sol	PrIn	—	1–5	5.5–8.5 (1%)	2–12	—
Hydroxypropyl cellulose NF1	—	2	2.5	PrIn	—	5–8.0 (1%)	6–8	—
Hydroxypropyl methylcellulose USP	—	Sol	PrIn	—	0.5–5	5.5–8 (1%)	3–11	—
Magnesium aluminum silicate NF	—	PrIn	PrIn	—	0.5–10	9–10 (5%)	—	—
Methylcellulose USP	—	Sol	PrIn	—	—	5.5–8.0 (1%)	3–11	—
Pectin USP	—	20	PrIn	—	—	5% acidic	—	—
Poloxamer NF	—	Varies	Varies	—	10%–40%	6–7.4 (2.5%)	—	—
Polyethylene oxide NF	—	—	—	—	1%	—	—	—
Polyvinyl alcohol USP	—	FS	—	—	0.5–3.0	5–8 (4%)	—	—
Povidone USP	—	FS	FS	—	2–10	3.0–7.0 (5%)	—	—
Propylene glycol alginate NF	—	Sol	—	—	1–5%	—	3–6	—
Silicon dioxide NF colloidal	—	PrIn	IS	—	2–10	—	—	—
Sodium alginate NF	—	Sol (slowly)	PrIn	—	1–5	7.2 (1%)	4–10	Chlorocresol 0.1% Chloroxylenol 0.1% Parabens Benzoic acid (if acidic)
Tragacanth NF	—	PrIn	PrIn	—	—	5–6 (1%)	4–8	Benzoic acid (0.1%)

— = Not available.

physical stability of suspension dosage forms; they thicken while standing and stabilize the suspension and become thinner when shaken, which makes pouring and application easier.

Depending on the desired characteristics of the final formulation, one can select Newtonian or non-Newtonian flow properties and formulate accordingly. For example, a gel of Pluronic F-127 exhibits reverse thermal gelling. It is fluid at colder temperatures and becomes a gel at warmer temperatures. This type of product is good for application to the skin, where it sets up and delivers the drug over a longer time period.

Preparation Methods

Most viscosity-increasing agents are best dispersed by pouring the powder slowly and steadily into vigorously stirred water, with continued stirring during hydration. A second method is to mix the agent with another, water-soluble substance, such as sucrose, before adding it to water. A third method is to form a paste of the agent with a water-miscible liquid, such as alcohol or glycerin, before adding it to water. Some agents are best dispersed initially in hot water, with the remaining water added as cold or ice water. These methods will help minimize the clumping that can occur with polymers, making their preparation more difficult.

One characteristic of a good suspension is its resuspendability. The product can be observed over time for a determination of its settling and caking tendencies. In formulating the suspension, a pharmacist should ensure it is not too thick, because the product may be difficult to pour, especially if it has been refrigerated.

Quality Control

Quality control involves checking certain characteristics of the suspension, including weight and volume, extent of settling, ease of dispersibility, appearance, odor, and pourability. The measured and observed characteristics should be documented, and, if possible, the product should be periodically checked for these characteristics.

The amount of settling can be measured by allowing the product to sit for a day and then measuring the height of the settled particles. If necessary, formulation changes can be made to reduce the amount of settling. Measuring the height of the settled particles in different batches of the same product can serve as a general guide in determining the consistency of preparation.

Packaging, Storage, and Labeling

Suspensions should be packaged in tight containers that have an opening large enough to easily pour a viscous liquid. Sufficient headspace should be allowed for ease of shaking.

These preparations should be stored at room temperature or refrigerated, depending on the physicochemical characteristics of the active drug and the supporting matrix.

The instruction "Shake Well Before Using" or "Shake Well Before Taking" should always appear on the label of a suspension preparation. In addition, these preparations should be labeled for internal or external use.

Stability

Suspension dosage forms should be observed for the following physical attributes: uniformity, settling, caking, crystal growth, and difficulty in resuspending, as well as mold or bacterial growth, odor, and loss of volume. Suspensions are less susceptible to chemical degradation than are solutions, but if water is present, they generally have a short beyond-use date.

For water-containing oral suspensions that are prepared from ingredients in solid form and stored at cold temperatures, beyond-use dates are no later than 14 days after preparation; for topical preparations, beyond-use dates are no later than 30 days after preparation. This period can be extended if valid scientific information is available to support greater stability, as discussed in Chapter 6 of this book.

Patient Counseling

Patients should be instructed to always shake the suspension before taking or applying it. They should also be instructed on how to shake suspensions—shake vigorously or mix using a rolling action. Patients should be counseled on the proper storage of suspensions and the proper method for measuring doses.

Sample Formulations

℞ Spironolactone Suspension

Spironolactone	200 mg	Active
Cetylpyridinium chloride, monohydrate	10 mg	Surfactant
Potassium sorbate	150 mg	Preservative
Xanthan gum	200 mg	Thickener
Magnesium aluminum silicate	1 g	Suspending Aid
Citric acid, anhydrous	60 mg	Acidifier
Sucrose	20 g	Sweetener
Purified water	qs 100 mL	Vehicle

1. Calculate the quantity of each ingredient required for the prescription.
2. Accurately weigh or measure each ingredient.
3. Place the spironolactone powder in a mortar and add the cetylpyridinium chloride, which has previously been dissolved in 15 mL of purified water. Mix to form a paste.
4. Place 20 mL of purified water in a beaker on a magnetic stirrer, and stir. Sprinkle the xanthan gum on the stirred water.
5. Add the stirred xanthan gum mixture to the mortar containing the spironolactone mixture, and mix well.
6. Dissolve the potassium sorbate in 50 mL of purified water. Place this solution on a magnetic stirrer, and stir.
7. Sprinkle the magnesium aluminum silicate on the stirred water prepared in step 6, and ensure it is thoroughly dispersed.
8. Add the sucrose and citric acid to the mixture prepared in step 7, using heat if necessary; cool to room temperature.
9. Add the spironolactone and xanthan gum mixture prepared in step 5 to the mixture prepared in step 8.
10. Add sufficient purified water to volume, and mix well.
11. Package and label the product.

℞ Progesterone Oral Suspension

Progesterone, micronized	4 g	Active
Glycerin	5 mL	Cosolvent
Methylcellulose 1% solution	50 mL	Vehicle/Thickener
Flavored syrup	qs 100 mL	Vehicle

1. Calculate the quantity of each ingredient required for the prescription.
2. Accurately weigh or measure each ingredient.
3. Place the progesterone powder in a mortar, and wet with the glycerin to obtain a thick, smooth paste.
4. Slowly add the methylcellulose solution to the paste while triturating.
5. Pour the mixture into a graduated cylinder.
6. Add small quantities of flavored syrup to the mortar and mix, and then add these portions to the graduated cylinder.
7. After transferring all the material to the graduated cylinder, add sufficient flavored syrup to volume, and mix thoroughly.
8. Package and label the product.

℞ Progesterone Enema

Progesterone, micronized	20 g	Active
Povidone	10 g	Thickener
Purified water	qs 100 mL	Vehicle

1. Calculate the quantity of each ingredient required for the prescription.
2. Accurately weigh or measure each ingredient.
3. Wet the povidone with about 15 mL of water to form a paste.
4. Using a magnetic stirrer, add about 60 mL of water and stir until a clear solution is obtained.
5. Add the micronized progesterone, and mix well.
6. Add the remaining water to volume, and mix thoroughly.
7. Package and label the product.

Xanthan Gum Suspension Vehicle

Xanthan gum	300 mg	Thickener
Sodium saccharin	100 mg	Sweetener
Aspartame	200 mg	Sweetener
Propylene glycol	5 mL	Cosolvent
Syrup or other preserved vehicle	qs 100 mL	Preserved Vehicle

1. Calculate the required quantity of each ingredient for the total amount to be prepared.
2. Accurately weigh or measure each ingredient.
3. Place the xanthan gum, sodium saccharin, and aspartame in a mortar, and triturate the ingredients, using a pestle.
4. Add the propylene glycol, and make a smooth paste.
5. Add the syrup in small portions, and then pour into a graduated cylinder, rinsing the mortar into the cylinder until 100 mL of suspension is prepared.
6. Mix the suspension well.
7. Package and label the product.

℞ Wound Care Mixture

Phenol	200 mg	Active
Zinc oxide	12 g	Astringent
70% Ethanol, Calcium hydroxide solution	aa qs 100 mL	Vehicle

1. Calculate the quantity of each ingredient required for the prescription.
2. Accurately weigh or measure each ingredient.
3. Prepare 100 mL of the vehicle, using equal parts of 70% ethanol and calcium hydroxide solution (lime water).
4. Dissolve the phenol in about 75 mL of the vehicle prepared in step 3.
5. Sprinkle the zinc oxide powder on the phenol–vehicle mixture.
6. Add additional vehicle to the zinc oxide–phenol mixture to make 100 mL of suspension. (Discard the remainder of the vehicle.)
7. Package and label the product.

Sugar-Free Suspension Structured Vehicle USP

Xanthan gum	200 mg	Thickener
Saccharin sodium	200 mg	Sweetener
Potassium sorbate	150 mg	Preservative
Citric acid	100 mg	Acidifier
Sorbitol	2 g	Sweetener
Mannitol	2 g	Sweetener
Glycerin	2 mL	Cosolvent
Purified water	qs 100 mL	Vehicle

1. Calculate the required quantity of each ingredient for the total amount to be prepared.
2. Accurately weigh or measure each ingredient.
3. Place 30 mL of purified water in a beaker on a hot plate or stirrer.
4. Using moderate heat, stir to form a vortex, and slowly sprinkle the xanthan gum into the vortex.
5. In a separate beaker, dissolve the saccharin sodium, potassium sorbate, and citric acid in 50 mL of purified water.
6. Using moderate heat, incorporate the sorbitol, mannitol, and glycerin into this mixture.
7. Add to the xanthan gum dispersion prepared in step 4.
8. Add sufficient purified water to volume, and mix well.
9. Package and label.

℞ Metronidazole Benzoate 400 mg/5 mL Oral Suspension

Metronidazole benzoate	8 g	Active
Glycerin	qs	Levigating Agent/Cosolvent
Flavoring	qs	Flavoring
Suspension structured vehicle or sugar-free suspension structured vehicle or commercial oral liquid vehicles	qs 100 mL	Flavoring

1. Calculate the quantity of each ingredient required for the prescription.
2. Accurately weigh or measure each ingredient.
3. Mix the metronidazole benzoate powder with sufficient glycerin to form a smooth paste.
4. Add the flavoring, and mix well.
5. Add sufficient suspension vehicle to volume, and mix well.
6. Package and label the product.

℞ Misoprostol 0.001% and Lidocaine 0.5% Oral Rinse

Misoprostol	1 mg	Active
Lidocaine hydrochloride	500 mg	Active
Methylparaben	200 mg	Preservative
Glycerin	10 mL	Cosolvent/Levigating Agent
Cherry flavoring, anhydrous	10 µL	Flavoring
Syrup	40 mL	Vehicle
Sodium carboxymethylcellulose 0.25% solution	qs 100 mL	Vehicle

1. Calculate the quantity of each ingredient required for the prescription.
2. Accurately weigh or measure each ingredient, and obtain and pulverize five 200-µg misoprostol tablets.
3. Dissolve the methylparaben in the glycerin, and add the lidocaine hydrochloride, pulverized misoprostol tablets, and cherry flavoring.
4. Add the syrup and sufficient sodium carboxymethylcellulose 0.25% solution to volume, and mix well.
5. Package and label the product.

Rx Stomatitis Preparations (100 mL)

Ingredient	Kaiser	Kraemer	Powell	Reynolds	Stanford	T-N-D-D	Ingredient
Tetracycline 25 mg/mL suspension	50 mL		8 mL	50 mL	48 mL		Active
Nystatin oral suspension	12 mL	30 mL	4.8 mL	12 mL	12 mL		Active
Hydrocortisone powder	46 mg		20 mg	46 mg	46 mg		Active
Purified water	qs 100 mL				qs 100 mL		Vehicle
Dyclonine 1% solution		22.5 mL					Active
Lemon oil		0.25 mL					Flavoring
Glycerin		qs 100 mL					Vehicle
Diphenhydramine 2.5 mg/mL elixir			qs 100 mL				Active
Chlorpheniramine 0.4 mg/mL syrup				qs 100 mL			Active
Chlorpheniramine 4 mg tablets					#5		Active
Tetracycline						1.25 g	Active
Nystatin						1,666,667 units	Active
Diphenhydramine HCl						125 mg	Active
Dexamethasone						333 µg	Active
Xanthan gum						200 mg	Thickener
Aspartame						200 mg	Sweetener
Saccharin sodium						100 mg	Sweetener
Flavoring						qs	Flavoring
Simple syrup						qs 100 mL	Vehicle

(Note: Empty cell indicates ingredient is not present.)

1. Calculate the quantity of each ingredient required for the prescription.
2. Accurately weigh or measure each ingredient.
3. Select the appropriate method of preparation:
   - Kaiser: Mix the hydrocortisone powder with a small amount of the tetracycline suspension until smooth. Slowly add the remaining tetracycline suspension, mix in the nystatin suspension, and add sufficient purified water to volume and mix well.
   - Kraemer: Add the lemon oil to about 100 mL of glycerin followed by the dyclonine solution and nystatin oral suspension. Add sufficient glycerin to volume, and mix well.
   - Powell: Mix the hydrocortisone powder with a small amount of the tetracycline suspension. Add the remainder of the tetracycline suspension followed by the nystatin oral suspension and the diphenhydramine elixir, and mix well.
   - Reynolds: Mix the tetracycline suspension and nystatin suspension. Slowly add the hydrocortisone (previously dissolved in 15 mL of ethanol) with constant stirring. Add sufficient chlorpheniramine syrup to volume, and mix well.
   - Stanford: Thoroughly pulverize the chlorpheniramine tablets, and blend in the hydrocortisone powder. Add the tetracycline suspension in portions with thorough mixing followed by the nystatin oral suspension. Add sufficient purified water to volume, and mix well.
   - T-N-D-D: Blend the tetracycline, nystatin, diphenhydramine hydrochloride, dexamethasone, xanthan gum, aspartame, and saccharin sodium powders, and mix well. Add 90 mL of simple syrup, in portions, with thorough mixing after each addition. Add the desired flavoring, and mix well. Add sufficient simple syrup to volume, and mix well.
4. Package and label the product.

℞ Bi-Est 0.25 mg/drop in Oil Suspension

Estradiol	0.2 mg/drop	Active
Estrone	0.05 mg/drop	Active
Saccharin	100 mg	Sweetener
Tangerine oil (flavoring)	qs	Flavoring
Sesame oil	qs	Vehicle

1. Accurately determine the number of drops per milliliter depending on the dropper and container being used. Using a dropper, count the number of drops to make a volume of 2 mL. Divide by 2 to get the number of drops per mL.
2. This formula calls for 0.25 mg of Bi-Est per drop. To determine the quantity of each of the estrogens needed per milliliter, multiply the concentration (estradiol 0.2 mg and estrone 0.05 mg per drop) by the number of drops per milliliter. Multiply result by the number of milliliters to be prepared to determine the quantity for the prescription.
3. Accurately weigh or measure each of the ingredients.
4. Mix the estradiol and estrone in a suitable oil, such as sesame oil. Add the saccharin and tangerine oil, and mix well. Add additional sesame oil to volume, and mix well.
5. Package and label the product.

℞ Progesterone 100 mg/mL Sublingual Drops

Progesterone, micronized	1 g	Active
Silica gel, micronized	200 mg	Thickener
Saccharin	100 mg	Sweetener
Flavoring (mild)	qs	Flavoring
Almond oil or peanut oil	qs 10 mL	Vehicle

1. Calculate the quantity of each ingredient required for the prescription.
2. Accurately weigh or measure each ingredient.
3. Mix the progesterone, silica gel, and saccharin in a mortar.
4. Add a small quantity of the vehicle (oil) to make a paste.
5. Add the flavoring, and mix well.
6. Add sufficient vehicle to volume, and mix well.
7. Package and label the product.

℞ Minoxidil 5% and Finasteride 0.1% Topical Liquid

Minoxidil	5 g	Active
Finasteride	100 mg	Active
Propylene glycol	20 mL	Vehicle/Penetration Enhancer
Ethanol 95%	70 mL	Vehicle/Penetration Enhancer
Purified water	qs 100 mL	Vehicle

1. Calculate the quantity of each ingredient required for the prescription.
2. Accurately weigh or measure each ingredient; count out the number of finasteride (Proscar) tablets.
3. Thoroughly pulverize the finasteride tablets, add to the ethanol, mix well, and filter.
4. To the filtrate, add the propylene glycol and minoxidil.
5. Mix well until all ingredients are dissolved.
6. Add sufficient purified water to volume, and mix well.
7. Package and label the product.

Emulsions

Definitions and Types

Emulsions are heterogeneous systems consisting of at least one immiscible liquid that is intimately dispersed in another liquid in the form of droplets, or globules, whose diameters generally exceed 0.1 µm. Emulsions are also defined as thermodynamically unstable mixtures of two essentially immiscible liquids with an emulsifying agent to hold them together. The process of combining these ingredients is termed *emulsification.*

An emulsion consists of a dispersed phase (internal phase or discontinuous phase), a dispersion medium (external phase or continuous phase), and a third component, known as an emulsifying agent. The diameter of the dispersed-phase globules is generally in the range of about 0.1 to 10 µm, although some can be as small as 0.01 µm or as large as 100 µm.

Emulsions are used as a dosage form whenever two immiscible liquids must be dispensed in the same preparation. Ordinarily, the mixture has both a polar and a nonpolar component, each of which is a liquid. When the dispersed phase is nonpolar (oil) and the dispersion medium is polar (water), the emulsion is known as an oil-in-water (o/w) emulsion. When the dispersed phase is water and the dispersion medium is oil, the emulsion is the water-in-oil (w/o) type. Generally, emulsions for internal use are the o/w type; those for external use can be either type. Water-in-oil emulsions are insoluble in water, are not water washable, will absorb water, are occlusive, and can be greasy. Conversely, o/w emulsions are miscible with water, are water washable, will absorb water, are nonocclusive, and are nongreasy.

Creams are opaque, soft solids or thick liquids consisting of medications that are dissolved or suspended in water-removable (i.e., vanishing cream) or emollient bases. They are intended for external application and can be either type of emulsion. The term *cream* is often applied to soft, o/w, cosmetically acceptable types of preparations. Creams are usually applied to moist, weeping lesions because they have a somewhat drying effect in that the lesions' fluids are miscible with the aqueous external phase of creams.

Lotions are fluid emulsions or suspensions designed for external application. They have a lubricating effect and thus are applied to intertriginous areas, that is, areas where the skin rubs together, such as between the fingers, between the thighs, or under the arms.

Historical Use

The term *emulsion* is derived from the word "emulsus." The verb associated with this word, "emulgere," means "to milk out." Emulsion originally referred to the milky liquid extracted from almonds but in time was used to refer to any milky fluid. Although emulsions still have a milky appearance, the term now commonly refers to a dispersion of immiscible liquids.

Applications

Topical creams and lotions are popular forms of emulsions for external use. Internally, emulsions are used to dispense oily and aqueous drugs together, to mask the taste of unpleasant oily drugs, and sometimes to enhance the absorption of selected drugs. Emulsions containing high caloric oil can be administered intravenously to severely debilitated patients.

Composition

Emulsions generally contain three components: a lipid phase, an aqueous phase, and an emulsifier. A compounding pharmacist has the greatest flexibility in the choice of an emulsifier. Common emulsifiers are listed in Table 19-1.

Preparation

Emulsions do not form spontaneously when liquids are mixed. Rather, they require energy input, such as mechanical agitation, ultrasonic vibration, or heat, to break up the liquids, thereby increasing the surface area of the internal phase.

Emulsions can be prepared by both manual and mechanical methods. These methods can involve the use of a mortar and pestle, a bottle for shaking, beakers, an electric mixer or a mechanical stirrer, a hand homogenizer, and sonifiers. A mortar and pestle can be used with both the English and the Continental methods of emulsification, which are described below. For best results, the mortar should have rough surfaces to help shear the liquid into small globules.

The English method, also called the wet gum method, relies on the use of mucilages or dissolved gums. The ratio of oil:water:emulsifier often is 2–4:2:1 for forming the primary emulsion, as shown in Table 19-2. The mucilage is made by adding a small quantity of water to the hydrocolloid (e.g., acacia) and then triturating the mixture until uniform. Oil is added in small quantities by using rapid trituration. The resulting mixture will be thick and viscous. More water is added slowly, and the emulsion is triturated rapidly until complete.

TABLE 19-1 Emulsifiers and Stabilizers for Use in Emulsions

Carbohydrates	*Surfactants*
Acacia	Anionic
Agar	Cationic
Chondrus	Nonionic
Pectin	*Solids*
Tragacanth	Aluminum hydroxide
Proteins	
Casein	Bentonite
Egg yolk	Magnesium hydroxide
Gelatin	
High Molecular Weight Alcohols	
Cetyl alcohol	
Glyceryl monostearate	
Stearyl alcohol	

TABLE 19-2 Component Ratios for Preparation of Primary Emulsions

Oil	Acacia	Tragacanth
Fixed oils	4:2:1	40:20:1
Mineral oil	3:2:1	30:20:1
Linseed oil	2:2:1	20:20:1
Volatile oils	2:2:1	20:20:1

The Continental method, known as the dry gum method, involves rapid mixing of the hydrocolloid with the oil for a short time, after which the water is added all at once with rapid trituration. When a snapping sound is heard, the primary emulsion has formed. More water is then added slowly with rapid trituration until the emulsion is complete. The ratio of oil:water:emulsifier for preparing the primary emulsion is generally about 4:2:1.

The bottle method (shaking) is another approach to preparing emulsions that contain volatile oils and other nonviscous oils. This method eliminates the splashing problem that sometimes occurs when a mortar and pestle are used. The bottle method, which is a variation of the dry gum method, involves mixing the powder (emulsifier) and oil in a bottle and then shaking the bottle with short, rapid movements. The required quantity of water is added all at once, and the mixture is again shaken rapidly to form the primary emulsion (4:2:1 ratio). If more water is required, it is added in small amounts, with the bottle shaken after each addition. The oil and gum should *not* be allowed to remain in contact too long, as the gum can imbibe the oil and partially waterproof the powder.

The beaker method is often used with synthetic emulsifying agents. The prescription ingredients are generally divided into two separate phases: oil and water. Each phase is heated individually to about 60°C to 70°C, if needed. The internal phase is then stirred into the external phase. Finally, the preparation is removed from the heat and stirred gently and periodically until it has cooled (congealed).

A mechanical stirrer (mixer) with various impellers can be used to prepare an emulsion. The unit's propeller should be placed directly into the system to be emulsified. Mixers are available commercially and can be found in department stores and gourmet kitchen stores (Figure 19-1).

Hand homogenizers function by forcing the mixture of liquids through a small inlet orifice at a high pressure. This shearing action causes the globules to break up.

Pluronic lecithin organogels (PLO gels) are liposomal emulsions commonly prepared by placing one phase in one syringe (large enough to hold the total quantity of formula) and attaching it to another identical syringe containing the second phase by using a luer-to-luer adapter. The mixing occurs by forcing the contents of one syringe into the other and then reversing the procedure. Emulsification occurs owing to the shear stress when the mixture is forced through the small orifice as it moves from one syringe to the other. When mixing is complete, one syringe is completely filled, the luer-to-luer connector is removed, and a syringe cap is placed on the syringe. To fill smaller syringes, one can simply replace the large syringe with a small syringe, fill the contents into the smaller syringe, and repeat the process.

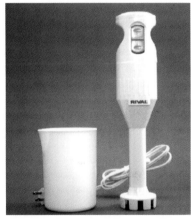

FIGURE 19-1 Two-speed mixer.

Compounding Multiple Emulsions (Water-in-Oil-in-Water, Oil-in-Water-in-Oil)

Multiple emulsions can be prepared by emulsifying an emulsion into a second external phase. An example would be combining a w/o emulsifier (sorbitan monooleate) with liquid petrolatum and adding this to an aqueous phase to form a w/o emulsion, followed by dispersion in an aqueous solution of an o/w emulsifying agent (Tween 80) to form a final water-in-oil-in-water (w/o/w) emulsion. Similarly, an oil-in-water-in-oil (o/w/o) emulsion can be prepared. Potential applications include detoxification, drug targeting or localization, prolonged-action dosage forms, and use in cosmetics.

Incorporating Materials into a W/O Emulsion

Oils and insoluble powders can be incorporated directly into an emulsion by using a pill tile and spatula or a mortar and pestle. A levigating agent may be needed if large amounts of insoluble powders are required for the formulation. In many w/o emulsions, sufficient emulsifying agent is available to emulsify a larger quantity of the aqueous solution of the drug, which can be incorporated by using a pill tile with a spatula, a mortar and pestle, or gentle heat from a water bath. When using heat, a pharmacist should ensure that the preparation is not held at a high temperature for too long, because some loss of water can occur. This loss of water would change the volume of the preparation. Adding oily ingredients usually poses no problem. Some crystalline drugs may need to be dissolved in oil before being incorporated, if possible. In this case, using the base form rather than the salt form of the drug may be necessary. Adding water to these emulsions is difficult unless an excess quantity of the emulsifier is present.

Incorporating Materials into an O/W Emulsion

A pill tile and spatula or a mortar and pestle are also used to incorporate insoluble powders and aqueous solutions into emulsions. Using a levigating agent, such as glycerin or propylene glycol, may be advisable when mixing the insoluble powder with the emulsion. Crystalline materials should be dissolved in a small quantity of water before they are added to the emulsion. Water-soluble materials should also be dissolved in a small amount of water before the solution is incorporated into the base. Because there is usually an excess of emulsifying agent, a small quantity of oil can be incorporated directly into the base. However, if larger amounts of oil are required, adding a small quantity of an o/w surfactant to help disperse the oil uniformly in the vehicle may be necessary. Generally, adding water-soluble ingredients is easy.

Using heat to incorporate an ingredient into an o/w vehicle can cause the preparation to lose water. Thus, one must work quickly. If water is lost, the volume of the preparation will change; moreover, if it is a semisolid, it may tend to become stiff and waxy. (See Box 19-1 for additional suggestions.)

BOX 19-1 Hints for Compounding Emulsions

Suggestions for compounding emulsions are as follows:

- Dissolving the oil-soluble ingredients in the oil phase and the water-soluble ingredients in the aqueous phase is advisable.
- Light, rapid trituration is more effective than heavy, slow trituration when using a mortar and pestle.
- Under a given set of conditions, an o/w emulsion can be more easily produced with glass equipment, whereas w/o emulsions can be more easily prepared with water-repellent plastic equipment. This ease of preparation could be related to the wettability of the external phase when it comes in contact with the surface of the equipment.
- Water and oil phases should be added slowly under constant agitation.
- If heat is used, the aqueous phase should be a few degrees warmer than the oil phase.
- The viscosity of emulsions generally increases with their aging.
- The greater the volume of the internal phase, the greater is the apparent viscosity.
- There is a linear relationship between emulsion viscosity and the viscosity of the continuous phase.

Physicochemical Considerations

A pharmacist must consider a number of factors before compounding an emulsion, including the purpose and route, whether internal or external, of the drug; the concentration of the active drug; the liquid vehicle; the physicochemical stability of the drug; and any preservatives, buffers, solubilizers, emulsifying agents, viscosity enhancers, colors, and flavorings.

Two immiscible liquids in contact with each other will tend to maintain as small an interface as possible. Consequently, mixing these liquids together will be difficult. If the liquids are shaken together, spherical droplets will form because the liquids tend to maintain as small a surface area as possible. There will be interfacial tension between the two liquids. With the addition of a surfactant, the liquids will become miscible because the molecules of the agent will tend to be oriented between the two phases, with the polar ends in the polar phase and the nonpolar ends in the nonpolar phase.

An emulsifying agent makes the globules less likely to coalesce, or join together to form larger globules, which would eventually cause the two liquids to separate. The stability of an emulsion depends on the properties of the emulsifier and the film it forms where the two phases interface. This film, which should form rapidly during the emulsification process, should be both tough and elastic.

Emulsifying agents aid in forming emulsions through three mechanisms: (1) reduction of interfacial tension, as described above, (2) formation of a rigid interfacial film, and (3) formation of an electrical double layer. If the concentration of the emulsifier is sufficiently high, a rigid film can form between the immiscible phases. This film can act as a mechanical barrier to the coalescence of the globules. An electrical double layer minimizes coalescence by producing electrical forces that repulse approaching droplets.

Emulsifying agents can be divided into three categories: (1) surfactants, (2) hydrophilic colloids, and (3) finely divided solid particles. Surfactants are adsorbed at oil:water interfaces to form monomolecular films, resulting in a decrease in interfacial tension, whereas hydrophilic colloids form multimolecular films that surround the dispersed particles. The finely divided solid particles are adsorbed at the interface between the two liquid phases of the globules and create a film of particles around the dispersed globules. As can be noted, the one common feature of each of these agents is that they form a film. Examples of agents that can be used in emulsions can be found in Table 19-1.

Hydrophile–Lipophile Balance

The hydrophile–lipophile balance (HLB) system is used to describe the characteristics of a surfactant. The system consists of an arbitrary scale to which HLB values are experimentally determined and assigned. If the HLB value is low, the number of hydrophilic groups on the surfactant is small, which means it is more lipophilic (oil soluble) than hydrophilic (water soluble). For example, according to Table 19-3, Span 80 has an HLB value of 4.3 and is oil soluble. If the HLB value is high, there are a large number of hydrophilic groups on the surfactant, which makes it more hydrophilic (water soluble) than oil soluble. Tween 20, for example, has an HLB value of 16.7 and is water soluble. The HLB ranges of various types of surfactants are listed in Table 19-4. Table 19-5 shows physicochemical characteristics of wetting and solubilizing agents.

Antifoaming agents include alcohol, castor oil, ether, and some surfactants. These agents dissipate foam by destabilizing the air:liquid interface, which allows the liquid to drain away from the air pocket.

TABLE 19-3 Hydrophile–Lipophile Balance (HLB) Values of Emulsifiers

Commercial Name	Chemical Name	HLB Value
Acacia	Acacia	12.0/8
Arlacel 83	Sorbitan sesquioleate	3.7
Brij 30	Polyoxyethylene lauryl ether	9.7
Glyceryl monostearate	Glyceryl monostearate	3.8
Methocel 15 cP	Methylcellulose	10.5
Myrj 45	Polyoxyethylene monostearate	11.1
Myrj 49	Polyoxyethylene monostearate	15.0
Myrj 52	Polyoxyl 40 stearate	16.9
PEG 400 monooleate	Polyoxyethylene monooleate	11.4
PEG 400 monolaurate	Polyoxyethylene monolaurate	13.1
PEG 400 monostearate	Polyoxyethylene monostearate	11.6
Pharmagel B	Gelatin	9.8
Potassium oleate	Potassium oleate	20.0
Sodium lauryl sulfate	Sodium lauryl sulfate	40
Sodium oleate	Sodium oleate	18
Span 20	Sorbitan monolaurate	8.6
Span 40	Sorbitan monopalmitate	6.7
Span 60	Sorbitan monostearate	4.7
Span 65	Sorbitan tristearate	2.1
Span 80	Sorbitan monooleate	4.3
Span 85	Sorbitan trioleate	1.8
Tragacanth	Tragacanth	13.20
Triethanolamine oleate	Triethanolamine oleate	12
Tween 20	Polyoxyethylene sorbitan monolaurate	16.7
Tween 21	Polyoxyethylene sorbitan monolaurate	13.3
Tween 40	Polyoxyethylene sorbitan monopalmitate	15.6
Tween 60	Polyoxyethylene sorbitan monostearate	14.9
Tween 61	Polyoxyethylene sorbitan monostearate	9.6
Tween 65	Polyoxyethylene sorbitan tristearate	10.5
Tween 80	Polyoxyethylene sorbitan monooleate	15.0
Tween 81	Polyoxyethylene sorbitan monooleate	10.0
Tween 85	Polyoxyethylene sorbitan trioleate	11.0
N/A	Diethylene glycol monolaurate	6.1
N/A	Ethylene glycol distearate	1.5
Pluronic F-68	Poloxamer	17.0
Lauroglycol	Propylene glycol monostearate	3.4
N/A	Sucrose dioleate	7.1

N/A = not applicable.

Emulsifying agents are surfactants that reduce the interfacial tension between oil and water, thereby minimizing the surface energy through the formation of globules. *Wetting agents,* however, aid in attaining intimate contact between solid particles and liquids.

Detergents used in cleaning reduce surface tension and wet a surface as well as any foreign material. When a detergent is used, the foreign material will be emulsified, foaming can occur, and the foreign material will then wash away.

Surfactants can act as solubilizing agents by forming micelles. For example, a surfactant with a high HLB would be used to increase the solubility

TABLE 19-4 Hydrophile–Lipophile Balance (HLB) Ranges of Surfactants

	HLB Range	Surfactants
Low	1–3	Antifoaming agents
	3–6	Emulsifying agents (w/o)
	7–9	Wetting agents
	8–18	Emulsifying agents (o/w)
	13–16	Detergents
High	16–18	Solubilizing agents

TABLE 19-5 Physicochemical Characteristics of Wetting and Solubilizing Agents

Item	Physical State	Solubility		Container Specifications
		Water	Alcohol	
Benzalkonium chloride	Gel	VS	VS	T
Benzethonium chloride	Solid	Sol	Sol	T, LR
Cetylpyridinium chloride	Solid	VS	VS	W
Docusate sodium	Solid	SpS	FS	W
Nonoxynol-9	Liquid	Sol	Sol	T
Octoxynol-9	Liquid	Misc	Misc	T
Poloxamer(s)	Solid	FS	FS	T
Polyoxyl 35 castor oil	Liquid	VS	Sol	T
Polyoxyl 40 hydrogenated castor oil	Paste	VS	Sol	T
Polyoxyl 10 oleyl ether	Semisolid/ Liquid	Sol	Sol	T
Polyoxyl 20 cetostearyl ether	Solid	Sol	Sol	T
Polyoxyl 40 stearate	Solid	Sol	Sol	T
Polysorbate 20	Liquid	Sol	Sol	T
Polysorbate 40	Liquid	Sol	Sol	T
Polysorbate 60	Liquid/Gel	Sol	—	T
Polysorbate 80	Liquid	VS	Sol	T
Sodium lauryl sulfate	Solid	FS	—	W
Sorbitan monolaurate	Liquid	IS	—	T
Sorbitan monooleate	Liquid	IS	—	T
Sorbitan monopalmitate	Solid	IS	[a]	W
Sorbitan monostearate	Solid	[b]	—	W
Tyloxapol	Liquid	Misc	—	T

— = Not available.
[a]Sorbitan monopalmitate is soluble in warm absolute alcohol.
[b]Sorbitan monostearate is dispersible in warm water.

of an oil in an aqueous medium. The lipophilic portion of the surfactant would entrap the oil in the lipophilic (interior) portion of the micelle. The hydrophilic portion of the surfactant surrounding the oil globule would, in turn, be exposed to the aqueous phase.

An HLB value of 10 or higher means that the agent is primarily hydrophilic, whereas an HLB value of less than 10 means it is lipophilic. For example, Spans have HLB values ranging from 1.8 to 8.6, which is indicative of oil-soluble or oil-dispersible molecules. Consequently, the oil phase will predominate, and a w/o emulsion will be formed. Tweens have HLB values that range from 9.6 to 16.7, which is characteristic of water-soluble or water-dispersible molecules. Therefore, the water phase will predominate, and o/w emulsions will be formed.

TABLE 19-6 Hydrophile–Lipophile Balance (HLB) Values for Lipid Materials Used in O/W Emulsions

Lipid Material	Required HLB W/O	Required HLB O/W
Beeswax	4	9–12
Carbon tetrachloride		16
Carnauba wax	12	
Castor oil	6	14
Cetyl alcohol		15
Cottonseed oil	5	6–10
Kerosene		14
Lanolin, anhydrous	8	10–12
Lauric acid		15–16
Lauryl alcohol		14
Methyl silicone		11
Mineral oil, light/heavy	5	11–12
Oleic acid		17
Olive oil	6	14
Paraffin wax	4	10–11
Petrolatum	5	7–12
Stearic acid	6	15
Stearyl alcohol		14

Blending of Surfactants

Often a blend of emulsifiers produces a more stable emulsion than does the use of a single emulsifier with a correctly calculated HLB. Because the HLB numbers are additive, the HLB value of a blend can be readily calculated. Table 19-6, which lists the required HLB values for some common lipid materials, will aid a pharmacist in preparing o/w emulsions.

Surfactants can be blended by direct ratios and proportions. For example, if 20 mL of an agent with an HLB value of 9.65 is required, then two surfactants, one with an HLB value of 8.6 and one with an HLB value of 12.8, can be blended in a 3:1 ratio. The following quantities of each surfactant will be required:

$\frac{3}{4} \times 8.6 = 6.45 \ (15 \ mL)$

$\frac{1}{4} \times 12.8 = 3.20 \ (5 \ mL)$

Total HLB $= 9.65 \ (20 \ mL)$

To calculate the HLB required for the emulsifier in the formulation shown below, the following method is used:

	% of Oil Phase	Required HLB	Portion of HLB
Petrolatum	25 g	56 (25 g/45 g) × 8	= 4.5
Cetyl alcohol	20 g	44 (20 g/45 g) × 15	= 6.7
Emulsifier	2 g		
Preservative	0.2 g		
Pure water	qs ad 100 g		

Approximate HLB value for emulsifier $= 4.5 + 6.7 = 11.2$

Preserving an Emulsion

Because emulsions will support microbiological growth, contamination can occur during the preparation stage or during use. To minimize contamination, one should keep the work area and equipment clean; every attempt should be made to produce an uncontaminated preparation. However, if the preparation is going to be stored for any length of time, a preservative may have to be added.

A preservative must be nontoxic, stable, compatible, and inexpensive. In addition, it must have an acceptable taste, odor, and color. It should also be effective against a wide variety of bacteria, fungi, and yeasts.

The preservative should be concentrated in the aqueous phase because bacterial growth will normally occur there. Additionally, because the nonionized form of the preservative is more effective against bacteria than the ionized form, most of the preservative should be in the nonionized state. To be effective, the preservative must be neither bound nor adsorbed to any agent in the emulsion or the container. Preservatives can partition into the oil phase and lose their effectiveness. Examples of preservatives that are often used in emulsions are shown in Table 19-7. The parabens (methylparaben, propylparaben, butylparaben) are considered to be some of the most satisfactory preservatives for emulsions.

Oils and fats can become rancid, which causes the preparation to have an unpleasant odor, appearance, and taste. Antioxidants can prevent rancidity. Table 19-8 lists examples of antioxidants used in emulsions.

TABLE 19-7 Preservatives Used in Emulsions

Preservative	% Concentration
Alcohol	15
Benzoic acid, sodium benzoate (pH $\leq$ 4)	0.05–0.1
Benzyl alcohol (pH > 5)	1–4
Chlorobutanol[a]	0.5
Imidazolidyl urea (Imidurea)	0.05–0.5
Mercurials	0.005
Organic mercurials	
Phenylmercuric nitrate	0.002–0.004
Phenylmercuric acetate	0.002–0.004
Thimerosal	0.005–0.02
Parabens[b]	
Methylparaben	0.05–0.3
Propylparaben	0.02–0.2
Butylparaben	0.02–0.2
Quaternary ammonium compounds	
Benzalkonium chloride	0.002–0.1
Sorbic acid (pH < 6)	0.1–0.2

[a]Chlorobutanol needs a pH < 5; it will also sorb to plastic.
[b]Parabens are generally used in pairs, have low water solubility and poor taste, and may degrade at a pH > 8. Use at pH 4–8.

Flavoring an Emulsion

When selecting an appropriate flavoring agent, a pharmacist should consider the dispersion medium (external phase) of the emulsion. For example, if a flavoring oil is used and most of the oil partitions into the internal phase as an o/w emulsion, the flavor will be reduced in strength. Oils can be incorporated by using small quantities of surfactants. Usually, surfactants with HLB values of 15 to 18 are used, often in conjunction with a surfactant with an HLB value of 8 to 12. As a general rule, three to five times as much surfactant as oil (flavoring) is necessary to ensure solubilization. For best results, the oil should be mixed with the surfactants before it is added to the aqueous phase. Because this technique can cause the flavoring to lose some of its potency, another approach is to use a cosolvent system to incorporate the flavoring. The use of ethanol, glycerin, or some appropriate solvent often provides acceptable results.

TABLE 19-8 Agents Used as Antioxidants in Emulsions

Ascorbic acid

Ascorbyl palmitate

Butylated hydroxyanisole

Butylated hydroxytoluene

Gallic acid

4-Hydroxymethyl-2,6-*di-tert-*butylphenol

Propyl gallate

Sulfites

L-Tocopherol

Determining the Type of Emulsion

A pharmacist should know whether an emulsion is o/w or w/o in case other ingredients must be added. Determining the type of emulsion can be accomplished by some simple tests, including the drop dilution test, dye solubility test, electrical conductivity test, and filter paper test. The drop dilution test is based on the principle that an emulsion is miscible with its external phase. This test is performed by simply dropping a small quantity of the emulsion onto a surface of water. If the drop is miscible with the water, it will spread, indicating that water is the external phase (i.e., an o/w emulsion). The dye solubility test is based on the principle that a dye disperses uniformly throughout an emulsion if it is soluble in the external phase. This test is performed by adding a small quantity of a water-soluble dye (powder or solution) to the emulsion. If the dye diffuses uniformly throughout the emulsion, water is the external phase (i.e., an o/w emulsion). The principle underlying the electrical conductivity test is that water conducts an electric current and oils do not. Generally, o/w emulsions tend to conduct electricity better than do w/o emulsions, if the required equipment is available. The filter paper test involves putting a drop of emulsion on a clean piece of filter paper. If the drop spreads rapidly into the filter paper, it is an o/w emulsion, because water (the external phase) tends to spread more rapidly throughout the filter paper than does oil. Table 19-9 lists some commercial emulsion bases and indicates whether they are o/w or w/o emulsions.

Quality Control

Quality control involves both observing physical attributes and checking calculations. The final volume of the prepared emulsion should be confirmed with the prescription. The physical appearance and smell should be noted and recorded. Observations should include the color of the emulsion and a description of the size of the globules. A microscope can be used to study a portion of the emulsion so that an approximate range of globule sizes can be recorded. The emulsion should be checked for signs of creaming, coalescence, and mold or bacterial growth. Emulsions are subject to chemical degradation, especially when aqueous vehicles are used.

TABLE 19-9 Commercial Emulsion Bases

Product	Type	Emulsifier
Allercreme Skin Lotion	O/W	Triethanolamine stearate
Almay Emulsion Base	O/W	Fatty acid glycol esters
Cetaphil	O/W	Sodium lauryl sulfate
Dermovan	O/W	Fatty acid amides
Eucerin	W/O	Wool wax alcohols
HEB Cream Base	O/W	Sodium lauryl sulfate
Keri Lotion	O/W	Nonionic emulsifiers
Lubriderm	O/W	Triethanolamine stearate
Neobase	O/W	Polyhydric alcohol esters
Neutrogena Lotion	O/W	Triethanolamine lactate
Nivea Cream	W/O	Wool wax alcohols
pHorsix	O/W	Polyoxyethylene emulsifiers
Polysorb Hydrate	W/O	Sorbitan sesquioleate
Velvachol	O/W	Sodium lauryl sulfate

Packaging, Storage, and Labeling

Packaging emulsions in tight containers to minimize the evaporation of water from the preparation is important. If the preparation is a liquid, the container should have sufficient headspace to allow shaking of the preparation. Oral liquids should be packaged in bottles that have an opening large enough to allow easy pouring of the preparation. Squeeze bottles work fine for topical liquid emulsions, whereas tubes or pump containers work well for viscous creams.

Emulsions should be stored at room temperature or refrigerated. They should be protected from temperature extremes. Their labels should include the instruction "Shake Well."

Stability

Beyond-use dates for water-containing formulations are no later than 14 days for oral preparations when stored at cold temperatures or 30 days for topical preparations compounded from ingredients in solid form when stored at room temperature. These dates can be extended if there is valid scientific information to support stability, as discussed in Chapter 6 of this book.

The stability of an emulsion can be enhanced by (1) decreasing the globule size of the internal phase, (2) obtaining an optimum ratio of oil to water, and (3) increasing the viscosity of the system. Because the oil-to-water ratio (concentration of active ingredient:oil) is frequently determined by the referring health care provider, a compounding pharmacist's efforts to enhance the emulsion's stability are directed at the other two factors.

If the size of the globule is reduced to less than 5 μm, the stability and dispersion of the emulsion will increase. This reduction can be accomplished both with the shearing action of a mortar and pestle and with a homogenizer.

The optimum phase:volume ratio is generally obtained when the internal phase is about 40% to 60% of the total quantity of the preparation. As the percentage of the internal phase increases, the viscosity of the preparation will also increase. A linear relationship exists between the viscosity of the emulsion and the viscosity of the continuous or external phase. The viscosity of an emulsion generally increases on aging.

Enhancing the viscosity of the external phase will tend to enhance the stability of the emulsion. To improve the viscosity, a pharmacist can add a substance that is soluble in or miscible with the external phase of the emulsion. In the case of o/w emulsions, hydrocolloids can be used, whereas for w/o emulsions, waxes and viscous oils as well as fatty alcohols and fatty acids are appropriate.

Of major importance to a compounding pharmacist is the physical stability of the emulsion. The emulsion is stable when it retains its original appearance, odor, color, and other physical properties and when no creaming or coalescence occurs.

Creaming

Creaming occurs when the globules flocculate and concentrate in one specific part of the emulsion. This action creates an unsightly preparation and causes the drug to be distributed unevenly. In o/w emulsions, creaming can be identified when one sees the oil globules gather and rise to the top. This situation occurs because the oil is generally less dense than the water phase. Creaming is easily reversible because the dispersed globules are still surrounded by the protective film. In some cases, shaking can redistribute the emulsion.

Three methods are used to minimize creaming: (1) enhance the viscosity of the external aqueous phase, (2) reduce the size of the globules to a very fine state with a homogenizer, and (3) adjust the densities of both the internal and the external phases so that their densities are the same. Thus, neither phase would tend to rise to the top or settle at the bottom.

Coalescence

Unlike creaming, coalescence (i.e., breaking) is an irreversible process because the film that surrounds the individual globules is destroyed. Altering the viscosity may help stabilize globules and minimize their tendency to coalesce. An optimum viscosity can be determined experimentally.

Another factor is the phase:volume ratio, or the ratio of the internal volume to the total volume of the preparation. The maximum phase:volume ratio that can be achieved is 74%, if one assumes that the particles are perfectly spherical. In general, a phase:volume ratio of about 50%, which approximates loose packing of spherical particles (i.e., a porosity of 48% of the total bulk volume of a powder), yields a reasonably stable emulsion.

Phase Inversion

Phase inversion occurs when an emulsion inverts from one form to another, that is, from o/w to w/o or from w/o to o/w. Phase inversion, which is the basis for the Continental method of emulsion preparation described earlier, can result in the formation of a better emulsion. Monovalent cations tend to form o/w emulsions, whereas divalent cations tend to form w/o emulsions. If sodium stearate is used to form an o/w emulsion and then a calcium salt is added to form calcium stearate, the emulsion inverts from an o/w to a w/o type. The Continental method uses a small proportion of water in the presence of a large proportion of oil. The nucleus of the initial emulsion, or primary emulsion, is the w/o type; however, when water is added in small quantities, the emulsion inverts to an o/w type.

Patient Counseling

A patient should be instructed on how to shake the emulsion and how to measure the required dose. Instruction should also be provided on the proper recapping and storage of the bottle, as well as the way to determine if the emulsion has become physically unstable.

Sample Formulations

℞ Ivermectin 0.8% Cream Rinse

Ivermectin	480 mg	Active
Polyethylene glycol 300	10 mL	Levigating Agent
Hair conditioner/cream rinse	qs 60 mL	Vehicle

1. Calculate the quantity of each ingredient required for the prescription.
2. Accurately weigh or measure each ingredient.
3. Add the ivermectin powder to the polyethylene glycol 300 and mix well.
4. Incorporate sufficient commercial cream rinse preparation to make 60 mL, and mix well.
5. Package and label the product.

(Note: Most hair conditioners and cream rinses are o/w emulsions.)

℞ Dry Skin and Massage Lotion

Safflower oil	30 mL	Active
Glycerin	20 mL	Vehicle/Solvent
Rose oil (or other oil)	2 mL	Aroma
Polysorbate 80	2 mL	Emulsifier
Benzyl alcohol	1 mL	Preservative
Purified water	qs100 mL	Vehicle

1. Calculate the quantity of each ingredient required for the prescription.
2. Accurately measure each ingredient.
3. Mix the safflower oil, rose oil, and polysorbate 80.
4. Mix the glycerin with the benzyl alcohol, and add 45 mL of purified water to form the aqueous phase.
5. Add the oil–polysorbate 80 mixture to the aqueous phase, and mix well.
6. Use a hand homogenizer or a high-speed mixer, if available, to enhance the emulsification process.
7. Package and label the product.

Foams

Pharmaceutical foams are not new but have been gaining in popularity. The use of foam technology now delivers a range of topical active agents, including corticosteroids; sunscreening compounds; and antibacterial, antifungal, and antiviral agents. In addition to the distinct application advantages and improved patient compliance with foams, a real reason for the rapid growth of topical foam technology is that foams are elegant and aesthetically and cosmetically appealing products that provide an alternative to ointments, creams, lotions, and gels in the highly competitive dermatological market. (See Table 20-1.) Foams can be compounded to take advantage of the uniqueness and applicability of this dosage form in medication administration. As an example, for the treatment of inflamed skin conditions such as sunburn and eczema, topical foams are preferred because they can be spread more easily and thereby minimize the amount of rubbing required to distribute the formulations.

Definitions and Types

Definitions

A foam is a preparation that comprises gas bubbles distributed in a liquid; the liquid contains the drug substance and suitable excipients. Foams are intended for application to the skin or mucous membranes.

Foams are examples of disperse systems (a type of colloid). In general, gas is present in a large amount that is divided into bubbles of many different sizes (polydisperse) separated by liquid regions that may form films, thinner and thinner when the liquid phase is drained out of the system films.

Rapid evaporation of foam ingredients can influence the rate of drug penetration into the skin because the rate of drug penetration is proportional to its degree of saturation in the vehicle at the vehicle–skin interface. As a result of evaporation of the solvent, there is a cooling effect on the skin, especially inflamed skin.

Medicated foams are emulsions containing a dispersed phase of gas bubbles in a liquid continuous phase containing an active pharmaceutical ingredient (API). They are packaged in either pressurized containers or special dispensing devices and are intended for application to

TABLE 20-1 Desirable Characteristics and Advantages of Foams

Minimal or lack of greasiness, oiliness, or tackiness
Creation of a pleasant feeling after application
Easy use on hair-bearing skin
Easy application to mucosal areas and to sensitive or highly inflamed skin
Easy spreading on a skin surface
Minimal shiny residual look
Rapid absorption and penetration without any greasy residue
Substantial absorption following rubbing onto the skin

the skin or mucous membranes. A medicated foam is actually formed at the time of application to the affected body site. Surfactants are present to ensure the distribution of the gas in the liquid and to stabilize the form. Medicated foams usually have a fluffy, semisolid consistency and can be formulated to break down into a liquid quickly or to remain as foam to ensure prolonged contact.

The European Pharmacopoeia describes a medicated foam as a formulation consisting of a large amount of gas dispersed in a liquid generally containing one or more active substances, a surfactant ensuring their formation, and various other excipients. Medicated foams intended to treat severely injured skin or open wounds must be sterile.

Aerosol foams containing numerous drugs are commercially available. They are generally water miscible and nongreasy and include those that are applied topically or dermally, vaginally, rectally, and, possibly, nasally. An example of a commercial product is rectally administered Cortifoam that contains hydrocortisone acetate 10% in a base containing propylene glycol, emulsifying wax, polyoxyethylene-10-stearyl ether, cetyl alcohol, methylparaben, propylparaben, trolamine, purified water, and inert propellants.

Types

Foams include pharmaceutical and cosmetic preparations as follows:

- Quick-breaking foams are thermally unstable and collapse on exposure to skin temperature. A typical example is the hydroalcoholic foams.
- Lathering soapy foams are stable when formed and increase in volume when rubbed (shaving foam).
- Breakable foams are stable at skin temperature but collapse and spread easily when a mild shear force is applied. These are very good for dermatological and mucosal tissue application.
- Aqueous foams contain a large percentage of water and may be alcohol free.
- Hydroalcoholic foams contain varying percentages of alcohol.

Composition

Foams generally are composed of hydrophilic and hydrophobic solvents or liquids, cosolvents, emollients, foaming agents, foam adjuvants, gelling agents, water, miscellaneous agents, and propellants.

Hydrophilic Solvents

Water is a primary solvent in most foam systems. The creation of a foamable composition with low water content is not easy and usually requires very high concentrations of a foaming surfactant system. Examples of hydrophilic solvents include azone, caprylic acid, diethylene glycol, dimethylacetamide, dimethylformamide, dimethyl sulfoxide (DMSO), dioxolane, di-terpenes, ethylene glycol, glycerin, hexylene glycol, lauric acid, lauryl alcohol, limonene, l-menthol, myristyl alcohol, polyethylene glycols, propylene glycol, terpenes, and terpineol.

Hydrophobic Solvents

Hydrophobic solvents are described as materials with a solubility in purified water at room temperature of about 1 g/1000 mL or less and are liquid at room temperature. Examples include borage seed oil, canola oil, cod liver oil, coconut oil, corn oil, cottonseed oil, docosahexaenoic acid, eicosapentaenoic acid, evening primrose oils, flaxseed oil, gamma-linoleic acid, linoleic acid, linolenic acid, mineral oil, olive oil, omega-3 and omega-6 fatty acids, salmon oil, sesame oil, soybean oil, sunflower oil, triglyceride oil, wheat germ oil, and some essential oils.

Cosolvents

Solvents and sometimes cosolvents are the primary constituents of topical foams. Depending on the solvent or combination of solvents (cosolvents) employed, topical foams can be either aqueous or nonaqueous, that is, containing no or little water. In most cases, topical foams are water based because the generation of nonaqueous foams is more difficult. Examples of water-miscible cosolvents include combinations of ethanol, glycerin, isopropanol, polyethylene glycol, and propylene glycol.

Emollients

Emollients are agents that can be used to soften the skin or soothe irritated skin or mucous membranes. Examples include acetylated lanolin alcohol, cetyl acetate, cetyl lactate, cetyl ricinoleate, diisopropyl adipate, diisopropyl dimerate, glyceryl oleate, hexylene glycol, isopropyl isostearate, isopropyl palmitate, isostearic acid derivatives, maleated soybean oil, myristyl myristate, phenyl trimethicone, propylene glycol, octyl dodecanol, octyl hydroxystearate, octyl palmitate, tocopheryl acetate, tocopheryl linoleate, triisocetyl citrate, wheat germ glycerides, and mixtures.

Silicone Oil

Silicone oils are known for their skin-protective properties and may be used as a hydrophobic solvent. Generally, examples are silicone oil at a 2%–5% concentration.

Foaming Agents

Foaming agents are amphiphilic substances; the hydrophilic part relates to their solubility in water and the hydrophobic part arranges to minimize that portion's contact with the water and leads to its orientation at the air–water interface and the formation of micelles in the bulk of the liquid phase. Foaming agents may include many different surface-active agents, including anionic, cationic, nonionic, ampholytic, amphoteric, and zwitterionic surfactants or combinations.

When a foaming agent is adsorbed into the air–water interface, the surface tension of water is lowered and the surface pressure is increased. For stability of the foam, the concentration of the foaming agent in an adsorbed layer is most important. In a homologous series of foaming agents, the maximum foaming ability occurs at a concentration about equal to the critical micelle concentration. The combination of two different foaming agents may or may not lead to increased foam stability.

Examples of foaming agents include Brij 38, Brij 52, Brij 56, isoceteth-20, laureth-4, lecithin, Myrj 45, Myrj 49, Myrj 59, polyglyceryl-4 isostearate, polyoxyethylene (20) sorbitan monostearate (Tween 60), polyoxyethylene (2) sorbitan monooleate (Tween 80), sodium lauryl sulfate, sorbitan laurate, sorbitan monolaurate, sorbitan palmitate, and triethanolamine lauryl sulfate.

However, in terms of pharmaceutical application, surfactants are the most common foaming agents. Both ionic and nonionic surfactants can be used, but the former are known for their skin irritancy and thus nonionic surfactants are preferred, particularly when the target area of treatment is infected or inflamed.

Foam Adjuvants

Foam adjuvants are included to improve the stability and reduce the specific gravity of the foamed composition; they may increase the foaming capacity of the surfactants. They can include fatty alcohols, fatty acids, and their mixtures. Examples include arachidyl alcohol, behenyl alcohol, cetyl alcohol, oleyl alcohol, stearyl alcohol, arachidic acid, behenic acid, hexadecanoic acid, octacosanoic acid, and stearic acid.

Gelling Agents

Gelling agents are present for the creation and stabilization of the foam, having a fine bubble structure so the foam does not readily collapse on release. They are usually included at less than 1% of the composition and will aid in increasing viscosity. Examples include acrylic acid/ethyl acrylate copolymers, carboxymethyl cellulose, carboxyvinyl polymers, carrageenan gum, egg albumin, gelatin agar, guar gum, hydroxyethyl cellulose, hydroxypropyl methylcellulose, hydroxypropyl guar gum, locust bean gum, polymethacrylic acid polymers, polyvinyl alcohol, polyvinylpyrrolidone, quince seed extract, sodium alginate, sodium caseinate, starch, tragacanth gum, and xanthan gum.

Miscellaneous Agents

When foam compositions are used to administer chemically unstable topical therapeutic agents (e.g., ascorbic acid), a stabilizer (e.g., flavonoids) can be added to the formulation to ensure that the active agent is not degraded before dose application. In addition, topical foams can also incorporate a cooling agent (e.g., menthol), a warming agent (e.g., polyhydric alcohols), or a soothing agent (e.g., aloe vera) to generate a unique sensation or sensation-modifying effect on application.

In addition, other excipients can be incorporated, depending on the active agent and the required foam characteristics. For example, when formulating a foam containing the ionizable drug minoxidil, used for hair loss treatment, a pharmacist can use an acid to enhance the drug's solubility or to maintain the pH of the formulation at a most favorable range in order to enable the maximum amount of drug to be formulated.

Excipients in a Sample Foam

The commercial product Verdeso (Desonide) 0.05% Foam illustrates the different categories of excipients. It contains the following excipients: citric acid, cetyl alcohol, cyclomethicone, isopropyl myristate, light mineral oil, white petrolatum, polyoxyl 20 cetostearyl ether, potassium citrate, propylene glycol, sorbitan monolaurate, phenoxyethanol, and purified water.

Preparation

A foam may contain one or more APIs, surfactants, aqueous or nonaqueous liquids, and the propellants. Typical preparation methods include (1) pressure-filled containers and pressurized aerosols, (2) airspray foam pump, (3) whipping or shaking (i.e., mechanical agitation of a liquid or a solution), and (4) bubbling (i.e., injection of a stream of gas or liquid or the mixture into a liquid). We will discuss methods 2, 3, and 4.

Airspray Foam Pump

The airspray foam pump creates foam without the use of gas propellants. It allows mixing of the liquid with air, resulting in foam generation. These are relatively simple systems to use, and the viscosity of the liquids may need to be altered for greater efficiency. In fact, one relatively simple method is to dilute a lotion vehicle with preserved water, add the API, and package the mixture in the pump system. This device enables compounding pharmacists to extemporaneously prepare foamed dosage forms. These pumps are available from compounding supply companies.

Whipping or Shaking

Whipping, also called beating or shaking, is accomplished with different devices that agitate a liquid in order to form an interface with a gas phase. The volume of air incorporated usually increases with an increase in the beating intensity. High viscosity liquids do not produce stable foams. During whipping, each air bubble undergoes severe mechanical stress and a more rapid coalescence occurs during foam generation than in a standing foam. The mechanical stress produces smaller bubbles from larger ones. This technique is widely used in the food industry (whip cream, desserts, toppings).

Shaking is rarely used because it produces low foam volumes after a long generation time. The resulting foam is based on the frequency and amplitude of shaking, the volume and shape of the container, and the volume and viscosity of the liquid.

Bubbling

Bubbling is the injection of gas through narrow openings into a foamable liquid. It is reproducible and gives uniform bubble sizes. The foam volume produced using this technique is dependent on the total amount of foaming agent and the solution being bubbled.

Miscellaneous

The gas generation method can use effervescent formulations for gas production. When the ingredients come in contact with water or mucosal secretions, gas is generated, resulting in foam production. This method is used in preparing vaginal and rectal foams and tablets.

Physicochemical Considerations

A *foam booster* is a substance that enhances foam formation and includes fatty acid alcohol amides, such as oleic acid diethanolamide, coco fatty acid diethanolamide, and polycarboxylic acid poly diethanolamide, which are normally used at a 5% concentration because higher concentrations may become irritating. The addition of some polymers (such as cellulose derivatives and xanthan gum) can be used to increase foam stability.

Foam destroyers are agents that will decrease the stability of a foam. Foam destroyers include small oil droplets that spread on the foam lamellae, thin the lamellae, and result in breakage. These include oils, alcohols, and organic solvents that are normally poorly soluble in water. They orient themselves at the surface, which leads to an increase in surface pressure and a reduction of the elasticity of the surface film produced by the foaming agent; this results in rupture of the lamella or film. Foam inhibitors generally have an affinity for the interface in preference to the foaming agents and prevent foam generation. Foam inhibitors include some electrolytes as well as poorly wettable solid particles.

Quality Control

Quality control assessment can include weight and volume, pH, specific gravity, active drug assay, color, globule size range, rheological properties and pourability, physical observation, and physical stability (discoloration, foreign materials, gas formation, mold growth).

Packaging, Storage, and Labeling

Foams formulated with flammable components should be appropriately labeled. Labeling indicates that before dispensing, a foam drug product is shaken well to ensure uniformity. The instructions for use must clearly note special precautions that are necessary to preserve sterility. In the absence of a metering valve, delivered volume may be variable.

Stability

The stability of foams involves consideration of two factors: predose application (i.e., inside the container) and postdose application (i.e., outside the container). Also, a pharmacist may not be aware of the link between the foam structure inside the canister and the foam stability on application.

Foam stability is oftentimes difficult to predict. Although many studies have been conducted, researchers have had extreme difficulty in developing a general theory related to foam stability because both dynamic and static factors are involved. Basically, if a film or lamella between two bubbles ruptures, the bubbles coalesce, as a result of a number of different processes that may be occurring, including Ostwald ripening, gravitational separation (creaming, bubbles rising, and drainage), and Brownian motion. When bubbles are formed, changes occur. The pressure in smaller bubbles is greater than in larger bubbles, resulting in dissolution of the smaller bubbles into larger ones by diffusion of the gas (air). Also, with a difference in the density between the phases, gravitational and capillary forces cause a flow of the continuous liquid around the air bubbles, resulting in the air bubbles moving toward the top and the liquid flowing downward. This gradient can be stabilized with the adsorption of a foaming agent from the bulk solution.

Foams with a higher gas volume fraction are more stable because liquid drainage and creaming is delayed. Also, higher viscosities can delay the drainage and creaming activity. Arabic gum, methylcellulose, and similar hydrophilic materials of high molecular weight will tend to increase foam stability because of increased viscosity. In addition, temperature can affect stability by altering bulk viscosity. The use of macromolecules that orient at the surface can provide steric stabilization and hinder the coalescence of bubbles.

The assigned beyond-use dates for foams generally would be, in the absence of documented stability information, 30 days, according to Chapter <795>, Pharmaceutical Compounding—Nonsterile Preparations, of the *United States Pharmacopeia*.

Patient Counseling

Patient counseling topics can include storage, use, and disposal of foams. A patient should be instructed to protect the preparation from heat and generally to avoid refrigeration. The foam should be stored at room temperature and out of direct sunlight. For use, the area to be covered needs to be clean and dry. A patient should not apply an excess of foam, but only what is needed to cover the area appropriately. If the skin is intact, the foam can be rubbed in; if it is abraded, the foam should only be applied and not rubbed. A protective cover can be added as directed. The container should be stored away from the reach of children. An empty container should be disposed of in the trash. If the container is not used and is no longer needed, the contents should be discarded appropriately and the container rinsed and then discarded in the trash.

Sample Formulations

℞ Iodine Foam in Airspray Foam Pump

Iodine	1%	Active
Purified water	64.3%	Vehicle
Glycofurol	30%	Vehicle/Gel
Stearyl alcohol	1%	Thickener/Emulsifier
Sucrose stearate	1%	Thickener/Dispersant
Sodium lauryl sulfate	1%	Surfactant/Emulsifier
Cocamidopropyl betaine	0.5%	Emulsifier
Hydroxypropyl methylcellulose	0.8%	Thickener
Xanthan gum	0.4%	Thickener

1. Calculate the quantity of each ingredient required for the prescription.
2. Accurately weigh or measure each ingredient.
3. Dissolve the iodine in a mixture of glycofurol and stearyl alcohol, heating to about 60°C until homogenous.
4. Disperse the hydroxypropyl methylcellulose in one-third of the purified water that has been preheated to 80°C.
5. Add the sucrose stearate to the mixture in step 4, and mix well.
6. Using the remaining two-thirds of purified water at room temperature, add the xanthan gum, sodium lauryl sulfate, and cocamidopropyl betaine to the mixture in step 5, and mix continuously for 15 minutes with vigorous stirring.
7. Add the iodine mixture carefully to the aqueous mixture, and stir for an additional 5 minutes for complete homogeneity.
8. Cool the mixture to room temperature, place into bottles, and label.

℞ Foamable Carrier Formed by Whipping or Shaking

Propylene glycol	82%	Vehicle/Solvent
Laureth-4	2%	Emulsifier
Glyceryl stearate	2%	Emulsifier
Polyethylene glycol-100 stearate	2%	Emulsifier
Polyethylene glycol 4000	10%	Vehicle/Thickener
Hydroxypropyl cellulose	2%	Thickener

1. Calculate the quantity of each ingredient required for the prescription.
2. Accurately weigh or measure each ingredient.
3. Warm the propylene glycol to about 50°C, and dissolve all the ingredients.
4. Cool the solution to room temperature.
5. Agitate or whip the solution until it foams and the desired bubble size is obtained.
6. Package and label the product.

℞ Diclofenac Foam with Aerosol Propellants

Mineral oil	6%	Vehicle
Isopropyl myristate	6%	Emulsifier
Stearyl alcohol	1%	Emulsifier/Thickener
Xanthan gum	0.3%	Thickener
Methocel K100M	0.3%	Thickener
Tween 80	1%	Emulsifier
Myrj 49	3%	Emulsifier
Cocamidopropyl betaine	0.5%	Emulsifier
Diclofenac sodium	1%	Active
Methylparaben	200 mg	Preservative
Propylparaben	50 mg	Preservative
Propellant	8%	Propellant
Purified water	qs 100%	Vehicle

1. Calculate the quantity of each ingredient required for the prescription.
2. Accurately weigh or measure each ingredient.
3. Aqueous phase: Dissolve the gelling agent and surface-active agent in water with agitation. Heat the solution to 50°C–70°C. Add the water-soluble active ingredient with agitation.
4. Oil phase: Heat the mineral oil to the same temperature used in the aqueous phase, add the methylparaben and propylparaben, and mix well.
5. Add the warm oil phase to the warm aqueous phase with agitation, followed by homogenization.
6. Allow the mixture to cool to room temperature.
7. Add the mixture to an aerosol container together with the propellant, and seal.
8. Label the product.

℞ Minoxidil 50 mg/mL Topical Foam

Minoxidil	5 g	Active
Espumil Foam Base	qs 100 mL	Vehicle

1. Calculate the quantity of each ingredient required for the prescription.
2. Accurately weigh or measure each ingredient.
3. Weigh the required quantity of minoxidil, and bring final volume with Espumil Foam Base in a beaker.
4. Heat the solution to 50°C on a hotplate, stirring for approximately 10 minutes.
5. Transfer the contents to a plastic foam-activating bottle, and store at room temperature.
6. Label the product.

℞ Effervescent Foam Breakup Tablet

Sucrose	3 g	Sweetener/Vehicle
Citric acid	120 mg	Acidifier
Sodium bicarbonate	100 mg	Alkalizer
Mannitol	3 g	Sweetener/Vehicle
Polyethylene glycol 3350	1 g	Binder/Lubricant
Flavoring	qs	Flavoring

1. Calculate the quantity of each ingredient required for the prescription.
2. Accurately weigh or measure each ingredient.
3. Place the ingredients in a mortar, and mix well.
4. Place the required quantity of powder into molds, and set on sieve or other holder.
5. Heat the molds at 90°C for 10 minutes, remove to a refrigerator for 10 minutes, and then allow to cool to room temperature.
6. Package and label the product.

℞ Effervescent (Foaming) Metoclopramide and Aspirin Granules

Metoclopramide HCl	236 mg	Active
	(Equiv. to 200 mg base)	
Aspirin	6 g	Active
Citric acid (Hydrous)	49.8 g	Acidifier
Sodium bicarbonate	44 g	Alkalizer

1. Calculate the quantity of each ingredient required for the prescription.
2. Accurately weigh or measure each ingredient.
3. Thoroughly mix the powders.
4. Place the mixture in a flat-bottom glass container (Pyrex cake or similar), and spread out with a flat spatula.
5. Place the container in a 300°C oven, and monitor carefully.
6. When the citric acid begins to lose its water, the mass will stick together and the powder should be gently moved around to form granules.
7. After the water has been released and the powder formed into small granules, sieve through a No. 8- or No. 10-mesh sieve.
8. Cool the mixture to room temperature, and package in a tight container.
9. A 5-g measuring device can be used to measure the dose of granules.
10. Package and label the product.

(Note: When ready to administer the preparation, place the granules in a small glass of water where they will effervesce [foam]. When the effervescence slows down, the mixture can then be administered.)

℞ Drug *X* mg Mini Marshmallow

Drug	*x*	Active
Stevia	200 mg	Sweetener
Peppermint/wintergreen blend	qs	Flavor
Alcohol 95%	qs 100 mL	Solvent
Mini marshmallows	qs	Vehicle

1. Calculate the quantity of each ingredient required for the prescription.
2. Accurately weigh or measure each ingredient.
3. Dissolve the drug, stevia, and peppermint/wintergreen blend in sufficient alcohol to volume.
4. Prepare the solution so that the required amount of drug is in about 50–100 µL of solution.
5. Using a calibrated micropipette, deliver the required volume of drug solution to each mini marshmallow, and allow to air dry.
6. Package and label the product.

(Note: As an option, each mini marshmallow can be halved before administration.)

Chapter 21

Ointments, Creams, and Pastes

Topical Forms

Topical dosage forms have been used throughout human history; for instance, ointments are mentioned many times in the Bible. These dosage forms, which include salves, ointments, pastes, and compresses, are used to deliver a drug topically to the skin to treat various disorders.

Topically applied pharmaceuticals have three main functions: (1) to protect the injured area from the environment and permit the skin to rejuvenate; (2) to provide skin with hydration or to produce an emollient effect; and (3) to convey a medication to the skin for a specific effect, either topically or systemically (transdermals). If the dosage form is a semisolid, the volume of drug that penetrates the skin is determined by (1) the amount of pressure applied and the vigor with which the semisolid is rubbed, (2) the surface area covered, (3) the condition of the skin, (4) the base used, and (5) the use of occlusive dressings.

Transdermal Forms

Transdermal drug delivery involves the passage of therapeutic quantities of drug substances through the skin and into the general circulation for systemic effects. Numerous manufactured drug products (gels, creams, patches, ointments, etc.) are on the market and are routinely compounded using different technologies for enhancing the amount of drug delivered through the skin. Evidence of actual percutaneous drug absorption may be found through (1) measurable blood levels of the drug, (2) detectable excretion of the drug or its metabolites in the urine, and (3) clinical response of a patient to the therapy; not all three may necessarily occur in every situation. Transdermal drug delivery is considered ideal when the drug migrates through the skin to the underlying blood supply without buildup in the dermal layers.

Mechanisms of Transdermal Delivery

Percutaneous absorption of a drug generally results from direct penetration of the drug through the stratum corneum (SC), a 10- to 15-μm thick layer of flat, partially desiccated nonliving tissue. The SC is composed of approximately 40% protein (mainly keratin) and 40% water, with the balance being lipid, principally as triglycerides, free fatty acids, cholesterol, and phospholipids. The lipid content is concentrated in the extracellular phase of the SC and, to a large extent, forms the membrane surrounding the cells. Because a drug's major route of penetration is through the intercellular channels, the lipid component is an important determinant in the first step of absorption. Once through the SC, drug molecules may pass through the deeper epidermal tissues and into the dermis. When the drug reaches the vascularized dermal layer, it becomes available for absorption into the general circulation.

The SC, as keratinized tissue, behaves as a semipermeable artificial membrane, and drug molecules penetrate by passive diffusion. It is the major rate-limiting barrier to transdermal drug transport. Over most of the body, the SC has 15 to 25 layers of flattened corneocytes with an overall thickness of about 10 μm. The rate of drug movement across this layer generally depends on the drug's concentration and aqueous solubility and the oil–water partition coefficient between the SC and the vehicle. Substances with both aqueous and lipid solubility characteristics are good candidates for diffusion through the SC, epidermis, and dermis.

Factors Involved in Transdermal Delivery

Not all drug substances are suitable for transdermal delivery. Among the factors playing a part in percutaneous absorption are the physical and chemical properties of the drug, including its molecular weight, solubility, partition coefficient, dissociation constant (pK_a), the nature of the carrier vehicle, and the condition of the skin. Although general statements applicable to all possible combinations of drug, vehicle, and skin condition are difficult to draw, most research findings may be summarized as follows:

- Generally, the amount of drug absorbed per unit of surface area per time interval increases with an increase in the concentration of the drug in the dosage form.
- The larger the area of application, the larger is the quantity of drug absorbed.
- The drug should have a greater physicochemical attraction to the skin than to the formulation vehicle so that the drug will leave the vehicle in favor of the skin. Some solubility of the drug in both lipids and water is thought to be essential for effective percutaneous absorption. In essence, the aqueous solubility of a drug determines the concentration presented to the absorption site, and the partition coefficient influences the rate of transport across the absorption site. Drugs generally penetrate the skin better in their nonionized form. Nonpolar drugs tend to cross the cell barrier through the lipid-rich regions (transcellular route), whereas polar drugs favor transport between cells (intercellular route).
- Drugs with molecular weights of 100 to 800 and adequate lipid and aqueous solubility can permeate skin. The ideal molecular weight of a drug for transdermal drug delivery is believed to be 400 or less.
- Hydration of the skin generally favors percutaneous absorption. The dosage form often acts as an occlusive moisture barrier through which sweat cannot pass, thereby increasing skin hydration.
- Percutaneous absorption appears to be greater when the dosage form is applied to a site with a thin horny layer than with a thick one.
- Generally, the longer the medicated application is permitted to remain in contact with the skin, the greater is the total drug absorption.

Some drugs have an inherent capacity to permeate the skin without chemical enhancers. However, when this is not the case, chemical permeation enhancers may render an otherwise impenetrable substance useful in transdermal drug delivery. Penetration enhancers facilitate the absorption of drugs through the skin. Some of these ingredients have a direct effect on the permeability of the skin, whereas others augment percutaneous absorption by increasing the thermodynamic activity of the penetrant, thus creating a greater concentration gradient across the skin. A chemical skin penetration enhancer increases skin permeability by reversibly altering the physicochemical nature of the SC to reduce its diffusional resistance. Among the alterations are increased hydration of the SC or a change in the structure of the lipids and lipoproteins in the intercellular channels through solvent action or denaturation, or both.

Definitions and Types

Ointments are semisolid preparations that are applied externally to the skin or mucous membranes. Ointments soften or melt at body temperature; they should spread easily and should not be gritty.

Creams are opaque, soft solids or thick liquids for external application. Creams consist of medications dissolved or suspended in water-soluble or vanishing cream bases and can be either a water-in-oil (w/o) or an oil-in-water (o/w) type of emulsion. The term *cream* is most frequently applied to soft, cosmetically acceptable types of preparations.

Pastes are thick, stiff ointments that ordinarily do not flow at body temperature and thus protectively coat the areas to which they are applied. They usually contain at least 20% solids.

Historical Use

The Greek word *miron* and the Latin word *unguentum* were combined to form the modern word *ointment*. Early ointments were primarily oils that were used as anointing preparations. Changes in early ointment preparations resulted in the development of pastes (preparations with a high content of solids), cerates (preparations with a high content of waxes), and creams (emulsified ointments).

Applications

The decision to use an ointment, a paste, a cream, or a lotion (emulsion) depends not only on how much skin penetration of the medication is desired, but also on the characteristics of the skin to which the product is being applied. For example, ointments (oleaginous bases) are generally used on dry, scaly lesions because their emollient properties will aid in rehydrating the skin. They also stay on the skin longer. Ointments are formulated as topical, rectal, and ophthalmic preparations. Pastes are topical preparations that are usually applied to an area that requires protection. Creams are typically applied to moist, weeping lesions because they have a drying effect in that the lesions' fluids are miscible with the aqueous external phase of creams. Creams are formulated as topical, rectal, and vaginal preparations. Because of their lubricating effect, lotions are generally applied to intertriginous areas, that is, areas where the skin rubs together, such as between the fingers, between the thighs, or under the arms. Because of these considerations, a pharmacist should not substitute one of these dosage forms for another without the consent of the prescriber.

Topical ointment bases have traditionally been classified in two different ways: by the degree of skin penetration (Table 21-1) and by the relationship of water to the composition of the base (Table 21-2). Transdermals are a new category of topically applied, penetrating ointments, creams, and gels.

TABLE 21-1 Ointment Bases Classified by Skin Penetration

Base Type	Skin Penetration?	Example Bases
Epidermic[a]	None or very little	Oleaginous
Endodermic[b]	Into the dermis	Absorption
Diadermic[c]	Into and through the skin	Emulsion, water soluble

[a]Epidermic refers to the external layer of the skin, or epidermis.
[b]Endodermic refers to the internal layer of the skin, or dermis.
[c]Diadermic refers to going through the skin.

TABLE 21-2 Ointment Bases Classified in Relation to Water

Base Type	Characteristics	Examples
Oleaginous	Insoluble in water	White petrolatum
	Not water washable	White ointment
	Will not absorb water	
	Emollient	
	Occlusive	
	Greasy	
Absorption	Insoluble in water	Hydrophilic petrolatum
	Not water washable	Aquabase
	Anhydrous	Aquaphor
	Can absorb water	
	Emollient	
	Occlusive	
	Greasy	
W/O emulsion	Insoluble in water	Cold cream
	Not water washable	Lanolin, hydrous
	Will absorb water	Hydrocream
	Contains water	Eucerin
	Emollient	Nivea
	Occlusive	
	Greasy	
O/W emulsion	Insoluble in water	Hydrophilic ointment
	Water washable	Dermabase
	Will absorb water	Velvachol
	Contains water	Unibase
	Nonocclusive	
	Nongreasy	
Water soluble	Water soluble	Polyethylene glycol ointment
	Water washable	
	Will absorb water	
	Anhydrous or hydrous	
	Nonocclusive	
	Nongreasy	

Composition

In addition to the active drug, ingredients in topical preparations can include stiffeners, oleaginous components, aqueous components, emulsifying agents, humectants, preservatives, penetration enhancers, and antioxidants. Some of these ingredients are discussed in greater detail in the "Preparation" and "Physicochemical Considerations" sections later in this chapter.

Stiffeners generally include waxes that have high melting points (e.g., white wax). The waxes blend into oleaginous bases to enhance the viscosity of a preparation.

Humectants, such as glycerin, propylene glycol, or polyethylene glycol (PEG) 300, can be added to a preparation to decrease the evaporation rate of water from the preparation, especially just after its application to the skin.

Penetration (absorption) enhancers are agents that can interact sufficiently with the active drug and the SC to increase the rate of penetration of the drug through the skin.

Antioxidants, such as butylated hydroxytoluene, are sometimes required to delay the rate of rancidification of selected bases.

Preparation

Most of the techniques discussed here are directed toward incorporating ingredients into commercially prepared bases. If a base must be extemporaneously prepared from individual ingredients, the principles discussed in Chapter 19 apply in addition to those discussed in this chapter.

Manual Methods of Preparation

Manual methods of ointment preparation primarily involve using a pill tile and spatula or a mortar and pestle. Ointment pads and various hard, clean surfaces have also been used. Ointment pads, however, can absorb moisture and tear unless one works quickly. The surface used must be clean and nonshedding and should provide for ease of mixing. The advantage of a pill tile is its use for both particle size reduction and mixing of the ointment. Pill tiles are easy to clean and should allow no carryover of materials from one preparation to the next. In some situations, mixing in a plastic bag is convenient and less messy.

Mechanical Methods of Preparation

To prepare large quantities of ointments, pharmacists may want to invest in mixers, which range from hand-held propeller types to kitchen mixers with paddles or blades. In fact, if regular supply sources do not have the type of equipment desired, a pharmacist may find it at gourmet kitchen shops, which are excellent sources of unusual equipment. Electronic mortars and pestles (the Unguator) are gaining widespread acceptance and offer the advantage of mixing and dispensing in the same container.

Preparation of Oleaginous Bases

White petrolatum and white ointment are examples of oleaginous bases. Official *United States Pharmacopeia/National Formulary (USP/NF)* ointment bases are shown in Table 21-3. An example of an extemporaneously prepared prescription using an oleaginous base is 5% sulfur in white petrolatum.

The preparation of an oleaginous-based ointment is rather simple. After obtaining the desired quantities of the individual ingredients, a pharmacist finely pulverizes the powder on a pill tile with a spatula. When incorporating insoluble powders by using a levigating agent,

TABLE 21-3 Characteristics and Packaging of Official USP/NF Ointment Bases

Vehicle	Melting Point (°C)	Specific Gravity	Container
Diethylene glycol monoethyl ether	—	0.991	T
Lanolin	38–44	0.932–0.945[a]	W
Ointment, hydrophilic	—	—	T
Ointment, white	—	—	W
Ointment, yellow	—	—	W
Polyethylene glycol ointment	—	—	W
Petrolatum	38–60	0.815–0.880[b]	W
Petrolatum, hydrophilic	—	—	W
Petrolatum, white	38–60	0.815–0.880[b]	W
Rose water ointment	—	—	T, LR
Squalane	—	0.807–0.810	T
Vegetable oil, hydrogenated, type II	20–50	—	T

— = Not available.
[a]At 15°C.
[b]At 60°C.

the pharmacist should follow the technique of geometric dilution to ensure that the active ingredient is thoroughly mixed with the vehicle. For example, a few drops of mineral oil can be used to levigate sulfur before it is mixed with white petrolatum. The sulfur–mineral oil mixture would be mixed with an equal quantity of white petrolatum. Then more white petrolatum equal in quantity to the new mixture would be added, and the process repeated until all of the white petrolatum has been added. A small quantity of the melted base can also be used as a levigating agent. Examples of levigating agents are shown in Table 21-4.

Heat should be used in preparing a base containing ingredients with high melting points. Generally, a water bath or direct heat is used. Water baths are used for low-temperature applications, whereas direct heat is used for preparations that require higher temperatures. When using direct heat (a hot plate), a pharmacist must be careful not to scorch the preparation. Microwaves can be used either to heat the formulation directly or to heat the water for preparing a water bath. Using a microwave with a carousel will minimize the occurrence of hot spots—areas with high temperatures caused by uneven heating. When heat is used, materials with the highest melting points are placed in a container that has been set on the heat source. The container is heated until the materials melt. The rest of the ingredients are then added according to their decreasing melting points, beginning with the highest and moving

TABLE 21-4 Levigating Agents Used in Preparing Ointments

Agent	Specific Gravity
Aqueous Systems and O/W Dispersions	
Glycerin	1.25
Polyethylene glycol 400	1.13
Propylene glycol	1.04
Oleaginous Systems and W/O Dispersions	
Castor oil	0.96
Cottonseed oil	0.92
Mineral oil, heavy	0.88
Mineral oil, light	0.85
Tween 80	—

— = Not available.

downward. The product is thoroughly mixed and then cooled. During the cooling process, the product is stirred occasionally; however, cooling should not be too rapid because the product can become lumpy. When cool, the product is packaged and labeled.

Oleaginous bases are often used to prepare pastes. Heat makes the preparation process easier by allowing a high percentage of powders to be introduced into the base. The product must be stirred thoroughly during the cooling process, however, to prevent the solids from settling.

Stiffening Agents

Many pharmaceutical preparations require adjustment of the viscosity, or stiffness, to produce the characteristics that can make them useful and acceptable to patients. Ointments, creams (emulsions), medication sticks, pastes, suppositories, and other dosage forms can require stiffening agents. Generally, stiffening agents have higher melting points (usually greater than about 50°C but less than about 100°C) and, when blended with materials with lower melting points, will raise the lower melting point materials to within an acceptable range for patient use. Excessive quantities, however, will result in a product that will not melt or soften appropriately and is stiff or grainy.

The term *stiffening agents* is ordinarily applied to oleaginous ingredients, such as those in Table 21-5. Their incorporation into dosage forms usually involves the use of heat. Generally, a pharmacist should have the different phases of a product heated to approximately the same temperature before combining them to prevent premature solidification, which might occur if, for example, a melt of a wax is poured into a cool aqueous mixture. When combining materials with different melting points, melting the material with the highest melting point first and then adding the lower melting point materials as the temperature is lowered is often best. This approach eliminates the need to bring all materials up to the melting point of the highest ingredient. Stiffening agents for ointments are listed in Table 21-5.

Preparation of Absorption Bases

If a w/o emulsifying agent is added to an oleaginous base, an absorption base is formed. Examples of these bases include hydrophilic petrolatum, Aquabase, and Aquaphor. Examples of prescriptions include 1% hydrocortisone incorporated into Aquabase and 3% crude coal tar/3% polysorbate 80 in Aquabase.

Ointments using an absorption base can be prepared by using the same techniques as for an oleaginous base, that is, incorporation directly into the base or with the use of heat. Other options, however, depend on the material(s) to be incorporated.

Levigation can be used to incorporate a water-insoluble powder. For absorption bases, such as Aquabase or Aquaphor, the choice of the levigating agent depends on where the drug should be, that is, in the external phase or in the internal phase if water is going to be added to the base. In the latter case, alcohol, glycerin, propylene glycol, or water can generally be used and should be taken up into the internal phase of the finished product. Mineral oil can be used if the ingredient should stay in the continuous phase of the product.

Before a water-soluble ingredient is added, it should be dissolved in a small quantity of water. The water can then be incorporated into the base by using either a pill tile and spatula or a mortar and pestle. If large quantities of water or an aqueous solution are to be incorporated, using heat can be the best approach. Adding an additional emulsifying agent and a preservative may be necessary. The preservative would be needed because water will usually support microbial growth. Another alternative would be to assign a short expiration date, such as 2 weeks. The base can be melted by using a water bath, after which the aqueous phase is added by stirring. The final product should be stirred continuously during cooling.

TABLE 21-5 Physical Properties of USP/NF Stiffening Agents

Substance	Melting Range (°C)	Flashpoint Range (°C)	Density (g/mL)	Solubility				
				Water	Alcohol	Chloroform	Ether	Fixed Oils
Castor oil, hydrogenated	85–88	316	1.023	IS	Sol	Sol		
Cetostearyl alcohol	48–55	150	0.820	PrIn	FS		Sol	
Cetyl alcohol	46–52		0.907	PrIn	PrIn	Sol	Sol	Misc
Cetyl esters wax	43–47		0.830	PrIn	PrIn	Sol		Sol
Hard fat	27–44			PrIn	SlS	FS	FS	
Paraffin				IS	IS	FS	FS	FS
Synthetic paraffin						SlS		
Stearyl alcohol	55–60	191	0.812	PrIn	Sol	Sol	Sol	Sol
Wax, emulsifying	50–54	>55	0.940	IS	Sol	FS	FS	
Wax, white	62–65	245–258	0.955	PrIn	SpS	Sol	FS	Sol
Wax, yellow	62–65	245–258	0.955	PrIn	SpS	Sol	FS	Sol

Preparation of W/O Emulsion Bases

Water-in-oil emulsion bases can be prepared by adding water to an absorption base. Commercial preparations are also available, including Eucerin, Hydrocream, Nivea, and cold cream. An example of an extemporaneous preparation is 2% miconazole in Hydrocream.

Oils and insoluble powders can be incorporated directly by using a pill tile and spatula or a mortar and pestle. A levigating agent may be needed if large amounts of insoluble powders are required. If Hydrocream or Eucerin is used as the base, the levigating agent should be miscible with the oil phase (i.e., mineral oil). In many of the w/o emulsion bases, however, sufficient surfactant is available to further emulsify a reasonable quantity of an aqueous solution of a drug, which can be incorporated by using a pill tile with a spatula or a mortar and pestle or using gentle heat from a water bath. When using heat, a pharmacist should ensure that the preparation is not held at a high temperature for too long, because a loss of water can occur. This loss results in a thicker ointment or cream.

Preparation of O/W Emulsion Bases

Oil-in-water emulsion bases are usually elegant preparations and are known as "vanishing cream" preparations because they disappear, or vanish, on application. These bases include Dermabase, Velvachol, and hydrophilic ointment USP (United States Pharmacopeia). Various concentrations of retinoic acid, urea, or triamcinolone have been included in these bases as extemporaneous preparations.

Insoluble powders and aqueous solutions can be incorporated by using a pill tile and spatula or a mortar and pestle. Water-soluble materials can be added by dissolving the powder in a small quantity of water and incorporating the solution into the base. A small quantity of an oil can be directly incorporated into the base, because there is usually excess emulsifying agent. If a larger amount of an oil is required, adding a little o/w surfactant to help the oil disperse uniformly throughout the vehicle may be necessary.

If an o/w emulsion base, such as Dermabase or Velvachol, is used, the levigating agent should be alcohol, glycerin, PEG 300 or 400, propylene glycol, water, or some liquid that is miscible with water.

If heat is used to incorporate an ingredient into an o/w vehicle, a pharmacist must work quickly because water can be lost rather rapidly from the product. This loss could make the product stiff and waxy, thereby causing it to lose its elegant character.

To prevent an o/w emulsion from drying too rapidly on the skin, a pharmacist can add a humectant such as glycerin, PEG 300 or 400, propylene glycol, or 70% sorbitol to the formulation in a concentration of about 2% to 5%.

Preparation of Water-Soluble Bases

PEG 400 (600 g) and PEG 3350 (400 g) are examples of water-soluble bases. Incorporating 20% benzocaine into any of these bases yields a satisfying ointment that can be easily removed by washing. Water-soluble ingredients can be dissolved in a small quantity of water and mixed with the base by using a pill tile and spatula or a mortar and pestle. Insoluble powders can be levigated with a small quantity of glycerin, PEG 300, or propylene glycol and then mixed with the base. To enhance stability, a pharmacist should mix an intermediate solvent such as glycerin or propylene glycol with oils before they are incorporated into a water-soluble base. If large quantities of water or aqueous solutions are to be added, the use of gentle heat or a water bath to prepare the product can be preferable. For additional suggestions on preparing these dosage forms, see Box 21-1.

BOX 21-1 Hints for Compounding Ointments, Creams, and Pastes

Suggestions for compounding ointments, creams, and pastes are as follows:

Ointments
- Two or more ointments can be combined by mixing them in a plastic bag.
- Ointments can be transferred directly from plastic bags into tubes by cutting one corner of the plastic bag and squeezing the contents into the ointment tube or jar. This method makes cleanup very easy.
- A few drops of mineral oil or other suitable solvent can enhance the workability of drugs that build up electrostatic forces, such as sulfur.
- Volatile solvents should not be used in levigating powders, because the solvent will evaporate and leave crystals of drug.
- When oil and aqueous phases are mixed together, heating the aqueous phase a few degrees higher than the oil phase before mixing is helpful. The aqueous phase tends to cool faster than the oil phase.
- Ointments should be cooled to just a few degrees above solidification before they are poured into tubes or jars. This cooling will minimize layering of the ointment in the packaging.
- Heat softens ointments and makes filling jars and tubes easier. Heating must be done cautiously to prevent stratification of the ingredients.
- When a base is being prepared, the ingredient with the highest melting point should be melted first, and then the heat should be gradually reduced. The remaining ingredients should be added in the order of the highest to lowest melting point until a uniform mixture is obtained. This process will enhance the stability of the final product, because it ensures that the ingredients are exposed to the lowest possible temperature during preparation.
- If a water-containing base is used and the drug is water soluble, the drug should be dissolved in a minimum quantity of water before incorporating it into the base.

Creams
- Whether an emulsion is o/w or w/o can be determined by placing a drop of the emulsion on the surface of water. If the drop spreads out, it is the o/w type because the external phase of the emulsion is miscible or continuous with water. If the emulsion remains in a ball, it is probably the w/o type and immiscible.
- If no active drugs are present, creams can be softened by heating in a microwave for a short time at a low power setting.
- Adding a humectant, such as glycerin, PEG 300 or 400, propylene glycol, or sorbitol 70% to a cream will minimize evaporation. These humectants can be added in a 2% to 5% concentration.
- Use of low heat in preparing creams will minimize evaporation of water.
- Hand-held homogenizers can aid in preparing emulsions.
- Generally, the smaller the globule size, the more stable will be the emulsion.
- Before volatile oils are added, cooling the preparation is best. Temperatures of less than 78°C work well with many bases. If alcoholic solutions of flavors are to be added, the preparation should be cooled below the boiling point of alcohol before their addition.
- The quantity of surfactant required to prepare a good emulsion is generally about 0.5% to 5% of the total volume.

(continued)

BOX 21-1 Hints for Compounding Ointments, Creams, and Pastes *(Continued)*

- Lotions can often be prepared from creams (o/w emulsions) by diluting the cream with water or an aromatic water such as rose water. To do this successfully, a pharmacist usually must add the water slowly while stirring continuously. However, this process will also dilute the preservative, which could lead to bacterial growth. Therefore, a short beyond-use date should be assigned to the preparation.

Pastes
- Levigating agents are generally not used in preparing pastes that are characterized by relatively high percentages of solids. The easiest method of preparing pastes involves the fusion technique (heat). Heat improves the workability of pastes.
- Products prepared by using fusion should be cooled before they are placed in tubes or jars. If poured while hot, they tend to separate on cooling. They should be cooled to the temperature at which they are viscous fluids and then poured into containers.
- If a product is too stiff and difficult to apply, a pharmacist should decrease the concentration of the waxy components.

General Considerations
- Insoluble materials need to be in a very fine state of subdivision before incorporation into the base or vehicle.
- Levigating agents must be compatible with the vehicle used.
- When insoluble powders are incorporated by using a levigating agent, the technique of geometric dilution should be used to ensure thorough mixing of the active ingredient with the vehicle.
- When incorporating soluble powders, a pharmacist should use solvents that have low vapor pressure (e.g., water, glycerin, and propylene glycol). Generally, volatile solvents should not be used, especially in oleaginous bases, because the solvent may evaporate and the drug may, in turn, be crystallized out in the base and cause irritation on application to the skin.
- Before adding volatile ingredients, whether flavorings or active drugs, the product should be slightly cooled. The melt should still be fluid, but not hot, to allow uniform mixing without evaporative loss of ingredients. Temperatures less than 78°C work well with many bases, but lower temperatures would be required if alcohol and volatile materials were present.
- When working with aqueous systems, a pharmacist should use heat for as short a time and at as low a temperature as feasible. This will minimize the quantity of water lost through evaporation.
- If a product is too stiff and difficult to apply, a pharmacist should try decreasing the concentration of the waxy components.
- Generally, drugs can be incorporated into ointments, creams, and pastes easily on a pill tile with a spatula. If large quantities of solids are to be incorporated, using heat to melt the base before incorporating the drug may be advisable.
- For maximum stability, the product should be kept anhydrous, if possible.
- Unless otherwise instructed, when a pharmacist is adding several powders to a topical vehicle, adding the powders one at a time with thorough mixing after each addition is best. This action ensures maximum stability and uniformity of the final product.

Physicochemical Considerations

Problems involved in ointment preparation include drug degradation, discoloration, separation of ointment components, and development of a rancid odor. To check for potential incompatibilities, a pharmacist should refer to appropriate information sources. Because potent products are now being used topically, preparing an ineffective product can be expensive and wasteful.

One potential problem involves Plastibase (Squibb). In compounding a preparation containing this product, a pharmacist should not apply heat, because Plastibase will not regain its viscosity upon cooling. Plastibase is a shock-cooled product consisting of mineral oil gelled with polyethylene.

Penetration Enhancers

Absorption enhancers facilitate the absorption of drugs through the skin. These excipients have attracted more attention in the general scientific literature as the transdermal route of administration has grown popular. Some of these materials appear to have a direct effect on the permeability of the skin, whereas others augment percutaneous absorption by increasing the thermodynamic activity of the penetrant, thus creating a greater concentration gradient across the skin. Absorption enhancers that have a direct effect can be either common or not-so-common chemicals, including solvents, surfactants, and chemicals such as urea and N,N-diethyl-m-toluamide.

More than 275 chemical compounds have been cited in the literature as skin penetration enhancers. The selection of a permeation enhancer for pharmaceuticals should be based not only on its efficacy in enhancing skin permeation, but also on its dermal toxicity (low) and its physicochemical and biologic compatibility with the system's other components. Chemical penetration enhancers include acetone, dimethylacetamide, dimethylformamide, dimethyl sulfoxide, ethanol, laurocapram (Azone), oleic acid, polyethylene glycol, polysorbates, propylene glycol, sodium lauryl sulfate, and others. See Table 21-6 for examples of penetration enhancers.

Because of its occlusive nature, water is the most prevalent absorption enhancer, even in anhydrous systems. The classic absorption enhancer is dimethyl sulfoxide. Other solvents, such as laurocapram (Azone), have been shown to be quite effective, even in concentrations below 5%, because they are retained in the SC for a period of time, which prolongs their effect. Surfactants also function as absorption enhancers, but their usefulness is limited because they can cause irritation. Examples of absorption enhancers used in ointments and creams are shown in Table 21-6.

Water Repellents

Silicon-containing personal care products were introduced in 1950 with Revlon's Silicare. The use of silicone in topical preparations continues to expand, in part because of the safety benefits and positive performance characteristics. The silicones lubricate without feeling oily, reduce stickiness and the tacky sensation associated with many lotions and creams, provide water-repelling characteristics, and enhance and stabilize foams. A list of official water-repelling agents is shown in Table 21-7.

Preservation

Unless water is present in the product, incorporating a preservative into an ointment is usually unnecessary. If the product does contain water, however, as in the case of emulsion bases, a preservative normally is needed. Selecting a preservative and determining the

TABLE 21-6 Examples of Absorption-Enhancing Agents

Water

Alcohols: benzyl alcohol, butanol, 2-butanol, decanol, ethanol, hexanol, methanol, nonanol, octanol, pentanol, 2-pentanol, propanol

Fatty alcohols: caprylic, cetyl, decyl, lauryl, 2-lauryl, linolenyl, linoleyl, myristyl, oleyl, stearyl

Fatty acids: capric, caproic, caprylic, heptanoic, isosteric, isovaleric, lauric, myristic, neodecanoic, neoheptanoic, neononanoic, neopentanoic, oleic, pelagonic, stearic, trimethylhexanoic, valeric

Fatty acid esters, aliphatic: isopropyl myristate, isopropyl *n*-butyrate, isopropyl *n*-decanoate, isopropyl *n*-hexanoate, isopropyl palmitate, octyldodecyl myristate

Alkyl: butyl acetate, diethyl sebacate, ethyl acetate, ethyl oleate, methyl acetate, methyl propionate, methyl valerate

Polyols: butanediol, diethylene glycol, dipropylene glycol, ethylene glycol, glycerol, hexanetriol, pentanediol, polyethylene glycol, propanediol, propylene glycol, triethylene glycol

Alkyl methyl sulfoxides: decylmethyl sulfoxide, dimethyl sulfoxide, tetradecyl methyl sulfoxide

Pyrrolidones: *N*-(2-hydroxyethyl) pyrrolidone, *N*-methyl-2-pyrrolidone, 2-pyrrolidone

Anionic surfactants: docusate sodium, sodium laurate, sodium lauryl sulfate

Cationic surfactants: benzalkonium chloride, cetylpyridinium chloride, quaternary ammonium salts

Amphoteric surfactants: alkylbetamines, cephalins, lecithins

Nonionic surfactants: diglycerides, monoglycerides, triglycerides; poloxamers; Miglyol; Spans; Tweens

Bile salts: sodium cholate; sodium salts of taurocholic, desoxycholic, glycolic acids

Organic acids: citric acid, salicylic acid, succinic acid

Amides: diethanolamide, diethyltoluamide, dimethylacetamide, dimethyldecamide, dimethyl-formamide, dimethyloctamide, triethanolamide, urea

TABLE 21-7 Characteristics of Official USP/NF Silicones[a]

Silicone	Nominal Viscosity (centistoke)	Specific Gravity	Refractive Index
Cyclomethicone NF	—	—	—
Dimethicone	20	0.946–0.954	1.3980–1.4020
	100	0.962–0.970	1.4005–1.4045
	200	0.964–0.972	1.4013–1.4053
	350	0.965–0.973	1.4013–1.4053
	500	0.967–0.975	1.4013–1.4053
	1000	0.967–0.975	1.4013–1.4053
	12,500	—	1.4015–1.4055
	30,000	0.969–0.977	1.4010–1.4100
Silicone USP	575	0.967	1.402

— = Not available.
[a]All require tightly closed containers.

required concentration can be difficult. Chapter 19 of this book provides additional information on preserving this type of product.

Commercial Bases Used in Compounding

There are many commercially available bases that can be used in compounding; in fact, they are too numerous to mention here but can easily be found.[1] These bases include those for general topical and transdermal use, specialty bases for pain management, bases for hormone replacement therapy, and so on. Once a compounding pharmacist selects a satisfactory base and becomes familiar with its characteristics, the pharmacist is generally wise to continue using it instead of constantly trying something new with unknown clinical effects related to drug release, stability, and so on.

When selecting a base, a pharmacist must be aware of its composition in case of a patient's allergies and so on. Also, the pharmacist must evaluate both the physicochemical and the clinical characteristics of the base and its compatibility with the active drugs that are to be incorporated.

Quality Control

Quality control involves checking the final preparation for the following characteristics: final weight, visual appearance, color, odor, viscosity, pH, homogeneity and phase separation, particle size distribution, and texture. A pharmacist should document the observations as a preparation record.

Packaging, Storage, and Labeling

Ointments can generally be packaged in tubes and jars. Creams can be packaged in tubes and jars and in syringes, applicators, and pump dispensers. Because of their high viscosity, pastes are generally dispensed in jars. Minimizing the headspace in a container is best for decreasing both the loss of water and the tendency toward rancidity. Pump dispensers, tubes, syringes, push-button plastic jars, and applicators are generally preferable to standard jars because the latter tend to become contaminated easily. Figure 21-1 shows some of the devices commonly used to package these dosage forms.

Ointments should generally be kept at room temperature and away from excessive heat. Labeling should be appropriate for the mode of administration.

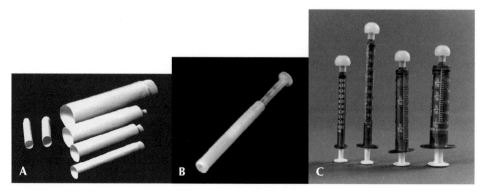

FIGURE 21-1 Packaging devices for ointments and creams. A: collapsible plastic ointment tubes; B: calibrated vaginal cream applicator; C: syringes with tip caps.

Stability

Ointments are relatively stable, especially if they are in an oleaginous, anhydrous absorption base or an anhydrous, water-soluble base. If water is present, as in the emulsion bases, the product is often less stable. Both physical stability (appearance, feel, odor, and color) and chemical stability (the active drug and the base ingredients) must be considered. Because the base ingredients are relatively stable, the stability of the active drug is a major determinant of the product's overall stability. In projecting a beyond-use date, one can usually look at commercial products containing the active drug to find a reasonable approximation. Being conservative in establishing the beyond-use date for an extemporaneous preparation is always best, especially if water is present, because water supports microbial growth. Usually, only a 30-day supply should be dispensed if the preparation contains water and lacks a preservative.

Ointments are best packaged in tubes or in syringes, if feasible. Such packaging leaves minimal space for air, and the product can be kept clean during administration. Ointment jars, although widely used, expose the preparation to air when opened and to microbial contamination, particularly when ointment is removed with the fingers. One way to lessen contamination is to use an implement similar to a tongue depressor to remove the required quantity of ointment from a jar for application. Pharmacies that prepare large quantities of ointments often use plastic tubes and a tube sealer.

To determine the stability of an ointment, a pharmacist should observe such physical attributes as changes in consistency and separation of a liquid, formation of granules or grittiness, and drying. Creams should be observed for emulsion breakage, crystal growth, shrinkage resulting from water loss, and gross microbial contamination. Ointments and emulsions are susceptible to chemical degradation, especially when water is present. Information on chemical stability can be obtained from the literature or from other appropriate sources. Beyond-use dates for topical formulations are no later than 30 days for products prepared from ingredients in solid form. These dates can be extended if valid scientific information is available to support the stability of the product, as discussed in Chapter 6 of this book. If a manufactured product is used to prepare nonaqueous liquids or anhydrous preparations, the beyond-use date is 25% of the time remaining on the product's expiration date or 6 months, whichever is earlier. If the product is prepared from United States Pharmacopeia or National Formulary grade substances, a beyond-use date of 6 months is appropriate unless evidence is available to support other dating.

Patient Counseling

Counseling about the proper application of ointments, creams, and pastes depends on the dosage form, active ingredients, and desired therapeutic outcomes. Usually, only a thin film of an ointment or a cream should be applied. Unless otherwise indicated, a patient removes a sufficient quantity from the container, applies it, and gently rubs it into the affected area. Patients should be instructed not to wash the area for a few hours so the drug will have sufficient time to take effect. Pastes often are placed on an area but not rubbed in, because of their viscosity. Pastes are usually used for a protectant effect and should not be removed until indicated. Creams (o/w) can be removed relatively easily by using warm water and, if necessary, soap. Removal of ointments and pastes requires warm water, soap, and some mechanical action. If the area is covered (e.g., by clothing), use of a protective pad to prevent the preparation from being removed by the clothing may be advisable. Usually, continuing use of the preparation for a short while after the symptom or injury has been resolved is best. Unless otherwise indicated, ointments, creams, and pastes should be stored at room temperature away from children, heat, and direct sunlight.

BOX 21-2 Advantages of Transdermal Drug Delivery

Transdermal drug delivery has the following advantages:

- Administration avoids gastrointestinal drug absorption difficulties caused by gastrointestinal pH; enzymatic activity; and drug interactions with food, drink, and other orally administered drugs.
- Delivery provides a substitute for oral administration of medication when that route is unsuitable, as with vomiting and diarrhea.
- Administration avoids the *first-pass effect,* that is, the initial pass of a drug substance through the systemic and portal circulation following gastrointestinal absorption, possibly avoiding the deactivation by digestive and liver enzymes.
- Delivery is noninvasive, avoiding the inconvenience of parenteral therapy.
- Extended therapy is provided with a single application, improving compliance over other dosage forms requiring more frequent dose administration.
- Activity of drugs having a short half-life is extended through the reservoir of drug in the therapeutic delivery system and its controlled release.
- Drug therapy may be terminated rapidly by removal of the application from the surface of the skin.

BOX 21-3 Disadvantages of Transdermal Drug Delivery

The disadvantages of transdermal drug delivery are as follows:

- Only relatively potent drugs are suitable candidates for transdermal drug delivery because of the natural limits of drug entry imposed by the skin's impermeability.
- Some patients develop contact dermatitis at the site of application from one or more of the system components, necessitating discontinuation.

Transdermal delivery has numerous advantages, as shown in Box 21-2, as well as some disadvantages, as shown in Box 21-3. In addition, a number of discussion and counseling points for patients with regard to transdermals are shown in Box 21-4.

BOX 21-4 What a Patient Needs to Know

A patient needs to know the following:

- Percutaneous absorption may vary with the site of application. The patient should be advised of the importance of using the recommended site and rotating locations within that site. Rotating locations is important to allow the skin to regain its normal permeability after being occluded and to prevent skin irritation. Skin sites may be reused after 1 week.
- Application should be to clean, dry skin and not to oily, irritated, inflamed, broken, or callused skin.

(continued)

BOX 21-4 What a Patient Needs to Know (Continued)

- Use of skin lotion should be avoided at the application site, because lotions affect skin hydration and can alter the partition coefficient between the drug and the skin.
- The drug should be placed at a site that will not subject it to being rubbed off by clothing or movement (as the belt line) or onto another person or pet.
- The patient or caregiver should be instructed to cleanse the hands thoroughly before and after applying the drug. Care should be taken not to rub the eyes or touch the mouth during handling of the system.
- If the patient exhibits sensitivity or intolerance to the drug or if undue skin irritation results, the patient should seek reevaluation.
- For gels, the patient should be counseled about the proper application of the gel, the way to handle and store the package, and the need to keep the package tightly closed.
- For creams and ointments, counseling for proper application may differ depending on the dosage form, active ingredients, and desired therapeutic outcomes.
- Generally, only a thin film of a preparation is required. A sufficient quantity is removed from the container, applied, and then gently rubbed into the area, unless otherwise indicated.
- A glove can be worn during application. Otherwise, hands must be washed before and after the application to remove any medication from the hands.
- The patient should be instructed not to wash the area for a few hours in order for the drug to have sufficient time to have an effect. If the area is covered by clothing, for example, using a protective pad over the area to prevent the preparation from being removed by the clothing may be advisable.
- Usually, continuing use of the preparation for a short while after resolution of the symptoms or injury is best, depending on the specific situation.

Sample Formulations

Bases

 White Ointment

White wax	50 g	Base/Thickener
White petrolatum	950 g	Base

1. Calculate the required quantity of each ingredient for the total amount to be prepared.
2. Accurately weigh or measure each ingredient.
3. Put the white wax in a suitable container, and melt the wax, using a water bath.
4. Add the white petrolatum, and mix until uniform.
5. Cool the mixture, package, and label.

Hydrophilic Petrolatum

Cholesterol	30 g	Emulsifier
Stearyl alcohol	30 g	Thickener/Emulsifier
White wax	80 g	Thickener
White petrolatum	860 g	Base

1. Calculate the required quantity of each ingredient for the total amount to be prepared.
2. Accurately weigh or measure each ingredient.
3. Place the stearyl alcohol, white wax, and white petrolatum in a suitable container, and melt the ingredients, using a water bath.
4. Add the cholesterol, and stir until the mixture is blended completely.
5. Remove the mixture from the bath, and stir until congealed.
6. Package and label the product.

Cold Cream

Cetyl esters wax	125 g	Emulsifier
White wax	120 g	Thickener
Mineral oil	560 g	Base
Sodium borate	5 g	Emulsifier
Purified water	190 mL	Base

1. Calculate the required quantity of each ingredient for the total amount to be prepared.
2. Accurately weigh or measure each ingredient.
3. Reduce the cetyl esters wax and the white wax to small pieces, and melt the pieces, using a water bath.
4. Add the mineral oil, and continue heating the mixture until it reaches 70°C.
5. Dissolve the sodium borate in the purified water, which has been warmed to 70°C. Add the warm mixture gradually to the melted oleaginous mixture.
6. Remove the mixture from the heat, and stir rapidly and continuously until the mixture has congealed.
7. Package and label the product.

Hydrophilic Ointment

Methylparaben	0.25 g	Preservative
Propylparaben	0.15 g	Preservative
Sodium lauryl sulfate	10 g	Surfactant/Emulsifier
Propylene glycol	120 g	Humectant
Stearyl alcohol	250 g	Thickener/Emulsifier
White petrolatum	250 g	Base
Purified water	qs 1000 g	Base

1. Calculate the required quantity of each ingredient for the total amount to be prepared.
2. Accurately weigh or measure each ingredient.
3. Melt the stearyl alcohol and the white petrolatum, using a steam bath. Warm the mixture to about 75°C.
4. Dissolve the other ingredients in the purified water, and warm the mixture to 75°C. Add this mixture to the stearyl alcohol–white petrolatum mixture.
5. Remove the mixture from the heat, and stir rapidly and continuously until the mixture has congealed.
6. Package and label the product.

Polyethylene Glycol Ointment

Polyethylene glycol 3350	400 g	Base
Polyethylene glycol 400	600 g	Base

1. Calculate the required quantity of each ingredient for the total amount to be prepared.
2. Accurately weigh or measure each ingredient.
3. Heat the polyethylene glycols to 65°C, using a water bath.
4. Mix the ingredients well, remove from heat, and stir until the mixture has congealed.
5. Package and label the product.

Ingredient-Specific Formulations

℞ Anthralin 1% in Lipid Crystals Cream

Anthralin	1 g	Active
Glyceryl laurate	7 g	Emulsifier
Glyceryl myristate	21 g	Emulsifier
Citric acid	1 g	Acidifier
Sodium hydroxide	140 mg	Alkalizer
Purified water	qs 100 g	Base

1. Calculate the quantity of each ingredient required for the prescription.
2. Accurately weigh or measure each ingredient.
3. Heat the glyceryl laurate and glyceryl myristate to about 70°C, and incorporate the anthralin powder.
4. Heat the citric acid and sodium hydroxide in 70 mL of purified water to 70°C.
5. Add the oil phase (step 3) to the aqueous phase (step 4), mix well, and continue heating at 70°C for 15 minutes.
6. Cool the mixture to about 40°C.
7. Slowly continue cooling the mixture, with stirring, to room temperature; this is a controlled cooling step.
8. Package and label the product.

(Note: Use glass or plastic equipment when working with this preparation; avoid contact with metal utensils.)

℞ Bismuth Iodoform Paraffin Paste (BIPP)

Bismuth subnitrate	25 g	Active
Iodoform	50 g	Active
Mineral oil (sterilized)	25 g	Vehicle

1. Calculate the quantity of each ingredient required for the prescription.
2. Accurately weigh or measure each ingredient.
3. If the mineral oil is not already sterile, sterilize it using dry heat.
4. Mix the powders with the mineral oil to form a smooth paste.
5. Package and label the product.

℞ Estradiol Vaginal Cream

Estradiol	200 mg	Active
Glycerin	qs	Levigating Agent
Hydrophilic ointment	100 g	Vehicle

1. Calculate the quantity of each ingredient required for the prescription.
2. Accurately weigh or measure each ingredient.
3. Levigate the estradiol powder with a few drops of glycerin.
4. Incorporate the hydrophilic ointment or other suitable o/w vehicles geometrically, mixing until uniform.
5. Package and label the product.

(Note: Commercial o/w vehicles can be used, and the quantity of estradiol is variable.)

℞ Progesterone 10% Topical Cream

Progesterone, micronized	10 g	Active
Glycerin	5 mL	Humectant/Solvent
Oil-in-water cream vehicle	qs 100 g	Vehicle

1. Calculate the quantity of each ingredient required for the prescription.
2. Accurately weigh or measure each ingredient.
3. Add the glycerin to the micronized progesterone, and form a smooth paste.
4. Incorporate the cream vehicle geometrically, and mix until uniform.
5. As an option, run the mixture through a roller ointment mill.
6. Package and label the product.

℞ Protective Hand Cream (100 g)

Dimethicone	4 g	Active
Stearic acid	6 g	Thickener/Emulsifying Agent
Cetyl alcohol	1.5 g	Thickener/Emulsifying Agent
Mineral oil, light	2.2 g	Base
Triethanolamine	1.5 g	Alkalizer
Glycerin	1.8 g	Humectant
Methylparaben	200 mg	Preservative
Purified water	82.8 g	Vehicle

1. Calculate the quantity of each ingredient required for the prescription.
2. Accurately weigh or measure each ingredient.
3. Mix the dimethicone, stearic acid, cetyl alcohol, and light mineral oil in a container, and heat to about 75°C.
4. Mix the triethanolamine, glycerin, methylparaben, and purified water in a separate container, and heat to about 75°C.
5. Add the oil phase (step 3) to the aqueous phase (step 4), and cool, stirring until the mixture congeals and is at room temperature.
6. Package and label the product.

℞ Testosterone 2% Ointment

Testosterone propionate	2 g	Active
White petrolatum	98 g	Vehicle

1. Calculate the quantity of each ingredient required for the prescription.
2. Accurately weigh or measure each ingredient.
3. Mix the testosterone propionate with a few drops of mineral oil.
4. Add the white petrolatum geometrically, and mix until uniform.
5. Package and label the product.

℞ Testosterone:Menthol Eutectic Ointment (2% Testosterone)

| Testosterone:menthol eutectic mixture | 4.33 g | Active |
| Hydrophilic petrolatum/Aquabase/Aquaphor | 95.67 g | Base |

1. Calculate the quantity of each ingredient required for the prescription.
2. Accurately weigh each ingredient.
3. Mix the testosterone:menthol eutectic mixture with a small quantity of the base.
4. Incorporate the remaining base into the drug mixture geometrically, and thoroughly mix.
5. Package and label the product.

The testosterone:menthol eutectic mixture can be prepared as follows:

Testosterone	31.6 g	Active
Menthol	68.4 g	Active
Methyl alcohol	qs	Solvent

1. Use sufficient methyl alcohol to dissolve both the testosterone and the menthol.
2. Allow the alcohol to evaporate while occasionally stirring the mixture. The alcohol can take a day or two to evaporate to dryness.
3. After the mixture dries, pulverize it thoroughly, and store it in a tight, light-resistant container.

Reference

1. *Drug Facts and Comparisons 2016.* St. Louis, MO: Wolters Kluwer; 2015:3332–41.

Chapter 22

Gels

One of the most versatile delivery systems that can be compounded is the pharmaceutical gel. Gels are an excellent drug delivery system for various routes of administration and are compatible with many different drug substances. Gels containing penetration enhancers are especially popular for administering anti-inflammatory and antinauseant medications. They are relatively easy to prepare and are quite efficacious.

Definitions and Types

According to the *United States Pharmacopeia/National Formulary (USP/NF)*, *gels* or *jellies* are semisolid systems consisting of suspensions made up of either small inorganic particles or large organic molecules interpenetrated by a liquid. If the gel mass consists of a network of small discrete particles, the gel is classified as a two-phase system. In a two-phase system, if the particle size of the dispersed phase is large, the product is referred to as a *magma*. Single-phase gels consist of large organic molecules or macromolecules uniformly distributed throughout a liquid in such a manner that no apparent boundaries exist between the dispersed macromolecules and the liquid. Single-phase gels can be made from synthetic macromolecules or from natural gums (mucilages). The continuous phase is usually aqueous but can also be alcoholic or oleaginous.

Gels are semirigid systems in which the movement of the dispersing medium is restricted by an interlacing three-dimensional network of particles or solvated macromolecules of the dispersed phase. A high degree of physical or chemical cross-linking can be involved. The increased viscosity caused by the interlacing and consequential internal friction is responsible for the semisolid state. A gel can consist of twisted, matted strands often bound together by stronger types of van der Waals forces to form crystalline and amorphous regions throughout the system (e.g., tragacanth and carboxymethylcellulose [CMC]).

Some gel systems are as clear as water in appearance; others are turbid because their ingredients may not be completely molecularly dispersed or they may form aggregates, which disperse light. The concentration of the gelling agents is typically less than 10%, usually in the 0.5% to 2% range.

To appeal to the consumer, gels should have clarity and sparkle. Most gels act as absorption bases and are water washable, water soluble, water absorbing, and greaseless. Gels should maintain their viscosity and character over a wide range of temperatures.

Applications

Gels can be used to administer medications orally, topically, intranasally, vaginally, and rectally. They can serve as ointment bases; examples are Plastibase and mineral oil gels made with aluminum monostearate.

Nasal absorption of drugs from gels has been extensively investigated. Some reports on drugs administered in nasal methylcellulose gels, such as propranolol, show that the drug is better absorbed through the nose than after oral administration. In the future, many more drugs may be administered in the form of nasal gels.

Composition and Classification Systems

Gels are categorized according to two classification systems. One system divides gels into inorganic and organic; the other, into hydrogels and organogels. Table 22-1 provides examples of both classification systems. *Inorganic gels* are usually two-phase systems, whereas *organic gels* are generally single-phase systems.

Examples of gelling agents are acacia, alginic acid, bentonite, carbomer, CMC sodium, cetostearyl alcohol, colloidal silicon dioxide, ethylcellulose, gelatin, guar gum, hydroxyethyl cellulose, hydroxypropyl cellulose, hydroxypropyl methylcellulose, magnesium aluminum silicate, maltodextrin, methylcellulose, polyvinyl alcohol (PVA), povidone, propylene carbonate, propylene glycol alginate, sodium alginate, sodium starch glycolate, starch, tragacanth, and xanthan gum.

Hydrogels contain ingredients that are either dispersible as colloids or soluble in water; they include organic hydrogels, natural and synthetic gums, and inorganic hydrogels. For example, bentonite is an inorganic hydrogel that has been used as an ointment base in concentrations of about 10% to 25%. In high concentrations, hydrophilic colloids form semisolid gels, also referred to as *jellies*. Sodium alginate has been used to produce gels that serve as ointment

TABLE 22-1 Classification and Description of Gels

Class	Description	Examples
Inorganic gels	Usually two-phase system	Aluminum hydroxide gel, bentonite magma
Organic gels	Usually single-phase system	Carbomer, tragacanth
Hydrogels (jellies)	Inorganic	Alumina, bentonite, silica, Veegum
	Natural and synthetic gums	Pectin, sodium alginate, tragacanth
	Organic	Carboxymethylcellulose sodium, methylcellulose, Pluronic F-127
Organogels	Hydrocarbon type	Mineral oil/polyethylene gel, petrolatum, Plastibase/Jelene
	Animal and vegetable fats	Cocoa butter, lard
	Soap base greases	Aluminum stearate with heavy mineral oil gel
	Hydrophilic organogels	Carbowax bases (polyethylene glycol ointment)

bases; in concentrations greater than 2.5% and in the presence of soluble calcium salts, a firm gel, stable at pH 5 to 10, is formed. Methylcellulose, hydroxyethylcellulose, and CMC sodium are among the commercially available cellulose products that can be used in ointments. They are available in several viscosities: usually high, medium, and low.

Organogels include the hydrocarbons, animal and vegetable fats, soap base greases, and hydrophilic organogels. The hydrocarbon type includes Jelene, or Plastibase, a combination of mineral oils and heavy hydrocarbon waxes with a molecular weight of about 1300. Petrolatum is a semisolid gel consisting of a liquid component together with a protosubstance and a crystalline waxy fraction. The crystalline fraction provides rigidity to the structure, whereas the protosubstance, or gel former, stabilizes the system and thickens the gel. The hydrophilic organogels, or polar organogels, are soluble to about 75% in water and are completely washable. They look and feel like petrolatum and are nonionic and stable.

Jellies are a class of gels in which the structural coherent matrix contains a high proportion of liquid, usually water. They are commonly formed by adding a thickening agent such as tragacanth or CMC to an aqueous solution of a drug substance. The resultant preparation is usually clear and has a uniform, semisolid consistency. Jellies are subject to bacterial contamination and growth; thus, most are preserved with antimicrobials. Jellies should be stored in tightly closed containers to prevent evaporation of the water and drying of the preparation.

Some substances, such as acacia, are termed *natural colloids* because they are self-dispersing in a dispersing medium. *Artificial colloids* are materials that require special treatment for prompt dispersion; this can involve fine pulverization to colloidal size with a colloid mill or a micropulverizer.

An interesting product, a *xerogel,* can be formed when the liquid is removed from a gel, leaving only the framework. Examples include gelatin sheets, tragacanth ribbons, and acacia tears.

Preparation

The characteristics of the gelling agents determine the techniques used in their preparation. Because carbomer gels are used extensively in gel preparations, techniques for preparing aqueous dispersions of these resins are presented first, followed by a general discussion of techniques for preparing other gelling agents.

Aqueous Dispersions of Carbomer Resins

Carbomer resins are primarily used in aqueous systems, although other liquids can be used as well. In water, a single particle of carbomer will wet rapidly, but, like many other powders, carbomer polymers tend to form clumps of particles when dispersed haphazardly in polar solvents. As the surfaces of these clumps solvate, a layer is formed that prevents rapid wetting of the interior of the clumps. When this occurs, the slow diffusion of solvent through the solvated layer determines the mixing or hydration time. To achieve the fastest dispersion of the carbomer, a pharmacist should take advantage of the small particle size of the carbomer powder by slowly adding it into the vortex of a liquid that is being stirred rapidly. Almost any device, such as a simple sieve, that can sprinkle the powder on the rapidly stirred liquid is useful. A metallic screen will help not only by reducing the particle size, but also by diffusing static charge buildup. Generally, the higher the agitation rate of the liquid, the better, but extremely high-shear mixers should not be used, because they can break down the polymers and reduce gel viscosity. Propeller or turbine-type mixers running about 800 to 1200 rpm work well. Variable-speed mixers are especially desirable to reduce vortexing when the mixture begins to thicken, and they will incorporate less air into the gel. The propeller should be located close to the bottom of the mixing vessel to minimize incorporating air into the preparation. The small-particle-size powder should be slowly sprinkled over the rapidly agitated water to prevent clumping. Once the powder is incorporated, continued stirring for 10 to 15 minutes at reduced speed is recommended to avoid entrapment of excess air.

A neutralizer is added to thicken the gel after the carbomer is dispersed. Sodium hydroxide or potassium hydroxide can be used in carbomer dispersions containing less than 20% alcohol. Triethanolamine will neutralize carbomer resins containing up to 50% ethanol. Other neutralizing agents include sodium carbonate, ammonia, and borax.

Air bubbles incorporated into the gel should be removed before the neutralizing agent is added. Otherwise, the air will remain entrapped in the preparation. Air bubbles can be removed by using an ultrasonic unit or by allowing the preparation to stand. A pharmacist may need to acidify the gel, remove the air, and neutralize it again. For this procedure, hydrochloric and phosphoric acids should be used in an amount equal to 0.5% of the weight of the carbomer present, *not* the total weight of the preparation. These acids will not produce the significant salt levels on neutralization that might occur with other acids (e.g., citric or lactic acid).

Equipment cleanup after preparation of carbomer formulations is facilitated by the use of warm water containing salt, a commercial detergent, and sufficient sodium hydroxide or ammonium hydroxide to raise the pH to 11 or higher. If the material has dried, the equipment can be soaked in water before this cleaning solution is used. Carbomer resin powders do not support growth of bacteria, mold, or fungi while in powder form. When they are present in aqueous systems, however, mold and some bacteria can grow. Table 22-2 lists commonly used preservatives and their compatibility with carbomer resins. When added to an aqueous system, 0.1% methylparaben or propylparaben is an acceptable preservative and does not affect the resin's efficiency. Carbomer resins are anionic and can decrease the efficiency of some of the cationic agents.

Other Gelling Agents
Alginic Acid
Alginic acid can be dispersed in water that is vigorously stirred for approximately 30 minutes. Premixing with another powder or with a water-miscible liquid aids in the dispersion process.

Bentonite
Bentonite is added to nonagitated water by sprinkling small portions on the surface of hot water. Each portion is allowed to hydrate and settle in the container. The mixture is allowed

TABLE 22-2 Preservative Compatibility with Carbomer Gels

Preservative	Concentration	Appearance	Compatible?
Benzalkonium chloride	0.01%	Clear	Yes
	0.1%	Cloudy	No
Sodium benzoate	0.01%	Clear	Yes
	0.1%	Cloudy	No
Methylparaben	0.18%	Clear	Yes
Propylparaben	0.02%	Clear	Yes
Thimerosal	0.01%	Clear	Yes
	0.1%	Clear	Yes

to stand for 24 hours, with occasional stirring. The mixture is thoroughly agitated the next day. Glycerin or a similar liquid can be used to prewet the bentonite before mixing with water.

Carboxymethylcellulose Sodium
CMC sodium is soluble in water at all temperatures. The sodium salt of CMC can be dispersed with high shear in cold water before the particles can hydrate and swell to sticky gel grains agglomerating into lumps. Once the powder is well dispersed, the solution is heated with moderate shear to about 60°C for fastest dissolution.

Colloidal Silicon Dioxide
Colloidal silicon dioxide (fumed silica) will form a gel when combined with L-dodecanol and n-dodecane. These gels are prepared by adding the silica to the vehicle and sonicating for about 1 minute to obtain a uniform dispersion. The preparation is then sealed and stored overnight at about 40°C to complete gelation. This gel is more hydrophobic in nature than the others.

Gelatin Gels
Gelatin gels are prepared by dispersing the gelatin in hot water, and then cooling the mixture. An alternative method is to moisten the gelatin with about 3 to 5 parts of an organic liquid that will not swell the polymer, such as ethyl alcohol or propylene glycol, and then add the hot water and allow the mixture to cool.

Methylcellulose
Methylcellulose is a long-chain, substituted cellulose that can be used to form gels in concentrations up to about 5%. Because methylcellulose hydrates slowly in hot water, the powder is dispersed with high shear in about one-third of the required amount of water at 80°C to 90°C. Once the powder is finely dispersed, the rest of the water is added, with moderate stirring to cause prompt dissolution. Cold water or ice should be used at this point. Anhydrous alcohol or propylene glycol can be used to help prewet the powders. Maximum clarity, fullest hydration, and highest viscosity will be obtained if the gel is cooled to 0°C to 10°C for about 1 hour. A preservative should be added. A 2% solution of methylcellulose 4000 has a gel point of about 50°C.

Polyvinyl Alcohol
PVA is used at concentrations of about 2.5% in preparing various jellies that dry rapidly when applied to the skin. Borax is a good agent that will gel PVA solutions. For best results, PVA should be dispersed in cold water, followed by hot water. It is less soluble in cold water.

Tragacanth
Tragacanth gum tends to form lumps when added to water; therefore, aqueous dispersions are prepared by adding the powder to vigorously stirred water. As noted earlier, ethanol, glycerin, or propylene glycol can be used to prewet the powder. Other powders can be mixed with the tragacanth while dry and then added to the water.

General Preparation Techniques
The active drug can be added before or after the gel is formed. If the active drug does not interfere with the gelling process, adding it before gelling is best because the drug will be more easily and uniformly dispersed. If the active drug does interfere with gelling, it should

be added after gelling occurs, although more effort is required and air can be incorporated into the preparation.

One easy method of preparation is to place the gel and the active drug in a plastic bag, which is then kneaded to thoroughly mix the drug. After the preparation is mixed, scissors can be used to snip off one corner of the bag, and then the preparation can be squeezed into the dispensing container; this is similar to the method used for decorating cakes.

When powdered polymers are added to water during gel preparation, they can form temporary gels that slow the dissolution process. As water diffuses into these loose clumps of powder, their exteriors frequently turn into clumps of solvated particles encasing dry powder. The clumps of gel dissolve quite slowly because of their high viscosity and the low diffusion coefficient of the macromolecules. Using glycerin or another liquid as a wetting or dispersing agent minimizes this occurrence.

Aqueous polymer solutions, especially of cellulose derivatives, are stored for approximately 48 hours after dissolution to promote full hydration, maximum viscosity, and clarity. If salts are to be added, a pharmacist should add them at this point rather than dissolving them in water before adding the polymer; otherwise, the solutions may not reach their full viscosity and clarity.

Additional suggestions for preparing this dosage form are given in Box 22-1.

BOX 22-1 Hints for Compounding Gels

Suggestions for compounding gels are as follows:

- In gel preparation, premixing some gelling agents with other powders often aids the dispersion process.
- Adding alcohol to some gels decreases their viscosity and clarity.
- When mixers of any type are used for preparing a gel, the propeller should be kept at the bottom of the container, and formation of a vortex should be avoided to minimize incorporating air into the product.
- In gel preparation, all agents should be dissolved in the solvent or vehicle before the gelling agent is added.
- Any entrapped air in carbomer dispersions should be removed before the thickening agent is added. Air bubbles can be removed by allowing the product to stand for 24 hours or by placing it in an ultrasonic bath. A silicone antifoam agent can be helpful.
- pH is important in determining the final viscosity of carbomer gels.
- Gelatin gels can be prepared by dispersing the gelatin in hot water and then cooling the gel. The procedure can be simplified by (1) mixing gelatin powder with an organic liquid in which it will not swell, such as ethyl alcohol or propylene glycol; (2) adding the hot water; and (3) cooling the gel.
- Tragacanth gels can be prepared by adding the powder to vigorously stirred water. Ethanol, glycerin, or propylene glycol can be used to prewet the powder. Other powders can be mixed with the tragacanth while dry, before it is added to the water.
- Generally, natural gums should hydrate for about 24 hours to form the best homogeneous gel or magma.

Physicochemical Considerations

The characteristics of gels and jellies include imbibition, swelling, syneresis, and thixotropy.

Imbibition is the taking up of a certain amount of liquid by a gel without a measurable increase in volume. *Swelling* is the taking up of a liquid by a gel with an increase in volume. Only those liquids that solvate a gel can cause swelling. The swelling of protein gels is influenced by pH and the presence of electrolytes.

Syneresis is the contraction of a gel caused by the interaction between particles of the dispersed phase. This interaction becomes so great that, on standing, the dispersing medium is squeezed out in droplets, causing the gel to shrink. Syneresis is a form of instability in aqueous and nonaqueous gels. The solvent phase is thought to separate because of the elastic contraction of the polymeric molecules; as swelling increases during gel formation, the macromolecules become stretched and the elastic forces expand. At equilibrium, the restoring force of the macromolecules is balanced by the swelling forces, determined by the osmotic pressure. If the osmotic pressure decreases, such as on cooling, water can be squeezed out of the gel. The syneresis of an acidic gel from *Plantago albicans* seed gum can be decreased by adding electrolytes, glucose, and sucrose and by increasing the gum concentration. pH has a significant effect on the separation of water. At low pH, marked syneresis occurs, possibly because of suppression of ionization of the carboxylic acid groups, loss of hydrating water, and formation of intramolecular hydrogen bonds. These conditions would reduce the attraction of the solvent for the macromolecule.

Thixotropy is a reversible gel–sol formation with no change in volume or temperature. It is considered a type of non-Newtonian flow.

These characteristics play a role in how some agents form a gel or, once formed, remain in this dosage form. This is illustrated in the following discussions of mechanisms of gel formation and the specific physicochemical properties of common gelling agents.

Mechanisms of Gel Formation

As a hot colloidal dispersion of gelatin cools, the gelatin macromolecules lose kinetic energy. With reduced kinetic energy, or thermal agitation, the gelatin macromolecules are associated through dipole–dipole interaction into elongated or threadlike aggregates. The size of these association chains increases to the extent that the dispersing medium is held in the interstices among the interlacing network of gelatin macromolecules, and the viscosity increases to that of a semisolid. Gums, such as agar, algin, Irish moss, pectin, and tragacanth, form gels by the same mechanism as gelatin.

Polymer solutions tend to cast gels because the solute consists of long, flexible chains of molecular thickness that can become entangled, attract each other by secondary valence forces, and even crystallize. Cross-linking of dissolved polymer molecules also causes these solutions to gel. The reactions produce permanent gels, held together by primary valence forces. Secondary valence forces are responsible for reversible gel formation. For example, gelatin will form a gel when its temperature is lowered to about 30°C, the gel point, but aqueous methylcellulose solutions will gel when heated above about 50°C because the polymer is less soluble in hot water and precipitates. Lower temperatures, higher concentrations, and higher molecular weights promote gelation and produce stronger gels. The reversible gelation of gelatin will occur at about 25°C for 10% solutions, 30°C for 20% solutions, and 32°C for 30% solutions. Gelation is rarely observed for gelatin above 34°C, and, regardless of concentration, gelatin solutions do not gel at 37°C. The gelation temperature, or gel point, of gelatin is highest at the isoelectric point. Some water-soluble polymers have the property of thermal gelation; that is, they gel on heating, whereas natural gums gel on cooling. The thermal gelation is reversed on cooling.

Inorganic salts will compete with the water present in a gel and cause gelation to occur at lower concentrations. This process is usually reversible, and the gels will re-form when water is added. Alcohol can cause precipitation or gelation because alcohol is a nonsolvent or precipitant, lowering the dielectric constant of the medium and tending to dehydrate the hydrophilic solute. Alcohol lowers the concentrations at which electrolytes salt out hydrophilic colloids. Phase separation through the addition of alcohol can cause coacervation.

Properties of Common Gelling Agents

Alginic Acid

Alginic acid is obtained from seaweed that is found throughout the world, and the prepared formulation is a tasteless, practically odorless, white to yellowish-white, fibrous powder. It is used in concentrations between 1% and 5% as a thickening agent in gels. It swells in water to about 200 to 300 times its own weight without dissolving. Cross-linking with increased viscosity occurs when a calcium salt, such as calcium citrate, is added.

Bentonite

Bentonite, a naturally occurring hydrated aluminum silicate, can be used to prepare gels. Aqueous bentonite suspensions retain their viscosity above pH 6 but are precipitated by acids. Alkaline materials, such as magnesium oxide, increase gel formation. Alcohol in significant amounts can precipitate bentonite, and, because bentonite is anionic, the antimicrobial efficacy of cationic preservatives can be reduced. Bentonite exhibits thixotropy; it can form a semirigid gel that reverts to a sol when agitated. The sol will re-form to a gel on standing.

Carbomer

Carbomer (Carbopol) resins were first described in the professional literature in 1955 and are currently used in a variety of pharmaceutical dosage systems, including controlled-release tablets, oral suspensions, and topical gels. The *USP/NF; British Pharmacopoeia;* United States Adopted Names Council; and Cosmetic, Toiletry and Fragrance Association have adopted the generic name *carbomer* for the Carbopol family of resins. Carbomer resins are allyl pentaerythritol–cross-linked, acrylic acid–based polymers, which have a high molecular weight and are modified with C10 to C30 alkyl acrylates. They are fluffy, white, dry powders with large bulk densities, 2% maximum moisture, and pK_a of 6.0 ± 0.5. The pH of 0.5% and 1% aqueous dispersions is 2.7 to 3.5 and 2.5 to 3, respectively. There are many carbomer resins, with viscosity ranges from 0 to 80,000 cP. pH is important in determining the viscosity of carbomer gels. The resins commonly used in a compounding pharmacy are listed in Table 22-3.

Carbomers 910, 934, 934P, 940, and 1342 are official in the *USP/NF.* Carbomer 910 is effective at low concentrations when low viscosity is desired and is frequently used for producing stable suspensions. It is the least ion sensitive of these resins. Carbomer 934 is highly effective in thick formulations such as viscous gels. The two alternative resins, carbomers 2984 and 5984, are polymerized in ethyl acetate/cyclohexane in place of benzene. Carbomer 934P is similar to 934 but is intended for oral and mucosal contact applications and is the most widely used carbomer in the pharmaceutical industry. In addition to its use for thickening, suspending, and emulsifying in both oral and topical formulations, the 934 polymer is also used to provide sustained-release properties in the stomach and the intestinal tract for commercial preparations. Carbomer 940, or 980, its cosolvent alternative, is the most efficient of all the carbomer resins and has good nondrip properties. Carbomer 1342 and its cosolvent analogue, 1382, provide pseudoplastic rheology, which is quite effective in

TABLE 22-3 Properties of Carbomer Pharmaceutical Resins

Product	Viscosity (cP)[a]	Properties and Uses
Carbomer 907	0–3000	Very water soluble; good lubricity at low viscosity; a "linear" polymer that is not cross-linked
Carbomer 910 NF	3000–7000	Effective in low concentrations; good ion tolerance
Carbomer 934 NF	30,500–39,400	Good stability at high viscosity; good for thick formulations, such as medium to high viscosity gels, emulsions, and suspensions; good for zero-order release of preparations, such as oral and muco-adhesive applications; excellent for transdermals and topicals
Carbomer 2984	45,000–80,000	
Carbomer 5984	25,000–45,000	
Carbomer 934P NF	29,400–39,400	
Carbomer 974P NF	29,400–39,400	
Carbomer 940 NF	40,000–60,000	Excellent thickening efficiency at high viscosities and very good clarity; produces sparkling clear water or hydroalcoholic topical gels
Carbomer 980 NF	40,000–60,000	
Carbomer ETD 2001	45,000–65,000	
Carbomer 941 NF	4000–11,000	Produces sparkling clear gels with low viscosity; good stabilizer for emulsions; effective in moderately ionic systems; more efficient than Carbomers 934 and 940 at low to moderate concentrations
Carbomer 981 NF	4000–11,000	
Carbomer ETD 2050	3000–15,000	

[a]These are typical viscosities of a 0.5% solution, pH 7.5, except for Carbomer 907, which is a 4.0% solution.

preparing pourable suspensions and stable emulsions and makes them especially good for preparations containing dissolved salts. Carbomer 974P NF differs from carbomer 934P NF in that ethyl acetate rather than benzene is used in its preparation. Carbomers 980 NF and ETD 2001 differ from carbomer 940 NF in that cosolvents are used in place of benzene for their preparation. Such is also the case with carbomers 981 NF and ETD 2050 versus carbomer 941 NF.

Adding alcohol to prepared carbomer gels can decrease their viscosity and clarity. To overcome the loss of viscosity, a pharmacist may need to increase the concentration of carbomer; the amount will vary depending on the pH of the preparation. A preparation at pH 5.5 that goes from 0% to 50% alcohol requires an increase of 0.5% carbomer; similarly, an increase of 0.35% carbomer is required at pH 8.2 when alcohol content increases from 20% to 40%. Also, gel viscosity depends on the presence of electrolytes and the pH. Generally, a maximum of 3% electrolytes can be added before a rubbery mass forms. Overneutralization will result in decreased viscosity, which cannot be reversed by adding acid. Maximum viscosity and clarity occur at pH 7, but acceptable viscosity and clarity begin at pH 4.5 to 5 and extend to pH 11.

Cross-linked carbomer resins can swell in water up to 1000 times their original volume to form gels when exposed to a pH environment above 4 to 6. Because the pK_a of these polymers is about 6, the carboxylate groups on the molecules ionize, resulting in repulsion between the negative particles of the polymer backbone, which contributes to the swelling of the polymer. Determining the molecular weight of the carbomers is difficult. Although the average molecular weights of the polymerized resins are on the order of about 500,000, the actual molecular weight of the cross-linked resin is in the billions.

Other Gelling Agents
CMC in concentrations of 4% to 6% of the medium viscosity grades can be used to produce gels; glycerin can be added to prevent drying. Precipitation can occur at pH values of less

than 2; CMC is most stable at pH 2 to 10, with maximum stability at pH 7 to 9. It is incompatible with ethanol.

CMC sodium dispersions are sensitive to pH changes because of the carboxylate group. The viscosity of the preparation is decreased markedly below pH 5 or above pH 10.

Colloidal silicon dioxide can be used to prepare transparent gels when used with other ingredients of similar refractive index. Colloidal silicon dioxide adsorbs large quantities of water without liquefying. The viscosity is largely independent of temperature. Changes in pH can affect the viscosity; it is most effective at pH values up to about 7.5. At a pH greater than 10.7, the viscosity-increasing properties are reduced, and, at these higher levels, the silicon dioxide dissolves to form silicates with no viscosity-increasing properties.

Magnesium aluminum silicate, Veegum, in concentrations of about 10%, forms firm, thixotropic gels. The material is inert and has few incompatibilities but is best used above pH 3.5. It can bind to some drugs and limit their availability.

Methylcellulose mixtures that contain high concentrations of electrolytes will have viscosity problems. The electrolytes will salt out the macromolecules and increase their viscosity, ultimately precipitating the polymer.

Plastibase and Jelene are each a mixture of 5% low molecular weight polyethylene and 95% mineral oil. The polymer is soluble in mineral oil above 90°C, close to its melting point. When cooled below 90°C, the polymer precipitates and causes gelation. A network of entangled and adhering insoluble polyethylene chains immobilizes the mineral oil. This network probably extends into small crystalline regions. This gel can be heated to about 60°C without a substantial loss of consistency.

Poloxamer, or Pluronic, gels are made from selected forms of polyoxyethylene–polyoxypropylene copolymers in concentrations ranging from 15% to 50%. Poloxamers generally are white, waxy, free-flowing granules that are practically odorless and tasteless. Aqueous solutions of poloxamers are stable in the presence of acids, alkalies, and metal ions. However, they do support mold growth and should be preserved. Commonly used poloxamers include the 124 (L-44 grade), 188 (F-68 grade), 237 (F-87 grade), 338 (F-108 grade), and 407 (F-127 grade) types, which are freely soluble in water. The "F" designation refers to the flake form of the preparation. The trade name Pluronic is used in the United States by BASF Corporation for pharmaceutical- and industrial-grade poloxamers. Pluronic F-127 has low toxicity and good solubilizing capacity and optical properties; thus, it is a good medium for topical drug delivery systems.

Povidone, in the higher molecular weight forms, can be used to prepare gels in concentrations up to about 10%. It has the advantage of being compatible in solution with a wide range of inorganic salts, natural and synthetic resins, and other chemicals. It can also increase the solubility of a number of poorly soluble drugs.

Propylene glycol alginate is used as a gelling agent in concentrations of 1% to 5%, depending on the specific application. The preparations are most stable at a pH of 3 to 6 and should contain a preservative.

Sodium alginate can be used to produce gels in concentrations up to 10%. Aqueous preparations are most stable between pH 4 and 10; below pH 3, alginic acid is precipitated. Sodium alginate gels for external use should be preserved, for example, with 0.1% chloroxylenol or the parabens. If the preparation is acidic, benzoic acid can be used. High concentrations will result in increased viscosity up to a point at which the sodium alginate is salted out; this point occurs at about 4% with sodium chloride.

Tragacanth gum has been used to prepare gels that are most stable at pH 4 to 8. These gels must be preserved with either 0.1% benzoic acid or sodium benzoate or a combination of 0.17% methylparaben and 0.03% propylparaben. These gels can be sterilized by autoclaving.

Liqua-Gel (Paddock) is a liquid lubricating gel that is water soluble and nongreasy. It can be used to dissolve or suspend a variety of topically applied dermatologic agents. Liqua-Gel contains purified water, propylene glycol, glycerin, hydroxypropyl methylcellulose, and potassium sorbate. Sodium phosphate and boric acid are used to buffer the gel to a pH of about 5. Diazolidinyl urea, methylparaben, and propylparaben are included as preservatives. Liqua-Gel is a clear, colorless, viscous gel with a faint characteristic odor and has a viscosity of about 80,000 cP at 25°C.

Quality Control

A pharmacist should follow standard quality control procedures. These procedures involve checking the appearance, uniformity, weight or volume, viscosity, clarity, pH, and smell of the gels.

Packaging, Storage, and Labeling

Gels generally should be stored in tight containers at refrigerated or room temperatures. This dosage form is commonly dispensed in tubes, jars, squeeze bottles, or pump dispensers (Figure 22-1). Some gels can be dispensed in applicators or syringes. The labels should include the instruction to keep containers tightly closed.

Carbomer resins are quite hygroscopic and should be stored in tight containers, away from moisture and extreme temperatures. Moisture does not affect the efficiency of the resins, but high levels make them more difficult to disperse and weigh accurately. Autoclaving appears to have no effect on the viscosity or pH of the prepared gels. Aqueous dispersions of carbomer that have not been neutralized can be stored as stock solutions at concentrations up to 5%.

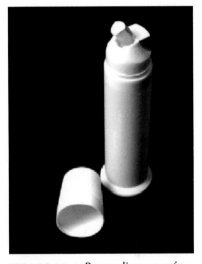

FIGURE 22-1 Pump dispenser for creams and gels.

Glass, plastic, or resin-lined containers are recommended for storage of carbomer preparations. Aluminum tubes should be used only when a preparation has a pH less than about 6.5. With other metallic materials, a pH of about 7.7 or greater is preferred.

Stability

Gels should be observed for such physical characteristics as shrinkage, separation of liquid from the gel, discoloration, and microbial contamination. Many gels will not promote bacterial or mold growth, nor will they prevent it. Consequently, they should be autoclaved or should contain preservatives. Table 22-2 lists a number of preservatives and concentrations that have been used in preparing gels. Gelling agents in the dry state are usually not a problem.

Beyond-use dates for water-containing oral gels stored at cold temperatures are no later than 14 days; for water-containing topical gels, they are no later than 30 days at room temperature for formulations prepared from ingredients in solid form. These dates can be extended if valid scientific information is available to support the stability of the formulation, as discussed in Chapter 6 of this book.

Patient Counseling

Patients should be counseled about the proper application of the gel. They should be instructed on the way to handle and store the package, as well as the need to keep it tightly closed.

Sample Formulations

℞ Amitriptyline Hydrochloride 2% and Baclofen 2% in Pluronic Lecithin Organogel

Amitriptyline hydrochloride	2 g	Active
Baclofen	2 g	Active
Ethoxydiglycol	5–10 mL	Solvent/Levigating Agent
Lecithin:isopropyl palmitate 1:1 solution	22 mL	Vehicle
Pluronic F-127 20% gel	qs 100 mL	Vehicle

1. Calculate the quantity of each ingredient required for the prescription.
2. Accurately weigh or measure each ingredient.
3. Combine the amitriptyline hydrochloride and baclofen powders.
4. Add sufficient ethoxydiglycol to form a smooth paste.
5. Add the lecithin:isopropyl palmitate 1:1 solution, and mix well.
6. Add sufficient Pluronic F-127 gel to volume, and mix well.
7. Package and label the product.

Bentonite Magma

Bentonite	50 g	Suspending/Gelling Agent
Purified water	qs 1000 mL	Vehicle

1. Calculate the required quantity of each ingredient for the total amount to be prepared.
2. Accurately weigh the bentonite powder.
3. Sprinkle the bentonite on 800 mL of hot (80°C–90°C) purified water, remove from heat, and allow to hydrate for 24 hours, stirring occasionally.
4. Increase the amount of purified water to make 1000 mL. If a mechanical blender is used, place approximately one-half of the water in the blender. Add the bentonite–water solution while the blender is in operation. Add more purified water to make the volume of 1000 mL, and operate the blender for 10 minutes.
5. Package and label the product.

℞ **Buspirone Hydrochloride 2.5 mg/0.1 mL in Pluronic Lecithin Organogel**

Buspirone hydrochloride	2.5 g	Active
Ethoxydiglycol	10 mL	Solvent/Levigating Agent
Lecithin:isopropyl palmitate 1:1 solution	22 mL	Vehicle
Pluronic F-127 20% gel	qs 100 mL	Vehicle

1. Calculate the quantity of each ingredient required for the prescription.
2. Accurately weigh or measure each ingredient.
3. Mix the buspirone hydrochloride with the ethoxydiglycol to form a smooth paste.
4. Add the lecithin:isopropyl palmitate 1:1 solution, and mix well.
5. Add sufficient Pluronic F-127 20% gel to make 100 mL, and mix thoroughly using a shear mixing method.
6. Package and label the product.

℞ **Capsaicin 0.075%, Ketamine Hydrochloride 2%, and Ketoprofen 10% in Pluronic Lecithin Organogel (100 mL)**

Capsaicin	75 mg	Active
Ketamine hydrochloride	2 g	Active
Ketoprofen	10 g	Active
Ethoxydiglycol	10 mL	Solvent/Levigating Agent
Lecithin:isopropyl palmitate 1:1 solution	22 mL	Vehicle
Pluronic F-127 30% gel	qs 100 mL	Vehicle

1. Calculate the quantity of each ingredient required for the prescription.
2. Accurately weigh or measure each ingredient.
3. Combine the capsaicin, ketamine hydrochloride, and ketoprofen powders.
4. Add sufficient ethoxydiglycol to form a smooth paste.
5. Add the lecithin:isopropyl palmitate 1:1 solution, and mix well.
6. Add sufficient Pluronic F-127 30% gel to volume, and mix well.
7. Package and label the product.

℞ Clear Aqueous Gel with Dimethicone

Purified water	59.8%	Vehicle
Carbomer 934	0.5%	Thickener
Triethanolamine	1.2%	Alkalizer
Glycerin	34.2%	Vehicle
Propylene glycol	2.0%	Vehicle
Dimethicone copolyol	2.3%	Active
Sodium hydroxide	1%	Alkalizer

1. Calculate the quantity of each ingredient required for the prescription.
2. Accurately weigh or measure each ingredient.
3. Disperse the carbomer 934 in 20 mL of purified water.
4. Adjust the pH of the dispersion to 7 by adding sufficient 1% sodium hydroxide solution (about 12 mL is required), and then add enough purified water to bring the volume to 40 mL.
5. Add the other ingredients, and mix well. (Note: Dimethicone copolyol is included to reduce the stickiness associated with glycerin.)
6. Package and label the product.

℞ Dexamethasone 1.2%, Lorazepam 0.1%, Haloperidol 0.1%, Diphenhydramine Hydrochloride 2.4%, and Metoclopramide Hydrochloride 2.4% in Pluronic Lecithin Organogel

Dexamethasone	1.2 g	Active
Lorazepam	100 mg	Active
Haloperidol	100 mg	Active
Diphenhydramine hydrochloride	2.4 g	Active
Metoclopramide hydrochloride	2.4 g	Active
Ethoxydiglycol	10 mL	Solvent/Levigating Agent
Lecithin:isopropyl palmitate 1:1 solution	22 mL	Vehicle
Pluronic F-127 20% gel	qs 100 mL	Vehicle

1. Calculate the quantity of each ingredient required for the prescription.
2. Accurately weigh or measure each ingredient.
3. Mix the powders together.
4. Incorporate the ethoxydiglycol to form a smooth paste.
5. Add the lecithin:isopropyl palmitate 1:1 solution, and mix well.
6. Add sufficient Pluronic F-127 20% gel to make 100 mL, and mix thoroughly, using a shear mixing method.
7. Package and label the product.

℞ Estradiol 0.5 mg/mL Topical Gel

Estradiol	50 mg	Active
70% Isopropyl alcohol	71 mL	Solvent/Vehicle
Carbomer 940	500 mg	Thickening Agent
Triethanolamine	670 mg	Alkalizing Agent
Purified water	28 mL	Vehicle

1. Calculate the quantity of each ingredient required for the prescription.
2. Accurately weigh or measure each ingredient.
3. Dissolve the estradiol in the 70% isopropyl alcohol.
4. Slowly add the carbomer 940 to this mixture, stirring constantly. A blender or high-speed mixer can be used.
5. Add the triethanolamine to the purified water.
6. Add the triethanolamine solution to the alcohol solution by slowly stirring. Mix thoroughly until the gel is formed. (Note: Slow stirring minimizes the introduction of air into the product.)
7. Package and label the product.

℞ Estradiol 2 mg/mL Vaginal Gel

Estradiol	200 mg	Active
Polysorbate 80	1 g	Surfactant
Methylcellulose 2% gel	99 g	Vehicle

1. Calculate the quantity of each ingredient required for the prescription.
2. Accurately weigh or measure each ingredient.
3. Levigate the estradiol with the polysorbate 80.
4. Geometrically add the methylcellulose 2% gel, and mix thoroughly.
5. Package and label the product.

Rx Ketamine Hydrochloride, Lidocaine Hydrochloride, and Ketoprofen in Pluronic Lecithin Organogel

Ketamine hydrochloride	10 g	Active
Lidocaine hydrochloride	5 g	Active
Ketoprofen	10 g	Active
Ethoxydiglycol	10 g	Levigating Agent
Polysorbate 80	5 g	Surfactant
Span 80	5 g	Surfactant
Potassium sorbate	200 mg	Preservative
Sorbic acid	200 mg	Preservative
Lecithin:isopropyl palmitate 1:1 solution	22 g	Vehicle
Poloxamer F127 30% gel	qs 100 g	Vehicle

1. Calculate the quantity of each ingredient required for the prescription.
2. Accurately weigh or measure each ingredient.
3. Combine all the powders, and mix with the ethoxydiglycol.
4. Incorporate the polysorbate 80 and Span 80, and mix well.
5. Add the lecithin:isopropyl palmitate 1:1 mixture, and mix well.
6. Incorporate the mixture into the poloxamer F127 30% gel, and mix well.
7. Package and label the product.

Rx Ketoprofen 5% in Pluronic Lecithin Organogel

Ketoprofen	5 g	Active
Ethoxydiglycol	10 mL	Solvent/Levigating Agent
Lecithin:isopropyl palmitate 1:1 solution	22 mL	Vehicle
Pluronic F-127 20% gel	qs 100 mL	Vehicle

1. Calculate the quantity of each ingredient required for the prescription.
2. Accurately weigh or measure each ingredient.
3. Mix the ketoprofen with the ethoxydiglycol to form a smooth paste.
4. Add the lecithin:isopropyl palmitate 1:1 solution, and mix well.
5. Add sufficient Pluronic F-127 20% gel to make 100 mL, and mix thoroughly, using a shear mixing method.
6. Package and label the product.

℞ Lidocaine Hydrochloride 4%–Epinephrine Hydrochloride 0.05%–Tetracaine Hydrochloride 0.5% Topical Gel

Lidocaine hydrochloride	4 g	Active
Epinephrine hydrochloride	50 mg	Active
Tetracaine hydrochloride	500 mg	Active
Ascorbic acid	1.7 g	Acidifier
Hydroxyethylcellulose (5000 cP)	1.75 g	Thickener
Preserved water	qs 100 mL	Vehicle

1. Calculate the quantity of each ingredient required for the prescription.
2. Accurately weigh or measure each ingredient.
3. Dissolve the lidocaine hydrochloride, epinephrine hydrochloride, tetracaine hydrochloride, and ascorbic acid in about 95 mL of preserved water.
4. Slowly, using a magnetic stirrer to form a vortex, sprinkle the hydroxyethylcellulose onto the surface of the moving water, allowing the particles to be wetted before adding additional powder. (Note: This action will help prevent clumping and speed up the gelling process.)
5. Add sufficient preserved water to volume, and mix well.
6. Package and label the product.

℞ Lidocaine Hydrochloride 2%, Misoprostol 0.003%, and Phenytoin 2.5% Topical Gel for Decubitus Ulcers

Lidocaine hydrochloride	2 g	Active
Misoprostol 200 μg tablets	#15	Active
Phenytoin	2.5 g	Active
Hydroxyethylcellulose	2 g	Thickener
Methylparaben	200 mg	Preservative
Glycerin	10 mL	Levigating Agent
Purified water	qs 100 mL	Vehicle

1. Calculate the quantity of each ingredient required for the prescription.
2. Accurately weigh or measure each ingredient; obtain the 15 tablets of misoprostol.
3. Pulverize the tablets to a fine powder, and blend in the remaining powders.
4. Add the glycerin, and make a smooth paste.
5. Slowly incorporate sufficient purified water to volume with mixing.
6. Package and label the product.

Liquid–Solid Emulsion Gel

Gelatin solution:

Gelatin, 200 bloom	8 g	Gelling Agent
Phosphate buffer (pH 7)	qs 40 mL	Vehicle

Gel preparation:

Gelatin solution	40 mL	Vehicle
Long-chain alcohol	10 g	Emulsifier

(Note: Liquid–solid emulsion gels can be prepared from gelatin and a selection of an alcohol from a homologous series [e.g., decanol, dodecanol, octanol, nonanol, or undecanol].)

1. Calculate the required quantity of each ingredient for the total amount to be prepared.
2. Accurately weigh or measure each ingredient.
3. Formulate the aqueous gelatin base such as 20% (weight/weight) 200 bloom gelatin in phosphate buffer (pH 7). Mature the gelatin–water mixture for about 1 hour at room temperature, and then melt at 60°C.
4. Leave the molten gel at 60°C for another 2 hours to allow air bubbles to escape.
5. Preheat 10 g of the long-chain alcohol to 60°C, add to 40 g of the heated molten aqueous gel, and stir at high speed for about 2 minutes.
6. Add the drug to the appropriate phase.
7. Pour the molten mixture onto a plate or between two plates to set, or cast.
8. Cut out circular or other shaped portions of the gel, and apply to the skin to release the enclosed drug.

℞ **Lorazepam 1 mg/mL in Pluronic Lecithin Organogel**

Lorazepam	100 mg	Active
Ethoxydiglycol	10 mL	Solvent/Levigating Agent
Lecithin:isopropyl palmitate 1:1 solution	22 mL	Vehicle
Pluronic F-127 20% gel	qs 100 mL	Vehicle

1. Calculate the quantity of each ingredient required for the prescription.
2. Accurately weigh or measure each ingredient.
3. Mix the lorazepam with the ethoxydiglycol to form a smooth paste.
4. Add the lecithin:isopropyl palmitate 1:1 solution, and mix well.
5. Add sufficient Pluronic F-127 20% gel to make 100 mL, and mix thoroughly, using a shear mixing method.
6. Package and label the product.

Lubricating Jelly Formula

Methylcellulose 4000 cP	0.8%	Thickener
Carbomer 934	0.24%	Thickener
Propylene glycol	16.7%	Vehicle
Methylparaben	0.015%	Preservative
Sodium hydroxide	qs pH 7	Alkalizer
Purified water	qs ad 100%	Vehicle

1. Calculate the required quantity of each ingredient for the total amount to be prepared.
2. Accurately weigh or measure each ingredient.
3. Disperse the methylcellulose in 40 mL of hot purified water (80°C–90°C).
4. Chill the mixture overnight in a refrigerator.
5. Disperse the carbomer 934 in 20 mL of purified water.
6. Adjust the pH of the dispersion to 7 by adding sufficient 1% sodium hydroxide solution (about 12 mL is required), and then add enough purified water to bring the volume to 40 mL.
7. Dissolve the methylparaben in the propylene glycol.
8. Carefully mix the methylcellulose, carbomer 934, and propylene glycol fractions to avoid incorporating air.
9. Package and label the product.

Methylcellulose Gels

Methylcellulose 1500 cP	1%–5%	Thickener
Purified water	qs 100%	Vehicle

1. Calculate the required quantity of each ingredient for the total amount to be prepared.
2. Accurately weigh or measure each ingredient.
3. Add the methylcellulose to about 50 mL of boiling purified water, and disperse well.
4. Add the remaining purified water, ice cold, to bring the volume of the gel to 100 mL.
5. Stir the mixture until uniform and thickened.
6. Package and label the product.

℞ Niacinamide 4% Acne Gel

Niacinamide	4 g	Active
Carbopol 940	600 mg	Thickener
Propylene glycol	20 mL	Vehicle/Cosolvent
Ethoxydiglycol	2 mL	Levigating Agent
Trolamine	3–4 drops	Alkalizer
Preserved water	73 mL	Vehicle

1. Calculate the quantity of each ingredient required for the prescription.
2. Accurately weigh or measure each ingredient.
3. Dissolve the niacinamide in the ethoxydiglycol and the preserved water.
4. Mix the Carbopol 940 with the propylene glycol.
5. Incorporate the solution from step 3 into step 4, and mix well.
6. Add the trolamine slowly with thorough mixing until the desired viscosity is obtained.
7. Package and label the product.

℞ Piroxicam 0.5% in an Alcoholic Gel (100 g)

Hydroxypropylcellulose	1.75 g	Thickener
70% Isopropyl alcohol	98.25 mL	Vehicle
Propylene glycol	4.1 mL	Levigating Agent
Polysorbate 80	1.7 mL	Surfactant
Piroxicam 20 mg capsules	25 capsules	Active

(Note: Piroxicam powder can be used if available.)

1. Calculate the quantity of each ingredient required for the prescription.
2. Accurately weigh or measure each ingredient.
3. Make the hydroxypropylcellulose gel by mixing the hydroxypropylcellulose in the 70% isopropyl alcohol until a clear gel results.
4. Make a paste with the piroxicam powder (from capsules), the propylene glycol, and the polysorbate 80.
5. Using geometric dilution, add enough hydroxypropylcellulose gel to the paste to make 100 g of the preparation.
6. Package and label the product.

(Note: Use an alcoholic water mixture, such as 70% isopropyl alcohol, or a gel may not form.)

Pluronic Lecithin Organogel (PLO) Gel

Lecithin and isopropyl palmitate liquid	20 mL	Vehicle
(Note: See preparation instructions below.)		
Pluronic F-127 20% gel	80 mL	Vehicle

1. Calculate the required quantity of each ingredient for the total amount to be prepared.
2. Accurately weigh or measure each ingredient.
3. Mix the two viscous liquids together well. A number of mixing techniques can be used, including using plastic bags, pushing the ingredients back and forth between two syringes fitted with a syringe adapter, and simply mixing in a mortar with a pestle. Minimize the incorporation of air.

The lecithin and isopropyl palmitate liquid is prepared as follows:

Soy lecithin, granular	10 g	Vehicle
Isopropyl palmitate NF	10 g	Vehicle
Sorbic acid	0.2 g	Preservative

1. Calculate the required quantity of each ingredient for the total amount to be prepared.
2. Accurately weigh or measure each ingredient.
3. Add the soy lecithin granules and the sorbic acid powder to the isopropyl palmitate liquid and allow to set overnight.
4. Mix by rolling or gentle agitation. Do not shake. Because the density of the isopropyl palmitate is about 0.855, a volume of 11.7 mL can be measured.

Poloxamer (Pluronic) Gel Base

Poloxamer F-127 NF	20–50 g	Thickener
Potassium sorbate NF	0.2 g	Preservative
Purified water/buffer	qs 100 mL	Vehicle

1. Calculate the required quantity of each ingredient for the total amount to be prepared.
2. Accurately weigh or measure each ingredient.
3. Add the powders and water to a bottle, and shake well.
4. Store in a refrigerator so that the gel will form.
5. Package and label the product.

℞ **Promethazine Hydrochloride 25 mg/mL Pluronic Lecithin Organogel**

Promethazine hydrochloride	2.5 g	Active
Ethoxydiglycol	5 mL	Solvent/Levigating Agent
Lecithin:isopropyl palmitate 1:1 solution	22 mL	Vehicle
Pluronic F-127 20% gel	qs 100 mL	Vehicle

1. Calculate the quantity of each ingredient required for the prescription.
2. Accurately weigh or measure each ingredient.
3. Mix the promethazine hydrochloride with the ethoxydiglycol to form a smooth paste.
4. Add the lecithin:isopropyl palmitate 1:1 solution, and mix well.
5. Add sufficient Pluronic F-127 20% gel to make 100 mL, and mix thoroughly, using a shear mixing method.
6. Package and label the product.

℞ **Scopolamine Hydrobromide 0.25 mg/0.1 mL Pluronic Lecithin Organogel**

Scopolamine hydrobromide	250 mg	Active
Soy lecithin:isopropyl palmitate 1:1 solution	25 mL	Vehicle
Buffer solution (pH 5)	2.5 mL	pH Adjustment
Pluronic F-127 gel, 20% dispersion	qs 100 mL	Vehicle

1. Calculate the quantity of each ingredient required for the prescription.
2. Accurately weigh or measure each ingredient.
3. Dissolve the scopolamine hydrobromide in the pH 5 buffer solution.
4. Add the soy lecithin:isopropyl palmitate 1:1 solution, and mix well.
5. Add sufficient 20% Pluronic F-127 gel to make 100 mL, and mix thoroughly.
6. Package and label the product.

Starch Glycerite

Starch	100 g	Thickener
Benzoic acid	2 g	Preservative
Purified water	200 g	Vehicle
Glycerin	700 g	Vehicle

1. Calculate the required quantity of each ingredient for the total amount to be prepared.
2. Accurately weigh or measure each ingredient.
3. Rub the starch and benzoic acid in the water to form a smooth mixture.
4. Add the glycerin, and mix well.
5. Heat the mixture to 140°C, applying constant, gentle agitation until a translucent mass forms. (Note: The heat ruptures the starch grains and permits the water to reach and hydrate the linear and branched starch molecules that trap the dispersion medium in the interstices to form a gel.)
6. Package and label the product.

Rx Vancomycin Gel (Vancomycin Paste, Vanc Paste)

Vancomycin	500 mg	Active
Aspartame	200 mg	Sweetener
Flavoring	qs	Flavoring
Sodium benzoate	200 mg	Preservative
Methylcellulose 2% gel	100 mL	Vehicle

1. Calculate the quantity of each ingredient required for the prescription.
2. Accurately weigh or measure each ingredient.
3. In a mortar, add a small quantity of the methylcellulose 2% gel to the vancomycin, aspartame, and sodium benzoate powders, and mix well.
4. Add the flavoring agent, and mix well.
5. Add additional methylcellulose 2% gel to almost reach 100 mL.
6. Transfer mixture to a previously calibrated container, add methylcellulose 2% gel to volume, and mix well.
7. Package and label the product.

Chapter 23

Ophthalmic, Otic, and Nasal Preparations

In this chapter, compounded preparations are grouped by route of administration—ophthalmic, otic, and nasal—rather than by dosage form, using the same sections as previous chapters.

Ophthalmic Preparations

Definitions and Types

Ophthalmic solutions are sterile, free from foreign particles, and prepared especially for instillation into the eye. *Ophthalmic suspensions* are sterile liquid preparations that contain solid particles in a vehicle suitable for instillation into the eye. *Ophthalmic ointments* are sterile preparations designed for application to the eye; they have an ointment base and may or may not include an active drug.

Historical Use

One of the early treatments of eye conditions with a liquid involved the use of the juice of a liver. This was one of the earlier preparations stemming from observations that applying substances topically to the eye was effective. In this case, the vitamin A content of the juice was effective in treating the condition. Throughout history, various plant extracts have been prepared and used for eye conditions. Current vehicles for ophthalmic liquids include primarily sterile, buffered aqueous systems that contain preservatives.

Eye "salves" were prepared during the time of the early Roman Empire by *medici ocularii*, or men who specialized in preparing such salves. One such preparation was described on a piece of green steatite as containing "crocus of Lucius Vallatinus for affectations of the eyes." Evidence exists that ophthalmic ointments were used throughout the Roman Empire, even in outlying areas such as Scotland. Ointments that were developed later used oils and fats as their vehicles. More recently, the petrolatums were used as vehicles for these ophthalmic preparations.

Applications

Ophthalmic preparations are used to treat allergies, bacterial and viral infections, glaucoma, and numerous other eye conditions. The eye is constantly exposed to the atmosphere, dust, pollutants, allergens, bacteria, and foreign bodies. When the eye's natural defensive mechanisms are compromised or overcome, an ophthalmic preparation, in a solution, suspension, or ointment form, may be indicated. Solutions are used most often to deliver a drug to the eye. Although solutions have a relatively short duration of action, they spread easily over the globe and cover well. Suspensions have a slightly longer duration of action because the particles will usually settle in the lower conjunctival sac and release the drug as the particles dissolve. Ointments have an even longer duration of action. The ointment spreads over the eye and into the conjunctival sac. The active drug is released slowly as the vehicle is slowly removed from the eye.

Composition

In addition to the active drugs, ophthalmic preparations contain a number of excipients, including vehicles, buffers, preservatives, tonicity-adjusting agents, antioxidants, and viscosity enhancers. Ingredients used in the formulation process must be nonirritating to and compatible with the eyes.

Preparation

All preparation must be done in a clean air environment by a qualified aseptic compounding pharmacist. The pharmacist must ensure that all the ingredients are of the highest grade that can be reasonably obtained. Box 23-1 lists the steps involved in preparing ophthalmic solutions, suspensions, and ointments. General Chapter <797>, Pharmaceutical Compounding—Sterile Preparations, of the *United States Pharmacopeia/National Formulary* provides more information.[1]

Ophthalmic ointments must be prepared so that they are nonirritating to the eye, permit diffusion of the drug, and retain the activity of the drug for a reasonable period of time when stored properly. White petrolatum is the base primarily used for ophthalmic ointments. Aqueous solutions of the drug can be incorporated by using an absorption base, as long as it does not irritate the eye. One example is anhydrous lanolin mixed with white petrolatum. A pharmacist must be aware that surfactants used to make absorption bases can cause eye irritation. Powders incorporated in the preparation must be micronized and sterilized to ensure that the final preparation is not gritty and thus is nonirritating.

The size of the particles in an ophthalmic suspension must be small enough that they do not irritate or scratch the cornea. The micronized form of the drug is required. Ophthalmic suspensions must be free from agglomeration or caking.

Physicochemical Considerations

In preparing ophthalmic solutions, a pharmacist must consider the general physicochemical parameters: clarity, tonicity, pH and buffers, and sterility. The addition of excipients such as preservatives, antioxidants, and viscosity enhancers, as well as potential incompatibilities between these excipients and active drugs, should be considered.

Clarity

Ophthalmic solutions must be free from foreign particles. Filtration is usually used to remove these particles and to achieve clarity of the solution. Polysorbate 20 and polysorbate 80, in a maximum concentration of 1%, can be used to achieve clarity.

BOX 23-1 Preparation of Ophthalmic Formulations

Solutions
1. Accurately weigh or measure each ingredient.
2. Dissolve the ingredients in about three-fourths of the quantity of sterile water for injection, and mix well.
3. Add sufficient sterile water for injection to volume, and mix well.
4. Take a sample of the solution, and determine the pH, clarity, and other quality control factors.
5. Package and label the product.
6. If a large number of solutions are to be prepared, select a random sample to be assayed and checked for sterility.

Suspensions
1. Accurately weigh or measure each ingredient.
2. Dissolve the ingredients in about three-fourths of the quantity of sterile water for injection, and mix well.
3. Add sufficient sterile water for injection to volume, and mix well.
4. Take a sample of the solution, and determine the pH and other quality control factors.
5. Package the product in a suitable container.
6. If a large number of suspensions are to be prepared, select a random sample to be assayed.

Ointments
1. Accurately weigh or measure each ingredient.
2. Sterilize each ingredient by a suitable method.
3. Using aseptic technique, mix the ingredients with the sterile vehicle.
4. Take a sample of the ointment, and determine the quality control factors.
5. Package and label the product.
6. If a large number of ointments are to be prepared, select a random sample to be assayed and checked for sterility.

Tonicity

For comfort during administration, many dosage forms must be isotonic with body fluids. This is especially true of parenterals, ophthalmics, and nasal solutions. Pain and irritation at the site of administration can occur if the formulation is either hypertonic or hypotonic.

The tonicity of solutions is a colligative property; it depends primarily on the number of dissolved particles in solution (i.e., $KCl \rightarrow K^+ + Cl^-$, two particles). In addition to osmotic pressure, colligative properties include changes in vapor pressure, boiling point, and freezing point. *Osmotic pressure* is the pressure that must be applied to a more concentrated solution just to prevent the flow of pure solvent into the solution through a semipermeable membrane.

Biologic systems are compatible with solutions having similar osmotic pressures (i.e., an equivalent number of dissolved species). For example, red blood cells, blood plasma, and 0.9% sodium chloride solution contain approximately the same number of solute particles per unit volume and are termed *iso-osmotic* and *isotonic*. If solutions do not contain the same number of dissolved species (i.e., they contain more [hypertonic] or fewer [hypotonic]), then the composition of the solution may need to be altered to bring them into an acceptable range. An osmol (Osm) is related to a mole (gram molecular weight) of the molecules or ions in solution. One mole of glucose (180 g) dissolved in 1000 g of water has an osmolality of 1 Osm, or 1000 mOsm/kg of water. One mole of sodium chloride (23 + 35.5 = 58.5 g) dissolved in 1000 g of water has an osmolality of almost 2 Osm or 2000 mOsm because sodium chloride dissociates into almost two particles per molecule. In other words, a 1-molal solution of sodium chloride is equivalent to a 2-molal solution of dextrose.

Normal serum osmolality values are in the vicinity of 285 mOsm/kg (often expressed as 285 mOsm/L), with a range of about 275 to 300 mOsm/L. Pharmaceutical preparations should be close to this value to minimize discomfort when applied to the eyes or nose or when injected.

Lacrimal fluid is isotonic, or equivalent in tonicity to 0.9% sodium chloride solution. However, the eye can tolerate values as low as 0.6% and as high as 1.8% sodium chloride equivalency. Some ophthalmic solutions will be hypertonic because of the high concentration of the drug substance. Others will be hypotonic and will require adjustment into the proper tonicity range; sodium chloride, boric acid, and dextrose are commonly used for this purpose. The ideal tonicity is 300 mOsm/L; however, a range of 200 to 600 mOsm/L is acceptable. Hypotonicity can be easily addressed by a compounding pharmacist, but hypertonicity can be addressed only when decreasing the concentration of some components of the formulation is possible.

Pharmacists can use the sodium chloride equivalent method to calculate the quantity of solute that must be added to render a hypotonic solution of a drug isotonic. A sodium chloride equivalent is defined as the amount of sodium chloride that is osmotically equivalent to 1 g of the drug. For example, the sodium chloride equivalent of ephedrine sulfate is 0.23 (i.e., 1 g of ephedrine sulfate is equivalent to 0.23 g of sodium chloride). Chapter 7 of this book provides examples of this calculation. Table 23-1 lists agents used to adjust tonicity.

pH and Buffering

Ophthalmic solutions are ordinarily buffered at the pH of maximum stability for the drug(s) they contain. Buffers are included to minimize any change in pH that can occur during the storage life of the drug, such as from carbon dioxide absorption from the air or absorption of hydroxyl ions from a glass container. Minimizing changes in pH is important because they can affect the solubility and the stability of drugs. Buffer systems should be designed to maintain pH throughout the expected shelf life of the preparation. The buffer capacity should be

TABLE 23-1 Characteristics of Agents Used to Adjust Tonicity

Agent	Solubility (mL)[a]			Sodium Chloride Equivalent (E1%)	Iso-osmotic Concentration (%)	Volume Needed (mL)[b]	Packaging
	Water	Ethanol	Glycerin				
Dextrose	1	100	—	0.16	5.51	6	W
Glycerin	Misc	Misc	Misc	—	2.6	11.7	T
Mannitol	5.5	—	—	—	—	—	W
Potassium chloride	2.8	—	—	0.76	1.19	25.3	W
Sodium chloride	2.8	—	10	1.0	0.9	—	W

— = Not available.
[a]Volume required to dissolve 1 g of the drug.
[b]Volume of water added to 300 mg of the agent to produce an isotonic solution.

low enough that when the ophthalmic solution is dropped into the eye, the buffer system of the tears will rapidly bring the pH of the solution back to that of the tears. Thus, a pharmacist should use a concentration of buffer salt that is effective but as low as possible. Generally, a buffer capacity of less than 0.05 is desired; pH in the range of 4 to 8 is considered optimum.

Sterility

Ophthalmic solutions must be sterile. Sterility is best achieved by sterile filtration, which involves using a sterile membrane filter with a pore size of 0.45 μm or 0.2 μm and filtering into a sterile container. Other methods of sterilizing ingredients or components of ophthalmics include dry heat, steam under pressure (autoclaving, Figure 23-1), and gas sterilization with ethylene oxide.

Preservatives

Because most ophthalmic solutions and suspensions are prepared in multiuse containers, they must be preserved. The preservative must be compatible with the active drug as well as with all the other excipients in the preparation. Common preservatives for ophthalmic preparations are shown in Table 23-2.

Antioxidants

Antioxidants may be required for some active drug ingredients. Table 23-3 lists a number of antioxidants that can be used in ophthalmic preparations.

Viscosity Enhancers

If an ophthalmic solution is viscous, the preparation will remain in the eye longer and will thereby allow more time for drug absorption and effect. For this reason, viscosity enhancers are used. The most common is methylcellulose, generally in a concentration of about 0.25% if the 4000 cP grade is used. If methylcellulose is autoclaved, it will come out of solution; however, it can be redispersed after cooling, especially if placed in a refrigerator. Solution viscosity ranging from 25 to 50 cP is common with hydroxypropyl methylcellulose, methylcellulose, or polyvinyl alcohol. Maintaining the clarity of the solution with all these enhancers is important. Additives that increase viscosity are shown in Table 23-4.

Incompatibilities

Because zinc salts can form insoluble hydroxides at a pH above 6.4, a vehicle of boric acid solution can be used. Boric acid solution has a lower pH (about pH 5) and a slight buffering action.

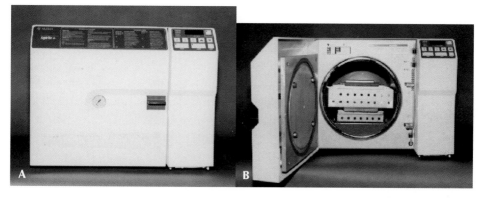

FIGURE 23-1 Microprocessor-controlled sterilizer/autoclave. A: exterior view; B: interior view.

TABLE 23-2 Preservatives Used in Ophthalmic, Otic, and Nasal Preparations

Preservative	Usual Concentration (%)	Concentration Range (%)	Maximum Concentration (%)[a]	Incompatibilities
Chlorobutanol			0.5	
Quaternary ammonium compounds	0.01	0.004–0.02		Soaps, anionic materials, salicylates, nitrates
Benzalkonium chloride			0.013	
Benzethonium chloride			0.01	
Organic mercurials		0.001–0.01		Certain halides with phenyl-mercuric acetate
Phenylmercuric acetate			0.004	
Phenylmercuric nitrate			0.004	
Thimerosal			0.01	
Parahydroxybenzoates			0.1	Adsorption by macro-molecules

[a]The U.S. Food and Drug Administration Advisory Review Panel on OTC Ophthalmic Drug Products (1979) lists these concentrations for preparations that have direct contact with the eye tissues and not for ocular devices such as contact lens products.

Nitrates or salicylates are incompatible with solutions of benzalkonium chloride. Therefore, benzalkonium chloride should be replaced with 0.002% phenylmercuric nitrate.

Sodium chloride cannot be used to adjust the tonicity of silver nitrate solutions because silver chloride would precipitate. Instead, sodium nitrate should be used to adjust the tonicity, and phenylmercuric nitrate can be used as the preservative in this situation.

TABLE 23-3 Antioxidants Used in Ophthalmic and Nasal Preparations

Antioxidant	Usual Maximum Concentration (%)
Ethylenediaminetetraacetic acid	0.1
Sodium bisulfite	0.1
Sodium metabisulfite	0.1
Thiourea	0.1

TABLE 23-4 Viscosity Enhancers for Ophthalmic Preparations

Additive	Usual Maximum Concentration (%)
Hydroxyethylcellulose	0.8
Hydroxypropyl methylcellulose	1.0
Methylcellulose	2.0
Polyvinyl alcohol	1.4
Polyvinylpyrrolidone	1.7

Quality Control

A compounding pharmacist should follow standard quality control procedures. These procedures include checking sterility, clarity, appearance, pH, and volume or weight. Sterility can be checked by plating a sample of the preparation on an agar plate and checking for microbial growth. If this procedure is not feasible, samples of the formulation can be sent to a laboratory for testing.

Packaging, Storage, and Labeling

Ophthalmic solutions should be packaged in sterile dropper bottles. Individual doses can also be placed in sterile syringes without needles. Generally, these preparations should be stored at either room or refrigerated temperature. They should not be frozen. Ophthalmic preparations should be labeled "For the Eye," "Do Not Touch the Eye or Eyelid," "Store as Indicated," and "Dispose after [appropriate date]."

Stability

Water-containing formulations for topical use made from ingredients in solid form should have beyond-use dates of 30 days when stored at cold temperatures. If nonaqueous liquids are prepared with a manufactured product, the recommended beyond-use date is no later than 25% of the time remaining until the product's expiration date or 6 months, whichever is earlier. These recommended dates can be extended if valid scientific information is available to support the stability of the preparation, as discussed in Chapter 6 of this book.

Patient Counseling

Patients should be instructed on how to administer drops or ointments to the eye. Specifically, they should be cautioned not to allow the tip of the dropper or ointment tube to touch any part of the eye. They should be instructed to allow the drug to fall freely into the eye and not to allow the drug to touch the eye and then be drawn back into the bottle. See Box 23-2 for additional suggestions.

BOX 23-2 Hints for Administration of Ophthalmic Preparations

Suggestions for the administration of ophthalmic preparations are as follows:

- The normal volume of tear fluid in the eye is about 10 µL. The volume of an average drop is 25 to 50 µL. Consequently, only 1 drop should be administered to the eye at one time.
- If more than 1 drop or more than one drug is to be administered, a patient or caregiver should wait at least 5 minutes between doses to allow the drug to be distributed and absorbed.
- Immediately after instilling a drop into the eye, placing pressure on the lacrimal sac for a minute or two will help decrease systemic absorption of the drug that occurs when the drug is removed by the nasolacrimal duct and swallowed, thereby entering the gastrointestinal tract.
- An advantage of ophthalmic suspensions is that they dissolve slowly and remain in the cul-de-sac longer.
- Ophthalmic ointments provide maximum contact between the drug and the eye because they are cleared quite slowly (0.5% per minute) from the eye.
- The size of a drop delivered can vary with the angle of the dropper and the size of the dropper orifice.

Sample Formulations
Vehicles

The steps listed for solutions in Box 23-1 should be followed to prepare these vehicles.

Isotonic Sodium Chloride Solution

Sodium chloride USP	0.9 g	Tonicity Adjuster
Benzalkonium chloride	1:10,000	Preservative
Sterile water for injection	qs 100 mL	Vehicle

Three buffer solutions have been suggested for certain drugs when they are prepared as ophthalmic solutions. These drugs have been divided into three classes and are listed with the recommended buffer solution for that class.

Buffer Solution IA

Boric acid USP	1.9 g	Buffer
Benzalkonium chloride	1:10,000	Preservative
Sterile water for injection	qs 100 mL	Vehicle

The following drugs in Class IA can be placed in Buffer Solution IA, which has a pH of about 5:

- Cocaine
- Dibucaine
- Neostigmine
- Phenacaine
- Piperocaine
- Procaine
- Tetracaine
- Zinc

Buffer Solution IB

Boric acid USP	1.9 g	Buffer
Sodium sulfite, anhydrous	0.1 g	Antioxidant
Phenylmercuric nitrate	1:50,000	Preservative
Sterile water for injection	qs 100 mL	Vehicle

Some drugs can be incompatible with Buffer Solution IA because of an incompatibility with benzalkonium chloride. Buffer Solution IB contains a different preservative, phenylmercuric nitrate. Sodium sulfite has been added to prevent discoloration or oxidation of some of the drugs in this category. Drugs that are incompatible in Buffer Solution IA but can be prepared by using Buffer Solution IB include the following Class IB drugs:

- Epinephrine
- Phenylephrine
- Physostigmine

Buffer Solution II

Sodium acid phosphate, anhydrous	0.56 g	Buffer
Disodium phosphate, anhydrous	0.284 g	Buffer
Sodium chloride USP	0.5 g	Tonicity Adjuster
Disodium edetate	0.1 g	Chelating Agent
Benzalkonium chloride	1:10,000	Preservative
Sterile water for injection	qs 100 mL	Vehicle

Drugs in Class II that can be prepared in Buffer Solution II include the following:

- Atropine
- Ephedrine
- Homatropine
- Pilocarpine

Ingredient-Specific Preparations

Artificial Tears Solution

Polyvinyl alcohol	1.5%	Thickener
Povidone	0.5%	Thickener
Chlorobutanol	0.5%	Preservative
0.9% Sodium chloride solution	qs	Vehicle

1. Calculate the required quantity of each ingredient for the total amount to be prepared.
2. Accurately weigh or measure each ingredient.
3. Dissolve all ingredients in the sterile 0.9% sodium chloride solution.
4. Filter the solution through a 0.2-μm filter into a sterile ophthalmic container.
5. Package and label the product.

Cocaine Hydrochloride Ophthalmic Solution

Cocaine hydrochloride	5 g	Active
Ethylenediaminetetraacetic acid	10 mg	Chelator
Benzalkonium chloride	10 mg	Preservative
Sterile 0.9% sodium chloride solution	qs 100 mL	Vehicle

1. Calculate the quantity of each ingredient required for the prescription.
2. Accurately weigh or measure each ingredient.
3. Dissolve the cocaine hydrochloride, ethylenediaminetetraacetic acid, and benzalkonium chloride in sufficient sterile 0.9% sodium chloride solution to make 100 mL.
4. Filter the solution through a sterile 0.2-μm filter into a sterile container.
5. Package and label the product.

℞ Cyclosporine Ophthalmic Solution

Cyclosporine 10% oral solution	2%	Active
Corn oil or olive oil	qs	Vehicle

1. Calculate the quantity of each ingredient required for the prescription.
2. Accurately weigh or measure each ingredient.
3. Use alcohol to clean the container to be used for mixing the oral cyclosporine 10% solution and oil.
4. Clean a commercial container of cyclosporine 10% solution with alcohol; open the container, and place it in a laminar-airflow hood for about 24 hours to allow the alcohol to evaporate.
5. Add four volumes of corn oil or olive oil with one volume of the 10% cyclosporine oral solution to the previously cleaned container, and mix thoroughly.
6. Filter the solution through a 0.2-μm filter into a sterile, dry ophthalmic container.
7. Package and label the product.

℞ Ophthalmic Decongestant Solution

Phenylephrine hydrochloride	0.125%	Active
Polyvinyl alcohol	1.4%	Thickener
Disodium edetate	0.05%	Chelator
Sodium acetate	0.1%	Buffer
Monobasic sodium phosphate	0.1%	Buffer
Dibasic sodium phosphate	0.05%	Buffer
Sodium thiosulfate	0.1%	Antioxidant
Sterile water for injection	qs 100%	Vehicle

1. Calculate the quantity of each ingredient required for the prescription.
2. Accurately weigh or measure each ingredient.
3. Dissolve all the ingredients in sterile water for injection.
4. Filter the solution through a sterile 0.2-μm filter into a sterile container.
5. Package and label the product.

Ophthalmic Lubricant

White petrolatum	55%	Vehicle
Mineral oil	41.5%	Vehicle
Lanolin alcohol	2%	Vehicle
0.9% Sodium chloride injection	1.5%	Vehicle

1. Calculate the required quantity of each ingredient for the total amount to be prepared.
2. Accurately weigh or measure each ingredient.
3. Mix the white petrolatum, mineral oil, and lanolin alcohol together, using a water bath.
4. Sterilize the mixture with dry heat.
5. Using aseptic technique, cool the sterile mixture in a laminar-airflow hood.
6. Incorporate the sterile 0.9% sodium chloride injection, and mix.
7. Package the solution in sterile containers.

℞ Tobramycin-Fortified Ophthalmic Solution

| Tobramycin ophthalmic solution | 5 mL | Active |
| Tobramycin injection, 80 mg/2 mL | 1 mL | Active |

1. Calculate the quantity of each ingredient required for the prescription.
2. Prepare the formulation, using aseptic technique.
3. Accurately measure each ingredient.
4. Mix the ingredients well.
5. Package and label the product.

℞ Acetylcysteine 10% Ophthalmic Solution

Acetylcysteine	10%	2 g (10 mL of a 20% solution)	Active
Disodium edetate	0.025%	5 mg	Chelator
Chlorobutanol	0.5%	100 mg	Preservative
Artificial tears solution		qs 20 mL	Vehicle

(Note: Prepare solution in a clean air environment.)

1. Calculate the quantity of each ingredient required for the prescription.
2. Accurately weigh or measure each ingredient.
3. Place the chlorobutanol in a clean, previously sterilized beaker.
4. Add 9 mL of artificial tears solution.
5. Cover the solution, and stir (with a magnetic mixer with stir bar) until dissolved.
6. Add the disodium edetate to the solution.
7. Add 10 mL of 20% acetylcysteine oral inhalation solution.
8. Filter the solution through a 0.2-μm filter into a sterile ophthalmic container.
9. Package and label the product.

℞ Tropicamide–Hydroxyamphetamine Hydrobromide Ophthalmic Solution

Tropicamide	0.25%	250 mg	Active
Hydroxyamphetamine hydrobromide	1%	1 g	Active
Benzalkonium chloride	0.005%	5 mg	Preservative
Disodium edetate	0.5%	500 mg	Chelator
Sodium chloride		490 mg	Tonicity Adjuster
Sodium hydroxide or hydrochloric acid		To adjust pH to 4.2–5.8	pH Adjuster
Sterile water for injection		qs 100 mL	Vehicle

1. Calculate the quantity of each ingredient required for the prescription.
2. Accurately weigh or measure each ingredient.
3. Dissolve the solid ingredients in approximately 50 mL of sterile water for injection.
4. Add the benzalkonium chloride dilution to the solution, and mix well.
5. Add sufficient water to make about 90 mL, and mix well.
6. Adjust the pH to between 4.2 and 5.8, using the sodium hydroxide or hydrochloric acid.
7. Add sufficient sterile water for injection to make 100 mL.
8. Filter the solution through a 0.2-μm filter into sterile containers.
9. Package and label the product.

The benzalkonium chloride for this prescription can be prepared as follows:

1. Accurately measure 1 mL of 50% benzalkonium chloride solution.
2. Place in a 100-mL graduated cylinder.
3. Add sufficient sterile water for injection to make 100 mL, and mix well.
4. Remove 1 mL of the solution, which contains 5 mg of benzalkonium chloride, and add it to the solution containing the active drug.

℞ Cefazolin Ophthalmic Solution USP

Cefazolin sodium	350 mg	Active
Thimerosal	2 mg	Preservative
0.9% Sodium chloride injection	qs 100 mL	Vehicle

(Note: This formulation should be prepared in an aseptic working environment, using aseptic technique, by a validated aseptic compounding pharmacist.)

1. Calculate the quantity of each ingredient required for the prescription.
2. Accurately weigh or measure each ingredient.
3. Dissolve the cefazolin sodium and thimerosal in about 90 mL of the 0.9% sodium chloride injection.
4. Add sufficient 0.9% sodium chloride injection to volume, and mix well.
5. Sterilize solution by filtering through a sterile 0.2-μm filter into sterile ophthalmic containers.
6. Package and label the product.

℞ Interferon 10 × 10⁶ units/mL Ophthalmic Solution

Interferon alfa-2a	100×10^6 units	Active
Ammonium acetate	7.7 mg	Buffer
Benzyl alcohol	100 mg	Preservative
Human albumin	10 mg	Stabilizer
Sterile water for injection	qs 10 mL	Vehicle

1. Calculate the quantity of each ingredient required for the prescription.
2. Accurately weigh or measure each ingredient. Roferon-A can be used to provide the interferon alfa-2a. (Note: The final volume may need to be adjusted depending on the source of the interferon.)
3. Dissolve the ammonium acetate, benzyl alcohol, and albumin in about 8 mL of the sterile water for injection.
4. Add the interferon alfa-2a, and mix well.
5. Add sufficient sterile water for injection, and mix well.
6. Sterilize the solution by filtering through a sterile 0.2-μm filter into a sterile ophthalmic container.
7. Package and label the product.

℞ Lissamine Green 0.5% Ophthalmic Solution

Lissamine green	500 mg	Active
Sterile water for injection	25 mL	Vehicle
0.9% Sodium chloride injection	qs 100 mL	Vehicle

1. Calculate the quantity of each ingredient required for the prescription.
2. Accurately weigh or measure each ingredient.
3. Dissolve the lissamine green in the sterile water for injection.
4. Add sufficient sterile 0.9% sodium chloride injection to volume, and mix well.
5. Sterilize the solution by filtering through a sterile 0.2-μm filter into sterile containers.
6. Package and label the product.

℞ **Tobramycin Sulfate 0.3% and Diclofenac Sodium 0.1% Ophthalmic Solution (100 mL)**

Tobramycin sulfate injection	300 mg	Active
Diclofenac sodium	100 mg	Active
Sodium chloride	806 mg	Tonicity
Sterile water for injection	qs 100 mL	Vehicle

(Note: This formulation should be prepared in a laminar-airflow hood, using aseptic technique, by a validated aseptic compounding pharmacist.)

1. Calculate the quantity of each ingredient required for the prescription.
2. Accurately weigh or measure each ingredient. The tobramycin sulfate can be obtained from 7.5 mL of the tobramycin sulfate 40 mg/mL injection.
3. Dissolve the powders in sufficient sterile water for injection to make about 90 mL of solution.
4. Add the tobramycin sulfate injection, followed by sufficient sterile water for injection to 100 mL, and mix well. Adjust the pH to 7 to 8 if necessary.
5. Sterilize the solution by filtering through a sterile 0.2-μm filter into sterile containers.
6. Package and label the product.

Otic Preparations

Definitions and Types

Otic preparations can be in liquid, ointment, or powder dosage forms. Both *otic solutions* and *otic suspensions,* the liquid dosage forms, are prepared for instillation into the ear. Solutions are liquid preparations in which all ingredients are dissolved, whereas suspensions are liquid preparations containing insoluble materials. Solutions are also used for irrigating the ear. *Otic ointments* are semisolid preparations that are applied to the exterior of the ear. *Insufflations* are preparations made of finely divided powder that are administered to the ear canal. Insufflating a powder into the ear canal is not too common because the ear lacks fluids and a powder–wax buildup can occur.

Historical Use

Throughout history, medications have been administered to the ear for a local effect. Early otic preparations were applied by soaking materials, such as cloth, wood, or plants, in various oils or extracts from plants or animals and then placing the impregnated materials in the ear. A more recent method of applying otic preparations involves placing a liquid in the ear and inserting a cotton plug to keep the medication from draining out of the ear. This method is still used today, together with the use of ear irrigants, which clean debris from the ear. This debris is the cause of many otic infections.

Applications

Otic irrigating solutions, which can consist of surfactants, weak sodium bicarbonate, boric acid (0.5%–1%), or aluminum acetate solutions, can be warmed to about 37°C before instillation into the ear. These irrigating solutions can be used to remove earwax, purulent discharges of infection, and foreign bodies from the ear canal.

Otic suspensions can be used when a long duration of drug effect is desired or when the drug is not soluble in the vehicles commonly used in otic preparations.

Otic ointments are seldom used. Any ointment base can be used in their preparation, however, and they can include antibacterial, antifungal, or corticosteroid ingredients. These ointments are applied directly to the exterior portions of the ear.

Fine powders used as insufflations can serve as a repository for an antibacterial or antifungal agent. A small rubber or plastic bulb insufflator (powder blower or puffer) can be used to blow, or insufflate, the powder into the ear.

Composition

Categories of medications commonly used in the ear are local anesthetics, cleansing agents (peroxides), and anti-infective and antifungal agents. Also included are liquids for cleaning, warming, or drying the external ear and for removing any fluids that can be entrapped by local waxy buildup.

Vehicles used most often in otic preparations are glycerin, propylene glycol, and the lower-molecular-weight polyethylene glycols (PEGs), especially PEG 300. These vehicles are viscous and will adhere to the ear canal. Water and alcohol (ethanol and isopropyl) can be used as vehicles and solvents for some medications. However, because they moisten the ear canal, they are used primarily for irrigation; a therapeutic aim of these preparations is to keep the ear canal dry to minimize bacterial or fungal growth. Full-strength alcohol can be used. Vegetable oils, especially olive oil, are good vehicles. Mineral oil has been used as a vehicle for some antibiotics and anti-inflammatory medications. Otic ointments primarily contain petrolatum as a vehicle, whereas otic powders can contain talc or lactose as a vehicle.

Preparation

The method of formulating otic preparations is similar for all four dosage forms. The specific steps involved in preparing otic solutions, suspensions, ointments, and powders are listed in Box 23-3.

Physicochemical Considerations

Physicochemical considerations in developing otic preparations include solubility, viscosity, tonicity, surfactant properties, and preservatives. Although sterility is not generally a consideration, the preparations need to be clean.

Many drugs are soluble in the vehicles commonly used in these preparations. If a drug is insoluble in these vehicles, the preparation can be formulated as a suspension. Because most of these vehicles are relatively viscous agents, the addition of suspending agents may not be necessary.

The viscosity of the preparation is important for keeping the medication in the ear canal. If the preparation is too thin, the medication will drain from the ear. However, if the medication is too thick, it may not reach the inner recesses of the ear.

Hygroscopicity and tonicity are important in the preparation's ability to aid in withdrawing fluids from the immediate area of the ear. If the preparation is hypertonic, some fluid can be withdrawn from the ear, thereby releasing some of the pressure. If the preparation is hypotonic, however, some fluid may flow into the area.

Because many ear conditions are related to the difficulty of cleaning the ear, the presence of a surfactant in the preparation helps the medication spread out and aids in breaking up earwax. This allows for easier removal of any foreign material.

Many otic preparations are self-preserving because of the high concentration of glycerin, propylene glycol, or the like. If these agents are not present, adding a preservative to minimize

BOX 23-3 Preparation of Otic Formulations

Solutions
1. Accurately weigh or measure each ingredient.
2. Dissolve the ingredients in about three-fourths of the quantity of the vehicle, and mix well.
3. Add sufficient vehicle to volume, and mix well.
4. Take a sample of the solution, and determine the pH, clarity, and other quality control factors.
5. Package and label the product.

Suspensions
1. Accurately weigh or measure each ingredient.
2. Dissolve the ingredients in about three-fourths of the quantity of the vehicle, and mix well.
3. Add sufficient vehicle to volume, and mix well.
4. Take a sample of the suspension, and determine the pH and other quality control factors.
5. Package the product in a suitable container.
6. Label the product.

Ointments
1. Accurately weigh or measure each ingredient.
2. Mix each of the ingredients with the vehicle.
3. Take a sample of the ointment, and determine the quality control factors.
4. Package and label the product.

Powders
1. Accurately weigh or measure each ingredient.
2. Geometrically mix the powders together, starting with the powders present in the smallest quantity.
3. Take a sample of the powder, and determine the quality control factors.
4. Package and label the product.

the chance of introducing bacteria that might grow in an unpreserved preparation may be wise.

Quality Control

A compounding pharmacist should follow standard quality control procedures, checking the volume or weight, pH, viscosity, appearance, and odor of these preparations.

Packaging, Storage, and Labeling

Otic preparations should be packaged in dropper containers (Figure 23-2), puffers, or tubes appropriate for the preparation and method of administration. Generally, otic preparations should be stored at room or refrigerated temperatures. They should not

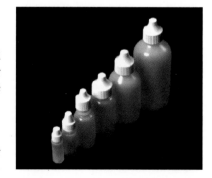

FIGURE 23-2 Dropper containers in various sizes (3 mL, 7 mL, 15 mL, 30 mL, 60 mL, 125 mL).

be frozen. These preparations should be labeled "For the Ear," "Discard after [appropriate date]," and "Use Only as Directed."

Stability

Water-containing formulations prepared from ingredients in solid form should have beyond-use dates of no later than 30 days when stored at cold temperatures. If nonaqueous liquids are prepared with a manufactured product, the recommended beyond-use date is no later than 25% of the time remaining until the product's expiration date or 6 months, whichever is earlier. These recommended dates can be extended if valid scientific information is available to support the stability of the preparation, as discussed in Chapter 6 of this book.

Patient Counseling

Patients should be instructed on how to apply drops to the ear from dropper bottles. They should be told to place a cotton or gauze pad in the ear to keep the liquid from escaping.

Sample Formulation

℞ Benzocaine Otic Solution

Benzocaine	200 mg	Active
Glycerin	qs 15 mL	Vehicle

1. Calculate the quantity of each ingredient required for the prescription.
2. Accurately weigh or measure each ingredient.
3. Dissolve the benzocaine in sufficient glycerin to make 15 mL of solution.
4. Package and label the product.

Nasal Preparations

Definitions and Types

Nasal solutions are prepared for administration either as drops or as sprays. *Nasal suspensions* are liquid preparations containing insoluble materials. *Nasal gels* and *ointments* are semisolid preparations for nasal application that can be used for either local or systemic effects. The gels are generally water soluble.

Historical Use

Collunaria is the term for early nasal preparations that contained various oils as the vehicles. When the harm from spraying or dropping mineral oil into the nose became apparent, preparation shifted to the use of aqueous vehicles. With some modifications, aqueous vehicles are used currently in these preparations. In recent years, the trend has been toward developing isotonic, preserved vehicles that do not interfere with the action of nasal cilia.

Applications

A number of drug substances can be prepared as nasal solutions to be administered as either drops or sprays; other dosage forms include nasal gels, jellies, or ointments. Some drugs are sufficiently volatile that they can be carried into the nose through an inhaler.

Composition

In addition to the active drugs, nasal preparations contain a number of excipients, including vehicles, buffers, preservatives, tonicity-adjusting agents, gelling agents, and, possibly, antioxidants. Ingredients used in the formulation process must be nonirritating and compatible with the nose.

Preparation
The methods used to formulate the four dosage forms of nasal preparations are similar. The steps to be followed in preparing nasal solutions, suspensions, ointments, and gels are listed in Box 23-4.

Physicochemical Considerations
A vehicle for a nasal solution should have a pH in the range of 5.5 to 7.5 and a mild buffer capacity. It should be isotonic, stable, preserved, and compatible with normal ciliary motion and ionic constituents of nasal secretions, as well as with the active ingredient. It should not modify the normal mucus viscosity.

pH and Buffering
Nasal preparations are ordinarily buffered at the pH of maximum stability for the drug(s) they contain. The buffers are included to minimize any change in pH that can occur during the storage life of the drug. Minimizing pH changes is important because they can affect the solubility and the stability of drugs. The buffer system should be designed to maintain the pH throughout the expected shelf life of the preparation, but with a low buffer capacity. Generally, pH in the range of 4 to 8 is considered optimum. Phosphate buffer systems are usually compatible with most nasal medications.

Tonicity Adjustment
The preferred agents for adjusting the tonicity of nasal solutions are sodium chloride and dextrose. Severely hypertonic solutions should be avoided. Nasal fluid is isotonic, or equivalent in tonicity to 0.9% sodium chloride solution. If tonicity is beyond the proper range, the nasal ciliary movement can slow or even stop. Tonicity values ranging from 0.6% to 1.8% sodium chloride equivalency are generally acceptable. If the solution of the active drug is hypotonic, adding a substance to attain the proper tonicity may be necessary. Sodium chloride, boric acid, and dextrose are commonly used for this purpose. A tonicity of 300 mOsm/L is ideal, although a range of 200 to 600 mOsm/L is acceptable.

Sterility
Nasal preparations are not required to be sterile.

Antioxidants
Antioxidants may be required for some active drug ingredients. Table 23-3 contains antioxidants that can be used in nasal preparations.

Other Excipients
Because most nasal preparations are prepared in multiuse containers, they must be preserved. The preservative used must be compatible with the active drug as well as with all other excipients in the preparation. Common preservatives that can be used for nasal preparations are shown in Table 23-2.

Quality Control
A compounding pharmacist should follow standard quality control procedures, including checks for tonicity, clarity (for solutions), pH, and volume or weight.

BOX 23-4 Preparation of Nasal Formulations

Solutions

1. Accurately weigh or measure each ingredient.
2. Dissolve the ingredients in about three-fourths of the quantity of sterile water for injection, and mix well.
3. Add sufficient sterile water for injection to volume, and mix well.
4. Take a sample of the solution, and determine the pH, clarity, and other quality control factors.
5. Package and label the product.
6. If a large number of solutions are to be prepared, select a random sample to be assayed and checked for sterility.

Suspensions

1. Accurately weigh or measure each ingredient.
2. Dissolve the ingredients in about three-fourths of the quantity of sterile water for injection, and mix well.
3. Add sufficient sterile water for injection to volume, and mix well.
4. Take a sample of the suspension, and determine the pH and other quality control factors.
5. Package the suspension in a suitable container, and label.
6. If a large number of suspensions are to be prepared, select a random sample to be assayed.

Ointments

1. Accurately weigh or measure each ingredient.
2. Sterilize each ingredient using a suitable method.
3. Using aseptic technique, mix each ingredient with the sterile vehicle.
4. Take a sample of the ointment, and determine the quality control factors.
5. Package and label the product.
6. If a large number of ointments are to be prepared, select a random sample to be assayed and checked for sterility.

Gels

1. Accurately weigh or measure each ingredient.
2. Dissolve the ingredients in about three-fourths of the quantity of sterile water for injection, and mix well.
3. Add the gelling agent, and mix well.
4. Add sufficient sterile water for injection to volume or weight, and mix well.
5. Take a sample of the gel, and determine the pH, clarity, and other quality control factors.
6. Package and label the product. (Note: Sterile 1-mL syringes that are preloaded with individual doses work well.)
7. If a large number of gels are to be prepared, select a random sample to be assayed.

Packaging, Storage, and Labeling

Containers for dispensing nasal preparations include dropper bottles, spray bottles (Figure 23-3), and syringes (for gels and ointments). Generally, these preparations should be stored at room or refrigerated temperature. They should not be frozen. These preparations should be labeled "For the Nose" and "Discard after [appropriate date]."

FIGURE 23-3 Nasal spray bottles in various sizes (15 mL, 20 mL, 30 mL).

Stability

Water-containing formulations prepared from ingredients in solid form should have beyond-use dates of no later than 30 days when stored at cold temperatures. If nonaqueous liquids are prepared with a manufactured preparation, the recommended beyond-use date is no later than 25% of the time remaining until the preparation's expiration date or 6 months, whichever is earlier. These recommended dates can be extended if valid scientific information is available to support the stability of the preparation, as discussed in the Chapter 6 of this book.

Patient Counseling

When systemic therapeutic drugs, such as dihydroergotamine mesylate or morphine sulfate, are to be administered, a pharmacist should calibrate a dropper or spray container to deliver a consistent and uniform dose. The patient should be taught how to use the dosage device properly.

Sample Formulations
Vehicle

 General Nasal Solution Vehicle

(pH 6.5 and isotonic)

Sodium acid phosphate, hydrous	0.65 g	Buffer
Disodium phosphate, hydrous	0.54 g	Buffer
Sodium chloride	0.45 g	Tonicity Adjuster
Benzalkonium chloride	0.05–0.01 g	Preservative
Distilled water	qs 100 mL	Vehicle

1. Calculate the required quantity of each ingredient for the total amount to be prepared.
2. Accurately weigh or measure each ingredient.
3. Dissolve the ingredients in about 75 mL of the distilled water.
4. Adjust the pH to 6.5 if necessary.
5. Add sufficient distilled water to make 100 mL.
6. Package and label the preparation.

Ingredient-Specific Preparations

℞ Atropine Sulfate 0.5% Nasal Solution

Atropine sulfate	500 mg	Active
Sodium chloride	835 mg	Tonicity Adjuster
Sterile water for injection	qs 100 mL	Vehicle

1. Calculate the quantity of each ingredient required for the prescription.
2. Accurately weigh or measure each ingredient.
3. Dissolve the atropine sulfate and the sodium chloride in about 95 mL of sterile water for injection.
4. Add sufficient water for injection to make 100 mL.
5. Package and label the product.

℞ Desmopressin Acetate Nasal Solution 0.033 mg/mL

Desmopressin solution 0.1 mg/mL	2.5 mL	Active
0.9% Sodium chloride solution	5 mL	Vehicle

1. Calculate the quantity of each ingredient required for the prescription.
2. Accurately weigh or measure each ingredient.
3. Mix the two solutions together, and stir well.
4. Package and label the product.

℞ Saline Nasal Mist

Sodium chloride	650 mg	Active
Monobasic potassium phosphate	40 mg	Buffer
Dibasic potassium phosphate	90 mg	Buffer
Benzalkonium chloride	10 mg	Preservative
Sterile water for injection	qs 100 mL	Vehicle

1. Calculate the quantity of each ingredient required for the prescription.
2. Accurately weigh or measure each ingredient.
3. Dissolve the ingredients in sufficient sterile water for injection to make 100 mL of solution.
4. Package the product in a nasal spray bottle, and label.

℞ Xylometazoline Hydrochloride Nasal Drops

Xylometazoline hydrochloride	100 mg	Active
Sodium chloride	850 mg	Tonicity Adjuster
Benzalkonium chloride	10 mg	Preservative
Sterile water for injection	qs 100 mL	Vehicle

1. Calculate the quantity of each ingredient required for the prescription.
2. Accurately weigh or measure each ingredient.
3. Dissolve all the ingredients in sufficient sterile water for injection to make 100 mL.
4. Package and label the product.

℞ Buprenorphine Hydrochloride 150 µg/100 µL Nasal Spray

Buprenorphine hydrochloride	150 mg	Active
Glycerin	5 mL	Cosolvent
Methylparaben	200 mg	Preservative
0.9% Sodium chloride injection	95 mL	Vehicle

1. Calculate the quantity of each ingredient required for the prescription.
2. Accurately weigh or measure each ingredient.
3. Dissolve the methylparaben in the glycerin.
4. Add the buprenorphine hydrochloride to the sodium chloride injection.
5. Add the methylparaben–glycerin solution (step 3) to the sodium chloride injection solution (step 4), and mix.
6. Package and label the product.

℞ Progesterone 2 mg/0.1 mL Nasal Solution

Progesterone	20 mg	Active
Dimethyl-β-cyclodextrin	62 mg	Solubilizing Agent
Sterile water for injection	1 mL	Vehicle
Hydrochloric acid or sodium hydroxide 10% solutions	Adjust to pH 7.4	pH Adjusters

1. Calculate the quantity of each ingredient required for the prescription.
2. Accurately weigh or measure each ingredient.
3. Dissolve the dimethyl-β-cyclodextrin in 0.9 mL of sterile water for injection.
4. Add the progesterone, and stir until dissolved.
5. Adjust the pH to 7.4 using either hydrochloric acid or dilute sodium hydroxide 10% solutions.
6. Add sufficient sterile water for injection to make 1 mL.
7. Package and label the product.

℞ Scopolamine Hydrobromide 0.4 mg/0.1 mL Nasal Solution

Scopolamine hydrobromide	400 mg	Active
Buffer solution (pH 5)	5 mL	Buffer
0.9% Sodium chloride solution	qs 100 mL	Vehicle

1. Calculate the quantity of each ingredient required for the prescription.
2. Accurately weigh or measure each ingredient.
3. Dissolve the scopolamine hydrobromide in about 50 mL of the 0.9% sodium chloride solution.
4. Add the pH 5 buffer, and mix well.
5. Add sufficient 0.9% sodium chloride solution to volume, and mix.
6. Package the product in a metering nasal spray container, and label.

℞ Fentanyl Citrate 25 µg/0.1 mL Nasal Spray (10 mL)

Fentanyl citrate	2.5 mg	Active
Methylparaben	10 mg	Preservative
Propylparaben	10 mg	Preservative
Propylene glycol	0.2 mL	Cosolvent
0.9% Sodium chloride solution	qs 10 mL	Vehicle

1. Calculate the quantity of each ingredient required for the prescription.
2. Accurately weigh or measure each ingredient.
3. Dissolve the methylparaben and propylparaben in the propylene glycol.
4. Dissolve the fentanyl citrate in about 9 mL of 0.9% sodium chloride solution.
5. Add the paraben mixture, and mix well.
6. Add sufficient 0.9% sodium chloride solution to volume, and mix well.
7. Package and label the product.

℞ Meperidine Hydrochloride 50 mg/mL Nasal Solution

Meperidine hydrochloride	5 g	Active
Phenol	200 mg	Preservative
Sterile water for injection	qs 100 mL	Vehicle

(Note: Metacresol 100 mg can be used in place of phenol as a preservative.)

1. Calculate the quantity of each ingredient required for the prescription.
2. Accurately weigh or measure each ingredient.
3. Place the meperidine hydrochloride powder and phenol crystals in a graduate.
4. Add sufficient sterile water for injection to volume, and mix well.
5. Package and label the product.

℞ Methylsulfonylmethane (MSM) 16% Nasal Solution (100 mL)

Methylsulfonylmethane	16 g	Active
Benzalkonium chloride	20 mg	Preservative
Purified water	qs 100 mL	Vehicle

1. Calculate the quantity of each ingredient required for the prescription.
2. Accurately weigh or measure each ingredient. (Note: Dilutions may be required to obtain the correct quantity of benzalkonium chloride.)
3. Dissolve the methylsulfonylmethane and benzalkonium chloride in sufficient purified water to make 100 mL, and mix well.
4. Package and label the product.

℞ Mupirocin 0.5% Nasal Drops (30 mL)

Mupirocin ointment (2%)	15 g	Active
0.9% Sodium chloride solution	qs 30 mL	Vehicle

1. Calculate the quantity of each ingredient required for the prescription.
2. Empty the contents of a 15-g tube of mupirocin (Bactroban) ointment into an appropriate graduated cylinder.
3. Add sufficient 0.9% sodium chloride solution to 30 mL.
4. Mix until uniform.
5. Package and label the product.

Reference

1. United States Pharmacopeial Convention. Chapter <797>, Pharmaceutical compounding—sterile preparations. In: *United States Pharmacopeia/National Formulary.* Rockville, MD: United States Pharmacopeial Convention; current edition.

Chapter 24

Inhalation Preparations

Inhalation has been used as a method of drug delivery throughout history, in forms such as aromatic perfumes or oils, burned incenses, and smoked leaves and herbs. Drugs can be introduced into the lungs quite easily by this method. A patient simply inhales a dose of a drug incorporated in a properly designed dosage form. The drug is then caught up in the flow of air and carried into the deep recesses of the pulmonary environment, that is, into the respiratory bronchioles and the alveolar region. Drugs for inhalation can be vapors, very fine powders, or solutions in the form of aerosols. Preparations administered by inhalation can produce either a local or a systemic effect. Drugs commonly administered for respiratory purposes include antitussives, bronchodilators, corticosteroids, expectorants, respiratory stimulants, surfactants, and therapeutic gases.

Drug administration by inhalation has many advantages, including rapid onset of action, bypass of the first-pass effect, and absence of drug degradation in the gastrointestinal tract. In addition, low dosages can be used, minimizing adverse reactions, and doses can be titrated easily. This route works well for as-needed dosing. It is a good alternative route for drugs that may chemically or physically interact with a patient's concurrent drugs and for drugs with erratic pharmacokinetics after oral or parenteral administration.

Definitions and Types

A wide range of dosage forms and methods of administering drugs by inhalation are available. They include aerosols, atomizers, inhalations, insufflations, metered-dose inhalers (MDIs), nebulizers, and vaporizers.

An *aerosol* is a colloidal dispersion of a liquid or solid internal phase in an outer gaseous phase. Examples of natural aerosols are mist (i.e., water/air) and dust (i.e., solid/air). The ultimate deposition of drugs prepared as inhalation aerosols depends on (1) the formulation; (2) the design of the components, the packaging, and the container; (3) the administration skills and techniques of a patient; and (4) the anatomic and physiologic status of the patient's respiratory system.

Both oral inhalation and nasopharyngeal medications can be administered as aerosols. They are commonly administered by manual sprays or from pressurized packages. Aerosol use has become so widespread that the term *aerosol* has come to mean a self-contained product that is sprayed, through the propelling force of either a liquefied or a compressed gas.

In the practice of pharmacy, pressure-packaged aerosol preparations consist of the active drug dissolved, suspended, or emulsified in a propellant or a mixture of a solvent and a propellant. Aerosol preparations are generally designed either for topical administration or for inhalation into the nasopharyngeal region or bronchopulmonary system. For pulmonary delivery, particles greater than 60 μm are usually deposited in the trachea; those greater than 20 μm are deposited between the trachea and the bronchioles but do not enter the bronchioles. Particles about 1 μm often remain airborne and are exhaled. Thus, particles need to be in the range of about 5 to 20 μm to reach the bronchioles. The largest group of oral aerosol products formulated as either solutions or suspensions is inhalation aerosols.

An *atomizer* is an instrument used to disperse a liquid in a fine spray. Many of the older pressure-type atomizers used Bernoulli's principle. When a stream of air moves at a high velocity over the tip of a dip tube, the pressure is lowered, which causes the liquid to be drawn into the airflow. The liquid is broken up into a spray as it is taken up into the air stream. For production of smaller droplets, a baffle, bead, or other device can be put in the flow to break the droplets into smaller droplets as they collide with the stationary device. These smaller droplets are then carried by the airflow into the inhaled stream of air. Many different configurations are available that use Bernoulli's principle. A finer spray can be obtained if a pressure atomizer is used. Currently, plastic spray bottles are similar to the pressure atomizers. When the plastic bottle is squeezed, the air inside is compressed, forcing the liquid up a dip tube into the tip. The liquid stream is mixed with air as it is emitted from the nozzle, thereby producing a spray.

Inhalations are preparations designed to deliver the drug into a patient's respiratory tree for local or systemic effect. Rapid relief is obtained when the vapors, mist, or droplets reach the affected area. The *United States Pharmacopeia/National Formulary* defines inhalations as "drugs or solutions or suspensions of one or more drug substances administered by the nasal or oral respiratory route for local or systemic effect."[1] The drugs can be nebulized to produce droplets sufficiently fine and uniform in size to reach the bronchioles. The patient can breathe the mist directly from the nebulizer of a face mask or tent. An intermittent positive-pressure breathing machine can be used to produce a contained environment to maximize the quantity of drug available for delivery to the lungs.

The *British Pharmacopoeia (BP)* defines inhalations as solutions or suspensions of one or more active ingredients that can contain an inert, suspended diffusing agent. These liquids are designed to release volatile constituents for inhalation, either when placed on a pad or when added to hot water. An example of the latter is adding 1 teaspoonful of benzoin inhalation BP to 1 quart of hot water and inhaling the vapors.

Inhalants are characterized by high vapor pressure and can be carried by an air current into the nasal passage where the drugs usually exert their effect. The device or container from which the inhalant is administered is called an inhaler. An inhaler consists of rolls of a fibrous material that has been impregnated with the drug, usually containing an aromatic substance in addition to an active substance. Inhalers are often cylindrical, with a cap in place to retard loss of the medication. A patient removes the cap and inserts the inhaler into a nostril. When the patient inhales, the air passes through the inhaler and carries the vapor of the medication into the nasal passage. An actual drug vapor is being delivered to the patient. For example, camphor, menthol, propylhexedrine, and tuaminoheptane inhalants are of this type. Another type, the amyl nitrite inhalant, is packaged with the drug contained in a thin glass ampul encased in gauze netting. When the product is squeezed and the glass ampul broken, the amyl nitrite is released, absorbed on the gauze netting, and inhaled by the patient.

Insufflations are powders administered with the use of a powder blower (or puffer) or insufflator. These devices can consist of a rubber bulb connected to a container and a delivery pipe. As the bulb is squeezed, air is blown into the container, creating turbulence. This turbulence causes the powder to fly around. Some of the fine particles are carried out with the air as it leaves the container through the delivery tube and are ready for inhalation. The puffer device consists of a plastic accordion-shaped container with a spout on one end. The powder is placed in the puffer, and, as the puffer is sharply squeezed, a portion of the powder is ejected from the spout into the air, where it is available for inhalation or application. In contemporary delivery systems, powders are delivered by various mechanical devices designed so that a patient breathes deeply to inhale the powder particles. The patient's inspiration provides the energy to spin a propeller that breaks up and distributes the particles as they are inhaled.

Metered-dose inhalers contain the drug, in the form of a solution or suspension, and a liquefied gas propellant with or without a cosolvent. MDIs commonly deliver a volume of 25 to 100 μL of liquid drug for inhalation.

Nebulae, or spray solutions, are intended for spraying into the throat and nose. Usually these are simple solutions, delivered from plastic spray bottles that work in much the same way as pressure atomizers. When the flexible plastic container is squeezed, the air is compressed, forcing the liquid in the container up through a dip tube into the tip where it mixes with a stream of air. Droplets are formed, depending on the geometry of the device and the pressure exerted by the patient squeezing the bottle.

A *nebulizer* was formerly described as a small, vacuum-type atomizer inside a chamber. Large droplets would strike the walls of the chamber, fall back, and be reprocessed. The smaller particles would be carried out of the unit in the air stream. The nebulizer would be placed in the mouth, and a patient would inhale while simultaneously squeezing the bulb. Electrically powered nebulizers are now used; the solution (usually less than 5 mL) is placed in the reservoir, and the mouthpiece or nosepiece is positioned for administration. To be suitable for administering inhalation solutions, nebulizers must produce droplets sufficiently fine and uniform in size (optimally 0.5 to 7 μm) so that the mist will reach the bronchioles. An advantage of the newer pressurized aerosols is that they produce a fine mist and more uniform doses than do the older manual nebulizers.

A *vaporizer* is an electrical device producing moist steam, either with or without medication, for inhalation. It is often used to soothe upper respiratory irritations but is relatively ineffective in providing medications to the deeper areas of the respiratory tract.

Historical and Future Use

One of the earliest ways to inhale drug products was to burn the material and inhale the smoke. In some cases, a natural vegetable product was dried, broken up, and burned; in others, an oil or another material was burned and its vapors were inhaled. A contemporary term for an age-old method of drug administration is *aromatherapy;* today, the term refers primarily to the use of volatile or aromatic oils that serve as room sprays, massage products, room fresheners, and even inhalants when placed in hot water.

Until recently, an asthma "cigarette" (Asthmador) containing a bronchodilator was available. The cigarette was smoked and inhaled, delivering the drug to the lungs. Recreational drugs such as tobacco, marijuana, and opium are used in the same way. Some recreational drugs are simply inhaled in the powder form, resulting in a rapid onset of action. The effectiveness of this route of drug administration is beyond question.

However, one problem with the use of inhalers for drug delivery has been the inability to determine the accuracy of the dose. This problem has been overcome in part with the advent of the newer MDIs, which administer the same volume of drug every time. Nevertheless, such methods fail to address the variability in a patient's rate of inspiration, breath holding, and expiration, which causes varying quantities of the drug to be absorbed.

In the past, inhalations were simple solutions of volatile medications, usually volatile oils, in alcohol or an alcoholic preparation. Often, compound benzoin tincture was used. A sample formulation is as follows:

Pine oil	5 mL	Active
Eucalyptus oil	5 mL	Active
Compound benzoin tincture	30 mL	Vehicle/Active

Sig: Add 1 teaspoonful to 1 pint of hot water. Inhale the vapor.

Other inhalations designed to be added to hot water were aqueous preparations containing a volatile oil, water, and light magnesium carbonate. The light magnesium carbonate served as a distributive or dispersing agent. The volatile material was distributed on the light magnesium carbonate, which was then mixed with the water. This mixture ensured that the oil was uniformly dispersed on shaking, because it was distributed throughout the mixture rather than remaining as a globule or being dispersed as large globules. The presence of the light magnesium carbonate did not interfere with the free volatilization of the oil when the product was added to hot water. If the oil would emulsify, it would actually retard volatilization. An approximate ratio of 100 mg of light magnesium carbonate to 0.2 mL of oil was used. A sample formulation is as follows:

Menthol	325 mg	Active
Eucalyptus oil	3.7 mL	Active
Light magnesium carbonate	2 g	Dispersing Agent
Purified water	qs 30 mL	Vehicle

Sig: Add 1 teaspoonful to 1 pint of hot water (not boiling). Inhale the vapor. Shake the bottle before using.

In the early 1950s, Riker Laboratories introduced the first contemporary pressurized aerosol dosage form. The Medihaler-Epi consisted of epinephrine hydrochloride in a hydro-alcoholic solvent system containing sorbitan trioleate as a dispersing agent and a fluorinated hydrocarbon propellant system. Today, these self-contained aerosol propellant systems generally contain up to about 30 mL of product in a small, stainless steel container fitted with a metered-dose valve. The four components include a product concentrate, propellant, container, and suitable dispensing or metering valve. Products available in this dosage form have included albuterol, beclomethasone dipropionate, dexamethasone sodium phosphate, epinephrine bitartrate, isoetharine mesylate, isoproterenol hydrochloride, metaproterenol sulfate, and triamcinolone acetonide.

Oral and nasal inhalation products are a promising means of administering many local and systemic drugs. Thus, pharmacists may have many opportunities to compound these preparations in the future. With their rapid onset of action, generally good stability profiles, easy titration, and simple formulation development, these preparations will continue to meet patient needs and their use will continue to grow.

Applications

Oral inhalants are most commonly used to deliver drugs directly to the airways and the lungs in the treatment of pulmonary disorders. Gases are administered by this method to provide anesthesia during surgery. Oral inhalants used for local treatment include preparations that suppress coughing, break up mucus, and treat fungal infections. Systemic agents administered by oral inhalation include antiasthmatic and anti-inflammatory agents and respiratory stimulants.

Composition

Solution aerosols are fairly simple to formulate if the active drug is soluble in the propellant system. If not, a suspension or an emulsion aerosol can be prepared. For oral inhalation, either solution or suspension aerosols are used. Table 24-1 gives examples of ingredients used in oral inhalations or nasal aerosol solutions.

Suspension aerosols have been used to formulate antiasthmatic agents, steroids, antibiotics, and other drugs. Potential problems include caking, agglomeration, particle size growth, and clogging of the valve systems. Table 24-2 gives examples of ingredients used in nasal aerosol solutions or suspensions.

Citric acid is often used in solution and suspension aerosols as an acidifying agent. Polysorbate 80 is used as an emulsifying and solubilizing agent. Sodium chloride and dextrose are used to adjust tonicity.

TABLE 24-1 Components of Oral Inhalation and Nasal Aerosol Solutions

Component	Example
Active ingredient	Ingredient appropriate for condition; soluble in vehicle
Solvent	Ethyl alcohol, propylene glycol, purified water
Surfactant	Polysorbate 80
Antioxidant	Ascorbic acid
Flavoring	Aromatic oils
Propellant	As needed

TABLE 24-2 Components of Nasal Aerosol Solutions or Suspensions

Component	Example
Active ingredient	Solubilized or suspended forms of appropriate ingredient for condition
Antioxidant	Ascorbic acid, bisulfites
Preservative	Benzalkonium chloride
Buffer	Phosphate buffer
Tonicity adjuster	Sodium chloride
Surfactant	Sorbitan esters
Vehicle	Purified water

Preparation

The steps that follow should be used in formulating most inhalation preparations in solution form. They should be used for the preparations in the "Sample Formulations" section of this chapter, because all are solutions.

1. Calculate the quantity of the individual ingredients required for the prescription.

2. Accurately weigh or measure each ingredient.
3. Dissolve the solids in about two-thirds of the volume of vehicle.
4. Add the liquid ingredients, and mix well.
5. Add sufficient vehicle to volume, and mix well.
6. Sterilize the solution by filtering through a sterile 0.2-μm filter system into sterile containers.
7. Package and label the product.

Physicochemical Considerations

In compounding, or formulating, preparations for oral or nasal inhalation, a pharmacist must consider the variables of particle size, solubility, vehicles, tonicity, pH, sterility, preservatives, viscosity, buffers, surfactants, and moisture content.

Particle Size

Generally, the particle size should be within the range of about 0.5 to 10 μm. The range should preferably be between about 3 and 6 μm if the inhaled drug is intended to penetrate to the small bronchioles and the lung alveoli for a rapid effect. Particles in this size range will deposit in the lung by gravitational sedimentation, inertial impaction, and diffusion into terminal alveoli by Brownian motion. For inhalation aerosols, particles of 5 to 10 μm are common, whereas for topical sprays, a range of 50 to 100 μm is typical.

Solubility

Active drugs that are soluble in the matrix and in the pulmonary fluids will have a rapid onset of action and ordinarily a shorter duration of action, compared with drugs that are somewhat less soluble in the matrix and in the pulmonary fluids. Drugs that are poorly soluble in the pulmonary fluids can irritate the lung tissue. When preparing a suspension, a pharmacist should select a vehicle in which the drug is not very soluble; this minimizes the particle size growth that results when a drug in solution crystallizes out onto the crystals that are present. Polymorphic forms of crystalline drugs should not be used for suspension aerosols. To enhance the stability of a suspension aerosol, the pharmacist should select a liquid phase with a density similar to that of the suspensoid, which will minimize the tendency to settle.

Vehicles

Sterile water for inhalation and 0.9% sodium chloride inhalation solution are commonly used vehicles to carry the drugs in inhalations. Some inhalations are simple solutions of nonvolatile or volatile medications in water or cosolvent mixtures. Small quantities of alcohol or glycerin can be used to solubilize ingredients.

Tonicity

Generally, inhalation solutions are best when they are isotonic with physiologic fluids, that is, equivalent to 0.9% sodium chloride or an osmolality of about 290 mOsm. The solution should be slightly hypotonic to enhance movement of the fluid and drug through the alveoli and into the tissue for more rapid absorption and therapeutic effect. If the solution were hypertonic, the fluid would tend to move from the alveoli into the pulmonary space to reach an isotonic equilibrium.

pH

A pH in the neutral range, similar to that of body fluids, should minimize any cough reflex that might occur if the pH were too low. However, the solubility and stability characteristics of the drug must be considered in establishing the pH.

Sterility

Inhalation solutions are required to be sterile. Compounded oral inhalation solutions should be sterilized to ensure that patients receive the best preparations available. Sterility can be easily accomplished by using 0.2-μm filtration systems designed for extemporaneous compounding (Figure 24-1).

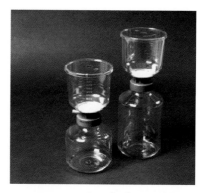

FIGURE 24-1 Sterile disposable vacuum filters (0.2-μm filter; 500-mL volume).

Preservatives

Any preparation that is not in unit-dose containers should contain a preservative, given the sterility requirement for this group of dosage forms. The minimum amount of preservative that is effective should be used; too high a concentration can initiate a patient's cough reflex. If the concentration of certain preservatives that are also surfactants is too high, foaming can result, which could interfere with delivery of the complete dose.

Viscosity

The viscosity of the external phase for most aerosol preparations is quite low; consequently, they are very sensitive systems. Evaporation, sedimentation, and an increase in particle size are processes that can occur and change rapidly.

Buffers

A buffer, if used, should be at low buffer strength to maintain the desired pH. It should not induce pH changes in a microenvironment in the pulmonary cavity.

Surfactants

Surfactants can be used as dispersing agents for suspensions, solubilizing agents to enhance the solubility of the drug, and spreading agents when the drug is deposited in the lungs. The sorbitan esters, especially sorbitan trioleate, can be used, as well as lecithin derivatives, oleyl alcohol, and others. The concentration of surfactants should be kept as low as possible to minimize foaming that might interfere with proper administration.

Moisture Content

For inhalation dispersion aerosols, the moisture content of all active and inactive ingredients should be kept extremely low. The ingredients should be anhydrous to minimize caking.

Quality Control

A compounding pharmacist should follow standard quality control procedures. Solutions should be checked for precipitation, discoloration, haziness, gas formation resulting from microbial growth, and final volume.

Packaging, Storage, and Labeling

Oral inhalation preparations should be packaged in individual sterile, unit-of-use containers. Generally, these preparations should be stored at either room or refrigerated temperature. These preparations should be labeled "Oral Inhalation Use Only. Not for Injection." Labeling should also contain detailed instructions for proper use of the preparation.

Stability

Beyond-use dates for water-containing formulations prepared from ingredients in solid form and stored at cold temperatures are no later than 14 days, if sterility tested. These dates are extended if valid scientific information supports the stability of the preparation, as discussed in Chapter 6 of this book.

Patient Counseling

A patient or caregiver should be thoroughly instructed on how to administer oral inhalation solutions. If the solution does not include a preservative, the patient should be instructed to discard any remaining solution in the individual dosage vials and in the device used for aerosolization.

Sample Formulations

The sample formulations given here are preservative free. The preparations should be packaged as single-use or unit-dose preparations. Formulations are provided for 100-mL quantities for ease of calculation. The formulas should be reduced or expanded according to the total quantity to be compounded. These solutions can be preserved by adding 4 mg of benzalkonium chloride per 100 mL of solution. (This amount would be 3 mL of a benzalkonium chloride 1:750 solution.) The steps listed in the "Preparation" section of this chapter apply to all the following formulations.

℞ Albuterol Sulfate 0.5% Inhalant Solution (preservative free)

Albuterol sulfate	500 mg	Active
Citric acid, anhydrous	100 mg	Acidifier
Sodium chloride	800 mg	Tonicity Adjuster
Sterile water for inhalation	qs 100 mL	Vehicle

℞ Albuterol Sulfate 2.7% Inhalant for Hand-Held Nebulizer (preservative free)

Albuterol sulfate	2.7 g	Active
Citric acid, anhydrous	100 mg	Acidifier
Sterile water for inhalation	qs 100 mL	Vehicle

℞ Beclomethasone Dipropionate 0.042% Nasal Solution (preservative free)

Beclomethasone dipropionate, monohydrate	43 mg	Active
Dextrose	5.4 g	Tonicity Adjuster
Polysorbate 80	1 mL	Surfactant
Hydrochloric acid (3%–5%)	Adjust to pH 7	pH Adjuster
Ethanol, 95%	13 mL	Cosolvent
0.9% Sodium chloride solution	qs 100 mL	Vehicle

℞ Cromolyn Sodium 1% Inhalation Solution (preservative free)

Cromolyn sodium	1 g	Active
Sterile water for inhalation	qs 100 mL	Vehicle

℞ Cromolyn Sodium 4% Inhalation Solution (preservative free)

Cromolyn sodium	4 g	Active
Sterile water for inhalation	qs 100 mL	Vehicle

℞ Flunisolide 0.025% Inhalation Solution (preservative free)

Flunisolide	25 mg	Active
Ethanol, 95%	2 mL	Cosolvent
0.9% Sodium chloride solution	qs 100 mL	Vehicle

℞ Ipratropium Bromide 0.02% Solution (preservative free)

Ipratropium bromide	20 mg	Active
Citric acid, anhydrous	50 mg	Acidifier
0.9% Sodium chloride solution	qs 100 mL	Vehicle

℞ Metaproterenol Sulfate 0.3% Solution (preservative free)

Metaproterenol sulfate	300 mg	Active
Citric acid, anhydrous	250 mg	Acidifier
0.9% Sodium chloride solution	qs 100 mL	Vehicle

℞ Metaproterenol Sulfate 0.6% Solution (preservative free)

Metaproterenol sulfate	600 mg	Active
Citric acid, anhydrous	500 mg	Acidifier
0.9% Sodium chloride solution	qs 100 mL	Vehicle

℞ Metaproterenol Sulfate 5% Concentrate (preservative free)

Metaproterenol sulfate	5 g	Active
Citric acid, anhydrous	500 mg	Acidifier
0.9% Sodium chloride solution	50 mL	Tonicity Adjuster
Sterile water for inhalation	qs 100 mL	Vehicle

℞ Terbutaline Sulfate 0.1% Inhalant Solution (preservative free)

Terbutaline sulfate	100 mg	Active
Citric acid, anhydrous	100 mg	Acidifier
0.9% Sodium chloride solution	qs 100 mL	Vehicle

℞ Albuterol–Cromolyn–Betamethasone for Inhalation (preservative free)

Albuterol sulfate	500 mg	Active
Cromolyn sodium	1 g	Active
Betamethasone sodium phosphate	250 mg	Active
Citric acid, anhydrous	100 mg	Acidifier
Sodium chloride	800 mg	Tonicity Adjuster
Sterile water for inhalation	qs 100 mL	Vehicle

Adjust pH to 6.8–7.0.

℞ Albuterol–Ipratropium for Inhalation (preservative free)

Albuterol sulfate	100 mg	Active
Ipratropium bromide	20 mg	Active
Citric acid, anhydrous	50 mg	Acidifier
Sterile water for inhalation	qs 100 mL	Vehicle

℞ Ipratropium–Metaproterenol–Betamethasone for Inhalation Concentrate (preservative free)

Ipratropium bromide	125 mg	Active
Metaproterenol sulfate	5 g	Active
Betamethasone sodium phosphate	250 mg	Active
Citric acid, anhydrous	100 mg	Acidifier
Sterile water for inhalation	qs 100 mL	Vehicle

Reference

1. United States Pharmacopeial Convention. Chapter <1151>, Pharmaceutical dosage forms. In: *United States Pharmacopeia/National Formulary.* Rockville, MD: United States Pharmacopeial Convention; current edition.

Chapter 25

Parenteral Preparations

Definitions and Types

A parenteral is a preparation that is administered to the body by injection. Because an injection bypasses the normal body defense mechanisms, parenteral formulations must be prepared with a higher degree of care and skill than is needed for routine oral or topical preparations. The finished preparation must be sterile, nonpyrogenic, and free from extraneous insoluble materials.[1,2] Because sterile formulations must be prepared under strict environmental conditions, they present a challenge to a compounding pharmacist.

Historical Use

In 1656, Sir Christopher Wren, a professor of surgery and a mathematician, used a syringe and pipe to inject opium, which had been dissolved in wine, into a dog. Two years later, in 1658, a solution was injected into a human by using a pig's bladder and a goose quill. Few advancements were made over the next 200 years, but by the middle of the 19th century, analgesics were being injected with greater frequency. When an antisyphilitic agent was found to be effective if given by injection but not if given by mouth, the use of injections expanded rapidly. In the mid-1920s, the need for sterility was recognized, and it became a requirement for injections. Today, parenterals must be free of both microorganisms and their byproducts such as endotoxins. Over the past 50 years, the use of parenteral products and their preparation by pharmacists have dramatically increased. This growth has been due to increases in available products, clean rooms, laminar-airflow (LAF) hoods, automated compounding equipment, and, especially, home health care.

USP Chapter <797>, Pharmaceutical Compounding— Sterile Preparations

A current copy of Chapter <797>, Pharmaceutical Compounding—Sterile Preparations, of the *United States Pharmacopeia/National Formulary (USP/NF)* should be obtained for detailed and up-to-date information.[3] The purpose of *USP* Chapter <797> is to describe the minimum practices and quality standards that are to be followed when a pharmacist prepares compounded sterile human and animal drugs (compounded sterile preparations, or CSPs). The practice standards are necessary to prevent harm, including death, to human and animal patients that could result from microbial contamination, excessive bacterial endotoxins, variability from the intended strength of correct ingredients, chemical and physical contaminants, and use of ingredients of inappropriate quality. The chapter applies to all individuals who prepare CSPs and to all places where CSPs are prepared.

USP Chapter <797> uses a risk-based approach that considers batch size, complexity of the compounding process, inherent nature of the drug being compounded, complexity of the compounding operation, and the length of time between the initiation of compounding and administration of the drug to a patient. The risk is obviously lower if the compounding is for an individual patient as compared to batch compounding for multiple patients. The risk assessment relates to risk categories that are used as a basis for the standards throughout the chapter, including the assignment of beyond-use dates, environmental monitoring, and so on.

The risk levels are intended to serve as a guide to the extent (both breadth and depth) of compounding performed at a facility. Assigning the appropriate risk category is the responsibility of the pharmacist in charge of the operations of the sterile compounding area. Contamination may result from solid and liquid matter from compounding personnel and objects, nonsterile components, inappropriate conditions within the restricted compounding environment, or prolonged presterilization procedures involving aqueous preparations. The chapter is not concerned with clinical administration and does not address the duration of administration of CSPs.

Organizationally, USP Chapter <797> is divided into the following sections: (1) Introduction and Scope; (2) Personnel Qualifications—Training, Evaluation, and Requalification; (3) Personal Hygiene and Personal Protective Equipment; (4) Buildings and Facilities; (5) Environmental Monitoring; (6) Cleaning and Disinfecting Compounding Areas; (7) Equipment and Components; (8) Sterilization and Depyrogenation; (9) SOPs [Standard Operating Procedures] and Master Formulation and Compounding Records; (10) Release Testing; (11) Labeling; (12) Establishing Beyond-Use Dates and In-Use Times; (13) Quality Assurance and Quality Control; (14) CSP Storage, Handling, Packaging, and Transport; (15) Complaint Handling and Adverse Event Reporting; (16) Documentation; (17) Radiopharmaceuticals as CSPs; a Glossary; and Appendices. The appendices include (1) Acronyms; and (2) Common Disinfectants Used in Health Care for Inanimate Surfaces and Noncritical Devices, and Their Microbial Activity and Properties.

Applications

The forms of parenteral preparations include standard injections (epidural, intradermal, intramuscular, intrathecal, intravenous [IV], subcutaneous), parenteral admixtures (combinations of two or more preparations mixed together), and parenteral nutrition products (products containing caloric sources such as carbohydrates, fats, and proteins). In addition, hospitals, physicians' clinics, and home health care providers use parenteral preparations in patient-controlled analgesia, antibiotic therapy, chemotherapy, and sclerotherapy. As one of the fastest-growing segments in health care today, home health care offers many opportunities for aseptic compounding.

Composition

In compounding parenteral admixtures, pharmacists must be cognizant of adjuvants such as vehicles, cosolvents, buffers, preservatives, antioxidants, inert gases, surfactants, complexation agents, and chelating agents.

Water is the most common vehicle used today. If a drug is not very water soluble, a number of cosolvents (ethyl alcohol, 1%–50%; glycerin, 1%–50%; polyethylene glycol [PEG], 1%–50%; propylene glycol, 1%–60%) can be used.

For maintenance of a desired solution pH for both solubility and stability, many preparations contain buffer systems. The buffer capacity (i.e., the resistance to change on the addition of either an acid or a base) is generally low so that these systems will not alter the pH of the body fluids on injection. Buffer systems are sufficiently strong, however, to resist changes in pH under normal storage and use.

TABLE 25-1 Preservatives Used in Parenteral Products

Agent	Usual Concentration (%)
Benzalkonium chloride	0.01
Benzethonium chloride	0.01
Benzyl alcohol	1.0–2
Chlorobutanol	0.25–0.5
Chlorocresol	0.1–0.3
Cresol	0.3–0.5
Metacresol	0.1–0.3
p-Hydroxybenzoate esters	
Butyl	0.015
Methyl	0.1–0.2
Propyl	0.02–0.2
Phenol	0.25–0.5
Phenylmercuric nitrate	0.002
Thimerosal	0.01

Preparations that are packaged in multiple-dose vials are required to contain a preservative to prevent the growth of microorganisms that may be introduced when the container is manipulated. However, the preservatives may not always be compatible with other drugs to which the drug may be added. For example, benzyl alcohol is incompatible with chloramphenicol sodium succinate, and the parabens and phenol preservatives are incompatible with amphotericin B, erythromycin, and nitrofurantoin. When bacteriostatic water for injection is used for reconstitution, selection of a product with a preservative that will be compatible with the solution is important. Preservatives must also be compatible with the container to which the preparation is added and with its closure. Table 25-1 provides a list of the preservatives used in parenteral products.

Antioxidants and inert gases are used to enhance stability. Table 25-2 lists antioxidants used in parenteral products and their usual concentrations.

Surfactants can be used to increase the solubility of a drug in an aqueous system. The presence of a surfactant could possibly result in an increase or decrease in the rate of drug degradation. Examples of surfactants include polyoxyethylene sorbitan monooleate (0.1%–0.5%) and sorbitan monooleate (0.05%–0.25%). Others are listed in Table 25-3.

Complexation and chelating agents can also be used to enhance solubility and stability. Ethylenediaminetetraacetic acid salts (0.01%–0.075%) are an example of these agents.

Preparation

All aseptic manipulations should be carried out by validated aseptic compounding pharmacists in a class 100 LAF hood (horizontal or vertical) enclosed within a class 10,000 clean room.[4] Only pharmacists who have been adequately trained should attempt to prepare sterile parenteral products. Personnel should be properly garbed, with attire appropriate for the risk level of the product to be prepared.

All items should be removed from their outer cartons before being placed on a clean cart or being manually carried into the clean room. A nonlinting wiper should be used to wipe the surfaces of the materials before their placement in the hood. At no time should any object come between the airflow of the high-efficiency particulate air (HEPA) cleaner filter and the critical site or the critical area. The critical site is the point of entry into a container, and the immediate environment surrounding the critical site is the critical area. Anything placed upstream from the critical area can contaminate the critical site. This situation occurs when the airflow washes over the item, removes any foreign material, and carries it into the critical site.

To compound sterile parenteral preparations, a pharmacist should carefully follow each step in Box 25-1. When withdrawing a drug from an ampul, the pharmacist should place the beveled side of the needle against the ampul wall to reduce the possibility of aspirating glass fragments along with the solution. The glass fragments will ordinarily be at the bottom of the ampul or floating on the surface of the drug. If the needle tip is placed at a position halfway down the ampul during withdrawal and the ampul is slowly rotated, the larger glass particles will often stick to the bottom of the ampul as it is turned more horizontally. If the pharmacist slowly moves the needle bevel down the side of the ampul to the shoulder and continues to rotate the ampul a little more, the remainder of the solution can be withdrawn, with the larger particles adhering to the bottom of the ampul and the smaller ones floating on the surface of the remainder of the solution. The pharmacist should then remove the needle from the ampul, replace it with a filter and a new needle, and inject the solution into the new container.

Withdrawing a solution from a vial can be easily done by injecting an equivalent amount of clean air into the vial. A pharmacist may need to do this stepwise by injecting a small portion of the air in the syringe into the vial, aspirating a portion of the liquid, rotating the vial and syringe so that the needle is pointing up, and injecting another portion of air into the vial. This process should be continued until all the solution is withdrawn.

TABLE 25-2 Antioxidants Used in Parenteral Products

Agent	Usual Concentration (%)
Ascorbic acid	0.01–0.5
Butyl hydroxyanisole	0.005–0.02
Cysteine	0.1–0.5
Monothioglycerol	0.1–1
Sodium bisulfite	0.1–1
Sodium metabisulfite	0.1–1
Thiourea	0.005
Tocopherol	0.05–0.5

TABLE 25-3 Solubilizing, Wetting, and Emulsifying Agents for Parenteral Products

Agent	Usual Concentration (%)
Dimethylacetamide	0.01
Dioctyl sodium sulfosuccinate	0.015
Ethyl alcohol	0.61–0.49
Ethyl lactate	0.1
Glycerin	14.6–25
Lecithin	0.5–2.3
PEG-40 castor oil	7–11.5
PEG 300	0.01–50
Polysorbate 20	0.01
Polysorbate 40	0.05
Polysorbate 80	0.04–4
Povidone	0.2–1
Propylene glycol	0.2–50
Sodium desoxycholate	0.21
Sorbitan monopalmitate	0.05

BOX 25-1 Compounding Sterile Parenteral Preparations

Sterile parenteral preparations should be compounded as follows:

1. Clean the work area of the laminar-airflow hood (LAF) thoroughly with a suitable sanitizing agent. A sterile 70% isopropyl alcohol spray or another equally effective disinfectant or cleaner should be used to wipe the internal surfaces. A water-based preparation should be used for the plastic side panels, because alcohol may discolor the plastic. Cleaning should begin at the innermost surface and advance outward (toward the operator) in a uniform line of movement. Nonlinting cloths should be used for this procedure. No solutions should ever be directed at the high-efficiency particulate air (HEPA) filter. After cleaning, allow the surface to dry before proceeding.
2. Place the items for one prescription at a time in the workspace of the LAF; avoid both bunching items and placing any item in the direct airflow pathway of another item.
3. Remove the packaging or wrapping from the necessary syringes, needles, bags, and the like and place them on the work area, also being cognizant of the air pathway and the critical site.
4. Remove the protective aluminum or plastic cap or seals from the containers. Using an appropriate sanitizing agent, such as 70% isopropanol or ethanol, clean the tops, stoppers, and ampul necks of the individual items.
5. Move the plungers on the syringes back and forth to loosen them.
6. If ampuls are used, break off the neck by breaking away the body.
7. Withdraw the medications from the ampuls or vials. If vials are used, injecting a volume of air equal to that of the medication to be removed may be necessary.
8. Filter the solution(s) during the withdrawal phase or the injection phase.
9. Use separate needles for the injection and withdrawal phases.
10. Place the medications in the appropriate container, vial, bag, or syringe.
11. Swirl the preparation to mix the medications after each addition.
12. After all medications are added and mixed, place an additive cap on the syringe or seal on the bag.
13. Label the product.
14. If necessary, place a colorless or amber overwrap on the preparation. Label the overwrap with a second, identical label.

In reconstituting a drug, a pharmacist is advised to inject the reconstitution fluid slowly into the vial and rotate or rock the vial for dissolution. If this process is done too rapidly, foaming can result, creating difficulty in measuring the desired volume of the drug. Drug solutions should be immediately labeled after reconstitution.

Physicochemical Considerations

Freezing
In facilities that do a lot of sterile compounding, a common practice is to reconstitute and prefill syringes and additive bags or vials. This process saves time; some manufacturers even provide frozen antibiotics that are ready to thaw and use. However, a pharmacist should not

indiscriminately freeze drugs and assume they are stable. The pharmacist should check the manufacturer's literature, drug information services, and stability literature before freezing additives. Because different freezers are set at different temperatures, monitoring the temperature is important. Some freezers can be set at −5°C to −20°C, but some preparations may require an ultrafreezer that reaches temperatures as low as −70°C to −80°C.

If drugs are frozen, they must be thawed and returned to room temperature before compounding. This should be done by hanging the bags or placing the vials or containers in a clean area and forcing room-temperature air over the units. Microwave thawing should generally not be used, nor should the bags be placed in hot or warm water baths or sinks. A second LAF hood works well for thawing preparations.

Sorption and Leaching

Another consideration in compounding parenteral preparations is sorption of the drug to the container, filters, stopper, administration sets, and the like. For example, chlorpromazine hydrochloride, clomethiazole edisylate, diazepam, hydralazine, insulin, promazine hydrochloride, promethazine hydrochloride, thiopental sodium, thioridazine hydrochloride, trifluoperazine dihydrochloride, and warfarin sodium have been shown to be lost from aqueous solutions during infusion through plastic IV administration sets.

In some circumstances, the drug preparation itself can extract substances from the container (i.e., leaching). For example, Taxol contains a solvent system that extracts diethylhexyl phthalate from plastic containers. Other types of containers and administration sets are available for administering Taxol.

Incompatibilities

pH, solubility, concentration, complexation, and light are among the factors that affect compatibility and stability of drug substances.

pH

The most important factor in parenteral incompatibilities is a change in the acid–base environment of the drug. The solubility and stability profiles of a drug can be critically related to pH. As a solution goes away from the pH of maximum solubility, the drug can precipitate out of solution. As the solution goes away from the pH of maximum stability, the drug can degrade more rapidly and have a short beyond-use date. The pH of 5% dextrose injection ranges from 3.5 to 6.5, depending on the free sugar acids present and formed during the sterilization process and preparation storage. This low pH must be considered to avoid incompatibilities with additives. For example, potassium, sodium, and related salts are usually more soluble at higher pH levels, but the free acids are formed at lower pH values and can be less soluble. Acid salts (e.g., hydrochlorides, sulfates) are more soluble at lower pH values, and basic drugs can precipitate out at higher pH levels. Generally, solutions of high pH are incompatible with solutions of low pH because of the relatively poor solubility of the free bases or free acids that are formed.

Solubility

Water is the most commonly used solvent in parenterals. When a compound is not soluble in water or is degraded in water, it can be dissolved in a nonaqueous solvent. A nonaqueous solvent must be nontoxic, nonirritating, nonsensitizing, and pharmacologically inactive. Also, the solvent must be in the proper viscosity range to permit easy injection. Ethanol, glycerin, low molecular weight PEGs, and propylene glycol have been used, among others. The effect of these cosolvent systems can be complicated and difficult to predict. In some cases, fixed oils (e.g., corn oil, cottonseed oil, peanut oil, sesame oil) can be used as solvents for parenterals, and these vehicles should be considered. Any preparation containing oils may be incompatible with the water-based parenterals.

Concentration
Some drug preparations are stable and compatible at certain concentrations but not at others. Detailed stability information should be consulted.

Complexation
Some materials, such as tetracycline in the presence of calcium ions, will complex and reduce the activity of the drug. Complexation can also be used to enhance the solubility of a drug (e.g., caffeine, sodium benzoate).

Light
Light-sensitive drugs, such as amphotericin B, B-complex vitamins, cisplatin, daunorubicin, doxorubicin, furosemide, NephrAmine (essential amino acid injection), and vitamin K, should be protected from light. In the case of admixtures, the drugs are removed from their protective environment and mixed in a new medium and new environment. They must be protected from light through use of a light barrier, such as foil or an amber overwrap, during both storage and administration.

Precautions
Precautions that can be taken to decrease the occurrence of incompatibilities include the following:

- Always use freshly prepared solutions. Solutions, if not used, should be discarded after 24 hours, or earlier as indicated.
- Store the solutions at room temperature during preparation, unless advised otherwise.
- Reconstitute solutions according to the manufacturer's instructions, unless advised otherwise. Some preparations may not be soluble or stable if not reconstituted as instructed.
- Use as few additives as possible in infusion fluids. Incorporating more additives increases the possibility of incompatibilities.
- Mix the solution thoroughly after each addition. This task will distribute the drugs throughout the entire solution and minimize the possibility of any interaction between areas of high concentrations of drugs.
- If one particular additive is a problem, dilute it before incorporating any other additives.
- Check all containers first for clarity of solution and complete dissolution of reconstituted products.
- During filtration, ensure that an active drug or an important excipient is not being removed. For example, if a drug precipitates out of solution because of pH or solvent problems, it can be filtered out; also, some preservatives, such as benzalkonium chloride, can be retained on membrane-type filters.
- Be aware of potential incompatibilities in advance. Use published compatibility charts, and prepare a compatibility notebook, adding observations as they occur.

If an incompatibility problem cannot be prevented, use a different administration technique such as (1) administering the problem drugs at staggered intervals so that they are physically separated, (2) using a heparin lock (intermittent injection site) for administration, (3) selecting an alternative site or route of administration, or (4) using a Y-site administration set and thoroughly flushing the line between the drugs so that the problem drugs do not come in contact with each other.

Quality Control

Quality control of parenterals should address sterility, pyrogenicity, particulate matter, and pH. Preparations should be checked for the volume or weight prepared. Quality assurance activities also include routine disinfection (see Appendix IX) and air quality testing, visual confirmation that compounding personnel are properly protecting the processes and preparations, review of all orders and ingredient packages to confirm correct identity and amounts, and visual inspection for leakage and for accuracy and thoroughness of labeling.[5,6]

Sterility and pH are discussed earlier in the chapter. Chapter 10 of this book discusses endotoxins and depyrogenation; interpretation of endotoxin testing endpoints can be difficult and should be done only by persons with appropriate training and experience. Detection of particulate matter and media-fill testing for sterility are discussed below.

A number of software products have been introduced to support sterile compounding activities. Among these are technology for the management of pharmacy workflow to ensure best practices in dose preparation and tracking and for the support for critical pharmacist dose-checking and verification activities. Guidance for evaluating software for use in the compounding pharmacy has been published.[7]

Particulate Matter

According to *USP/NF* Chapter <788>, Particulate Matter in Injections,[8]

> Particulate matter in injections and parenteral infusions consists of extraneous mobile undissolved particles, other than gas bubbles, unintentionally present in the solutions.

Particulate matter can consist of many different things, such as dust, glass, precipitate from drug incompatibility, rubber, cotton fibers, latex, and other insoluble objects.[9] Common sources of particulates include chemicals (undissolved substances, trace contaminants), solvent impurities, packaging components (glass, plastic, rubber, IV administration sets), environmental contaminants (air, surfaces, insect parts), processing equipment (glass, rubber, rust, stainless steel), fibers, and people (hair, skin). Particulate matter can be detected against a light or dark (or light and dark) background.[10]

The source of particulate contamination in sterile products or compounded sterile preparations can be anything that directly or indirectly comes in contact with the solution:[11]

- The solution itself and its ingredients
- Factors involved in the production process, such as the environment, equipment, and personnel
- The preparation's packaging
- Factors involved in preparing the formulation for administration (e.g., manipulation of the drug solution, the environment in which preparation takes place)

Particulate matter contamination of parenteral fluids and drugs is a potentially life-threatening health hazard. Adverse reactions to particulates introduced into the bloodstream may include vein irritation and phlebitis,[12] clinically occult pulmonary granulomas that are detected at autopsy, local tissue infarction, severe pulmonary dysfunction, occlusion of capillaries and arteries, anaphylactic shock, and death. The United States Pharmacopeial Convention (USP) has established an official test for particulate matter in preparations intended for IV use to ensure that unintended and nontherapeutic particulates do not exceed established limits.[8]

Particulate matter testing of injections for extraneous material should not be confused with determination of particle size in nonsoluble drugs. Particle size determination is often performed on nonsolution therapeutic entities, such as emulsions and suspensions, in which the particle size distribution is important.

Steps for visually inspecting injectable solutions for particulate matter are as follows:

1. Inspect the formulation immediately after preparation. If it is not dispensed immediately, it should be inspected again just before dispensing.
2. Inspect the contents, container, and closure during this procedure.
3. Make sure the container is free of any labels or attachments.
4. Remove any external particles with a dampened, nonlinting wiper.
5. Don clean, talc-free gloves.
6. Hold the container by its top, and carefully swirl its contents by rotating the wrist in a circular motion. Avoid vigorous swirling.
7. Any air bubbles that rise to the top can be disregarded.
8. Hold the container horizontally about 4 inches below the light source against a white and black background; slowly move the container back and forth between the white and the black parts of the background.
9. If no particles are noted, slowly invert the container and observe whether any heavy particles are on the bottom of the container or are sliding down the container walls.

Media-Fill Testing

Media-fill testing is used to check a compounding pharmacist's ability to perform aseptic compounding and manipulations. A testing procedure should be selected or designed to mimic the most difficult sterile compounding procedure that is conducted in the pharmacy. The test consists of manipulations with sterile media (for CSPs with low- and medium-risk levels) or with nonsterile media and a terminal sterilization procedure (for CSPs with high-risk levels). The test should be performed when the pharmacist is near the end of a working shift in order to mimic a worst-case scenario. The transfers with the media are performed using routine aseptic procedures, and the media are placed in an incubator and observed after 1 and 2 weeks for microbial growth. If growth occurs, the pharmacist should not formulate any sterile preparations until he or she has repeated and successfully completed the media-fill test.

Packaging

To ensure that the drug concentration, quality, and purity of CSPs are not altered, a pharmacist must use packaging materials that do not interact physically or chemically with the CSP.[13] An ideal container should do the following:

- Allow visual inspection of the contents
- Be chemically inert
- Not interact with the drug or drug additives

- Not contribute to particulate contamination
- Not allow for loss of the drug or solution
- Maintain the sterility and nonpyrogenicity of the contents before and during administration

IV bags and bottles do not meet all the criteria for an ideal container, but they are the only commercially available containers that come close to meeting these criteria. Plastic containers and IV administration sets used with CSPs present some challenges. Plasticizers, such as diethylhexyl phthalate (DEHP) and trioctyl trimellitate (TOTM), are used in the manufacture of these devices to make them soft and pliable. DEHP is the most commonly used plasticizer in IV solution bags. Certain additives used in IV admixture preparation can cause DEHP to be extracted from the bags and tubing into the solution. To address this problem, TOTM has been introduced and is used in many bags and administration sets. Medications that leach significant amounts of DEHP from polyvinyl chloride containers and administration sets include cyclosporine, docetaxel, fat emulsion, paclitaxel, propofol, tacrolimus, and teniposide.[14] In addition, some drugs may sorb to polyvinyl chloride containers and administration sets; these include amiodarone, calcitriol, diazepam, isosorbide dinitrate, lorazepam, nicardipine, nitroglycerin, propofol, quinidine gluconate, tacrolimus, and vitamin A.[14]

Storage and Labeling

The recommended storage temperature for CSPs depends on the specific preparation. Recommended storage temperatures can be room temperature (15°C–25°C), refrigerator temperature (2°C–8°C), frozen temperature (−20°C), or ultrafrozen temperature (down to −80°C).

Labeling for parenterals should, as a minimum, include the following:

- Patient's name and other appropriate identification information
- Solution and ingredient names, amounts, strengths, and concentrations
- Expiration or beyond-use date
- Administration instructions
- Auxiliary labeling
- Storage requirements
- Identification of the responsible pharmacist

Stability and Beyond-Use Dating

In the past, a beyond-use time of 24 hours was routinely placed on parenteral preparations because of the potential for microbiological contamination. Currently, with the use of clean rooms, LAF hoods, and the like, concern about maintaining sterility has largely been addressed. Furthermore, the 24-hour time limits were routine procedure in hospitals, where removal of a preparation from the nursing units was relatively simple if it had not been used. With ambulatory and home health care, however, medications may be dispensed to a patient or caregiver or a clinic and be stored for a few days before their actual administration. This practice has altered the way beyond-use times are assigned. Emphasis now appears to be placed on whether the drug is chemically and physically stable during the projected time for dispensing, storage, and administration, if one assumes that the formulation is prepared in a sterile manner.

Manufacturers' literature, the published literature, and other sources can be used to obtain information on the stability of a drug in a certain situation. The fact that a drug was found to be stable in 1000 mL of 5% dextrose injection does not mean that it will be stable when the same quantity is placed in 50 mL of 5% dextrose injection in an ambulatory drug delivery device; the storage and administration conditions are different and must be considered.[15]

The assignment of a beyond-use date is the responsibility of a pharmacist or compounding pharmacist. The current edition of the *USP/NF* must be consulted and appropriate standard operating procedures and documentation used.

Allowable Endotoxin Levels in Parenteral Preparations

Endotoxins are a subset of pyrogens that come from gram-negative bacteria. The terms *endotoxin* and *lipopolysaccharide* are often used interchangeably. However, to be more precise, endotoxins are the natural complex of lipopolysaccharides that occur in the outer layer of bilayered gram-negative bacterial cells, whereas lipopolysaccharides are the purified form used as a standard for quality control and research purposes.

Inadvertent administration of endotoxins to humans may result in a number of events, ranging from fever to a cascade of pathogenic responses to death. Responses can include irreversible and fatal septic shock, hypotension, lymphopenia, neutrophilia, and elevated levels of cortisol and C-reactive protein.

Endotoxins are potent, toxic, and very stable and are present in many pharmaceutical ingredients and on surfaces that come in contact with preparations formulated for parenteral administration. They are water soluble, will pass through 0.22-μm filters, are not destroyed by autoclaving, and are insoluble in organic solvents. Endotoxins are very difficult to eliminate in a final preparation. Therefore, procedures are directed at eliminating endotoxins during the preparation process.

The body can tolerate a certain load of endotoxins (measured as endotoxin units, or EU) without adverse results. The generally accepted endotoxin limit (EL) is defined as

$$EL = K/M$$

where K is the threshold human pyrogenic dose of endotoxin per kilogram of body weight per hour, which is 5 EU/kg for parenteral drugs (except those administered intrathecally) and 0.2 EU/kg for the intrathecal route of administration, and where M is the maximum recommended human dose per kilogram of body weight that would be administered in a single 1-hour period.

The EL, then, is equal to the threshold pyrogenic response (K in EU/kg) divided by the dose in the units by which it is administered (milliliters, units, or milligrams) per 70-kg person per hour. The delivery method (multiple or bolus doses) and other factors must also be considered.

To use the EL = K/M formula, a pharmacist must know the maximum endotoxin levels established for the drugs being prepared. The table[16] included in Appendix VII, derived from the USP/NF,[3] provides a handy reference. The most recent edition of that compendium should be consulted to determine if the information has been updated.

Pharmacists compounding high-risk sterile preparations from bulk substances need access to a calculator and a current *USP/NF* or an endotoxin limit table in order to calculate the endotoxin load for the preparation. (See Figure 25-1 for a worksheet and Appendix VII

Endotoxin Limit Worksheet

Patient Name _____ Date _____ Rx No. _____

Patient Weight (kg) _____

Nonintrathecal use: _____ kg × 5 EU/kg = _____ EU endotoxin limit/hour

Intrathecal use: _____ kg × 0.2 EU/kg = _____ EU endotoxin limit/hour

Drug Name	Dose/24 Hours	×	Endotoxin Level	=	Endotoxin Contribution	Volume of Drug Used
_____	_____	×	_____	=	_____	_____
_____	_____	×	_____	=	_____	_____
_____	_____	×	_____	=	_____	_____
_____	_____	×	_____	=	_____	_____
_____	_____	×	_____	=	_____	_____
_____	_____	×	_____	=	_____	_____
_____	_____	×	_____	=	_____	_____
_____	_____	×	_____	=	_____	_____
_____	_____	×	_____	=	_____	_____

Vehicle

_____	_____	×	_____	=	_____	_____
_____	_____	×	_____	=	_____	_____
_____	_____	×	_____	=	_____	_____
_____	_____	×	_____	=	_____	_____

TOTAL

_____ _____ × _____ = _____ _____

Total endotoxin contribution/Total volume = _____ EU/mL

_____ / _____ = _____ EU/mL

EU/mL/24 hours = Endotoxin load/hour

_____ / 24 = _____

FIGURE 25-1 Endotoxin limit worksheet.

for compendial requirements for bacterial endotoxins in sterile preparations.) The endotoxin load in compounded sterile preparations can be calculated as follows:[16,17]

1. Multiply the weight of the patient (in kilograms) times the allowable endotoxin units (EU) per kilogram [EU/kg] to obtain the endotoxin limit per hour for non-intrathecal or intrathecal medication delivery.
   5.0 EU/kg × Patient weight (kg) = Endotoxin limit per hour (nonintrathecal)
   or
   0.2 EU/kg × Patient weight (kg) = Endotoxin limit per hour (intrathecal)
2. Obtain the required information for the calculations from *USP/NF* or a current endotoxin limit table.
3. Determine the final volume of the preparation.

4. Input the information on the Endotoxin Limit Worksheet.
5. Determine the final endotoxin load.
6. Consider the route of administration, and determine if the calculated value exceeds the value in Step 1.
7. If the calculated value does not exceed the value in Step 1, the compound may be prepared.
8. If the calculated value exceeds the value in Step 1, check with the prescriber.

Patient Counseling

Patients should be instructed on the proper storage and use of any parenteral preparations placed in their care. They should be informed about the proper method of maintaining a sterile administration site and the handling of administration sets and equipment. Patients may need to be taught how to program ambulatory pumps and how to deal with emergencies. Also, the correct disposal of parenteral preparations, needles, syringes, and tubing should be discussed in detail, so that patients are aware of the harm that can result from improper disposal.

Sample Formulations

Ingredient-Specific Preparations

℞ Antiemetic Injection for Cancer Chemotherapy

Reglan 5 mg/mL	30 mL (150 mg)	Active
Ativan 2 mg/mL	0.5 mL (1 mg)	Active
Mannitol 25%	50 mL (12.5 g)	Active
Compazine 5 mg/mL	2 mL (10 mg)	Active
5% Dextrose injection	50 mL	Vehicle

(Note: This preparation should be prepared in an LAF hood by a validated aseptic compounding pharmacist using aseptic technique.)

1. Calculate the quantity of each ingredient required for the prescription.
2. Accurately measure or weigh each ingredient.
3. Add each ingredient in sequence to a 50-mL partial-fill IV piggyback bag of 5% dextrose injection, mixing thoroughly after each addition.
4. Label the product.

℞ Fentanyl and Bupivacaine Injection for Ambulatory Pump Reservoirs

Fentanyl citrate 20 µg/mL	40 mL	Active
Bupivacaine hydrochloride 0.125%	25 mL	Active
0.9% Sodium chloride injection	qs 100 mL	Vehicle

(Note: All procedures should be carried out in a clean air environment by a qualified aseptic compounding pharmacist.)

1. Calculate the quantity of each ingredient required for the prescription.
2. Aseptically withdraw 40 mL of fentanyl citrate injection (Sublimaze), and introduce into a reservoir.
3. Aseptically withdraw 25 mL of 0.5% bupivacaine hydrochloride injection, introduce into the reservoir, and mix well.
4. Aseptically withdraw 35 mL of 0.9% sodium chloride injection, and introduce into the reservoir, along with a few milliliters of air.
5. Rotate the reservoir so that the air bubble will mix the contents.
6. Position the reservoir so that the air bubble is near the exit port, and remove the air in the reservoir and tubing by withdrawing the solution up to the end of the port.
7. Clamp, package, and label the product.

℞ Doxorubicin Hydrochloride and Vincristine Sulfate Injection

Doxorubicin hydrochloride 2 mg/mL	83.5 mL	Active
Vincristine sulfate 1 mg/mL	3.5 mL	Active
0.9% Sodium chloride injection	qs 100 mL	Vehicle

(Note: All procedures should be carried out in a clean air environment by a qualified aseptic compounding pharmacist.)

1. Calculate the quantity of each ingredient required for the prescription.
2. Reconstitute the doxorubicin hydrochloride, if necessary, according to the manufacturer's directions.
3. Carefully measure the required volumes of the reconstituted doxorubicin hydrochloride solution and the vincristine sulfate injection.
4. Add the measured volumes of doxorubicin hydrochloride and vincristine sulfate injections to a sterile container.
5. Add 13 mL of 0.9% sodium chloride injection to the container, and mix well.
6. Withdraw the solution into a sterile syringe, and fill the required reservoir or administration device container.
7. Expel any excess air, and seal the container.
8. Package and label the product.

℞ Hydromorphone Hydrochloride 50 mg/mL Injection

Hydromorphone hydrochloride	2.5 g	Active
Bacteriostatic 0.9% sodium chloride injection	22.2 mL	Vehicle/Tonicity Adjuster
Bacteriostatic water for injection	qs 50 mL	Vehicle

(Note: All procedures should be carried out in a clean air environment by a qualified aseptic compounding pharmacist.)

1. Check the calibration on the balance to be used for weighing the hydromorphone hydrochloride.
2. Accurately weigh the 2.5 g of hydromorphone hydrochloride.
3. Place the powder in a previously sterilized graduated cylinder.
4. Accurately measure the required volume of bacteriostatic 0.9% sodium chloride injection, add to the hydromorphone hydrochloride powder, and mix well.
5. Add sufficient bacteriostatic water for injection to make 50 mL, and mix well. (Note: The same bacteriostatic agents should be used in both the bacteriostatic 0.9% sodium chloride solution and the bacteriostatic water for injection to maintain a proper bacteriostatic agent concentration.)
6. Withdraw the solution into a sterile 60-mL syringe.
7. Affix a sterile 0.22-μm filter to the end of the syringe.
8. Filter the solution into the desired reservoir for administration.
9. Package and label the product.

℞ Hydroxyprogesterone Caproate 250 mg/mL in Oil Injection

Hydroxyprogesterone caproate	25 g	Active
Benzyl benzoate	46 mL	Solvent
Benzyl alcohol	2 mL	Preservative
Castor oil	qs 100 mL	Vehicle/Solvent

1. Calculate the quantity of each ingredient required for the prescription.
2. Accurately measure or weigh each ingredient.
3. Dissolve the hydroxyprogesterone caproate in the benzyl benzoate.
4. Add the benzyl alcohol, and mix well.
5. Add sufficient castor oil to volume, and mix well.
6. Sterilize the solution by either sterile filtration or dry heat.
7. Package and label the product.

General Injection

℞ Hyaluronidase Injection

Hyaluronidase	15,000 units	Active
Sodium chloride	850 mg	Tonicity Adjuster
Edetate disodium	100 mg	Chelating Agent
Calcium chloride dihydrate	53 mg	Active
Thimerosal	10 mg	Preservative
Sodium phosphate monobasic, anhydrous	170 mg	Buffer
Sterile water for injection	qs 100 mL	Vehicle
Sodium hydroxide 1% solution	qs to pH 6.4–7.4	pH Adjustment

(Note: This preparation should be prepared in an aseptic working environment by a validated aseptic compounding pharmacist using aseptic technique.)

1. Calculate the quantity of each ingredient required for the prescription.
2. Accurately weigh or measure each ingredient.
3. Dissolve the sodium chloride, edetate disodium, calcium chloride dihydrate, and thimerosal in about 80 mL of sterile water for injection.
4. Add the hyaluronidase, and stir until dissolved.
5. Add the sodium phosphate monobasic, and stir until dissolved.
6. Dropwise, adjust the pH by using the sodium hydroxide 1% solution until a pH in the range of 6.4 to 7.4 has been obtained.
7. Add sufficient sterile water for injection to volume, and mix well.
8. Filter the solution through a sterile 0.22-μm filter into sterile vials.
9. Package and label the product.

Sclerotherapy Injections

℞ Sodium Chloride 20% Hypertonic Injection

Sodium chloride	20 g	Active
Sterile water for injection	qs 100 mL	Vehicle

(Note: This preparation should be prepared in an LAF hood by a validated aseptic compounding pharmacist using aseptic technique.)

1. Calculate the quantity of each ingredient required for the prescription.
2. Accurately weigh or measure each ingredient.
3. Dissolve the salt in sufficient sterile water for injection to volume.
4. Filter the solution through a sterile 0.22-μm filter into sterile vials.
5. Package and label the product.

℞ **Sodium Chloride 20% with Lidocaine Hydrochloride 0.5% Injection**

Sodium chloride	20 g	Active
Lidocaine hydrochloride	500 mg	Active
Sterile water for injection	qs 100 mL	Vehicle

(Note: This preparation should be prepared in an LAF hood by a validated aseptic compounding pharmacist using aseptic technique.)

1. Calculate the quantity of each ingredient required for the prescription.
2. Accurately weigh or measure each ingredient.
3. Dissolve the salts in sufficient sterile water for injection to volume.
4. Filter the solution through a sterile 0.22-μm filter into sterile vials.
5. Package and label the product.

℞ **Phenol 5% Aqueous Injection**

Phenol	5 g	Active
Glycerin	5 mL	Solvent
Edetate disodium	50 mg	Chelating Agent
Sodium bisulfite	100 mg	Antioxidant
Sterile water for injection	qs 100 mL	Vehicle

(Note: This preparation should be prepared in an LAF hood by a validated aseptic compounding pharmacist using aseptic technique.)

1. Calculate the quantity of each ingredient required for the prescription.
2. Accurately weigh or measure each ingredient.
3. Dissolve the edetate disodium in about 30 mL of the sterile water for injection.
4. Dissolve the sodium bisulfite in about 30 mL of the sterile water for injection.
5. Dissolve the phenol in the glycerin, and add about 30 mL of the sterile water for injection.
6. Combine the edetate disodium solution (step 3) and the sodium bisulfite solution (step 4), and add them to the phenol–glycerin solution (step 5).
7. Add sufficient sterile water for injection to volume, and mix well. (If the solution is cloudy, gentle heat will clear it.)
8. Filter the solution through a sterile 0.22-μm filter into sterile vials (or package in vials and autoclave).
9. Package and label the product.

℞ Phenol 2.5%, Dextrose 25%, and Glycerin 25% Aqueous Injection

Liquefied phenol	2.8 g (2.6 mL)	Active
Dextrose	25 g	Active
Glycerin	25 g	Solvent/Vehicle
Sterile water for injection	qs 100 mL	Vehicle

1. Calculate the quantity of each ingredient required for the prescription.
2. Accurately weigh or measure each ingredient.
3. Dissolve the dextrose in about 50 mL of the sterile water for injection.
4. Mix the liquefied phenol with the glycerin, and add about 25 mL of the sterile water for injection.
5. Add the dextrose solution (step 3) to the phenol–glycerin solution (step 4) with mixing, followed by a sufficient quantity of sterile water for injection to volume, and mix well.
6. Filter the solution through a sterile 0.22-μm filter into sterile vials (or package in vials and autoclave).
7. Package and label the product.

℞ Phenol 10% in Glycerin

| Phenol | 10 g | Active |
| Glycerin | qs 100 mL | Vehicle |

1. Calculate the quantity of each ingredient required for the prescription.
2. Accurately weigh or measure each ingredient.
3. Dissolve the phenol in the glycerin and mix well.
4. Filter the solution through a sterile 0.22-μm filter into sterile vials.
5. Package and label the product.

References

1. Akers MJ. Unique and special characteristics of sterile dosage forms. *Int J Pharm Compound.* 2014;18(6):479–84.
2. Akers MJ. Aseptic processing. *Int J Pharm Compound.* 2015;19(1):49–56.
3. United States Pharmacopeial Convention. Chapter <797>, Pharmaceutical compounding—sterile preparations. In: *United States Pharmacopeia/National Formulary.* Rockville, MD: United States Pharmacopeial Convention; current edition.
4. Akers MJ. Barrier isolator technologies in aseptic processing. *Int J Pharm Compound.* 2015; 19(4):315–20.
5. Akers MJ. Quality assurance and quality control, Part 1. *Int J Pharm Compound.* 2015;19(2):121–4.
6. Akers MJ. Quality assurance and quality control, Part 2. *Int J Pharm Compound.* 2015;19(3):215–21.
7. Robinson M. A technology guide for evaluating software tools to support sterile compounding and workflow management. *Int J Pharm Compound.* 2011;15(1):20–6.
8. United States Pharmacopeial Convention. Chapter <788>, Particulate matter in injections. In: *United States Pharmacopeia/National Formulary.* Rockville, MD: United States Pharmacopeial Convention; current edition.
9. Borchert SJ, Abe A, Aldrich DS, et al. Particulate matter in parenteral products: a review. *J Parenter Sci Technol.* 1986;40(5):212–41.

10. Allen LV Jr. Standard operating procedure for particulate testing for sterile products. *Int J Pharm Compound.* 1998;2(1):78.
11. Buchanan EC, Schneider PJ. *Compounding Sterile Preparations.* 2nd ed. Bethesda, MD: American Society of Health-System Pharmacists; 2005:20.
12. Dorris GG, Bivins BA, Rapp RP, et al. Inflammatory potential of foreign particulates in parenteral drugs. *Anesth Analg.* 1977;56(3):422–8.
13. Akers MJ. Sterile product packaging and delivery systems. *Int J Pharm Compound.* 2015;19(6): 491–500.
14. Rice SP. A review of parenteral admixtures requiring select containers and administration sets. *Int J Pharm Compound.* 2002;6(2):120–1.
15. United States Pharmacopeial Convention. Chapter <795>, Pharmaceutical compounding— nonsterile preparations. In: *United States Pharmacopeia/National Formulary.* Rockville, MD: United States Pharmacopeial Convention; current edition.
16. Allen LV Jr. Standard operating procedure: calculating the endotoxin load in compounded sterile preparations. *Int J Pharm Compound.* 2004;8(6):466–7.
17. Allen LV Jr. Quality-control analytical methods: allowable endotoxin levels in sterile preparations. *Int J Pharm Compound.* 2004;8(6):479–85.

Chapter 26

Biotechnology, Nanotechnology, and Pharmacogenomics

We hope ultimately to bring pharmacogenomics, a way in which to foster the personalizing of medicine, to every healthcare professional's prescription pad for the benefit of their patients and U.S. consumers.

—Janet Woodcock,
Deputy Commissioner for Operations,
U.S. Food and Drug Administration

The world of pharmaceuticals is changing rapidly as biotechnology continues to grow and nanotechnology appears on the horizon. Biotechnology is gaining in importance in extemporaneous pharmaceutical compounding, and nanotechnology and pharmacogenomics could drastically change the practice of pharmacy.

Biotechnology

Definitions and Types

Biotechnology has been variously defined as (1) a science that applies the techniques of engineering and technology to the study of any living organism; (2) the use of living organisms and their cellular, subcellular, and molecular components to produce useful substances; and (3) any technique that uses living organisms (or parts of organisms) to make or modify products or to improve plants or animals for beneficial use. By one definition, it is the use of living organisms to produce beneficial products as diverse as antibiotics, alcohol, and dairy products. It can even involve cloning, with insertion of genetic material into a host cell and development in a cell culture or a microorganism.

Historical Use

The use of biotechnology has been traced back more than 5000 years. People of ancient civilizations, such as the Mesopotamians and the Egyptians, added yeast to food substances and nutrients to produce beer.[1] Similar techniques were used later to produce wines, cheeses, and various other fermented products. However, health care products of biotechnology were not developed until the 19th century.

Deoxyribonucleic acid (DNA) was first isolated in 1869, and its chemical composition was delineated in the early 1900s. In 1953, James D. Watson and Francis H. C. Crick proposed that the structure of DNA was a double helix, that is, two strands of sugar and phosphate molecules coiled around each other, similar to the structure of a spiral staircase. The strands are connected by four bases: adenine, guanine, cytosine, and thymine. Adenine and thymine always pair up opposite each other; the same is true for guanine and cytosine. In each DNA molecule, the sequence of the paired bases has a specific pattern. The pattern constitutes the DNA message for maintaining cells and organisms and for developing the next generation of organisms.

DNA duplicates by cloning itself. By altering the cloning process and using DNA probes, lysing agents, strands, and other materials to recombine the various parts, scientists can modify DNA to produce a different protein than the one it was originally programmed to produce. This life technology, or biotechnology, results in products that can be used to diagnose and treat disease. A number of approaches to biotechnology that are of interest to industry may ultimately involve the compounding pharmacist, including (1) the production of pharmacologically active recombinant proteins or modified proteins; (2) the use of recombinant proteins to design pharmacologically active smaller molecules; (3) the manipulation of cells and tissues to accomplish a therapeutic effect; and (4) the production of transgenic bacteria or animals that can be used as so-called "factories" to produce human and animal pharmaceuticals. In the last case, the bacteria might possibly be encapsulated and implanted in humans to produce specific beneficial compounds.

Applications

The first proteins developed by recombinant DNA technology for pharmaceutical use were human insulin for treating diabetes and somatrem for treating human growth hormone deficiency in children. These products became available in 1982 and 1985, respectively. In 1986, two major biotechnology products came on the market: interferon alfa, used to treat hairy cell leukemia, and muromonab-CD3, used to prevent acute allograft rejection after renal transplantation. About a dozen recombinant DNA products were approved for marketing during the 1980s. Since then, more than 200 biotechnologically derived medications have been approved.[2]

Biotechnology drug preparations present compounding pharmacists with a lucrative new source of demand for their special expertise. Potential routes of delivery for these products include nasal, oral (buccal, mucosal, sublingual), parenteral (intramuscular, intravenous, subcutaneous), and transdermal routes and oral inhalation. Most biotechnology drug products cannot be administered orally (swallowed) because of their instability in the strong acid environment of the stomach and their low systemic absorption through the gastrointestinal mucosa.

Composition

Most of the biotechnology products are proteins, but some may soon be smaller peptidelike molecules. Proteins are inherently unstable molecules, and their degradation profiles can be quite complex. Biotechnology products differ from conventional small-molecule drug products in their method of preparation and in the potential problems presented in their formulation. Pharmacists involved in compounding with biologically active proteins will be interested in their stabilization, formulation, and delivery.

In working with biotechnologically derived drugs, a pharmacist must be cognizant of both the active drug constituent and the total drug-delivery system, or carrier. Protein drugs are extremely potent and are generally used in quite low concentrations. The bulk of most compounded preparations may be the excipients. In addition to the vehicle, buffers, and the like, stabilizers are often incorporated into these products. A number of different stabilizers can be used, including surfactants, amino acids, polyhydric alcohols, fatty acids, proteins, antioxidants, reducing agents, and metal ions. Table 26-1 describes agents used as stabilizers.

pH is one of the key factors in developing a stable product. The optimal pH range for a specific product can be achieved through the selection of appropriate physiologic buffers. Usually, buffer concentrations are in the range of 0.01 to 0.1 M. In general, an increase in the buffer concentration means an increase in pain on injection.

TABLE 26-1 Stabilizing Agents for Biotechnology Preparations

Class	Agent	Action
Amino acids	Alanine	Serves as a solubilizer
	Arginine	Serves as a buffer
	Aspartic acid	Inhibits isomerism
	Glycine	Serves as a stabilizer
	Glutamic acid	Serves as a thermostabilizer
	Leucine	Inhibits aggregation
Antioxidants	Ascorbic acid, cysteine hydrochloride, glutathione, thioglycerol, thioglycolic acid, thiosorbitol	Help stabilize protein conformation
Chelating agents	EDTA salts	Inhibit oxidation by removing aspartic acid, glutamic acid, and metal ions
Fatty acids	Choline, ethanolamine, phosphotidyl	Serve as stabilizers
Proteins	Human serum albumin	Prevents surface adsorption; stabilizes protein conformation; serves as a complexing agent and cryoprotectant
Metal ions	Ca^{++}, Ni^{++}, Mg^{++}, Mn^{++}	Help stabilize protein conformation
Polyhydric alcohols	Ethylene glycol	Serves as a stabilizer
	Glucose	Strengthens conformation
	Lactose	Serves as a stabilizer
	Mannitol	Serves as a cryoprotectant
	Propylene glycol	Prevents aggregation
	Sorbitol	Prevents denaturation and aggregation
	Sucrose	Serves as a stabilizer
	Trehalose	Serves as a stabilizer
Polymers	Polyethylene glycol, povidone	Prevent aggregation
Surfactants	Poloxamer 407	Prevents denaturation and stabilizes cloudiness
	Polysorbates 20 and 80	Retard aggregation

Chelating agents can be incorporated to bind trace metals such as copper, iron, calcium, and manganese. Ethylenediaminetetraacetic acid (EDTA) is commonly used at a concentration of about 0.01% to 0.05%.

Antioxidants are often incorporated because oxidation is one of the major factors in protein degradation. α-tocopherol, ascorbic acid, monothioglycerol, and sodium disulfide are frequently used at a concentration of about 0.05% to 0.1%.

Preservatives may be necessary. These could include benzyl alcohol (1.0% to 3.0%), chlorobutanol (0.3% to 0.5%), and phenol (0.3% to 0.5%).

Polyols are good stabilizers. They are commonly used in concentrations from 1% to 10%.

Tonicity-adjusting agents include dextrose and sodium chloride in concentrations necessary to achieve isotonicity with 0.9% sodium chloride solution, or approximately 290 mOsm/L.

Preparation

A general rule for working with biotechnology formulations is to keep procedures as simple as possible. Most manipulations are the same as those discussed in Chapters 10 and 25 of this book. Sterility must be maintained in any preparation of parenteral products, because most do not contain a preservative. The recommended approach is that only one dose be prepared from each vial or container to minimize contamination. Many times this is not practical, however, because specific manipulations are needed to meet patient needs. Facilities should be clean, and proper techniques should be used. A kit for testing aseptic technique in preparing for-

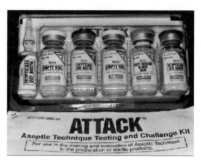

FIGURE 26-1 Aseptic technique testing and challenge kit.

mulations is available from equipment suppliers (Figure 26-1). At a minimum, a laminar-airflow hood should be used and appropriate attire worn. All equipment must be sterile. Any additive used in compounding parenteral drug products must be free of pyrogens; if a preparation becomes contaminated with pyrogens, it should be discarded. There are two special considerations in working with biotechnologically derived preparations—the use of filters and the sorption of these drugs to containers.

The use of filters in manipulating biotechnology products can result in some loss of the drug available to a patient. For example, muromonab-CD3 (Orthoclone OKT3) injection should be filtered with a low-protein-binding filter of 0.2 to 0.22 μm. Many biotechnology products should not be filtered at all. If a filtration device is part of the intravenous administration apparatus, biotechnology drugs should generally be administered distal to the site of the filter. Filters that have been shown to minimize protein adsorption are those made from polycarbonate, polysulfone, polyvinylidene difluoride, and regenerated cellulose. As a precaution, low-protein-binding filters should be used.

Sorption of proteins to containers can result in drug loss. This loss can be minimized either by the use of albumin or by siliconization. Adding about 0.1% albumin to the product can decrease the sorption of proteins to containers. If glass mixing vessels are used, the albumin solution should be added before the drug. If siliconization is used, a compounding pharmacist should prepare a silicon solution or emulsion and soak or rinse the glass vials in it. The drained vials should then be placed in an oven at about 250°C for 5 to 6 hours. This procedure will minimize protein adsorption to glass; it can be used for both the preparation equipment and the packaging containers.

Physicochemical Considerations

To retain a drug's biologic activity up to the time of administration to a patient, some factors associated with handling proteins must be considered: selecting an appropriate vehicle for drug delivery, individualizing dosages, administering drugs through novel drug-delivery systems, preparing drugs for delivery through these systems, monitoring their efficacy, and counseling patients on their use.

Some issues specific to protein pharmaceuticals are as follows:

- Their high molecular weight and potential for aggregation (i.e., a small change in structure can result in a change in activity)
- Their immunogenic potential, because some are produced by a fermentation-type process and proteins can co-purify with proteins
- The assignment of potency to the reference standards (when traditional pharmaceuticals are about 98% pure, these materials may be only 0.1% to 1% active, with their activity assigned by potentially variable assays)
- The use of micropipets, which can require frequent calibration
- The concern that constituted products can be less stable than lyophilized products
- The effect of agitation on a product's stability
- The possible interaction of the product with the inner wall of the glass vial and with the elastomeric closure
- The effectiveness of the preservative if a multidose product is mixed with other products

Physicochemical factors to be considered in compounding protein drug products include the structure of the protein drug, isoelectric point, molecular weight, solubility and factors affecting solubility (e.g., metal ions, pH, salts, surfactants), stability and factors affecting stability (e.g., freeze–thaw cycles, light, mechanical stress, metal ions, oxygen, pH, temperature), polymorphism, stereoisomers, filtration media compatibility, shear, and surface denaturation.

Solubility depends on a number of factors, including chemical structure, pH, and temperature. Proteins are generally more soluble in their native environment or medium or in a matrix that mimics their native environment, such as lipids, sodium chloride, trace elements, and other proteins in an aqueous medium. Before compounding these products, pharmacists must consider the ingredients' effects on the solubility of the active drug, especially because most of the products are currently administered parenterally. This task is critical because the actual drug is present in a small quantity and can go unnoticed if it precipitates. Sterile water for injection and 0.9% sodium chloride solution usually are good vehicles for use in a formulation.

The pH of the compound should be maintained close to the pH of the original approved, manufactured product; changes in pH can affect proteins in numerous ways. Chemical degradation rate constants are pH related, and hydrogen ion concentration can affect the actual structure of proteins (i.e., quaternary structure). Buffer systems may be needed in compounding; they should be prepared at the minimum buffer strength required to produce the most stable drug product.

Chemical instability of proteins is the modification of protein structures by bond formation or cleavage to yield a new compound. *Physical instability* generally involves changes in structure, conformation, or behavior in a particular environment. Stability, both chemical and physical, depends on pH, temperature, and agitation, as well as on the overall environment in which the drug is contained.

Sorption is a problem with colony-stimulating factors and with aldesleukin (Proleukin) at low concentrations. To minimize the sticking of the protein to the glass, adding about 0.1% albumin to the product to occupy the potential binding sites in the container may be helpful. Pharmacists must consider this problem before making any changes in packaging.

Agitation, which is frothing created by the physical decomposition of the protein, can adversely affect the product in two ways. First, frothing can cause difficulties in using a syringe to withdraw the required amount of drug from a vial. To avoid this problem, a compounding pharmacist should mix the product by rolling the vial in the hands or gently swirling it. Second, excessive agitation can cause changes in a protein's quaternary structure that often reduce or eliminate a drug's therapeutic activity. Some products, such as filgrastim (Neupogen) and sargramostim (Leukine), are reconstituted by directing a soft stream of diluent against the inside of the container wall. Others, such as recombinant tissue plasminogen activator (tPA; alteplase), are reconstituted by directing a stream of diluent directly into the product at the bottom of the vial.

Quality Control

A compounding pharmacist should follow standard quality control procedures. The compounded preparations can be tested for pH, final volume, sterility, and pyrogenicity and physically observed for clarity, presence of gas bubbles and particulate matter, and change in color.

Packaging

The container used for storage after compounding must be chosen carefully. For example, the manufacturer's directions for interleukin-2 (aldesleukin) suggest the use of a plastic bag because that type of dilution container enhances consistent drug delivery. Unless otherwise specified, USP (United States Pharmacopeial Convention) type I glass should be used for packaging when storage for extended time periods is indicated. A compounding pharmacist should be aware of the potential for sorption of the drug to the glass walls. The pharmacist should select closures and stoppers that are compatible and flexible; have low levels of particulates; and have few problems with adsorption, absorption, and permeation.

Storage and Labeling

The recommended storage temperature depends on the specific preparation. Recommended storage temperatures can be room temperature (15°C–25°C), refrigerator temperature (2°C–8°C), frozen temperature (−20°C), or ultrafrozen temperature (down to −80°C). Freezing does affect the activity of certain products; for instance, the activity of filgrastim decreases if it is frozen. Some products can retain potency at room temperature after reconstitution. Sargramostim retains potency for up to 30 days at 25°C. However, most manufacturers recommend refrigeration at 2°C to 8°C, regardless of the product's potency at room temperature.

The short shelf life of these products after reconstitution can be due to chemical or physical instability or to the fact that most do not contain preservatives. The manufacturer's recommendations or those validated by the published literature should be followed for products after they are reconstituted and manipulated. One example is tPA, which has been used in treating intraocular fibrin formation after a vitrectomy and in managing subconjunctival hemorrhage after glaucoma filtration surgery. The prepared solution is stable in a pH range of 5 to 7.5 and is incompatible with bacteriostatic agents. For compounding, the commercial product is reconstituted according to the manufacturer's directions, using sterile water for injection without preservatives to yield a concentration of 1 mg/mL. This solution is further diluted with 0.9% sodium chloride injection to yield a concentration of 25 µg/100 µL. Aliquots of 0.3 mL are withdrawn into 1-mL tuberculin syringes and capped. The syringes are stored in an ultrafreezer at −70°C. This product has been shown, by both bioassay and clinical use, to retain its activity for at least 1 year. This type of specific product information is not included in the manufacturer's label information and is usually obtained by reading the literature or by asking the manufacturer directly.

Stability

Physically, biotechnology products can degrade by aggregation, denaturation, and precipitation. Aggregation can be the result of covalent or noncovalent processes and can be either physical or chemical in nature. Aggregate formation can actually begin when primary particles are formed from protein molecules as a result of Brownian movement.

Denaturation can result from heat, cold, extreme pH values, organic solvents, hydrophilic surfaces, shear, agitation, mixing, filtering, shaking, freeze–thaw cycles, ionic strength, and other factors. Denaturation can be quite complex and can be either reversible or irreversible.

Precipitation can result from shaking, heating, filtration, pH, and chemical interactions. The first step in a precipitation process is generally aggregation. When the aggregates gain a sufficient size, they precipitate out of solution and are clearly evident. Precipitation can occur on membrane filters, in equipment, in tubing, and in contact with other equipment and supplies.

Patient Counseling

Patients should be aware of the importance of proper and careful handling of biotechnology drugs. They should be instructed on the proper preparation, administration, and disposal of these products.

Sample Formulation

℞ Tissue Plasminogen Activator (tPA) 25 µg/100 µL Ophthalmic Solution

Tissue plasminogen activator	20-mg vial	Active
Sterile 0.9% sodium chloride injection	60 mL	Vehicle/Tonicity Adjuster
Sterile water for injection	20 mL	Vehicle

1. Reconstitute a commercial 20-mg vial of tissue plasminogen activator (alteplase) according to the manufacturer's directions by adding 20 mL of sterile water for injection, without preservatives, to result in a 20 mg/20 mL (1 mg/mL) concentration.
2. Dilute this solution by adding 60 mL of sterile 0.9% sodium chloride injection to yield a concentration of 250 µg/mL, or 25 µg/100 µL.
3. Mix thoroughly, using gentle swirling or slow inversion of the container, or both.
4. Withdraw 0.3-mL aliquots into the desired number of 1-cc syringes, and cap syringes.
5. Place the syringes that are not going to be used immediately in a −70°C ultrafreezer.

Nanotechnology

Definitions and Development

Like biotechnology, *nanotechnology* has several definitions. It is the science of building machines that manipulate matter in the way the matter is created: one atom at a time. It is the art and science of building molecular structures so they are sufficiently large and complex to function as machines or devices; in essence, they are atomically precise, functional machine systems developed on the scale of the nanometer and built atom by atom, molecule by molecule.

Nanotechnology represents the convergence of computers, networks, and biotechnology to create products never before imagined. Nanodevices will likely be used in every industry, stretching the limits of what is possible. The arrival of nanotechnology in everyday life will not be a single, sudden transformational event; rather, it will emerge from a series of interrelated technologies and processes, all woven together and periodically crossing thresholds—the ultimate chemistry kit. Numerous Nobel Prize winners, billions of dollars in research throughout the world, myriad breakthroughs, competition among nations, and the U.S. National Nanotechnology Initiative have helped bring nanotechnology closer to fruition. Twenty years may pass, but nanotechnology will become as strategically important as oil or the invention of the computer. The creation of an ultrasmall world with tiny so-called "assemblers" and machines will propel businesses into unprecedented opportunities and may drastically alter the practice of pharmacy.

Nanotechnology will depend on the development of universal assemblers—nanoscale devices with robotic arms, under computer control, that will be able to grasp individual atoms and use them to assemble objects from the bottom up. The first assemblers will be programmed to reproduce themselves by the trillions. Their quality control will be near perfect, at a relatively low cost. Universal assemblers will be capable of being programmed to perform many functions, such as the following:

- Nanomachines or nanosurgeons may be able to repair cells, organs, or even DNA.
- "Smart" mouthwashes may be able to destroy harmful bacteria in the oral cavity and enhance oral hygiene.
- Cell-herding machines may stimulate rapid wound healing.
- Nanocruisers in the body may attack viruses and bacteria.
- Interactive medical libraries may be accessible by matchbook-size supercomputers.
- "Roto-rooters" may be used to remove cholesterol from veins.
- Nanites may restore youthful complexions and reverse organ breakdown.
- Assemblers may be able to construct bridges, automobiles, homes, and even spaceships.
- Machines may be able to maintain our physical bodies.
- Polymers of uniform lengths may be manufactured.
- Biochemically based nanocomputers and bioelectronic computers may be available.
- Blood products; artificial skin products; and bioartificial organs, blood vessels, and cartilage may be made on demand.
- Nanosensors that can reduce medical errors by monitoring the efficacy and side effects of prescription drugs from patients' homes may be available.

Nanomedicine and Nanopharmacy

If a breakthrough to a universal assembler occurs in the next 10 to 15 years, an entirely new field of nanomedicine and perhaps nanopharmacy will emerge by 2030. *Nanomedicine* has been defined as "monitoring, repair, construction, and control of human biological systems at the molecular level, using engineered nanodevices and nanostructures."[3] *Nanopharmacy* might be defined as "the preparation and delivery of ultrasmall pharmaceuticals, therapeutic substances, and delivery systems."

Nanopharmacy may involve the use of nanomotors. Such motors, consisting of ATPase (adenosine triphosphatase) molecules with a metallic substrate on one end and a chemical "propeller" on the other end, have already been created. As ATP (adenosine 5' triphosphate) breaks down, the biomotor moves. The motor may be able to compound tiny quantities of drugs and pump them directly to the target tissues, under the direction or programming of a pharmacist.

To help secure a distinct role for pharmacy in the new world of nanotechnology, pharmacists should keep up with developments in the field through reading and through participation in national organizations.

Pharmacogenomics

Definition

The terms *pharmacogenetics* and *pharmacogenomics* have often been used interchangeably, but each represents a different entity. Pharmacogenetics, a science for almost 50 years,[4] is defined as "the study of the effect of a medication as it relates to single or defined sets of genes."[5] It focuses on genetic polymorphisms that influence the structure or function of the protein for which the gene codes.[6] Pharmacogenomics, in contrast, "goes even further by identifying genes or whole genomes responsible for modifying an organism's response to drugs;"[7] it also includes the use of genomics in the search for new therapeutic targets.[8,9] Thus, pharmacogenomics is broader in scope than pharmacogenetics; it looks at "not only the molecular composition of genetic variants associated with drug response, but also the behavior of those variants, including how those genes affect drug receptor sites."[10]

Pharmacogenomics will change clinical practice. Individual patients' therapy will be based on their genetic makeup. Felix Frueh, formerly an official in the area of genomics at the U.S. Food and Drug Administration (FDA), has said that whereas medicine to date has taken a trial-and-error approach, treating everyone with the same dose, a pharmacogenomic-driven approach will mean individualizing or personalizing the dose for effective treatment.[11]

Pharmacogenomics offers the tools for prescribing personalized medicine that will improve treatment outcomes, decrease the occurrence of drug-related adverse effects, and ultimately reduce the cost of medical care. In essence, pharmacogenomics provides "the right dose of the right drug for the right indication for the right patient at the right time"— the goal of all compounding pharmacists.[12]

Benefits of Personalized Medicine

The reason each patient's unique genetic makeup directs his or her response to drug therapy is that genes encode enzymes, including drug-metabolizing enzymes (DMEs). Variations in gene sequencing cause DMEs to be expressed in different forms in different people. Thus, the same drug is processed differently in different people, with different effects.

Pharmacogenomic-based medical care will be streamlined and simplified. In theory, a one-time analysis of a patient's blood sample will yield a genetic blueprint that can be used to guide all subsequent drug treatment for that individual. Trial-and-error therapy will be avoided, and early treatment with the appropriate drug in the right dose will enable the cure or management of the health issue. Because overdosing and underdosing will be eliminated, the occurrence of adverse effects and the expenses related to their treatment will be greatly reduced. Nonresponders and those intolerant of a specific drug will never receive it.

With a physician's prescription and the patient's pharmacogenomic profile in mind, a compounding pharmacist will be able to prepare a customized medication in the patient's unique best dosage, free of undesirable fillers and additives, and in the most effective and acceptable form. This targeted treatment will be safer, less expensive overall, more effective, and less likely to cause adverse effects compared to today's treatment with its limited number of commercially prepared doses and one-size-fits-all prescribing.

Long championed by compounding pharmacists, the pharmacogenomic approach to care is now receiving attention from leading U.S. government and private organizations: the FDA Center for Drug Evaluation,[13] Centers for Disease Control and Prevention,[14,15] and American Medical Association.[16] As guardians of the public welfare, consumers' best interests, and economy of investment, these organizations have identified the potential of personalized drug treatment to improve outcomes while reducing the costs of therapy.

The chance of overreaction or underresponse to drug treatment is indeed high: drug-related adverse events cause more than 2 million hospitalizations and 100,000 deaths annually in the United States.[17] These figures underscore the value of genetically guided therapy. According to Bolonna and colleagues,[18] "The aim of pharmacogenomic research is to enable customized drug treatment by identifying variations within multiple candidate genes (those encoding drug-targeted neurotransmitter receptors, transporters, and metabolic enzymes) that are likely to confer the interindividual differences in drug response and development of drug-induced side effects." In their recent study of pharmacogenomics and drug development, Guo and colleagues[19] showed that "efficacy is increased and toxicity is reduced when a genetically guided dose adjustment strategy is utilized in a clinical trial." Weber and colleagues[20] estimated that only 50% to 75% of patients benefit from drug therapy. They predicted that data from the Human Genome Project "will result in drugs personalized to small, genetically defined groups of patients or even to individuals."

Applications

The potential applications of pharmacogenomics are many. Genotypically guided regimens are under investigation for the treatment of human immunodeficiency virus (HIV) infection,[21] non-small-cell lung cancer,[22] Alzheimer's disease,[23] childhood acute lymphoblastic leukemia,[24] cardiovascular disease,[25-27] and colon cancer.[28] Targeted drugs now commercially available include trastuzumab (Herceptin) for the treatment of breast cancer, cetuximab (Erbitux) for colorectal cancer, erlotinib (Tarceva) for lung cancer, imatinib mesylate (Gleevec) for chronic myelogenous leukemia, atomoxetine HCl (Strattera) for attention-deficit hyperactivity disorder, and mercaptopurine (6-MP, Purinethol) for leukemia.

Genomics is changing modern medicine. Physicians have long known that not all drugs are appropriate for all patients. Some medications are effective only in specific subpopulations (responders), and the early identification of responders dramatically improves the success of treatment.[29,30] Treating nonresponders puts those patients at unnecessary risk for adverse events, provides no benefit, and may delay treatment with an effective agent. For example, identifying women whose breast cancer is nonresponsive to Herceptin before initiating Herceptin treatment could direct the prescription of another drug that would be effective and could save thousands of dollars that might have been spent in failed treatment.

Pharmacogenomically guided medicine is the future of drug therapy. Analytically and clinically validated tests are now available for predicting an individual's genetic response to a particular drug and potentially reducing treatment-related adverse effects. FDA is encouraging the use of pharmacogenomics and is supporting its translation into personalized medicine. The one-size-fits-all model of drug treatment is truly outdated.

Being able to predict—before treatment is initiated—which patients will not respond to a particular drug or will suffer unacceptable adverse events and to identify the correct dosage in those who will benefit from therapy is invaluable. For example, there is now an approved diagnostic test to detect patients with variations in the gene for CYP2C9, which is involved in warfarin metabolism. Patients with variants in this gene metabolize warfarin more slowly than others and require lower doses; they can now begin warfarin therapy at lower dosages.

How Compounding Will Help

Physicians in the future are likely to ask the following questions[20] before prescribing a drug to manage or cure a patient's condition: Does this patient have normal target receptors for this drug? Does he or she metabolize this drug normally? Is the drug transported normally in this patient? The answers should be provided by pharmacogenomic testing and will lead to customized or personalized treatment.

For example, in the future, before a particular HIV medication is prescribed, a patient's genotype might possibly be identified to determine the safest, most effective medication and dose for that individual. Because there is no cure for HIV, medications used to treat that disease must be prescribed indefinitely, at considerable cost and with great potential for cumulative toxicity.[21] If the regimen is suboptimal, not only will the patient fail to receive the full benefit, but also the virus may become resistant, leading to the need for new, more complex, and more costly treatments.

As therapy is individualized, having specialists at the front line who can implement the drug regimens suggested by pharmacogenomic testing will be critical. A compounding pharmacist could play an important role in making those customized therapies available and adjusting them as needed during the course of treatment. The results of pharmacogenomic tests could enable compounding pharmacists to develop and record for each patient a profile of drug response, indicating abnormalities in target receptors or a genotype that interferes with drug metabolism.[11] From that information, an accurate dose could be prepared in a form most acceptable to that patient. Compounding pharmacists can offer truly individualized medicines, prepared from pure USP-quality bulk drug substances or from FDA-approved drugs, that will produce the optimal result for each patient's genotypic profile. Free of additives, dyes, and allergenic fillers, compounded medications can be easily adjusted in dose or dosage form as the patient's therapeutic needs change.

Future Trends in High-Technology Pharmacy Compounding

Although pharmacy has its roots in forms such as extracts, suppositories, and ointments, compounding pharmacy is growing with the times and incorporating new technology. Manual mortars and pestles are giving way to electronic mortars and pestles, ointment slabs to ointment mills, torsion balances to electronic balances, pipets to micropipets, handmade capsules to capsule machines, and syringes and needles to automated compounders for total parenteral nutrition.

Compounding pharmacy must continue to change as biotechnology, nanotechnology, pharmacogenomics, and other scientific advances offer new challenges and opportunities and as societal needs evolve. The future is likely to bring increasingly potent drugs and highly complex delivery systems. New dosage forms that would require pharmacy compounding might include antibody-based drug delivery systems; biological-based drug delivery systems; DNA probes; enzyme-controlled, release site–specific drug delivery systems; injected microcapsules (containing microorganisms prepared and maintained by a pharmacist); living cell therapies; prodosage forms, like prodrugs; and resealed erythrocytes (prepared by a pharmacist).

Delivery systems for weekly, monthly, and yearly delivery will increase in number and become more flexible and powerful. Feedback membrane drug sensors for drugs or body chemicals (e.g., blood glucose) are being developed to adjust the rate of drug delivery to the needs of a patient. Nanotechnology-produced micromolecular devices may be introduced into the bloodstream to modify, destroy, or prevent a disease process.

With these changes, pharmacists may become increasingly involved in the manipulation and administration of drugs and biologicals. If compounding pharmacists keep abreast of new technologies, the products and devices they can provide will be in demand, together with the associated educational and counseling activities.

References

1. Bush P. Overview of technology. *J Pharm Pract.* 1998;11(1):6.
2. Biotechnology Industry Organization. Biotechnology & health care. Available at: http://bio.org/healthcare/. Accessed November 11, 2011.
3. Frietas RA Jr. *Nanomedicine.* Austin, TX: Landes Bioscience; 1999.
4. Frueh FW, Gurwitz D. From pharmacogenetics to personalized medicine: a vital need for educating health professionals and the community. *Pharmacogenomics.* 2004;5(5):571–9.
5. Cooke GE. Pharmacogenetics of multigenic disease: heart disease as an example. *Vasc Pharmacol.* 2006;44(2):66–74.
6. Lerer B. Understanding pharmacogenetics. *Psychiatr Times.* 2003;20(5). Available at: www.psychiatrictimes.com/p030537.html. Accessed November 11, 2011.
7. Vaszar LT, Rosen GD, Raffin TA. Pharmacogenomics and the challenge to privacy. *Pharmacogenomics J.* 2002;2(3):144–7.
8. Norbert PW, Roses AD. Pharmacogenetics and pharmacogenomics: recent developments, their clinical relevance and some ethical, social, and legal implications. *J Mol Med.* 2003;81(3):135–40.
9. Meyer UA. Introduction to pharmacogenomics: promises, opportunities, and limitations. In: Licinio J, Wong M-L, eds. *Pharmacogenomics.* Weinheim, Germany: Wiley-VCH Verlag GmbH & Co. KgaA; 2002:1–8.
10. Barash CI. Ethical issues in pharmacogenetics. ActionBioscience.org; February 2001. Available at: www.actionbioscience.org/genomic/barash.html. Accessed November 11, 2011.
11. Vale J. Pharmacogenomics: the end of trial-and-error medicine. *Int J Pharm Compound.* 2007;11(1):59–65.
12. Frueh F. Personalized medicine: what is it? How will it affect health care? Paper presented at: 11th Annual Food and Drug Administration Science Forum. April 26, 2005. Washington, DC. Available at: www.fda.gov/downloads/Drugs/ScienceResearch/ResearchAreas/Pharmacogenetics/ucm085716.pdf.
13. Frueh FW, Goodsaid F, Rudman A, et al. The need for education in pharmacogenomics: a regulatory perspective. *Pharmacogenomics J.* 2005;5(4):218–20.
14. Moore CA, Khoury MJ, Bradley LA. From genetics to genomics: using gene-based medicine to prevent disease and promote health in children. *Semin Perinatol.* 2005;29(3):135–43.
15. Khoury MJ, Morris J. Centers for Disease Control and Prevention. Pharmacogenomics & public health: the promise of targeted disease prevention. Available at: www.cdc.gov/genomics/training/perspectives/factshts/pharmacofs.htm. Accessed November 11, 2011.
16. American Medical Association. Pharmacogenomics. Available at: www.ama-assn.org/ama/pub/category/2306.html. Accessed November 11, 2011.
17. Shastry BS. Pharmacogenetics and the concept of individualized medicine. *Pharmacogenomics J.* 2006;6(1):16–21.
18. Bolonna AA, Arranz MJ, Mancama D, et al. Pharmacogenomics—can genetics help in the care of psychiatric patients? *Int Rev Psychiatry.* 2004;16(4):311–9.
19. Guo Y, Shafer S, Weller P, et al. Pharmacogenomics and drug development. *Pharmacogenomics.* 2005;6(8):857–64.

20. Weber WW, Caldwell MD, Kurth JH. Edging toward personalized medicine. *Curr Pharmacogenomics.* 2003;1(3):193–202.
21. Haas DW. Will pharmacogenomic discoveries improve HIV therapeutics? *Top HIV Med.* 2005;13(3):90–5.
22. Bepler G. Using translational research to tailor the use of chemotherapy in the treatment of NSCLC. *Lung Cancer.* 2005;50(Suppl 1):S13–S14.
23. Cacabelos R. Pharmacogenomics and therapeutic prospects in Alzheimer's disease. *Expert Opin Pharmacother.* 2005;6(12):1967–87.
24. Cheng Q, Evans WE. Cancer pharmacogenomics may require both qualitative and quantitative approaches. *Cell Cycle.* 2005;4(11):1504–7. Epub 2005 Nov 8.
25. Rieder MJ, Reiner AP, Gage BF, et al. Effect of VKORC1 haplotypes on transcriptional regulation and warfarin dose. *N Engl J Med.* 2005;352(22):2285–93.
26. Kajinami K, Akao H, Polisecki E, et al. Pharmacogenomics of statin responsiveness. *Am J Cardiol.* 2005;96(9A):65–70.
27. Kajinami K, Okabayashi M, Sato R, et al. Statin pharmacogenomics: what have we learned, and what remains unanswered? *Curr Opin Lipidol.* 2005;16(6):606–13.
28. Allen WL, Johnston PG. Have we made progress in pharmacogenomics? The implementation of molecular markers in colon cancer. *Pharmacogenomics.* 2005;6(6):603–14.
29. Sze J, Prakash S. Human genetics, environment, and communities of color: ethical and social implications. *Environ Health Perspect.* 2004;112(6):740–5.
30. National Institutes of Health. Seventh Meeting of the Secretary's Advisory Committee on Genetics, Health, and Society. June 15, 2005. Available at: www.webconferences.com/nihsacghs/15_jun_2005.html. Accessed November 11, 2011.

Chapter 27

Special Populations and Preparations

The uniqueness of pharmacy compounding is the ability to prepare individualized medications for special populations, such as pediatric and hospice patients, patients experiencing pain, patients with diabetes, and patients of advanced age. This chapter gives a brief overview of opportunities to serve special populations. It also includes sample compounded formulations for natural, herbal, and dietary supplement products and iontophoresis solutions.

Pediatric Patients

Children's medications can be a challenge for physicians and pharmacists. Because most marketed drugs do not have U.S. Food and Drug Administration (FDA)–approved indications for pediatric use, physicians must prescribe them "off label." When drugs do not have labeled indications for children, drug manufacturers do not produce strengths and dosage forms appropriate for this patient population. Technological limitations are rarely the reason for the lack of pediatric formulations; rather, market conditions often dictate the types of drugs for which formulations suitable for children are made available. So, how can a child receive proper medical care when pharmaceutical resources are limited?[1]

Oral liquids, including emulsions, solutions, and suspensions, are the most commonly used dosage forms for pediatric patients. Other common dosage forms include chewing gums, flavored gelatins, flavored ices, gummy gels, lollipops, lozenges, puddings, and topical formulations.

When commercial liquid formulations are not available, extemporaneously prepared formulations are an option. The development and compounding of pediatric formulations, particularly those suitable for infants and young children, can be vexing for a dispensing pharmacist. A major problem in treating sick newborns is the lack of appropriate concentrations of various drugs for parenteral administration. Preparation of oral medicines for children is subject to much variation in U.S. hospitals, and there is little harmonization of formulations or information on the stability of preparations. Information was found to be inadequate or missing altogether in 63% and 26%, respectively, of articles reviewed; this deficiency highlights the difficulty of relying on published formulas.

Tablets and capsules are usually unsuitable for children under the age of 4 years, and available tablets may not be of appropriate strength for older children. Splitting or breaking tablets is common practice but does not result in accurate or uniform dosing. Choking by aspiration of tablets is associated with significant morbidity. Of the 41 childhood deaths resulting from aspiration examined in a report by the Consumer Product Safety Commission, 12% were reported to be due to aspiration of pills; the average age of these patients was 14.8 months.[2]

Much emphasis has been placed on the availability of liquid preparations for use in infants and small children. Liquid preparations are clearly needed for small infants, but for limited-resource pharmacies, they are not the dosage form of choice because of their weight and volume and the instability of formulations.

Bulk powders and sometimes tablets can be used in formulations when commercial products are not available. For example, lorazepam 2 mg/mL suspension can be compounded using lorazepam bulk powder. The commercial injection should not be used as a drug source in compounding for young children because of its high propylene glycol content; it can be toxic to newborns in high doses. If tablets are used, the concentration may need to be reduced to about 1 mg/mL because the excipients in the tablets thicken the suspension.

Taste is probably the primary factor influencing patient compliance. Children may not like the taste of masked formulations or may object to the bitter or metallic taste of nonmasked formulations. A pharmacist may find an advantage in preparing placebo taste samples and asking a child to select one, which gives the child a role in decision making about the therapy. The taste of a formulation involves factors such as flavoring, sweetener, pH, color, and mouthfeel. Preferences of both children and parents concerning flavor, palatability, and dosage forms are influenced by culture.

Variables that must be considered in preparing pediatric formulations include dose (concentration and quantity to be administered), stability (chemical, physical, and microbiological), taste, color, packaging, storage, and the necessary administration devices or techniques.

Sample Formulations

℞ Nystatin Frozen Ices (10 frozen ices)

Nystatin powder	2.5×106 units	Active
Sorbitol 70% solution	20 mL	Vehicle/Sweetener
Syrup	50 mL	Sweetener
Flavoring (banana or other, to taste)	5 mL	Flavoring
Purified water	qs 300 mL	Vehicle

(Note: Because ice cube trays and molds vary, one may need to calibrate the specific tray or mold being used and adjust the formula before actual preparation.)

1. Calculate the quantity of each ingredient required for the prescription.
2. Accurately weigh or measure the ingredients.
3. Add the nystatin powder to the sorbitol 70% solution, and mix thoroughly.
4. Add the syrup, flavoring, and purified water, and mix well.
5. Pour 30 mL into each cavity in an ice cube tray (with deep cubes) or an appropriate plastic sleeve, and place molds in a freezer for 1 or 2 hours.
6. Insert a stick (junior tongue depressor) into each frozen ice to serve as a handle, and continue freezing until frozen firmly.
7. Remove each frozen ice, package separately in a 6 in. × 9 in. sealable plastic bag, and label.

℞ Malathion 0.5% Topical Lotion for Head Lice

Malathion	500 mg	Active
Isopropyl alcohol 70%	68 mL	Vehicle
Lavender oil	30 drops	Fragrance
Bay and pine oils	3 drops	Fragrance
Ethyl alcohol 95%	qs 100 mL	Vehicle

(Note: Malathion fumes can be irritating to the mucous membranes of the nasal passages; therefore, this product should be prepared in a well-ventilated area or under an exhaust hood. Wear disposable gloves to prevent retaining the odor on the hands. This preparation can be used for treatment of resistant head lice, as well as scabies.)

1. Calculate the quantity of each ingredient required for the prescription.
2. Accurately weigh or measure the ingredients.
3. Disperse the malathion in the isopropyl alcohol 70%.
4. Add the fragrances, and mix well.
5. Add sufficient ethyl alcohol 90% to volume, and mix well.
6. Package and label the product.

Geriatric Patients

One of the greatest challenges in compounding is individualizing dosage forms for patients of advanced age. More than 85% of the older adult ambulatory population and more than 95% of the older adult institutionalized population receive prescription drugs. The average number of prescriptions for persons 65 years of age and older is approximately 13. Most dosage forms are created for adults and pediatric patients with little thought to this segment of the population, which takes a significant portion of drug products. The most common dosage form today is the tablet, which tends to hang on the back of the tongue or throat; capsules and coated tablets have less tendency to do so. For bedridden patients or patients with swallowing difficulties, other dosage forms must be considered. For example, baths, creams, flavored gelatins, gels, gummy gels, frozen ices, liquids, lollipops, lozenges, ointments, puddings, sprays, suppositories, or washes can be used. Commonly compounded preparations include gummy-type preparations, oral liquids, and soft lozenges.

Physical, emotional, or social difficulties can affect compliance in patients of advanced age. Despite the skin changes that accompany aging, transdermal administration is a reasonable alternative. For masking taste, mint and fruit flavors are popular among geriatric patients. Because older adult patients may not remember everything said during a counseling session, providing written instructions with every prescription is important. A pharmacist may need to develop patient leaflets for the more commonly compounded preparations for older adults.

Hospice and Pain Management Patients

Hospice is a multidisciplinary program that provides health, psychological, and social services to terminally ill patients and their families. Hospice is designed to serve patients who can no longer benefit from curative treatment; most patients have a life expectancy of less than 6 months. The concept of hospice can be traced to early Western civilization, when the term was used to describe a place of shelter and rest for weary or sick travelers on long journeys. It was first applied to specialized care for dying patients in

1967 at St. Christopher's Hospice in a London suburb. The first hospice program in the United States began in 1974; currently, more than 2,500 hospice programs serve more than 250,000 patients.

Some 60% to 70% of hospice patients have cancer and experience intractable pain, severe anxiety, and depression, as well as social, psychological, and financial concerns. The current thinking is that these patients should not be subject to a ceiling or maximum dosage of analgesics. Rather, analgesics should be provided on a scheduled basis, with supplemental doses as needed to provide adequate blood levels of the drug to ensure patient comfort. Antidepressants and anxiolytics are sometimes given to help relieve a patient's symptoms of depression and anxiety.

Hospice care deals with grief and grieving and can be accomplished either in an institutional environment or in a patient's home. Home hospice care has logistical, psychological, social, emotional, and financial benefits. In addition to pain management and palliative care, home hospice may include wound care and other services that enable the patient to maintain activities of daily living and basic functional skills.

Sample Formulations

℞ Morphine Sulfate 10, 25, and 50 mg/mL Injections (preservative free)

	10 mg/mL	25 mg/mL	50 mg/mL
Morphine sulfate	0.5 g	1.25 g	2.5 g
0.9% Sodium chloride injection	42.2 mL	30.6 mL	11.1 mL
Sterile water for injection	qs 50 mL	qs 50 mL	qs 50 mL

1. Calculate the quantity of each ingredient required for the prescription.
2. Accurately weigh the required quantity of morphine sulfate powder.
3. Place the morphine sulfate in a previously sterilized graduated cylinder.
4. Accurately measure the required volume of 0.9% sodium chloride injection, add to the morphine sulfate powder, and mix well.
5. Add sufficient sterile water for injection to volume, and mix well.
6. Filter the solution through a sterile 0.22-μm filter into the desired sterile reservoir or container for administration.
7. Package and label the product.

℞ Morphine Sulfate and Clonidine Hydrochloride Epidural Injection

Morphine sulfate	2 g	Active
Clonidine hydrochloride	1 mg	Active
0.9% Sodium chloride injection	69 mL	Vehicle/Tonicity Adjuster
Sterile water for injection	qs 100 mL	Vehicle

(Note: This preparation should be prepared in a laminar-airflow hood in a clean room by a validated, aseptic compounding pharmacist using strict aseptic technique.)

If the source of the ingredients is commercially available preservative-free injectable products, compound as follows:

1. Calculate the quantity of each ingredient required for the prescription.
2. Accurately measure the volume of each ingredient, and pour into the sterile reservoir or container. An air bubble can be injected and used to thoroughly mix the solution.
3. Remove the air from the reservoir, and tightly seal or close the outlet.
4. Package and label the product.

If the source of the ingredients is other than commercially prepared injections, compound as follows:

1. Calculate the quantity of each ingredient required for the prescription.
2. Accurately weigh the solid ingredients, preparing dilutions if necessary.
3. Accurately measure the volume of 0.9% sodium chloride injection.
4. Place the morphine sulfate, clonidine hydrochloride, and 0.9% sodium chloride injection in a clean graduated cylinder or suitable measuring vessel or device that has been suitably depyrogenated.
5. Add sufficient sterile water for injection to volume.
6. Filter the solution through a 0.2-μm sterile filter into a sterile reservoir, and tightly seal or close the outlet.
7. Package and label the product.

℞ **Ketamine Hydrochloride 10%, Gabapentin 6%, Baclofen 2%, Amitriptyline Hydrochloride 2%, and Clonidine Hydrochloride 0.1% in Pluronic Lecithin Organogel**

Ketamine hydrochloride	10 g	Active
Gabapentin	6 g	Active
Baclofen	2 g	Active
Amitriptyline hydrochloride	2 g	Active
Clonidine hydrochloride	100 mg	Active
Diethylene glycol monoethyl ether	10 mL	Levigating Agent
Polysorbate 80 (Tween 80)	1–2 mL	Emulsifier
Sorbitan oleate (Span 80)	1–2 mL	Emulsifier
Lecithin:isopropyl palmitate 1:1 solution	22 mL	Emulsifier
Pluronic F-127 30% gel	qs 100 mL	Vehicle

(Note: The lecithin:isopropyl palmitate 1:1 solution can be prepared by mixing 0.2 g of sorbic acid, 50 g of soy lecithin, and 50 g of isopropyl palmitate. The Pluronic F-127 gel can be prepared by mixing 0.2 g of potassium sorbate, 30 g of Pluronic F-127, and sufficient purified water to make 100 mL. Pluronic F-127 gel [30%; 100 mL] can be prepared by mixing 0.2 g of sorbic acid, 30 g of Pluronic F-127, and sufficient purified water to make 100 mL. The pH should be adjusted to about 4.5 for maximum effectiveness of the sorbic acid as a preservative. Dissolution can be easily accomplished by placing the gel in a sealed container in a refrigerator, with periodic agitation that does not incorporate air into the gel.)

1. Calculate the quantity of each ingredient required for the prescription.
2. Accurately weigh or measure each ingredient.
3. Mix the powders together.
4. Add the diethylene glycol monoethyl ether, and mix to form a smooth paste.
5. Add the lecithin:isopropyl palmitate 1:1 solution and the sorbitan oleate, and mix well.
6. Add the polysorbate 80, previously blended with about 20 mL of Pluronic F-127 30% gel, followed by sufficient additional Pluronic F-127 30% gel to volume, and mix thoroughly, using a mechanical shearing force.
7. Package and label the product.

Rx Promethazine Hydrochloride 50 mg/mL in Pluronic Lecithin Organogel

Promethazine hydrochloride	5 g	Active
Purified water	4 mL	Solvent
Lecithin:isopropyl palmitate 1:1 solution	22 mL	Emulsifier
Pluronic F-127 30% gel	qs 100 mL	Vehicle

(Note: Pluronic F-127 gel [30%; 100 mL] can be prepared by mixing 0.2 g of sorbic acid, 30 g of Pluronic F-127, and sufficient purified water to make 100 mL. The pH should be adjusted to about 4.5 for maximum effectiveness of the sorbic acid as a preservative. Dissolution can be easily accomplished by placing the gel in a sealed container in a refrigerator, with periodic agitation that does not incorporate air into the gel.)

1. Calculate the quantity of each ingredient required for the prescription.
2. Accurately weigh or measure each ingredient.
3. Dissolve the promethazine hydrochloride in the purified water.
4. Add this solution to about 70 mL of the Pluronic F-127 30% gel, and mix well.
5. Incorporate the lecithin:isopropyl palmitate 1:1 solution with shear mixing.
6. Add additional Pluronic F-127 30% gel to volume, and continue shear mixing.
7. Package and label the product.

Patients with Diabetes

Compounded preparations can enhance the lifestyle of patients with diabetes. The following topical formulations are examples.

Sample Formulations

℞ Foot Care Ointments for Patients with Diabetes

	Formula 1	Formula 2	Formula 3
Aquabase or Aquaphor	4 g		
Lanolin	1 g		1 g
Glycerin	1 g		
Wheat germ oil	1 g	1 g	
Cocoa butter		2 g	
Olive oil		1 g	
Cod liver oil			1 g
White petrolatum			2 g

Formula 1
1. Calculate the required quantity of each ingredient for the total amount to be prepared.
2. Accurately weigh or measure each ingredient.
3. Blend the wheat germ oil and glycerin with the lanolin.
4. Incorporate the mixture into the Aquabase or Aquaphor, and mix well.
5. Package and label the product.

Formula 2
1. Calculate the required quantity of each ingredient for the total amount to be prepared.
2. Accurately weigh or measure each ingredient.
3. Blend the wheat germ oil with the olive oil, and mix well.
4. Incorporate the mixture into the cocoa butter by using mild heat, if necessary, and mix well to yield a thick, fluid preparation.
5. Package and label the product.

Formula 3
1. Calculate the required quantity of each ingredient for the total amount to be prepared.
2. Accurately weigh or measure each ingredient.
3. Blend the cod liver oil with the lanolin.
4. Incorporate the white petrolatum, and mix well.
5. Package and label the product.

℞ Skin Ulcer Cream for Patients with Diabetes

Misoprostol	2.5 mg	Active
Phenytoin	2 g	Active
Ketoprofen	2 g	Active
Lidocaine	2 g	Active
Propylene glycol	qs	Levigating Agent
Oil-in-water emulsion base	qs 100 g	Vehicle

1. Calculate the quantity of each ingredient required for the prescription.
2. Accurately weigh or measure each ingredient.
3. Comminute 12.5 g of the 200 μg misoprostol tablets to a very fine powder.
4. Add sufficient propylene glycol to make a smooth paste.
5. Mix and comminute the other powders to a very fine powder.
6. Add sufficient propylene glycol to make a smooth paste, and combine with misoprostol–propylene glycol paste (step 4).
7. Incorporate the paste into a sufficient quantity of an oil-in-water emulsion base to make 100 g.
8. Package and label the product.

Dental Patients

Many opportunities are available for working with dentists. Special oral hygiene products, preoperative medications, and preparations used in dental surgical areas are only a few of the mixtures needed. A number of disease states can result in oral ulceration. Compounding dental mouth rinses from bulk powders (antibiotics, anti-inflammatory agents, and the like) has advantages over using commercial dosage forms. Each manufactured product has numerous ingredients that can contribute to compatibility or stability problems. Also, if a preservative is present but the commercial product is diluted by mixing it with other products, the preservative can be below its effective concentration. Active drugs can be incorporated into toothpastes and gels. For gum disease, antibiotics can be incorporated into a poloxamer gel (a reverse thermal gel) and applied to the gum line between the gum and the tooth. The poloxamer will thicken and release the drug over a longer time period than if a rinse or irrigation were used. Many options are available depending on a patient's condition and needs.

Sample Formulations

Mouthwash and Gargle

Cetylpyridinium chloride	100 mg	Active
Polysorbate 20	1 mL	Emulsifier
Spearmint oil	0.25 mL	Flavoring
Ethanol 95%	10 mL	Solvent
Sodium saccharin	100 mg	Sweetener
Sodium benzoate	200 mg	Preservative
Sorbitol 70% solution	10 mL	Sweetener
Purified water	qs 100 mL	Vehicle

1. Calculate the required quantity of each ingredient for the total amount to be prepared.
2. Accurately weigh or measure each ingredient.
3. Add the spearmint oil to the polysorbate 20, and mix well.
4. Add the ethanol 95%, and mix well.
5. In a separate container, add the cetylpyridinium chloride, sodium saccharin, and sodium benzoate to about 70 mL of purified water, followed by the sorbitol 70% solution.
6. Combine the ethanol solution (step 4) and the sorbitol solution (step 5), and mix well.
7. Add a few drops of food coloring if desired.
8. Add sufficient purified water to volume, and mix well.
9. Package and label the product.

Tooth Gel Vehicle

Glycerin	22 g	Vehicle
Carbopol 934	500 mg	Thickener
Purified water	25.2 mL	Vehicle
Tetrasodium pyrophosphate	250 mg	Active
Sodium saccharin	200 mg	Sweetener
Sodium benzoate	500 mg	Preservative
Sodium hydroxide 50% solution	0.4 mL	Alkalizer
Dicalcium phosphate dihydrate	48.76 g	Active
Sodium lauryl sulfate	1.2 g	Surfactant
Flavoring	1 mL	Flavoring

1. Calculate the required quantity of each ingredient for the total amount to be prepared.
2. Accurately weigh or measure each ingredient.
3. Add the tetrasodium pyrophosphate, sodium saccharin, sodium benzoate, sodium lauryl sulfate, and flavoring to the purified water.
4. Mix the Carbopol 934 with the glycerin.
5. Mix the tetrasodium pyrophosphate solution (step 3) and the Carbopol 934–glycerin solution (step 4) until uniform.
6. Add the sodium hydroxide 50% solution, and mix well.
7. Geometrically incorporate the dicalcium phosphate dihydrate into the gel vehicle.
8. Package and label the product.

⚗ Toothpaste Vehicle

Calcium pyrophosphate	45 g	Active
Sorbitol 70% solution	20 mL	Sweetener/Vehicle
Sodium lauryl sulfate	1.2 g	Surfactant
Sodium carboxymethylcellulose	600 mg	Thickening Agent
Sodium saccharin	100 mg	Sweetener
Peppermint oil	0.75 mL	Flavoring
Purified water	32.35 mL	Vehicle

1. Calculate the required quantity of each ingredient for the total amount to be prepared.
2. Accurately weigh or measure each ingredient.
3. Add the sodium lauryl sulfate, sodium saccharin, and peppermint oil to the purified water.
4. Add the sodium carboxymethylcellulose to the sorbitol 70% solution.
5. Mix the sodium lauryl sulfate solution (step 3) with the sodium carboxymethylcellulose–sorbitol solution (step 4) until uniform.
6. Geometrically incorporate the calcium pyrophosphate to form a paste.
7. Package and label the product.

℞ Dental Cavity Varnish

Camphor	70 g	Active/Vehicle
Prednisolone	1 g	Active
Parachlorophenol	26.5 g	Active/Vehicle
Metacresol acetate	2.5 g	Active

1. Calculate the quantity of each ingredient required for the prescription.
2. Accurately weigh or measure each ingredient.
3. Mix the camphor with the parachlorophenol.
4. Add the metacresol acetate.
5. Add the prednisolone, and mix well.
6. Package and label the product.

℞ Dental Chemical Curettage Agent

Sodium hydroxide	7.8 g	Active
Sodium hypochlorite solution	100 mL	Active/Vehicle
Sodium carbonate	19 g (approximate)	Active

1. Calculate the quantity of each ingredient required for the prescription.
2. Accurately weigh or measure each ingredient.
3. Using an ice bath to keep the solution cool, slowly dissolve the sodium hydroxide in the sodium hypochlorite solution.
4. Allow the solution to warm to room temperature.
5. Add the sodium carbonate until the solution is saturated. It may not take all of the sodium carbonate.
6. Package and label the product.

Dental Pressure-Indicating Paste

Zinc oxide ointment	53 g	Vehicle
White petrolatum	17 g	Vehicle
Mineral oil	25 g	Vehicle
White wax	5 g	Thickener
Flavoring	qs	Flavoring

1. Calculate the required quantity of each ingredient for the total amount to be prepared.
2. Accurately weigh or measure each ingredient.
3. Reduce the white wax to a fine state by grating.
4. Heat the grated wax until it melts, using a double boiler to eliminate scorching.
5. Heat the mineral oil and white petrolatum in a separate double boiler to a temperature near that of the melted wax.
6. Add the mineral oil–white petrolatum mixture slowly, in small increments, with continuous stirring to the melted wax.
7. After the two oleaginous liquids are thoroughly mixed, and while constantly stirring the mixture, add the zinc oxide ointment in small increments.
8. When the mixture is completely melted and displays a uniform, creamy white appearance, remove the heat and allow the mixture to cool.
9. If a volatile flavoring agent is used, such as lemon oil or peppermint oil, add it during cooling, just before solidification occurs.
10. Pour the paste while it is still slightly warm into the desired ointment jars, or allow it to solidify and, using a spatula, place it into appropriate containers.
11. Package and label the product.

Iontophoresis

Iontophoresis is a method of administering medications through the skin by using a small electric current. The applied current or voltage creates a potential gradient through the skin, inducing increased migration of ionic drugs into the skin by electrostatic repulsion at the active electrode; negative ions are delivered by the cathode and positive ions by the anode. A typical iontophoresis device consists of a battery, microprocessor controller, drug reservoir, and electrodes.

Advantages of iontophoresis include (1) controlled delivery rates (through variations in current density, pulsed voltage, drug concentration, and ionic strength); (2) elimination of gastrointestinal incompatibility, erratic absorption, and first-pass metabolism; (3) reduction in adverse effects and interpatient variability; (4) avoidance of the risks of infection, inflammation, and fibrosis associated with continuous injection or infusion, because this route is noninvasive; and (5) enhanced patient compliance with a convenient and non-invasive therapeutic regimen.

The clinical use of iontophoresis is increasing. Analgesics and anesthetics can be administered transdermally by this method for a local or systemic effect. Applications include iontophoretic administration of pilocarpine for use in the diagnosis of cystic fibrosis, treatment of excessive perspiration (hyperhidrosis), application of fluoride to the teeth, and local anesthesia and anti-inflammatory treatments with lidocaine and dexamethasone (Table 27-1). Drugs such as anesthetics, corticosteroids, and nonsteroidal anti-inflammatory drugs (NSAIDs) are commonly delivered via iontophoresis. Other drugs under study include

TABLE 27-1 Drugs Used in Iontophoresis

Drug Solution	Concentration (%)	Use and Indication	Polarity
Acetic acid	2–5	Calcium deposits, calcified tendinitis	Negative
Atropine sulfate	0.001–0.01	Hyperhidrosis	Positive
Calcium chloride	2	Immobile joints, myopathy, myospasm	Positive
Sodium chloride	2	Sclerolytic; adhesions, keloids, scar tissue	Negative
Potassium citrate	2	Rheumatoid arthritis	Negative
Copper sulfate	2	Astringent; fungus infection	Positive
Dexamethasone sodium phosphate	0.4	Arthritis, bursitis, Peyronie's disease, tendinitis, tenosynovitis	Negative
Diclofenac potassium	—	Anti-inflammatory effects	Negative
Diclofenac sodium	—	Anti-inflammatory effects	Negative
Diflunisal	—	Anti-inflammatory effects	Negative
Estriol	Varies	Acne scars	Positive
Etodolac	—	Anti-inflammatory effects	Negative
Fenoprofen calcium	—	Anti-inflammatory effects	Negative
Fentanyl citrate	Varies	Analgesic	Positive
Fluoride sodium	2	Desensitization of teeth	Positive
Gentamicin sulfate	0.8	Ear chondritis	Positive
Glycopyrronium bromide	0.05	Hyperhidrosis	Positive
Hyaluronidase	150 units/mL	Absorption enhancement; edema, lymphedema, scleroderma	Positive
Ibuprofen	—	Anti-inflammatory effects	Negative
Idoxuridine	0.1	Herpes simplex	Negative
Indomethacin sodium	—	Anti-inflammatory effects	Negative
Iodine ointment	4.7	Sclerolytic, antimicrobial; adhesions, fibrosis, scar tissue, trigger finger	Negative
Iron/titanium oxide	Varies	Skin pigmentation	Positive
Ketoprofen	—	Anti-inflammatory effects	Negative
Ketorolac tromethamine	—	Anti-inflammatory effects	Negative
Lidocaine hydrochloride (with or without epinephrine 1:50,000 to 1:100,000)	4	Skin anesthesia; trigeminal neuralgia	Positive
Lithium chloride	2	Gouty arthritis	Positive
Magnesium sulfate	2	Muscle relaxant, vasodilator; deltoid bursitis, low back spasm, myalgias, neuritis	Positive
Meladinine sodium	1	Vitiligo	Negative
Methylphenidate hydrochloride	Varies	Attention deficit disorder	Positive
Morphine sulfate	0.2–0.4	Analgesic	Positive

(continued)

TABLE 27-1 Drugs Used in Iontophoresis *(Continued)*

Drug Solution	Concentration (%)	Use and Indication	Polarity
Naproxen sodium	—	Anti-inflammatory effects	Negative
Pilocarpine hydrochloride	Varies	Sweat test for cystic fibrosis	Positive
Piroxicam	—	Anti-inflammatory effects	Negative
Poldine methylsulfate	0.05–0.5	Hyperhidrosis	Negative
Potassium iodide	10	Scar tissue	Negative
Sodium salicylate	2	Analgesic, sclerolytic; myalgias, plantar warts, scar tissue	Negative
Sulindac	—	Anti-inflammatory	Negative
Tretinoin	Varies	Acne scars	Positive
Water	100	Palmar, plantar, axillary hyperhidrosis	Positive/ Negative
Zinc oxide suspension	20	Antiseptic; dermatitis, ulcers, wound healing	Positive

— = Not available.

a number of analgesics, nicotine, drugs for human immunodeficiency virus infection and cancer, and insulin and other proteins. Iontophoresis is also useful in veterinary medicine (Table 27-2).

The solutions used for this procedure should contain only the active drug and sterile water for injection. Any additional agents would compete for the current and decrease the efficacy of the iontophoresis process. These formulations are simple to prepare and should be sterile and packaged in single-use containers.

TABLE 27-2 Drugs Used in Veterinary Iontophoresis

Drug Solution	Polarity
Nonsteroidal Anti-inflammatory Drugs	
Flunixin meglumine	Negative
Ketoprofen	Negative
Phenylbutazone	Negative
Corticosteroids—Anti-inflammatory Agents	
Betamethasone	Negative
Dexamethasone sodium phosphate	Negative
Prednisolone sodium succinate	Negative
Antibiotics	
Amikacin sulfate	Positive
Ceftiofur sodium	Negative
Gentamicin sulfate	Positive
Local Anesthetic	
Lidocaine hydrochloride	Positive

Sample Formulations

℞ Dexamethasone Sodium Phosphate 4 mg/mL for Iontophoresis

Dexamethasone sodium phosphate	400 mg	Active
Sterile water for injection	qs 100 mL	Vehicle

1. Calculate the quantity of each ingredient required for the prescription.
2. Accurately weigh the dexamethasone sodium phosphate powder.
3. Place in a suitable graduated cylinder, add sufficient sterile water for injection to volume, and mix well.
4. Filter the solution through a 0.2-μm sterile filter into a sterile container.
5. Package and label the product.

℞ Estriol Solution for Iontophoresis for Acne Scars

Estriol	300 mg	Active
Citric acid	100 mg	Acidifier
Sterile water for injection	100 mL	Vehicle

1. Calculate the quantity of each ingredient required for the prescription.
2. Accurately weigh the required quantity of estriol and citric acid.
3. Accurately measure the required quantity of sterile water for injection.
4. Dissolve the citric acid and estriol in the sterile water for injection.
5. Filter the solution through a 0.2-μm sterile filter into a sterile container.
6. Package and label the product.

℞ Ketorolac Tromethamine Solution for Iontophoresis

Ketorolac tromethamine	600 mg	Active
Sterile water for injection	100 mL	Vehicle

1. Accurately obtain the required quantity of ketorolac tromethamine (from tablets as necessary).
2. Accurately measure the required volume of sterile water for injection.
3. Dissolve the ketorolac tromethamine powder in the sterile water for injection.
4. Filter the solution to remove tablet excipients.
5. Filter the solution through a 0.2-μm sterile filter into a sterile container.
6. Package and label the product.

Phonophoresis

Definition

Phonophoresis, or ultrasound, consists of inaudible, acoustic high-frequency vibrations that may produce either thermal or nonthermal physiologic effects. Traditionally, it has been used for the purpose of elevating tissue temperatures and referred to as a deep-heating modality.

Ultrasound uses a high-frequency generator that provides an electrical current through a coaxial cable to a transducer contained within an applicator wand or device. The ultrasonic waves are produced by a piezoelectric crystal within the transducer that converts electrical energy to acoustic energy.

Ultrasound energy can travel through body tissues as a beam that is focused but non-uniform in intensity. The intensity depends on the quantity of energy delivered to the applicator or wand head. The energy used in medicine ranges from about 1 to 3 watts per square centimeter (W/cm²). The ultrasound device emits sound waves that are outside the normal human hearing range. The sound transducer head of the ultrasonic unit is generally set to emit energy at 1 MHz at 0.5 to 1 W/cm². Like regular sound waves, ultrasound waves can be reflected, refracted, and absorbed by the medium.

When ultrasound is used to drive molecules of a topically applied medication, the process is called phonophoresis.[3] Although the exact mechanism is not known, drug absorption may involve a disruption of the stratum corneum lipids, allowing the drug to pass through the skin. Thus, phonophoresis (therapeutic ultrasound, sonophoresis, ultrasonophoresis, ultraphonophoresis) is a combination of ultrasound therapy with topical drug therapy to achieve therapeutic drug concentrations at selected sites in the skin. It is widely used by physiotherapists.

Two different approaches are used for drug delivery. Originally, a drug-containing coupling agent was applied to the skin, immediately followed by the ultrasound treatment. Currently, the product is usually applied to the skin and a period of time is allowed for the drug to begin absorption into the skin before the ultrasound is applied. Drug penetration is most likely in the 1- to 2-mm depth range.

A coupling medium is needed to provide an airtight contact between the skin and the ultrasound head. It should form a slick, low-friction surface over which the ultrasound head can glide. In phonophoresis, the coupling medium can also serve as the drug vehicle. Agents used as coupling media include water-miscible creams, gels, and mineral oil. The pseudoplastic rheology exhibited by gels is advantageous, because gels are shear thinning, decreasing viscosity and friction when stress is applied.

Variables

Variables involved in phonophoresis include energy levels, cavitation, microstreaming, coupling efficiency and transmissivity of the vehicle, extent of skin hydration, use of an occlusive dressing after treatment, and type of drug.

Energy levels are attenuated as the ultrasound waves are transmitted through the tissues, because of either absorption of the energy by the tissues or dispersion and scattering of the wave. Ultrasound used for therapeutics is generally in the frequency range of 0.75 to 3.0 MHz; 1 MHz energy is transmitted through the more superficial tissues into the deeper tissues (3–5 cm) and is more useful in individuals with a higher percentage of body fat, and 3 MHz energy is absorbed more in the superficial tissues (1–2 cm). Delivery of ultrasound can be either thermal–continuous (producing more thermal heating; intensity of 1.0 to 1.5 W/cm² for 5 to 7 minutes) or nonthermal–pulsed (producing less heating; 0.8 to 1.5 W/cm² with a duty cycle of 20% to 60% for 5 to 7 minutes). Another variable affecting dosage is the energy of application; 0.1 to 0.3 W/cm² is regarded as low intensity, 0.4 to 1.5 W/cm² is medium intensity, and 1.6 to 3 W/cm² is high intensity. Treatment times generally range from 5 to 10 minutes.

Effects produced by ultrasound, other than heating, include cavitation and acoustic microstreaming. Cavitation involves the formation and collapse of very small air bubbles in a liquid in contact with ultrasound waves because of the pressure changes induced in the tissue fluids. Cavitation can cause increased fluid flow around these vibrating bubbles. Microstreaming, closely associated with cavitation, is a movement of fluids in one direction along cell boundaries as a result of the mechanical pressure wave in an ultrasonic field. Microstreaming results in efficient mixing by inducing eddies in small-volume elements of a liquid; this may enhance dissolution of suspended drug particles, resulting in a higher concentration of drug near the skin for absorption. Microstreaming can alter the structure and function of the cell membrane as a result of changes in permeability to sodium and calcium ions.

Tissue penetration in phonophoresis also is dependent on the impedance or acoustic properties of the media or the efficiency of the coupling agent. The vehicle containing the drug must be formulated to provide good conduction of the ultrasonic energy to the skin. The product must be smooth and not gritty, because it will be rubbed into the skin by the head of the transducer. It should be of relatively low viscosity for ease of application and ease of movement of the transducer head during the ultrasound process. Gels work very well. Emulsions have been used, but the oil:water interface in emulsions can disperse the ultrasonic waves, resulting in reduced intensity of the energy reaching the skin. Gels may cause some localized heating. Air should not be incorporated into the product, because air bubbles may disperse the ultrasound waves, resulting in heating at the liquid:air interface.

For efficient ultrasound and phonophoresis, the skin should be well hydrated. Lack of moisture impedes sound transfer. The skin can be rehydrated using a warm, moist towel for about 10 to 15 minutes before the treatment.

Finally, after the treatment is completed, an occlusive dressing will help maintain skin hydration, warmth, and capillary dilatation; it will also keep the drug (residing on the skin surface) in intimate contact with the skin for further absorption.

Hydrocortisone is the drug most often administered using phonophoresis, in concentrations ranging from 1% to 10%. Other drugs administered include betamethasone dipropionate, chymotrypsin alpha, dexamethasone, fluocinonide, hyaluronidase, iodine, ketoprofen, lidocaine, mecholyl, naproxen, piroxicam, sodium salicylate, and trypsin.

Sample Formulations

 Ultrasound Gels

	Carbopol Type	Hydroxyethyl cellulose
Carbopol 940 (0.65%)	650 mg	
Hydroxyethyl cellulose (3%)		3 g
Propylene glycol	5 mL	5 mL
Methylparaben	200 mg	200 mg
Sodium hydroxide 10% solution	qs	
Purified water	qs 100 mL	qs 100 mL

1. Calculate the required quantity of each ingredient for the total amount to be prepared.
2. Accurately weigh or measure each ingredient.
3. Dissolve the methylparaben in the propylene glycol.
4. Add the solution to about 90 mL of the purified water.

Carbopol Gel
5. Disperse the Carbopol 940 in the solution using rapid agitation.
6. Slowly, add about 1.5 mL of the sodium hydroxide 10% solution.
7. Mix slowly to form a smooth gel and to avoid incorporating air into the product.
8. Slowly, add additional sodium hydroxide 10% solution until a pH of 6.5–7 is obtained.
9. Add sufficient purified water to volume, and carefully mix.
10. Package and label the product.

Hydroxyethyl Cellulose Gel
5. Initially, disperse the hydroxyethyl cellulose in the solution using moderate agitation.
6. Then, mix slowly to form a smooth gel and to avoid incorporating air into the product.
7. Add sufficient purified water to volume, and carefully mix.
8. Package and label the product.

℞ **Corticosteroid Gels for Phonophoresis**

	Betamethasone Dipropionate 0.05% Gel	Dexamethasone sodium phosphate 0.4% Gel	Fluocinonide 0.1% Gel	Hydrocortisone 10% Gel
Active drug	77 mg (equiv. to 50 mg beta-methasone)	528 mg (equiv. to 400 mg dexamethasone)	100 mg	10 g
Propylene glycol	qs	qs	qs	qs
Ultrasound gel	qs 100 g	qs 100 g	qs 100 g	qs 100 g

1. Calculate the quantity of each ingredient required for the prescription.
2. Accurately weigh or measure each ingredient.
3. Mix the corticosteroid powder with sufficient propylene glycol to form a smooth paste.
4. Carefully add the ultrasound gel without incorporating air into the product.
5. Mix the gel until uniform.
6. Package and label the product.

℞ **Nonsteroidal Anti-inflammatory Drug Gels for Phonophoresis**

	Ketoprofen 2% Gel	Naproxen 5% Gel	Piroxicam 0.5% Gel	Sodium Salicylate 10% Gel
Active drug	2 g	5 g	500 mg	10 g
Propylene glycol	qs	qs	qs	qs
Ultrasound gel	qs 100 g	qs 100 g	qs 100 g	qs 100 g

1. Calculate the quantity of each ingredient required for the prescription.
2. Accurately weigh or measure each ingredient.
3. Mix the nonsteroidal anti-inflammatory drug powder with sufficient propylene glycol to form a smooth paste.
4. Carefully add the ultrasound gel without incorporating air into the product.
5. Mix the gel until uniform.
6. Package and label the product.

℞ Dexamethasone 1.5% and Lidocaine Hydrochloride 4% Ultrasound Gel

Dexamethasone sodium phosphate	1.98 g (equiv. to 1.5 g dexamethasone)	Active
Lidocaine hydrochloride	4 g	Active
Propylene glycol	10 mL	Solvent
Hydroxyethyl cellulose ultrasound gel	qs 100 g	Vehicle

1. Calculate the quantity of each ingredient required for the prescription.
2. Accurately weigh or measure each ingredient.
3. Mix the powders with the propylene glycol to form a smooth mixture.
4. Carefully add the ultrasound gel without incorporating air into the product.
5. Mix the gel until uniform.
6. Package and label the product.

℞ Iodine and Methyl Salicylate Ultrasound Ointment

Iodine	4 g	Active
Oleic acid	5 mL	Emulsifier/Emollient
Methyl salicylate	4 mL	Aroma
White petrolatum	qs 100 g	Vehicle

1. Calculate the quantity of each ingredient required for the prescription.
2. Accurately weigh or measure each ingredient.
3. Dissolve the iodine in the oleic acid and methyl salicylate.
4. Incorporate the white petrolatum, and stir until uniform.
5. Package and label the product. Protect the product from light.

℞ Zinc Oxide 2% Gel

Zinc oxide	20 g	Active
Pluronic F-127 30% gel	80 g	Vehicle

1. Calculate the quantity of each ingredient required for the prescription.
2. Accurately weigh or measure each ingredient.
3. Add the zinc oxide powder, previously comminuted, in small portions to the Pluronic F-127 30% Gel.
4. Mix the gel until uniform, being careful not to incorporate air into the product.
5. Package and label the product.

Supplements

The use of nutraceuticals continues to increase in our society. *Nutraceuticals* are defined by the American Nutraceutical Association as "naturally occurring dietary substances in pharmaceutical dosage forms." Thus, nutraceuticals include dietary supplements as defined by the Dietary Supplement Health and Education Act (DSHEA) of 1994, as well as comparable substances unintended for oral ingestion. The popularity of nutraceuticals is consumer driven, and pharmacists are often asked about the composition and use of these substances. Nutraceuticals covered under DSHEA have no published standards. United States Pharmacopeial Convention (USP) monographs are being developed for some of the substances, so any preparation containing those substances and bearing the USP designation must meet those standards. Because many of the commercial products do not meet USP standards, patients cannot be sure of their quality. However, some of the bulk drug substances are available as USP quality, so a compounding pharmacist can assure patients of the quality of the compounded nutraceuticals they are receiving.

Most compounding of natural preparations and nutraceuticals involves the capsule dosage form. When capsules are not desired, alcoholic or aqueous extracts can be prepared; these extracts can be flavored.

Sample Formulation

℞ Compounded Coenzyme Q_{10} 100 mg Capsules (#100)

Coenzyme Q_{10}	10 g	Active
Polyethylene glycol 4000	30 g	Diluent/Vehicle

1. Calculate the quantity of each ingredient required for the prescription.
2. Accurately weigh each ingredient.
3. Reduce particle size, if necessary, so both products have a similar particle size.
4. Thoroughly mix the powders until uniform.
5. Encapsulate the powders into 100 capsules, each weighing 400 mg and containing 100 mg of coenzyme Q_{10}.
6. Package and label the product.

Nasogastric Tube Administration

Compounding medications for administration through a feeding tube offers an opportunity for a pharmacist to use both physical chemistry knowledge and clinical skills in developing each formulation. The pharmacist must consider a number of issues in evaluating patients with feeding tubes and designing doses to minimize complications for these patients. The major issues are as follows:

- Types of feeding tubes
- Distal site considerations
- Vehicles for administration of solid drugs
- Withholding of nutrition for drug administration
- Selection of dosage forms for administration via a feeding tube

The size and dimensions of a feeding tube will affect the formulations used. Some feeding tubes are inserted through the nose and passed into the stomach. Nasogastric tubes are 24 to 36 inches long and have a small diameter (French 10 to 16). Feeding tubes that extend through the pylorus and into the jejunum are longer (30 to 55 inches) and generally have a smaller diameter (French 8 to 12). Long, thin tubes have a greater tendency to loop, kink, or form knots. Surgically placed tubes such as percutaneous endoscopic gastrostomy (PEG) tubes are short (3 to 4 inches) and have a wide diameter (French 6 to 20). Tubes surgically placed in the jejunum (percutaneous endoscopic jejunostomy, or PEJ tubes) are also short but generally have a narrower diameter.

The larger-diameter, shorter tubes—PEG and some PEJ tubes—are less likely to clog than the longer, smaller-bore tubes inserted through the nose into the stomach or jejunum. Medications that are compounded for nasally inserted jejunal tubes should be completely dissolved in solution, because any solid, even solids mixed as a suspension, will contribute to clog formation.

There are no commercially available liquid medications formulated for administration via feeding tubes. Oral liquid medications are formulated for administration to pediatric patients or patients with limited ability to swallow tablets. Usually these liquid medications are prescribed at a low concentration to allow a pediatric dose to be given as 5 mL; in addition, they generally are sweetened and have increased viscosity to improve palatability. Sweetening agents include sucrose, maltose, and sorbitol. Sorbitol is used extensively, because it has solubilizing effects as a polyalcohol in addition to enhancing viscosity to improve stability. One consideration in nasogastric tube administration is osmolarity. On the basis of osmolarity alone, a pharmacist can calculate the amount of free water to add to a liquid medication to improve tolerance by decreasing osmolarity. The osmolarity tolerable by the gastrointestinal tract is about 300 mOsm/L. The larger the volume of a dose, the more water is needed to dilute the dose to a tolerable level.

An alternative is to avoid all commercial liquid formulations and prepare a low-osmolarity solution by mixing the solid directly with water until it dissolves. In some cases, the addition of an acid will enhance solubility and allow effective delivery.[4]

Ketogenic Diet Considerations

The ketogenic diet is a treatment option for young children with refractory seizure disorders or inborn metabolic defects involving glucose metabolism that do not respond to conventional medication. It is a high-fat, low-carbohydrate, and low-protein diet designed to increase the body's dependence on fatty acids rather than glucose for energy. Most children stay on the diet for 2 to 3 years, after which they slowly resume a normal diet or a modified Atkins diet.

Pharmacists can play an invaluable role in patient care by researching and calculating the carbohydrate content of medications. A quick reference list is available.[5] Although the carbohydrate content of compounded liquids appears to be quite small, it can quickly add up, depending on the dose and the number of medications a patient is taking. For example, if a patient is taking a couple of compounded medications that contain 0.45 grams of carbohydrate per milliliter, and the doses are 5 mL four times daily, almost all of the patient's daily allowance of carbohydrates could be used. When a patient is in a deliberate state of starvation and malnutrition, saving as much of the carbohydrate allowance as possible for a small serving of a fruit or vegetable rather than a few teaspoonfuls of medicine is more desirable.

Excipient Alternatives for Special Populations

Patients with allergies or intolerances and those requiring special diets are among the groups that require formulations with special excipients. Potentially troublesome excipients include aspartame; chocolate; corn; dyes (tartrazine); gelatin; gluten; honey, lactose, milk, and other animal-derived ingredients; peanuts, soy, and other nuts; preservatives (benzoates, parabens); saccharin; and salicylates. In many cases, there are alternatives that can be used to compound an acceptable preparation for a patient.[6]

References

1. Giacoia GP, Taylor-Zapata P, Mattison D. Need for appropriate formulations for children: The National Institute of Child Health and Human Development—Pediatric formulations initiative, Part 1. *Int J Pharm Compound.* 2007;11(1):5–8.
2. Reilly JA, Walter MA. Consumer product aspiration and ingestion in children: analysis of emergency room reports to the national electronic injury surveillance system. *Ann Otol Rhinol Laryngol.* 1992;10(9):739–41.
3. Allen LV Jr. Basics of compounding; phonophoresis. *Int J Pharm Compound.* 2002;6(5):362–5.
4. Klang M. Recommendations for compounding medications for feeding tube administration. *Int J Pharm Compound.* 2010;14(4):276–82.
5. McElhiney LF, Cheng A, Meshberger L, et al. Calculating the carbohydrate content of compounded medications for patients on a ketogenic diet. *Int J Pharm Compound.* 2010;14(1):21–5.
6. Nagel-Edwards KM, Ko JY. Excipient choices for special populations. *Int J Pharm Compound.* 2008;12(5):426–30.

Compounding with Special Ingredients

Compounding with Balsams

Balsams used in pharmacy include benzoin, Peruvian balsam, storax, and tolu balsam. These are listed in Table 28-1 together with their botanical source. A number of substances have the name "balsam" but are not technically balsams; these are also listed in Table 28-1. Currently, in the United States Pharmacopeial Convention (USP) monographs, there appear to be only three official balsams, Benzoin USP, Storax USP, and Tolu Balsam USP, and one official USP preparation, Compound Benzoin Tincture USP. Also, the only National Formulary (NF) preparations are Tolu Balsam Syrup and Tolu Balsam Tincture. Of the four common balsams, Peruvian balsam and its common preparations are not official.

Balsams are defined as aromatic and usually oily and resinous substances flowing from various plants, either spontaneously or from an incision; any of several resinous substances containing benzoic or cinnamic acid and especially used in medicine; and preparations containing resinous substances and having a balsamic odor.

Characteristics

Benzoin is the balsamic resin obtained from *Styrax benzoin* Dryander or *Styrax parallelo-neurus* Perkins, known in commerce as Sumatra benzoin. It occurs as blocks or lumps of varying size composed of compacted tears, with a reddish brown, reddish gray, or grayish brown resinous mass. Siam benzoin occurs as compressed pebble-like tears of varying size and shape. Both varieties are yellowish to rusty brown externally and milky white on fracture. They are hard and brittle at ordinary temperatures, but when softened by heat, they have an aromatic and balsamic odor and an aromatic and slightly acrid taste.

Benzoin is used in protective applications for irritations of the skin. Benzoin tincture is principally used as an ingredient in external preparations such as skin lotions. For throat and bronchial inflammation, the tincture may be administered on sugar. The tincture and compound tincture sometimes are used in boiling water as steam inhalants for their expectorant and soothing actions in acute laryngitis and croup. In combination with zinc oxide, the tincture is used in baby ointments.

Compound benzoin tincture (Balsam of the Holy Victorious Knight, Commander's Balsam, Friar's Balsam, Jerusalem Balsam, Persian Balsam, Saint Victor's Balsam, Swedish

Balsam, Turlington's Balsam of Life, Turlington's drops, Vervain Balsam, Wade's Drops, and Ward's Balsam) has had more different Latin titles and synonyms since its origin in the 15th or 16th century than any other preparation. Many of these reflect its uses or its originators, introducers, or patrons, because it is portrayed as a nostrum as well as an item in the pharmacopeias of the past 300 years. It contains 74% to 80% ethanol. The tincture should be preserved in tight, light-resistant containers, avoiding exposure to direct sunlight and excessive heat.

TABLE 28-1 Examples of Balsams

	Botanical Source
Balsam	
Benzoin	(*Styrax*)
Peruvian balsam	(*Myroxylon*)
Storax	(*Liquidambar*)
Tolu balsam	(*Myroxylon*)
Nonbalsam	
Balm of Gilead	(*Populus* sect. *Tacamahaca*)
Balsam of Mecca	(*Commiphora gileadensis*)
Canada balsam	(*Abies balsamea*)
Copaiba balsam	(*Copaifera langsdorffii*)

Peruvian balsam (Balsam of Peru, Black Balsam, and Indian Balsam) occurs as a thick, deep brown or black transparent fluid that appears reddish brown in thin layers, and it is neither stringy nor sticky. It has a tenacious, very sweet, balsamic odor with vanilla-like nuances and a bitter, acrid taste with a persistent aftertaste. Peruvian balsam is used as a fixative in perfumes where a long-lasting sweetness is required. Although it is stable at room temperature, excessive heat and flames may cause instability. It should be packaged in a tight container and stored in a cool, well-ventilated area away from both sunlight and sources of ignition. Containers should be stored below 40°C and above freezing. It does not harden on exposure to air and has a specific gravity from 1.150 to 1.170. Peruvian balsam is nearly insoluble in water but is soluble in alcohol, chloroform, and glacial acetic acid and only partly soluble in ether and in solvent hexane.

Peruvian balsam is used as a local irritant and is a valuable dressing to promote the growth of epithelial cells in the treatment of indolent ulcers, wounds, and certain skin diseases. In addition, it is used in suppositories for hemorrhoids and in dry socket treatment in dentistry. It has a very mild antiseptic action because of its cinnamic and benzoic acids. Diluted with an equal part of castor oil, it has been used as an application to bedsores and chronic ulcers. It has also been used topically in the treatment of superficial skin lesions and pruritus. Peruvian balsam is used in the treatment of respiratory congestion as well as in aromatherapy.

Storax is a balsam obtained from the trunk of *Liquidambar orientalis* Miller, known in commerce as Levant Storax, or of *Liquidambar styraciflua* Linné, or American Storax (Fam. *Hamamelidaceae*). It occurs as a semiliquid, grayish to grayish-brown, sticky, opaque mass depositing on standing a heavy dark brown layer (Levant Storax) or a semisolid, sometimes solid mass, softened by gentle warming (American Storax). Storax is transparent in thin layers, has a characteristic odor and taste, and is more dense than water. It is incompletely soluble in an equal weight of warm alcohol or acetone and in ether with some insoluble residue usually remaining; it is insoluble in water. It should be preserved in well-closed containers.

Tolu balsam is a brown or yellowish-brown, plastic solid that is transparent in thin layers and brittle when old, dried, or exposed to cold temperatures. It has a pleasant, aromatic odor resembling that of vanilla, and a mild aromatic taste. It is soluble in alcohol and chloroform and in ether, sometimes with slight residue or turbidity; it is practically insoluble in water and in solvent hexane. Tolu balsam should be preserved in tight containers, avoiding exposure to excessive heat.

Compounding Considerations

Peruvian Balsam

Ointments containing both Peruvian balsam and sulfur present a problem in compounding, because the resinous part of the balsam tends to separate. This problem can be overcome by mixing the balsam with an equal amount of castor oil before incorporating it into the base or, alternatively, by mixing it with solid petroxolin (a mixture of liquid petrolatum and ammonia soap medicated and perfumed especially for use in ointments).

Peruvian balsam, if mixed directly with iodoform, gradually deodorizes it and forms a compound with it. An example is shown in the following formula.

℞ Guaiacol and Peruvian Balsam Capsules (#36)

Guaiacol carbonate	11.7 g	Active
Dionin	0.195 g	Active
Iodoform	2.34 g	Active
Eucalyptol	2.34 g	Active
Peruvian balsam	2.34 g	Active/Diluent
Magnesium oxide, light	4.7 g	Adsorbent

To slow the reaction between Peruvian balsam and iodoform, avoiding the direct mixing of these two drugs is best. A pharmacist should triturate the balsam with 4.7 g of light magnesium oxide before mixing with the other solid ingredients. The eucalyptol can be added next and thoroughly mixed, and then the mixture can be encapsulated.

Peruvian balsam is only slightly soluble in most oleaginous vehicles, and frequently, after incorporation with fats or lanolin, it separates from these bases. Recommended practice is to incorporate Peruvian balsam with petrolatum by using castor oil, generally in an amount equal to that of the balsam.

In hydrophilic ointment, 5% of Peruvian balsam can be easily incorporated to produce an elegant, stable, and therapeutically efficacious preparation.

Tolu Balsam

Tolu balsam is a tenacious, plastic mass at room temperature. For convenience in handling and weighing, recommended practice is to chill the balsam to render it brittle and easily broken into fragments of suitable size for use in preparing the tincture.

Tolu balsam syrup is used as a vehicle and is especially popular in remedies for coughs and colds. It is slightly alkaline and is not preserved. As the syrup ages, growth of molds can result in the development of an unpleasant odor resembling that of coal gas or benzene.

Sample Formulations

℞ Diaper Rash Ointment

Peruvian balsam	6.6 g	Active
Castor oil	13.2 mL	Solvent/Compounding Aid
Boric acid ointment	13.2 g	Active
Zinc oxide ointment	67 g	Active/Vehicle

1. Calculate the quantity of each ingredient required for the prescription.
2. Accurately weigh or measure each ingredient.
3. Mix the Peruvian balsam with the castor oil.
4. Levigate this mixture into the boric acid ointment.
5. Incorporate this mixture into the zinc oxide ointment geometrically, and mix well.
6. Package and label the product.

℞ Peruvian Balsam and Ichthammol Ointment

Castor oil	250 mL	Solvent/Compounding Aid
Peruvian balsam	250 g	Active
Ichthammol	250 g	Active
Petrolatum	qs 1000 g	Vehicle

1. Calculate the quantity of each ingredient required for the prescription.
2. Accurately weigh or measure each ingredient.
3. Mix the Peruvian balsam with the castor oil.
4. Incorporate the ichthammol, and mix well.
5. Incorporate the ichthammol mixture into sufficient petrolatum to final weight, and mix well.
6. Package and label the product.

℞ Peruvian Balsam and Trypsin Liquid

Peruvian balsam	8.7 g	Active
Trypsin 1:75	0.333 g	Active
Castor oil	87 mL	Solvent/Compounding Aid
Triton X-100	1 mL	Surfactant

1. Calculate the quantity of each ingredient required for the prescription.
2. Accurately weigh or measure each ingredient.
3. Combine the Trypsin 1:75 and the Triton X-100.
4. Add a portion of the castor oil, and mix well.
5. Add the Peruvian balsam, and mix well.
6. Add the remaining castor oil, and mix well.
7. Package and label the product.

℞ Peruvian Balsam Compound Powder

Peruvian balsam	5.51 g	Active
Zinc stearate	3.48 g	Thickener/Sorbent
Boric acid powder	1.5 g	Active/Sorbent
Talc	20 g	Sorbent
Isopropyl alcohol, anhydrous 99%	30 mL	Vehicle

1. Calculate the quantity of each ingredient required for the prescription.
2. Accurately weigh or measure each ingredient.
3. Mix the Peruvian balsam and isopropyl alcohol.
4. Add the zinc stearate, boric acid, and talc powders, and mix well.
5. Spread out the mixture on a large surface (pan or beaker), and allow the alcohol to evaporate.
6. Mix the powder thoroughly after it is dried, and pulverize into a fine powder.
7. Package and label the product.

℞ Peruvian Balsam, Zinc Oxide, Allantoin, and Starch Ointment

Peruvian balsam	4.5 g	Active
Zinc oxide	12 g	Active/Sorbent
Allantoin	2 g	Emollient/Vehicle
Castor oil	6 g	Solvent/Compounding Aid
Cornstarch	10 g	Sorbent/Vehicle
Quaternium-15	100 mg	Antimicrobial
White petrolatum	65.4 g	Vehicle

1. Calculate the quantity of each ingredient required for the prescription.
2. Accurately weigh or measure each ingredient.
3. Mix the Peruvian balsam and castor oil together.
4. In a separate container, geometrically mix the zinc oxide, allantoin, cornstarch, and quaternium-15.
5. Sift the powder through a coarse sieve.
6. Levigate the Peruvian balsam–castor oil mixture into the white petrolatum.
7. Incorporate the zinc oxide mixture (step 4) into the Peruvian balsam mixture (step 6), and mix until uniform.
8. Package and label the product.

℞ Tolu Balsam in Polyethylene Glycol Dental Paste

Tolu balsam	13 g	Active
Eugenol	13 g	Active
Benzocaine	1.15 g	Active
Chlorobutanol	1.15 g	Preservative
Polyethylene glycol 3350	50 g	Vehicle
Polyethylene glycol 4450	10.7 g	Vehicle
Stearyl alcohol	7.14 g	Vehicle
Polyethylene glycol 300	3.68 g	Vehicle

1. Calculate the quantity of each ingredient required for the prescription.
2. Accurately weigh or measure each ingredient.
3. Combine the Tolu balsam, eugenol, benzocaine, and chlorobutanol, and mix well to form a solution.
4. In a separate container, combine the polyethylene glycol 3350, polyethylene glycol 4450, polyethylene glycol 300, and stearyl alcohol, and melt to about 45°C–50°C.
5. Remove the mixture from heat, combine the Tolu balsam mixture (step 3) and the polyethylene glycol mixture (step 4), and mix well while cooling.
6. Package and label the product.

Compounding with Silicones

As early as 1946, methylchlorosilanes were presented as a method to treat glassware in order to prevent blood from clotting. Since that time, the application of silicones in pharmaceutical and medical applications has grown to their current use in many life-saving devices (pacemakers, hydrocephalic shunts) and pharmaceutical applications from tubing to excipients in topical formulations to adhesives for affixing transdermal drug delivery systems, as well as their use in products as active pharmaceutical ingredients (APIs), such as an antiflatulents. About 60% of today's skin care products now contain some type of silicone, which is considered safe and is known to provide a pleasant, silky, nongreasy touch and nonstaining effect.

Silicones exhibit many useful characteristics (see Table 28-2). The safety of these agents supports their numerous applications, as listed in Table 28-3, which shows that prolonged contact with the human body is involved in some of the indicated uses. The biocompatibility of silicones is due partially to their low chemical reactivity, low surface energy, and hydrophobicity. Several hundred products contain silicones, and they are used as APIs, but even more prominently as excipients.

Silicones are used mainly in creams, followed by gels and lotions for the treatment of acne fungal diseases or psoriasis. Their noncomedogenic nature probably accounts for their use in anti-acne formulations.

Types of Silicones

Because of their low liquid surface tension, silicones spread easily to form films over substrates, like skin, but also spread over their own absorbed film. Their viscoelastic behavior enables resin-reinforced silicones or partially cross-linked elastomers (gels) to have high-pressure-sensitive properties. Consequently, their gentle adhesive and pliability properties have led to their widespread use in securing patches or dressings to the skin.

TABLE 28-2 Characteristics of Silicones

Antiadhesive

Defoaming properties

No support for microbial growth

Elastomers (drug-release-control membrane)

Electrical insulator

Flexibility

Forming of watertight seals

High gas permeability

Liquid form

Low thermal conductivity

Low chemical reactivity

Low toxicity

Lubrication properties

Noncomedogenic

Nonsticking to some substances but very adherent to others

Properties not very temperature dependent

Release liner coatings for transdermal patch (release coating)

Resistant to oxygen, ozone, and sunlight

Skin-adhesive properties

Thermal stability ($-100°C$ to $250°C$)

Water repellent

The polydimethylsiloxanes are among the most widely used silicones; they have viscosities between 10 and 100,000 mPa-s. Because of their high molecular weight, they are not absorbed in the gastrointestinal tract and are excreted without being metabolized. They also are not absorbed through the skin. If they are inhaled as aerosols of oily or fatty-type materials into the alveolar regions of the lung, physical disturbances of the lining of the lung may occur.

Properties

The following are some of the characteristics that make the silicones so useful in pharmacy.

Occlusivity

Some silicones exhibit *occlusive* properties and still retain the silky touch usually associated with silicones. *Occlusivity* is a term comprising the adherent qualities of a product, such as a sunscreen, and its ability to be retained after the skin is exposed to water and perspiration. The term also relates to the persistence of the effect of a topically applied drug or cosmetic, as determined by the degree of physical and chemical bonding to the surface; resistance to removal or inactivation by sweating, swimming, bathing, and friction; and so on.

Substantivity

Silicone gums are highly substantive on the skin and can significantly improve the substantivity of an API. A film is formed after application, and the volatile is removed; this action helps maintain the API in close contact with the skin and prevent loss by abrasion

TABLE 28-3 Medical, Pharmaceutical, and Personal Care Uses of Silicones

Medical

Acne products

Debridement of necrotic tissues when enzymes are present

Delivery of antibiotics in gynecological capsules or creams

Filling materials in cushions to prevent pressure sores

Foam elimination in the stomach during endoscopy or in conjunction with barium sulfate during x-ray examination

Gel form use in bandages and dressings, breast implants, testicle implants, pectoral implants, contact lenses, and others

Main indication for skin diseases, mostly as creams, followed by gels and lotions, including for treatment of acne, fungal diseases, or psoriasis

Personal lubricants for use in medical procedures

Silicone oil to replace vitreous following vitrectomy, silicone intraocular lenses following cataract extraction, silicone tubes to keep nasolacrimal passage open following dacryocystorhinostomy, canalicular stents for canalicular stenosis, punctal plugs for punctal occlusion in dry eyes, silicone rubber in bands as an external tamponade in treating retinal detachment and anteriorly located break in rhegmatogenous retinal detachment

Prevention of skin ulceration around stoma

Scar treatment (keloid and hypertrophic)

Treatment of hemorrhoids, anal dermatoses, or itch relief

Decreased jerk reflex during injections when needles are coated with silicone fluids, thereby reducing pain

Pharmaceutical

Defoaming agents

Mold release agent

Control of foaming of liquids

Personal Care

Hair conditioners, shampoos, and hair gel products; reflection-enhancing and color-correcting hair products for increased shine and glossiness

Personal lubricants

Shaving products

Baby bottle nipples

Sunscreens, aiding in substantivity and staying on skin longer

and washing away. This substantivity can improve the contact of the skin with an API (e.g., ketoprofen) when dispensed from a silicone volatile-based spray. The drug-loaded film is more resistant to removal.

Rub-Off and Wash-Off Resistance
Silicones form hydrophobic films that are spreadable and substantive. These characteristics explain their high resistance to being washed or rubbed off.

Antifoaming
Simethicone (dimethicone; silicone oil), which has a low hydrophile–lipophile balance value, is used in oily dispersions in which a hypromellose polymer is used as the polymeric

emulsifier and surface stabilizer. Dimethicone is used to treat neonatal acid reflux that can result from milk protein froth formation in the stomach. The simethicones function by forming hydrophobic solids, destabilizing the aggregates or oil droplets that sit in an aqueous-thin liquid film and prevent continuity.

Pharmaceutical Silicones

Three primary types of polymers are used in pharmaceutical applications: polymers, elastomers, and pressure-sensitive adhesives. Silicones are used as excipients in fluids, gums, and gels for topical creams, ointments, and lotions because of some of their unique physicochemical and performance properties.

USP/NF silicones include cyclomethicone, dimethicone, and simethicone. Their use categories are (1) Adhesives—Dimethicone; (2) Antifoaming Agents—Dimethicone, Simethicone; (3) Emollients—Cyclomethicone, Dimethicone; and (4) Water-Repelling Agents—Cyclomethicone, Dimethicone, Simethicone. Some of the properties of cyclomethicone, dimethicone, and simethicone and their applications are discussed below.

Cyclomethicone $(C_2H_6OSi)_n$, with chemical name cyclopolydimethylsiloxane and USP therapeutic category "Pharmaceutic aid (wetting agent)," is a fully methylated cyclic siloxane containing repeating units $[-(CH_3)2SiO-]_n$ in which n is 4, 5, or 6 or a mixture of them. It is soluble in 95% ethanol, isopropyl myristate, isopropyl palmitate, mineral oil, and petrolatum (at 80°C); it is practically insoluble in glycerin, propylene glycol, and water. Cyclomethicone should be preserved in tight containers and exposure to excessive heat avoided.[1]

Cyclomethicone is used as an emollient, humectant, and viscosity-increasing agent. It is found primarily in topical pharmaceutical and cosmetic formulations such as water-in-oil creams. It has been an ingredient in cosmetic formulations at concentrations of 0.1% to 50% and is now the most widely used silicone in the cosmetics industry. Cyclomethicones are widely used in personal care because of their volatility, aesthetic, and safety profile.

Its high volatility and solvent properties make it suitable for use in topical formulations; with a low heat of vaporization, it has a dry feel when applied to the skin. Commercial names include Dow Corning 245 Fluid, Dow Corning 246 Fluid, and Dow Corning 345 Fluid.[2]

Dimethicone is a mixture of fully methylated linear siloxane polymers. It occurs as a clear, colorless, and odorless liquid. It is soluble in amyl acetate, benzene, chlorinated hydrocarbons, ether, ethyl acetate, isopropyl myristate, methyl ethyl ketone, mineral oil, n-hexane, petroleum spirits, toluene, and xylene. Dimethicone is very slightly soluble in isopropyl alcohol and insoluble in acetone, alcohol, glycerin, methanol, propylene glycol, and water. It has a density of 0.94 to 0.98.[3]

Dimethicone is used as a skin protectant, antifoaming agent, water-repelling agent, adhesive, and emollient. Also, it is a lubricant, hydrophobing agent, and prosthetic aid (soft tissue). Dimethicone is widely used in cosmetic and pharmaceutical formulations. In topical oil-in-water emulsions, it is added to the oil phase as an antifoaming agent. It is also used in topical barrier preparations because of its hydrophobic properties. In creams, lotions, and ointments, concentrations are between 10% and 30%. In oil-in-water emulsions, generally 0.5% to 5% concentrations are used.

If used for coating containers that come in contact with articles for parenteral use, dimethicone contains not more than 1.0 USP Endotoxin Unit/mL, equivalent to not more than 10 Endotoxin Units/mL of the dimethicone taken. It should be packaged in tight containers and labeled to indicate its nominal viscosity value. If intended for use in coating parenteral containers, it is so labeled.[4]

A thin film of dimethicone can be sterilized by dry heat at 160°C for at least 2 hours. Autoclaving should not be used for large quantities of dimethicone because the excess water will diffuse into the fluid and cause it to become hazy. Gamma irradiation may also be used but may cause cross-linking and an increase in the fluid's viscosity. Dimethicone is flammable and should not be exposed to flames or high heat.

Simethicone is a mixture of poly (dimethylsiloxane) and silicon dioxide where *n* in the graphic formula is 200 to 350; the molecular weight ranges from 14,000 to 21,000. It occurs as a translucent, gray, viscous fluid. The liquid phase is soluble in benzene, chloroform, and ether, but silicon dioxide remains as a residue in these solvents. Simethicone is insoluble in water and in alcohol. It boils at 35°C and has a specific gravity of 0.95 to 0.98. It is used as an antifoaming agent, water-repelling agent, and capsule and tablet diluent. Also, it is used as an antiflatulent (Gas-X, Mylanta Gas Relief, Infants' Mylicon Drops).[5]

When used in aqueous formulations, simethicone should be emulsified to ensure compatibility with the aqueous system and components. If untreated simethicone is added to water, it will float like an oil. It should not be used in formulations with a pH less than 3 or above 10, because it has a tendency to break the polydimethylsiloxane polymer. Also, it cannot be mixed with polar solvents and is incompatible with oxidizing agents. Up to 10 ppm of simethicone can be used in food products in the United States. Simethicone can be sterilized by dry heating for 4 hours at 160°C or by autoclaving.[6]

Compounding Considerations

A pharmacist should consider the following when compounding with silicones:

- Most silicones are hydrophobic and are soluble in nonpolar solvents.
- With the exception of silicone waxes, silicones are liquid at room temperature and heating is not necessary for formulation.
- Silicone waxes need to be melted or softened before being introduced into a formulation.
- Silicones are safe, but one must remember that the volatile silicones are flammable.
- Lower molecular weight siloxanes are often used because of their volatility and generally dry skin feel. The lowest molecular weight linear silicone is hexamethyl-disiloxane, with a viscosity of 0.48 mPa-s.
- The required hydrophile–lipophile balance for silicones for producing oil-in-water emulsions is as follows:

Dimethicone	9
Methyl silicone	11
Silicone oil	10.5

- The inclusion of silicone oils, such as dimethicone at 10%–20%, may permit the formulation of oil-in-water products that are effective.
- Silicone oils are known for their skin-protective properties and may be used as a hydrophobic solvent. Generally, an example is silicone oil at a 2%–5% concentration.
- With regard to films, the incorporation of polyethylene glycols or carboxymethyl-cellulose into a silicone allows the creation of pores with an elastomer to provide a path for the release of the hydrophilic active drug.

Types of Formulations Using Silicones

Silicone may be used in the following formulations:

- *Emulsions:* Both water-in-oil and oil-in-water emulsions can be compounded with silicone.
- *Gels:* Water-free gels can be compounded with up to 99% silicone. Hydrogels can accept a limited amount of silicone (usually up to 10%), but silicone gels do not have this limitation.

- *Ointments:* Most silicones are soluble in petrolatum, and ointments can be formulated with silicone to improve aesthetics. An example is petrolatum:cyclomethicone (75:25), which improves the afterfeel of an ointment after application to the skin.
- *Sprays:* Silicone volatile sprays are nonoily, noncooling, and nonstinging.
- *Sticks:* These can be formulated with silicone wax to improve spreadability.
- *Solutions:* Shampoos often contain antitangling (cyclomethicone/simethicone oil) agents as well as viscosity-enhancing agents, humectants, sequestering agents, coloring, and conditioners. The dimethicone acts as a wetting, smoothing, and occlusion aid as it intercalates within hair cuticles and reduces friction and hair breakage while maintaining color and gloss.

Sample Formulations
Capsules

℞ Simethicone and Magnesium Carbonate Capsules (#100)

Dextrose	1.6 g	Diluent
Simethicone powder 30% GS	26.6 g	Active
Magnesium carbonate	6.4 g	Diluent
Microcrystalline cellulose	12.8 g	Diluent
Magnesium stearate	500 mg	Lubricant
Dextrates	qs	Diluent

1. Calculate the quantity of each ingredient required for the prescription.
2. Accurately weigh or measure each ingredient.
3. Determine the quantity of dextrates required for the total number of capsules to be filled.
4. Blend the powders together until uniform, and encapsulate the mixture.
5. Package and label the product.

Creams

℞ Dimethicone Hand Cream (100 g)

Dimethicone	5 g	Active
Emulsifying Wax NF	15 g	Thickener/Emulsifier
Oleyl alcohol	4 g	Vehicle
Ethoxylated lanolin	5 g	Vehicle
Mineral oil, light	15 g	Vehicle/Oil Phase
Purified water	qs 100 g	Vehicle
Fragrance		Fragrance
Colorant		Colorant

1. Calculate the quantity of each ingredient required for the prescription.
2. Accurately weigh or measure each ingredient.
3. Mix the dimethicone, Emulsifying Wax NF, oleyl alcohol, ethoxylated lanolin, and light mineral oil, and heat to about 60°C to 65°C.
4. Add the purified water to final weight to the oil phase with stirring.
5. While stirring, allow cream to cool to about 30°C.
6. Add any colorant or fragrance.
7. Package and label the product.

℞ Dimethicone Hand Cream, Preserved (100 g)

Dimethicone	4 g	Active
Stearic acid	6 g	Thickener
Cetyl alcohol	1.5 g	Emulsifier
Mineral oil, light	2.2 g	Vehicle/Oil Phase
Triethanolamine	1.5 g	Alkalizer
Glycerin	1.8 g	Solvent
Methylparaben	200 mg	Preservative
Purified water	82.8 mL	Vehicle

1. Calculate the quantity of each ingredient required for the prescription.
2. Accurately weigh or measure each ingredient.
3. Mix the dimethicone, stearic acid, cetyl alcohol, and light mineral oil in a container, and heat to about 75°C.
4. Mix the triethanolamine, glycerin, methylparaben, and purified water in a separate container, and heat the mixture to about 75°C.
5. Add the oil phase (step 3) to the aqueous phase, and cool while stirring until the mixture congeals and is at room temperature.
6. Package and label the product.

℞ Hydroxyzine Dihydrochloride 10 mg/g and Dimethicone 50 mg/g Cream (100 g)

Hydroxyzine dihydrochloride	1 g	Active
Dimethicone	5 g	Active
Emulsifying Wax NF	15 g	Emulsifier
Oleyl alcohol	4 g	Vehicle/Emulsifier
Ethoxylated lanolin	5 g	Vehicle/Emulsifier
Mineral oil, light	15 g	Vehicle/Oil Phase
Purified water	qs 100 g	Vehicle

1. Calculate the quantity of each ingredient required for the prescription.
2. Accurately weigh or measure each ingredient.
3. Mix the dimethicone, Emulsifying Wax NF, oleyl alcohol, ethoxylated lanolin, and light mineral oil, and heat to about 60°C to 65°C.
4. Dissolve the hydroxyzine dihydrochloride in 20 mL purified water, and add to the oil phase with stirring.
5. Add purified water to final weight to the mixture with stirring while the cream is warm.
6. Cool the cream to about 30°C with stirring.
7. Package and label the product.

Rx Silicone Protective Cream (100 g)

Emulsifying Wax NF	15 g	Vehicle/Thickener
Oleyl alcohol	4 g	Emulsifier
Polyethylene glycol 75 lanolin	5 g	Emulsifier
Mineral oil, light	15 g	Vehicle/Oil Phase
Dimethicone	5 to 10 g	Active
Purified water	qs 100 g	Vehicle
Fragrance		Fragrance
Colorant		Colorant

1. Calculate the quantity of each ingredient required for the prescription.
2. Accurately weigh or measure each ingredient.
3. Mix the Emulsifying Wax NF, oleyl alcohol, polyethylene glycol 75 lanolin, light mineral oil, and dimethicone, and heat to 65°C.
4. Heat the purified water to 65°C.
5. Add the purified water to the oil phase while stirring.
6. Stir the mixture while cooling to 30°C.
7. Add fragrance or colorant, or both, as desired.
8. Package and label the product.

Gel

Rx Clear Aqueous Gel Base with Dimethicone (100 mL)

Carbomer 934	500 mg	Thickener
Triethanolamine	1.2 mL	Alkalizer
Glycerin	34.2 mL	Vehicle/Solvent/Humectant
Propylene glycol	2 mL	Solvent
Dimethicone	2.3 mL	Active
Purified water	qs 100 mL	Vehicle

1. Calculate the quantity of each ingredient required for the prescription.
2. Accurately weigh or measure each ingredient.
3. Disperse the carbomer in 20 mL of purified water, and allow to hydrate.
4. Add the triethanolamine, and bring the volume to 40 mL with purified water.
5. Add the glycerin, propylene glycol, and dimethicone to the aqueous solution, and mix well.
6. Add sufficient purified water to volume, and mix well.
7. Package and label the product.

Lotions

℞ **Aluminum Chlorohydrate 15% in Cyclomethicone 10% Lotion, Paraben and Odor Free (100 mL)**

Aluminum chlorohydrate dihydrate	15 g	Active
Propylene glycol	25 mL	Vehicle/Humectant
Triethanolamine	1 mL	Alkalizer
Purified water	12 mL	Vehicle
Oleic acid	1.5 g	Vehicle/Emulsifier
Polyethylene glycol 400 monostearate	10.5 g	Emulsifier
Cyclomethicone	10 mL	Active
Carbopol 934 3% gel	40 g	Thickener

1. Calculate the quantity of each ingredient required for the prescription.
2. Accurately weigh or measure each ingredient.
3. Mix the aluminum chlorohydrate dihydrate with the purified water, add the triethanolamine and propylene glycol, and heat to about 70°C.
4. Mix the oleic acid, polyethylene glycol 400 monostearate, and cyclomethicone, and heat to about 70°C.
5. Mix the aqueous phase and oil phase together, remove from heat, and continue to mix while cooling.
6. Incorporate the mixture into the Carbopol 934 3% gel, and mix well.
7. Package and label the product.

℞ **Benzocaine Lotion, Clear (10 g)**

Benzocaine	6.1 g	Active
Cyclomethicone	36.4 g	Active
Polypropylene glycol 15 stearyl ether	43.9 g	Emulsifier
Polypropylene glycol 10 cetyl ether	13.6 g	Emulsifier

1. Calculate the quantity of each ingredient required for the prescription.
2. Accurately weigh or measure each ingredient.
3. Heat the polypropylene glycol 15 stearyl ether and the polypropylene glycol 10 cetyl ether to about 50°C–60°C.
4. Incorporate the benzocaine followed by the cyclomethicone, and mix until clear.
5. Package and label the product.

℞ Cyclomethicone 10% Lotion (100 mL)

Propylene glycol	25 mL	Vehicle/Humectant
Triethanolamine	1 mL	Alkalizer
Purified water	12 mL	Vehicle/Solvent
Oleic acid	1.5 g	Vehicle/Emulsifier
Polyethylene glycol 400 monostearate	10.5 g	Emulsifier
Cyclomethicone	10 mL	Active
Carbopol 934 3% gel	40 g	Vehicle

1. Calculate the quantity of each ingredient required for the prescription.
2. Accurately weigh or measure each ingredient.
3. Mix the triethanolamine and propylene glycol with the purified water, and heat to about 70°C.
4. Mix the oleic acid, polyethylene glycol 400 monostearate, and cyclomethicone, and heat to about 70°C.
5. Mix the aqueous phase and oil phase together, remove from heat, and mix while cooling.
6. Incorporate the mixture into the Carbopol 934 3% gel, and mix well.
7. Package and label the product.

Ointment

℞ Dimethicone and Zinc Oxide Ointment (100 g)

Dimethicone	1 g	Active
Zinc oxide	10 g	Active
Cod liver oil	10 g	Active
Propylene glycol	10 g	Solvent/Levigating Aid
Benzyl alcohol	200 mg	Preservative
Fragrance	qs	Fragrance
White petrolatum	qs 100 g	Vehicle

1. Calculate the quantity of each ingredient required for the prescription.
2. Accurately weigh or measure each ingredient.
3. Mix the dimethicone, benzyl alcohol, and cod liver oil with the propylene glycol.
4. Using low heat, just melt the white petrolatum and incorporate the dimethicone mixture (step 3).
5. Remove the mixture from heat, and while still warm, incorporate the zinc oxide and fragrance.
6. Allow the ointment to cool.
7. Package and label the product.

Powder

℞ Simethicone 60 mg Instant Granules in Powder Packets (100 packets)

Simethicone	6 g	Active
Cremophor RH 40	5 g	Emulsifier
Copovidone	3 g	Thickening Agent
Ethanol	40 g	Compounding Aid
Sorbitol, crystalline	50 g	Vehicle/Sweetener
Fructose	50 g	Vehicle/Sweetener
Crospovidone	50 g	Viscosity Agent
Orange flavoring	500 mg	Flavoring

1. Calculate the quantity of each ingredient required for the prescription.
2. Accurately weigh or measure each ingredient.
3. Mix the copovidone and the ethanol.
4. Add the simethicone and Cremophor RH 40, and mix well.
5. In a separate container, mix the crystalline sorbitol, fructose, crospovidone, and orange flavoring.
6. Combine the simethicone mixture (step 4) and the crystalline sorbitol mixture (step 5) together, spread out on a baking dish, and allow to dry.
7. Fill powder into 100 individual powder packets, each weighing 2.04 grams.

Solution

℞ Clear Sunscreen Oil (100 g)

Cyclomethicone	16 g	Active
Isopropyl myristate	13 g	Emulsifier
Mineral oil	68 g	Vehicle
Octyldimethyl-p-aminobenzoic acid	3 g	Active

1. Calculate the quantity of each ingredient required for the prescription.
2. Accurately weigh or measure each ingredient.
3. Heat the mineral oil to about 50°C–60°C, and incorporate the other ingredients.
4. Package and label the product.

Sticks

℞ Antiperspirant Stick (100 g)

Stearic acid	15 g	Vehicle/Thickener
Cetyl alcohol	15 g	Vehicle/Emulsifier
Aluminum chlorohydrate	20 g	Active
Cyclomethicone	50 g	Active

1. Calculate the quantity of each ingredient required for the prescription.
2. Accurately weigh or measure each ingredient.
3. Heat the stearic acid and cetyl alcohol to 50°C–60°C.
4. Incorporate the aluminum chlorohydrate followed by the cyclomethicone, and mix until uniform.
5. Begin allowing the mixture to cool, and pour into stick molds.
6. Package and label the product.

℞ Clear-Stick Medication Base (100 g)

Sodium stearate	7 g	Vehicle
Alcohol 95%	65 mL	Vehicle
Propylene glycol	25 mL	Vehicle
Cyclomethicone	3 g	Active

1. Calculate the quantity of each ingredient required for the prescription.
2. Accurately weigh or measure each ingredient.
3. Melt the sodium stearate.
4. In a separate container, mix the alcohol 95%, propylene glycol, and cyclomethicone, and add to the melted sodium stearate with stirring.
5. Cool the mixture slightly, and pour into stick molds.
6. Package and label the product.

Troches

℞ Simethicone 80 mg Chewable Troches (100 troches)

Simethicone	8 g	Active
Sorbitol	40 g	Vehicle/Sweetener
Cellulose, microcrystalline	2 g	Mouthfeel
Menthol	200 mg	Flavoring
Polyethylene glycol troche base	qs	Base

1. Calculate the quantity of each ingredient required for the prescription.
2. Accurately weigh or measure each ingredient.
3. Determine the quantity of polyethylene glycol troche base required for the formulation.
4. Mix the simethicone, sorbitol, and menthol together.
5. Melt the polyethylene glycol troche base at about 60°C, and slowly incorporate the simethicone mixture (step 4).
6. With constant stirring, sprinkle on the microcrystalline cellulose, and mix well.
7. Pour the mixture into molds, and cool.
8. Package and label the product.

Compounding with Tars

Tar refers to the substance obtained from a variety of organic materials through destructive distillation. Tar can be produced from coal, peat, petroleum, or wood. It is a black mixture of hydrocarbons and free carbon. The ancient Greeks produced tar from wood. Production and trade in pine-derived tar was a major contributor to the economies of Northern Europe and Colonial America, particularly North Carolina. It was used mainly in preserving wooden vessels against rot.

Production

The heating, or dry distillation, of pine wood causes tar and pitch to drip away from the wood and leave charcoal. One specific method of early production of tar consisted of a kiln that was a hole in the ground with a slope that allowed discharge of the generated tar. Wood was split into finger-sized pieces, stacked very tightly, and covered with dirt and moss; oxygen was prevented from entering because a flame could result. On top of this pile, a fire was stacked and lit. After a few hours, the tar began to drip out and was collected.

Definitions and Descriptions

Generally, a tar is a dark, oily, viscous material, consisting mainly of hydrocarbons, produced by the destructive distillation of organic substances such as coal, peat, or wood. Table 28-4 lists a comparison of the different medical tars and their characteristics. The following are the USP definitions and therapeutic uses of the various tars.

Coal tar is a nearly black, viscous liquid that is heavier than water. It has a characteristic, naphthalene-like odor and produces a sharp, burning sensation on the tongue. It is slightly soluble in water, to which it imparts its characteristic odor and taste and a faintly alkaline reaction; partially soluble in acetone, alcohol, carbon disulfide, chloroform, ether, methanol, and solvent hexane; and soluble in benzene and nitrobenzene.

Coal Tar Topical Solution USP (LCD, Liquor Carbonis Detergens) is a 20% solution of coal tar in alcohol prepared with the aid of polysorbate 80.

TABLE 28-4 Comparison of USP Tars

Characteristic	Coal Tar	Juniper Tar	Pine Tar
Synonyms	Crude coal tar; gas tar; Pix Carbon; Pix Carbonis; Pix Lithanthracis; Pix Mineralis; prepared coal tar.	Cade oil, Harlem oil, Caparlem, and Empyreumatic oil of juniper. Juniper tar oil; Oleum Juniperi Empyreumaticum; Pix Caci; Pix Juniperi.	Pix Liquida; Pix Pini; Pyroleum Pini; wood tar.
Description	Coal tar occurs as a nearly black, viscous liquid, heavier than water, with a characteristic naphthalene-like odor and a sharp burning taste. On ignition, it burns with a reddish, luminous, and very sooty flame, leaving not more than 2% of residue. It contains benzene, toluene, naphthalene, anthracene, xylene, and other aromatic hydrocarbons; phenol, cresol, and other phenol bodies; ammonia, pyridine, and some other organic bases; and thiophene.	Juniper tar occurs as a dark brown, clear, thick liquid with a tarry odor and a faintly aromatic, bitter taste. Cade oil is distilled from the young twigs and wood of more mature plants. The oil is resinous and has a strange, wary smell that is even caustic and tarlike (because cresol forms the main constituent of creosote). The principal constituents are phenols (cresol, guaiacol), sesquiterpenes (cadinene), and terpenes.	Pine tar consists primarily of aromatic hydrocarbons, tar acids, and tar bases. Components of tar vary according to the pyrolytic process (e.g., method, duration, and temperature) and origin of the wood (e.g., age of pine trees, type of soil, and moisture conditions during tree growth). It is a very viscous, blackish brown liquid that is noncrystalline and translucent in thin layers, becoming granular or crystalline (because of the separation of pyrocatechin) and opaque with age. It has a peculiar odor (empyreumatic and aromatic) and a pungent taste. The solution is a pale yellowish brown color and has an acid reaction. With a dilute solution of ferric chloride, it yields a reddish color, and with a stronger solution, an olive-green color, owing to the presence of pyrocatechin (distinguishing it from juniper tar). Its principal constituents include turpentine, resin, guaiacol, creosol, methylcreosol, phenol, phlorol, toluene, xylene, and other hydrocarbons.

(continued)

TABLE 28-4 Comparison of USP Tars *(Continued)*

Characteristic	Coal Tar	Juniper Tar	Pine Tar
Solubility	It is only slightly soluble in water, to which it imparts its characteristic odor and taste and a faintly alkaline reaction; partially soluble by alcohol, acetone, methanol, solvent hexane, carbon disulfide, chloroform, or ether; soluble to the extent of about 95% by benzene; and soluble entirely by nitrobenzene with the exception of a small amount of suspended matter.	It is sparingly soluble in solvent hexane and very slightly soluble in water. One volume dissolves in nine volumes of alcohol. It dissolves in three volumes of ether, leaving only a slight, flocculent residue. It is miscible with amyl alcohol, chloroform, and glacial acetic acid.	It is slightly soluble in water; soluble in alcohol, chloroform, ether, acetone, glacial acetic acid, fixed and volatile oils, and solutions of caustic alkalies.
Color	Dark brown to black mobile liquid	Dark brown, more or less viscid liquid	Blackish brown
Odor	Characteristic pitch/tar odor	Smoky and empyreumatic odor	Peculiar odor that is empyreumatic and aromatic
Specific gravity	0.83–0.85	0.950–1.055	0.99
Flammability	Yes	Yes	Yes
Stability	It is stable under normal conditions of use.	It is volatile and stable under normal conditions of use.	It is stable, but avoid contact with strong oxidizing agents.
Packaging	Store in tight containers.	Preserve in tight, light-resistant containers, and avoid exposure to excessive heat.	Store in original container, tightly closed, away from oxidizing agents and foodstuffs and out of reach of children and animals.
Miscellaneous	Residue on ignition is not more than 2.0% from 100 mg.	Refractive index is 1.510 to 1.530.	

Juniper tar is a dark brown, clear, thick liquid, having a tarry odor and a faintly aromatic, bitter taste. It is sparingly soluble in solvent hexane and very slightly soluble in water. One volume dissolves in 9 volumes of alcohol; 1 volume dissolves in 3 volumes of ether, leaving only a slight, flocculent residue; and it is miscible with amyl alcohol, chloroform, and glacial acetic acid.

Pine tar is no longer an official product. It is a sticky material produced by the high-temperature carbonization of pine wood in anoxic conditions (dry distillation or destructive distillation). The wood is rapidly decomposed by applying heat and pressure in a closed container; the primary resulting products are charcoal and pine tar. The product is obtained by the destructive distillation of the wood of *Pinus palustris* Miller or of other species of *Pinus* Linné (Fam. *Pinaceae*). It consists of a resinous substance, to which is added a small quantity of turpentine, acetic acid, methyl alcohol, and various volatile empyreumatic substances. On distillation, four distinct classes of products are obtained: (1) an aqueous distillate; (2) a light, oily distillate; (3) a heavy, oily distillate; and (4) a black resinous mass, or pitch, which has the odor of tar and has been official in some pharmacopeias under the name Pix nigra.

Uses

Coal tar predates steroids and has been used in the treatment of skin diseases for more than a century. It has thousands of compounds, and only a fraction of these are identified. It has been used to help ease the itch in inflammatory skin diseases. Coal tar preparations appear to exert their antipsoriasis benefits by interfering with DNA (deoxyribonucleic acid) and thus slowing down skin cell growth and turnover. The long-term result is thinning of the psoriatic plaques.

Coal tar is found in dozens of over-the-counter psoriasis and dandruff shampoos, as well as creams, gels, and bath additives. Compounding pharmacists can mix crude coal tar (a black, thick paste) or coal tar solution (a 20% alcohol-based liquid) with different vehicles or commercial products, including steroid creams and ointments. One effective remedy for hand and foot psoriasis is a compounded combination of a steroid with 5% coal tar solution and 2% salicylic acid.

Coal tar is often used in combination with phototherapy, because it sensitizes the skin to ultraviolet radiation. Care should be taken to avoid excess sun exposure when using coal tar shampoos and other preparations. Coal tar products and preparations have been used for their antieczematic, antipsoriatic, and antiseborrheic properties. It is used as a local irritant in the treatment of chronic skin diseases.

Juniper tar has therapeutic categories of use in antieczematic, antipsoriatic, and antiseborrheic treatments. For example, Juniper oil in yellow beeswax and soft paraffin has been used as an ointment in the treatment of psoriasis and eczema.

Pine tar has been used in antieczematic, antipsoriatic, and antimicrobial treatments.

Side Effects and Dangers

Occasionally, coal tar products may cause a rash, burning sensation, or other manifestations of excessive irritation or sensitization. Because photosensitization may occur, the treatment area should be protected from sunlight. Coal tar should be kept away from the eyes and from raw, weeping, or blistered surfaces. Temporary discoloration of the skin may occur.

A concentration of 5% or greater coal tar is classified as a carcinogen by the World Health Organization's International Agency for Research on Cancer. It is in the same category as methoxsalen (used in PUVA therapy, or photochemotherapy, for psoriasis) and solar radiation, two other forms of psoriasis treatment. Alcoholic beverages and tobacco are also included in this category. The U.S. Food and Drug Administration considers 0.5% to 5% over-the-counter coal tar preparations safe for psoriasis.

Compounding with Tars

A pharmacist should consider the following when compounding with tars:

- Coal tar should be weighed in disposable weigh boats or in the mixing vessel, as appropriate.
- Coal tar, a thick, sticky liquid, is more conveniently weighed if it is in a collapsible tube instead of a bottle.
- Coal tar may be incorporated readily into Hydrophilic Ointment USP, yielding an excellent product of uniform consistency.
- A 20% bentonite gel added to zinc oxide paste and coal tar produces a satisfactory ointment if the preparation is not allowed to dry in the container.
- Alcohol solutions of coal tar or prepared coal tar, prepared with the aid of polysorbate, have been referred to as Liquor Picis Carbonis and Liquor Carbonis Detergens.
- In the preparation of compound tar ointment, heat should be discontinued before the addition of the rectified tar oil to prevent its volatilization, because it is the volatile oil obtained from the pine tar. The ointment is used as an antiseptic and stimulant in various skin diseases.
- Pine tar ointment is prepared by incorporation. It is a firm ointment, containing a larger percentage of wax. It contains 50% pine tar and is frequently diluted before use. It is used in diseases of the skin, such as psoriasis and eczema.
- The color of the final preparation varies with order of mixing in the following formula.

Zinc oxide	4 g
Crude coal tar	4 g
Starch	4 g
Petrolatum	qs 30 g

(Note: There is a difference of opinion as to how this prescription should be prepared. One method for producing a black or very dark green ointment is obtained by mixing the crude coal tar with the zinc oxide and then adding the other ingredients. In some cases, requests are made that the coal tar–zinc oxide mixture be allowed to stand for 24 hours before completion of the preparation. If the coal tar is mixed with the starch or the petrolatum and later added to the zinc oxide, the resulting mixture varies from a gray to a light green color. Some pharmacists consider the latter method to be irritating and valueless, but others actually prefer it.)

- If the following formula is prepared as written, a solid lump of material may result. The intent here is to use coal tar solution to form a satisfactory lotion.

Pix liquid	12 parts
Camphor	4 parts
Phenol	4 parts
Glycerin	4 parts
Zinc oxide	20 parts
Liquor Calcis	240 parts
M lotion	qs

- All three tars are soluble in alcohol, which should be considered in all procedures.
- If a tar and an alcohol are to be compounded together, a mixing order that will maintain the alcohol concentration as high as reasonable during the procedures should be used to aid in keeping the tar in solution.
- Utensils should be rinsed with alcohol before washing with detergent and water.
- As appropriate, tar-containing substances or preparations should *not* be poured down the sink because the drain will tend to clog.

Sample Formulations

℞ Coal Tar Ointment (1000 g)

Coal Tar	10 g	Active
Polysorbate 80	5 g	Emulsifier
Zinc oxide paste	985 g	Vehicle

1. Calculate the quantity of each ingredient required for the prescription.
2. Accurately weigh or measure each ingredient.
3. Blend the coal tar with the polysorbate 80, and incorporate that mixture with the zinc oxide paste.
4. Package and label the product.

℞ Coal Tar 90% Ointment

Coal tar, crude	90 g	Active
Paraffin wax	10 g	Thickener

1. Calculate the quantity of each ingredient required for the prescription.
2. Accurately weigh or measure each ingredient.
3. Heat the paraffin wax and crude coal tar while stirring until completely melted, and mix well.
4. Remove the mixture from heat, and continue to stir and mix until cooled.
5. Package and label the product.

℞ Compound Ointment of Coal Tar

Coal tar	5 g	Active
Zinc oxide	5 g	Active/Adsorbent
Starch	45 g	Adsorbent
Petrolatum	qs 100 g	Vehicle

1. Calculate the quantity of each ingredient required for the prescription.
2. Accurately weigh or measure each ingredient.
3. Triturate the zinc oxide and starch together until a uniform powder results.
4. Incorporate the powders into a portion of the petrolatum.
5. Mix the coal tar with the remainder of the petrolatum, and combine the two mixtures until uniform.
6. Package and label the product.

℞ Coal Tar Cream

Coal tar solution	8 mL	Active
Stearic acid	15 g	Thickener
Alcohol	12 mL	Solvent
Potassium hydroxide	700 mg	Alkalizer
Glycerin	5 mL	Solvent/Humectant
Purified water	qs 100 g	Vehicle

1. Calculate the quantity of each ingredient required for the prescription.
2. Accurately weigh or measure each ingredient.
3. Mix the coal tar solution and alcohol.
4. Heat the stearic acid to 80°C with 30 mL of purified water, and add the potassium hydroxide previously dissolved in water.
5. Remove the mixture from the heat, and stir until the stearic acid is completely saponified.
6. Add the glycerin and the coal tar solution–alcohol mixture (step 3), shaking or stirring continuously.
7. Add sufficient purified water to final weight, and stir until a uniform cream results.
8. Package and label the product.

℞ Coal Tar Aqueous Gel

Coal tar, crude	25 g	Active
Polysorbate 80	25 g	Emulsifier
Carbopol 940	5 g	Thickener
Xanthan gum	2.5 g	Thickener
Ethyl alcohol 70%	285 mL	Vehicle
Urea	10 g	Active
Purified water	qs 500 g	Vehicle

1. Calculate the quantity of each ingredient required for the prescription.
2. Accurately weigh or measure each ingredient.
3. Triturate the crude coal tar, polysorbate 80, xanthan gum, and urea together.
4. In a separate container, disperse the Carbopol 940 in the alcohol stirring very rapidly.
5. Combine the powder mixture (step 3) and the Carbopol 940–alcohol mixture (step 4), and add 150 mL of purified water and mix well.
6. Allow the mixture to hydrate to form a gel.
7. Add additional purified water to final weight, and mix well.
8. Package and label the product.

℞ Coal Tar Alcoholic Gel

Coal Tar Topical Solution USP	1 mL	Active
Ethyl alcohol 70% or isopropyl alcohol 70%	97.5 mL	Vehicle
Carbopol 940	500 mg	Thickener
Trolamine	qs to pH 6.5 to 7	Alkalizer

1. Calculate the quantity of each ingredient required for the prescription.
2. Accurately weigh or measure each ingredient.
3. Disperse the Carbopol 940 into the alcohol using rapid stirring.
4. Add the trolamine dropwise until a pH of about 6.5 to 7 is achieved.
5. Add the Coal Tar Topical Solution USP, and blend until smooth.
6. Package and label the product.

℞ Coal Tar Emulsion

Coal tar solution	20 mL	Active
Purified water	80 mL	Vehicle

1. Calculate the quantity of each ingredient required for the prescription.
2. Accurately weigh or measure each ingredient.
3. Mix the coal tar solution and purified water thoroughly.
4. Package and label the product.

(Note: This emulsion is diluted with about 10 volumes of water before use.)

℞ Coal Tar, Juniper Tar, and Pine Tar Bath Oil, Self-Emulsifying

Coal tar, crude	7 g	Active
Juniper tar	8 g	Active
Pine tar	8 g	Active
Polysorbate 80	qs 100 mL	Emulsifier

1. Calculate the quantity of each ingredient required for the prescription.
2. Accurately weigh or measure each ingredient.
3. Mix the crude coal tar, juniper tar, and pine tar in a beaker.
4. Slowly add the polysorbate 80, and mix thoroughly.
5. Package and label the product.

℞ Coal Tar Bath Oil

Coal tar, crude	2.5 g	Active
Brij 93	25 g	Emulsifier
Brij 35	5 g	Emulsifier
Lanolin oil	5 mL	Active
Docusate sodium	5 g	Emulsifier
Fragrance	qs	Fragrance
Polysorbate 80	7 mL	Emulsifier
Mineral oil, light	qs 100 mL	Vehicle

1. Calculate the quantity of each ingredient required for the prescription.
2. Accurately weigh or measure each ingredient.
3. Melt the Brij 35 and docusate sodium in light mineral oil heated to 50°C–60°C while stirring.
4. When the ingredients are dissolved, add the lanolin oil and mix.
5. Allow the mixture to cool.
6. In a glass mortar, triturate the crude coal tar, Brij 93, and polysorbate 80 until homogenous.
7. Gradually add the lanolin oil mixture (step 4) until uniform.
8. Add the fragrance, and mix well.
9. Package and label the product.

℞ Salicylic Acid and Coal Tar Shampoo

Salicylic acid	2 g	Active
Coal tar solution	4.25 g	Active
Brij 35	7.5 g	Emulsifier
Brij 700	5 g	Emulsifier
Ethyl alcohol	12 mL	Solvent
Benzalkonium chloride 50% solution	1 mL	Preservative/Surfactant
Isopropyl alcohol	4 mL	Solvent
Purified water	qs 100 mL	Vehicle

1. Calculate the quantity of each ingredient required for the prescription.
2. Accurately weigh or measure each ingredient.
3. Dissolve the Brij 35 and Brij 700 in 60 mL purified water, and mix until completely dissolved.
4. Dissolve the salicylic acid and coal tar solution in the ethyl and isopropyl alcohols.
5. Mix the Brij mixture (step 3) and the alcohol mixture (step 4), and add the benzalkonium chloride 50% solution.
6. Add sufficient purified water to volume, and mix well.
7. Package and label the product.

℞ Coal Tar and Hydrocortisone Lotion

Coal tar solution	7.2 mL	Active
Hydrocortisone	1.2 g	Active
Cetyl alcohol	4.8 g	Emulsifier
Lanolin, anhydrous	2.4 g	Vehicle/Emulsifier
Mineral oil, light	29 mL	Vehicle
Polysorbate 80	7.2 g	Emulsifier
Propylene glycol	24 mL	Solvent/Humectant
Purified water	qs 240 mL	Vehicle

1. Calculate the quantity of each ingredient required for the prescription.
2. Accurately weigh or measure each ingredient.
3. Mix the coal tar solution and hydrocortisone, add the propylene glycol, and mix well.
4. In a separate container, melt the cetyl alcohol, anhydrous lanolin, and light mineral oil at 55°C, and then add the polysorbate 80 and mix well.
5. Heat 150 mL of purified water to 60°C, and add to the melted base with stirring.
6. Add the coal tar mixture (step 3), and stir until uniformly dispersed.
7. Add sufficient purified water to final volume, and mix well.
8. Package and label the product.

℞ Coal Tar Topical Applicator Stick

Coal Tar Topical Solution USP	5 mL	Active
Propylene glycol	13.5 g	Vehicle
Sodium stearate	1.5 g	Vehicle

1. Calculate the quantity of each ingredient required for the prescription.
2. Accurately weigh or measure each ingredient.
3. Mix the propylene glycol with sodium stearate, and heat until dissolved at about 80°C–85°C.
4. Allow the mixture to cool to 60°C, and add the Coal Tar Topical Solution USP.
5. Turn off heat, and continue stirring until the mixture begins to thicken.
6. Pour the mixture into plastic applicator tubes.
7. Package and label the product.

℞ Coal Tar 30% Emulsion

Coal tar, crude	30 g	Active
Polysorbate 80	40 g	Emulsifier
Polysorbate 20	20 g	Emulsifier
Polysorbate 60	10 g	Emulsifier

1. Calculate the quantity of each ingredient required for the prescription.
2. Accurately weigh or measure each ingredient.
3. Triturate the crude coal tar with the polysorbate 80 and polysorbate 20 in a mortar.
4. Add the polysorbate 60, and continue to triturate until homogenous.
5. Package and label the product.

℞ Crude Coal Tar 2% in Nivea Oil

Coal tar, crude	2 g	Active
Polysorbate 80	7 mL	Emulsifier
Benzyl alcohol	6 mL	Solvent
Alkyl benzoate	8 mL	Vehicle
Nivea oil	qs 100 mL	Vehicle

1. Calculate the quantity of each ingredient required for the prescription.
2. Accurately weigh or measure each ingredient.
3. Blend the crude coal tar with the polysorbate 80.
4. Add the alkyl benzoate and benzyl alcohol, and mix thoroughly.
5. Add the Nivea Oil in increments, and mix thoroughly with each addition to obtain a homogenous emulsion.
6. Package and label the product.

℞ Juniper Tar Ointment

Juniper tar	10 g	Active
Zinc oxide ointment	90 g	Vehicle

1. Calculate the quantity of each ingredient required for the prescription.
2. Accurately weigh or measure each ingredient.
3. Incorporate the juniper tar into the zinc oxide ointment until uniform.
4. Package and label the product.

℞ Compound Juniper Tar Lotion

Juniper tar	19.5 g	Active
Castor oil	15 g	Solvent/Compounding Aid
Salicylic acid	3.25 g	Active
Alcohol	qs 100 mL	Vehicle

1. Calculate the quantity of each ingredient required for the prescription.
2. Accurately weigh or measure each ingredient.
3. Dissolve the salicylic acid in 50 mL of the alcohol.
4. Add the castor oil and juniper tar, add sufficient alcohol to final volume, and mix well.
5. Package and label the product.

℞ Solution of Pine Tar

Pine tar	1 g	Active
Monohydrated sodium carbonate	1 g	Emulsifier
Purified water	qs 100 mL	Vehicle

1. Calculate the quantity of each ingredient required for the prescription.
2. Accurately weigh or measure each ingredient.
3. Dissolve the monohydrated sodium carbonate in 95 mL of purified water heated to about 50°C.
4. Add the pine tar, and shake vigorously until the mixture is homogenous.
5. Set aside the mixture for 12 hours, and then filter.
6. Add sufficient purified water through the filter to final volume.
7. Package and label the product.

℞ Pine Tar Shampoo

Pine Tar	0.3 mL	Active
Polysorbate 80	2 mL	Emulsifier
Triethanolamine lauryl sulfate	20 mL	Emulsifier
Cocamide diethanolamine	2 g	Emulsifier/Thickener
Imidazolidinyl urea	200 mg	Preservative
Purified water	qs 100 mL	Vehicle

1. Calculate the quantity of each ingredient required for the prescription.
2. Accurately weigh or measure each ingredient.
3. Blend the pine tar with the polysorbate 80.
4. Add the triethanolamine lauryl sulfate and 60 mL of purified water.
5. Add the cocamide diethanolamine, and stir until clear.
6. Add sufficient purified water to final volume, and add the imidazolidinyl urea.
7. Mix the solution until uniform.
8. Package and label the product.

℞ Sulfur and Pine Tar Ointment

Storax	13 g	Active
Sulfur ointment	26 g	Active
Pine tar ointment	13 g	Active
Medicinal soft soap	13 g	Vehicle
Petrolatum	35 g	Vehicle

1. Calculate the quantity of each ingredient required for the prescription.
2. Accurately weigh or measure each ingredient.
3. Warm the storax, and incorporate it with the petrolatum.
4. Add the sulfur ointment, pine tar ointment, and medicinal soft soap, and mix thoroughly.
5. Package and label the product.

References

1. United States Pharmacopeial Convention. Cyclomethicone NF. *United States Pharmacopeia/ National Formulary.* Rockville, MD: United States Pharmacopeial Convention; current edition.
2. Guest RT. Cyclomethicone. In: Rowe RC, Sheskey PJ, Cook WG, Fenton ME. *Handbook of Pharmaceutical Excipients,* 7th edition. London: Pharmaceutical Press; 2012:234–5.
3. United States Pharmacopeial Convention. Dimethicone NF. *United States Pharmacopeia/National Formulary.* Rockville, MD: United States Pharmacopeial Convention; current edition.
4. Guest RT. Dimethicone. In: Rowe RC, Sheskey PJ, Cook WG, Fenton ME. *Handbook of Pharmaceutical Excipients,* 7th edition. London: Pharmaceutical Press; 2012:262–4.
5. United States Pharmacopeial Convention. Simethicone USP. *United States Pharmacopeia/National Formulary.* Rockville, MD: United States Pharmacopeial Convention; current edition.
6. Guest RT. Simethicone. In: Rowe RC, Sheskey PJ, Cook WG, Fenton ME. *Handbook of Pharmaceutical Excipients,* 7th edition. London: Pharmaceutical Press; 2012:7088–9.

Chapter 29

Veterinary Pharmaceuticals

Historically, veterinarians dispensed most of the drugs they used in practice. In recent years, this tradition has changed, and pharmacists are developing working relationships with local veterinarians. Veterinary compounding, consistent with the U.S. Food and Drug Administration (FDA) regulations for extralabel use of drugs, is the customized manipulation of an approved drug(s) by a veterinarian, or by a pharmacist on the prescription of a veterinarian, to meet the needs of a particular veterinary patient. Pharmacists who become involved in veterinary compounding should develop a basic knowledge of veterinary pharmacology to be able to choose the appropriate vehicle, preservative, flavoring agents, and the like to meet the animals' needs. Veterinary compounding is necessary for the following reasons:

- Lack of appropriate dosage size for an approved form
- Lack of formulation for the desired route of
  administration
- Increased compliance of animal (palatability, etc.)
- Lack of availability (recalls or no approved drug)
- Need for multiple injections in the absence of a
  compounded product
- Rapid changes in management and disease problems in veterinary medicine
- Problems associated with the treatment of a large number of animals with several
  drugs in a short period of time
- Cost-prohibitive factors associated with the extremely large volume of some
  parenterals required for large animals
- Need for previously prepared antidotes for use in cases of animal poisoning
- Need to minimize suffering, harmful stress, and mortality in animals

Author's Note: At the time of this writing, many changes are occurring in the regulatory aspect of compounding for veterinary patients. This chapter is based on the currently available information; the reader should check for updates with the U.S. Food and Drug Administration, American Veterinary Medical Association, United States Pharmacopeial Convention, and other agencies and organizations.

- Need to combat multiple and concurrent disease processes
- Desire to achieve an additive therapeutic effect when simultaneously administering two or more products
- Encouragement of compliance by animal owners or their agents who are instructed to administer two or more products as part of a treatment regimen
- Need to achieve an appropriate treatment regimen for the species, age, or size of the animal patient

In addition, compounding a medication for animals may be inappropriate for reasons such as the following:

- Lack of a valid veterinary client–patient relationship
- Availability of an FDA-approved product
- Use in food animals (except for euthanasia, antidotes, and situations in which valid withdrawal times are available if the animals enter the human food chain)
- Mass manufacturing
- Compounding from bulk active pharmaceutical ingredients when approved products or alternatives exist
- Facilitation of decreased cost
- Compounding of copies of commercially available drugs

Relationship between Pharmacists and Veterinarians

Veterinary pharmaceutical compounding presents unusual challenges and rewards. A veterinarian and a compounding pharmacist must use professional judgment and work together in deciding to compound a medication for an animal. The reader is urged to become thoroughly familiar with veterinary laws and regulations before attempting to compound for milk- or food-producing animals, because some of the compounded medications can inadvertently find their way to the dining table. Done properly, veterinary compounding provides a service to the consumer and many opportunities for the professionals involved.

Some pharmacists have become heavily involved in working with veterinarians in the treatment of animals large and small, regular and exotic. Animals are usually categorized as companion pets (dogs, cats, parakeets, parrots, and the like); pocket pets; household, recreational, and work animals (horses, oxen); and food animals (cattle, hogs, poultry). Some veterinarians have the opportunity to work with animals as varied as mink, alligators, llamas, alpacas, vicuña, ostriches, elephants, gorillas, tigers, sharks, and poisonous snakes.

Marketing to veterinarians is generally quite easy: most do not realize the potential for working with a compounding pharmacist and need only some vision and assistance. Most veterinarians have a wish list of desired medications and dosage forms. A compounding pharmacist can adjust the concentration of drugs and offer various routes of administration; this flexibility is invaluable. Attending veterinary meetings is an excellent way to become acquainted with veterinarians in an area. Understanding that some animals have greater tendencies to develop certain disorders than others, including guinea pigs (vitamin C deficiencies), ferrets (cancer), reptiles (respiratory problems), and birds (respiratory problems), is helpful. An interesting opportunity for compounding pharmacists is working with zoos. In recent years, pharmacists have developed preparations such as raspberry jam–containing metronidazole (for a chimpanzee), a cored apple containing a paste of drug and ground apple, a raspberry-flavored Carbopol gel, a capsule or tablet placed inside the rectum of a live anesthetized mouse (for a boa constrictor), a peanut butter–flavored gel, the use of processed cheese spread to cover bitter or tart-tasting medications like methimazole (for cats), and the application of prednisone in a Pluronic lecithin organogel to the inner ear of a cat. Other preparations have been beef- and fish-flavored troches (a blank is given first, followed by a medicated troche), banana cream–flavored troches for ferrets, and a fish-flavored paste applied to a cat's paw (blending of tuna in oil or water and then incorporation of the drug).

Veterinary Compounding Guidelines

To ensure that compounded medications are safe and therapeutic for animals but do not inadvertently enter the food chain, compounding pharmacists need to be aware of guidelines under which veterinarians practice. The Drug Compounding Task Force of the American Veterinary Medical Association (AVMA) drafted guidelines for pharmaceutical compounding, which were approved by the AVMA House of Delegates in July 1991 and amended by the AVMA Executive Board in November 1991. The following information[1] is intended to acquaint pharmacists with the guidelines.

    I. The resulting medicament is a restricted product that
        A. Must be used only by or on the order of a licensed veterinarian;
        B. Must be used only within the confines of a valid veterinarian–client–patient relationship and must follow the AVMA Guidelines for Supervising Use and Distribution of Veterinary Prescription Drugs;[2]
        C. May be used or dispensed only for the treatment or prevention of disease or to improve the health or welfare of the animal(s); and
        D. May be used only when a need has been established and products approved by FDA are not available or clinically effective.
    II. The veterinarian must use professional judgment consistent with currently acceptable veterinary medical practice to ensure the safety and efficacy of the medicament, including
        A. The safety for the target animal; and
        B. The avoidance of violative residues in meat, milk, or eggs when administered to a food-producing animal.
    III. The veterinarian must use professional judgment consistent with proper pharmaceutical and pharmacologic principles when compounding medicaments. The following points should be considered:
        A. The stability of the active ingredients;
        B. The physical and chemical compatibility of the ingredients;
        C. The pharmacodynamic compatibility of the active ingredients; and
        D. The composition of the active ingredients and diluents, to ensure that they are not contaminated with harmful substances or agents.
    IV. The prepared medicament must be properly labeled before being dispensed. Labeling practices include the following:
        A. When the medicament is administered by the veterinarian or is administered under his or her direct supervision, no label is required.
        B. When the medicament is dispensed according to the veterinarian's order, the product must have a complete, indelible, legible label attached. A complete label requires the following items:
            (1) Name and address of the attending veterinarian,
            (2) Date dispensed,
            (3) Medically active ingredients,

(4) Identity of animal(s) to be treated (i.e., species, class, group, or individual animal[s]),

(5) Directions for use,

(6) Cautionary statements, if needed, and

(7) Slaughter withdrawal times or milk-withholding times, if needed.

All of the preceding requirements are consistent with the AVMA Guidelines for Veterinary Prescription Drugs–Key Points,[2] the 2011 Revision of the Grade "A" Pasteurized Milk Ordinance,[3] and the document Extra-label Drug Use in Veterinary Medicine.[4] The following additional information can be included on a label:

(8) Disease conditions to be treated, and

(9) Expiration date.

V. Compounded medicaments must not be advertised or displayed to the public.

VI. When compounded medicaments are used, appropriate patient records must be maintained.

VII. When compounded medicaments are used in food-producing animals, appropriate drug residue tests, when available and practical, and other procedures for ensuring violative residue avoidance should be instituted. Extralabel (not in accordance with labeling) use of the following drugs and drug classes, whether compounded or commercial, in food-producing animals is prohibited:[1] chloramphenicol, clenbuterol, diethylstilbestrol, dimetridazole, dipyrone, fluoroquinolones (enrofloxacin, ciprofloxacin, sarafloxacin), furazolidone (except for approved topical use), glycopeptides (vancomycin), ipronidazole, metronidazole, nitrofurazone (except for approved topical use), nitroimidazoles (other), and sulfonamide drugs in lactating dairy cattle (except approved use of sulfadimethoxine).

In addition to these guidelines, AVMA states that the use of compounded drugs should be limited to (1) drugs for which both safety and efficacy of the compounded form have been demonstrated in the target species, (2) disease conditions for which response to therapy or drug concentration can be monitored, or (3) individual animals for which no other method or route of drug delivery is practical.

There are not enough FDA-approved drugs to treat the numerous species under the veterinary profession's care. The lack of an available drug for veterinary use might be due to a temporary interruption in the drug supply chain. Other reasons might be that no drug was ever approved (e.g., potassium bromide for the control of seizures) and that a human drug with beneficial use in animals has been withdrawn from the market (e.g., cisapride for treatment of feline megacolon).

A commercially available drug may be inadequate for use in compounding veterinary preparations because the concentration of active ingredients is inappropriate, resulting in an unacceptable dosage size, or because the commercial drug has excipients that are unsuitable. In addition, using a commercial drug product in compounding may have negative effects on the quality of the preparation (gels, creams, or syrups may be gritty and active ingredients may be unevenly dispersed). The approved drug may contain an ingredient that the animal cannot tolerate. Flavoring may not be able to mask the objectionable taste of an approved drug.

Regulatory Framework

From a regulatory standpoint, there are two types of veterinary compounding. The first type, compounding from FDA-approved veterinary and human drugs, is covered under the Animal Medicinal Drug Use Clarification Act of 1994 (AMDUCA). This act legalized extralabel use of drugs in animals under certain circumstances and likewise legalized this form of compounding. The second type, compounding from bulk drugs, is not covered under AMDUCA.

A *bulk drug* is an active ingredient (in unfinished form) intended for manufacture into finished dosage form drug products. FDA considers the use of bulk drugs illegal but exercises discretion if the provisions of its Compliance Policy Guide (CPG) for the Compounding of Drugs for Use in Animals are followed. The CPG states that veterinary compounding from raw chemicals must meet the following conditions, and a veterinarian is responsible for ensuring that these conditions exist:

1. A legitimate medical need is identified.
2. A need exists for an appropriate dosage regimen for the species, age, size, or medical condition of the animal.
3. No marketed, approved animal or human drug can be used as labeled or in an extralabel manner, or some other rare extenuating circumstance is present (e.g., the approved drug cannot be obtained in time to treat the animal[s] in a timely manner, or there is a medical need for different excipients).

Once those three determinations are made, compounding from bulk drugs should meet the following criteria:

1. A compounded product can be dispensed by a veterinarian in the course of his or her practice or by a pharmacist, who must have a prescription from the veterinarian.
2. A veterinarian should take measures to ensure that no illegal residues occur when a compounded product is used in food animals, an extended time period is assigned for withdrawal, and steps are taken to ensure assigned time frames are observed.
3. A pharmacist compounding for a veterinary patient must adhere to the National Association of Boards of Pharmacy Good Compounding Practices or to equivalent state regulation, except where provisions conflict with the CPG.
4. The label of a compounded veterinary prescription filled by a pharmacist should contain the following information:
   - Name and address of the veterinary practitioner
   - Active ingredient(s)
   - Date dispensed and expiration date (not to exceed length of prescribed treatment unless the veterinarian can establish the rationale for a later expiration date)
   - Directions for use, including the class and species to identify the animal(s), and the dose, frequency, route of administration, and duration of therapy
   - Cautionary statements specified by the veterinarian or the pharmacist, including all appropriate warnings to ensure safety of humans handling the drugs
   - The veterinarian's specified withdrawal and discard time(s) for meat, milk, eggs, or any food that might be derived from the treated animal(s) (Although the veterinarian is responsible for setting the withdrawal time, he or she can use relevant information provided by a pharmacist in setting the time.)
   - Name and address of the dispenser, serial number, and date of order or its filling
   - Any other applicable requirements of state or federal law

Veterinary prescription drugs are drugs restricted by federal law to use by or on the order of a licensed veterinarian. Any other drugs used in animals in a manner not in accordance with their labeling should be subjected to the same supervisory precautions that apply to veterinary prescription drugs. Veterinary prescription drugs can be prescribed only within the context of a valid veterinarian–client–patient relationship.

Any veterinary prescription filled by a pharmacist requires a prescription from a veterinarian. Veterinary prescription medication labels read, "Caution: Federal law restricts this drug to use by or on the order of a licensed veterinarian." This statement is the veterinary counterpart of the human legend and must appear on the label of all manufactured veterinary prescription products. Phrases such as "For veterinary use only" and "Sold to veterinarians only" do not refer to the drug's prescription status but rather to sales policies of companies.

Compounding Considerations

Compounding can be considered when no effective FDA-approved products exist for treatment of the disease or condition diagnosed by a veterinarian and when the failure to treat would result in a veterinary patient's suffering or death. Even if dosage forms are available, they can be inappropriate for one or more of the following reasons:

- Patient size
- Patient anatomy
- Patient physiology
- Patient safety
- Individual patient sensitivity or idiosyncrasy
- Patient stress or suffering from formulations that require multiple injections or administration of large volumes
- Danger to personnel who must deal with patients difficult to restrain

Veterinarians also may consider compounding to minimize adverse effects or to increase the effectiveness of therapy. For example, combining specific anesthetic agents increases the analgesic and muscle relaxant effects while reducing the total dose of anesthetics used; this practice lessens the adverse cardiac and respiratory effects. Combining intra-articular medications for single injection minimizes both the discomfort to the animal and the probability of introducing pathogenic microorganisms into the animal.

Finally, compounding can be considered in extreme situations wherein economic realities would preclude treatment with the approved product. In such situations, pain, suffering, or even death would result from failure to treat.

The future existence of FDA-approved veterinary drugs labeled for every therapeutic need is inconceivable. However, compounding for veterinary medicine will likely become more prevalent, as it has in human medicine, especially with the future introduction of biotechnologically derived products with limited stability.

Decision to Compound

A veterinary compounding pharmacist must ask the following questions when considering whether to compound a prescription for an animal:

- What is known about the physical and chemical compatibility of the drugs?
- What is known about the stability of these drugs—before, during, and after the compounding process?

- What is known about the pharmacodynamic compatibility of the active ingredients?
- What is the overall goal of the treatment of this animal?
- Are any similar products available commercially to treat the animal?
- What regulatory concerns may be involved?
- Is this animal a food animal?
- Will the drug treatment cause a residue problem?
- Is there any risk to personnel who handle the drug during compounding or during administration of the compounded form?

In making the decision to compound, a veterinary compounding pharmacist must be aware that in some cases, there are official formulas in the *United States Pharmacopeia (USP)* for veterinary patients. Table 29-1 contains a list of the official, tested formulas and the current *USP* should be checked for any changes and additions.

TABLE 29-1 Official Veterinary Formulas in the *USP*

Atenolol Compounded Oral Suspension, Veterinary
Benazepril Hydrochloride Compounded Oral Suspension, Veterinary
Buprenorphine Compounded Buccal Solution, Veterinary
Cisapride Compounded Injection, Veterinary
Cisapride Compounded Oral Suspension, Veterinary
Clopidogrel Compounded Oral Suspension
Cyclosporine Compounded Ophthalmic Solution, Veterinary
Doxycycline Compounded Oral Suspension, Veterinary
Enalapril Maleate Compounded Oral Suspension, Veterinary
Enrofloxacin Compounded Oral Suspension, Veterinary
Famciclovir Compounded Oral Suspension
Lansoprazole Compounded Oral Suspension
Marbofloxacin Compounded Oral Suspension, Veterinary
Methylene Blue Injection, Veterinary
Metronidazole Benzoate Compounded Oral Suspension
Pergolide Oral Suspension, Veterinary
Phenoxybenzamine Hydrochloride Compounded Oral Suspension
Piroxicam Compounded Oral Suspension
Potassium Bromide Oral Solution, Veterinary
Prednisolone Compounded Oral Suspension, Veterinary
Sodium Bromide Injection, Veterinary
Sodium Bromide Oral Solution, Veterinary
Spironolactone Compounded Oral Suspension, Veterinary
Tadalafil Compounded Oral Suspension
Tramadol Hydrochloride Compounded Oral Suspension, Veterinary
Voriconazole Compounded Ophthalmic Solution, Veterinary
Zonisamide Compounded Oral Suspension

Devices for Administering Medications

As with humans, a variety of dosage forms can be prepared for animals, using several different routes of administration. Except for the intramammary route of administration, the administration routes used in animals are the same as those for humans. A multitude of devices are available for delivering a specified dose of a medication or for administering the medication by one of the routes used most frequently in veterinary medicine: oral, topical, transdermal, parenteral, and nasal.

Oral Administration

Oral dosage forms present the greatest challenge in administering medications to animals. Some ingenious devices have been developed to meet this challenge. A brief description of the most commonly used devices is presented here.[5] For more detailed information, the reader is referred to Blodinger's *Formulation of Veterinary Dosage Forms* and other sources listed at the end of this chapter.

Balling guns are relatively simple devices that have a barrel through which passes a plunger capable of dislodging a bolus into the gullet of the animal.

Buoyant devices, which resemble large, floating tablets, allow the dosage form to float in the intestine and release the medication over an extended period of time. To allow it to float, the dosage form must have a specific gravity somewhat less than that of the animal's intestinal contents. Some of these devices also release carbon dioxide, which aids in keeping the dosage form afloat.

Drench syringes are either single- or multiple-dose devices that are capable of delivering preset volumes of liquid into the gullet.

Esophageal delivery devices are syringes and tubes that are usually designed to deliver the medication directly into the stomach.

Hollow bits have a hollowed-out area in which medications that have a heat-sensitive release matrix are placed. Saliva causes the medication to be released slowly through perforations in the surface of the bit. A confection is often included in the matrix. Hollow bits are used to administer medications to horses.

Liquid drench guns are either single- or multiple-dose devices that are capable of delivering oral solutions or suspensions of an aqueous or oily nature relatively quickly.

Paste dispensers include devices such as paste guns, paste syringes, squeeze bottles, and squeeze tubes that are capable of delivering a specified dose to an animal.

Powder drench guns are devices, usually spring loaded, that are capable of delivering the required amount of powder into the back portion of the mouth, where it usually adheres and is subsequently swallowed.

Rumen-lodging devices are incorporated into medications that have a controlled-release delivery system. These devices aid the product in sticking to the mucosal surface and allowing the medication to be released at the desired rate.

Water medication-metering devices provide a method of adding a medication to the water supply of numerous animals. The amount of medication released in the water depends on the average daily water intake of the animals. These devices are often used to administer antibloating surfactants, disinfectants, electrolytes, medications, vaccines, and wormers.

Miscellaneous oral dose dispensers include droppers, mineral dispensers, mouthpieces, nursers, and pump-type dispensers.

Topical Administration

Several devices have been developed to aid in ridding animals of parasites such as lice and fleas, protecting the animals from biting or stinging insects, and treating skin conditions caused by these organisms or other environmental factors. The following descriptions of topical administration devices were adapted from Blodinger.[5]

Aerosol dispensers are a convenient and effective means of applying medications.

Dust bags are used to apply powders to cattle as they brush up against or walk underneath the bags. These devices are especially useful for the topical application of insecticide powders to control flies and lice. The pore size of the bag allows for ease of application of the product.

Flea and tick collars generally use slow-release generators containing medications that either have a high vapor pressure or are designed as a solid solution so that the product will migrate from the collar over the body.

Percutaneous absorption drug-reservoir devices are drug-containing matrices that allow the drug to diffuse from the device into the animal's skin or onto the skin surface. These devices can be attached to the skin by an adhesive, clips, pins, or staples. Drug-impregnated bandages, films, and ear tampons have also been used.

Pour-on, spot-on applicators are ordinarily used to treat skin conditions or surface (hooves, horns) conditions of animals.

Spray race and dip applicators are long troughs with deep sides that are commonly used for dipping treatments. For safety and effectiveness, the length, width, and depth of the dipping bath must be adequate to immerse the animal completely without injuring it.

Teat dip applicators are cups in which medication is added to a depth sufficient to immerse the lower extremity of the teat. The cups are filled with medication and then lifted to the teat.

Transdermal Administration

The use of compounded transdermal medications is a milestone in veterinary drug therapy. Scientific evidence is lacking on the effectiveness of some of these dosage forms, but there is extensive clinical evidence of their safety and effectiveness. Table 29-2 provides information on veterinary drugs that have been administered transdermally.[6]

Parenteral Administration

Because injections can often be administered quickly from a safe distance, they are sometimes the easiest method of administering medications to animals. Several devices are available that allow administration of therapeutic agents from a safe distance. Further, using a syringe to administer a medication through an orifice or to place a sustained-release medication in a body cavity may be the only viable option for long-term treatment of some conditions. Several devices have been developed for administering these types of injections. The following descriptions of these and other parenteral administration devices are adapted from Blodinger.[5]

Single-dose syringes are often used when treating only one animal at a time. Disposable syringes as well as resterilizable syringes made of glass, nylon, or polypropylene are available. Both types of syringes are available in numerous sizes. Prefilled syringes in sterilized packs are also available.

Multiple-dose syringes are generally used to treat small herds when an automatic syringe is not required. As the name implies, the syringe barrel, which has a stepping plunger, can contain several doses, allowing a veterinarian to treat several animals without stopping to reload the syringe.

Automatic syringes, which are used to treat large herds, include the adaptable, chamber-fill, handle-fill, and specialized varieties.

Multicompartment syringes are used for unstable drug products that require the diluent to be added to the dry powder just before injection.

Pole-mounted syringes allow injectable formulations to be administered from a safe distance.

TABLE 29-2 Veterinary Drugs Considered for Transdermal Therapy

| Drug and Pharmacokinetics | Dose in Cats[a] | | | Target for Efficacy | Symptoms of Toxicity |
	Oral	Injectable	Maximum Starting TD Dose[b]		
Aminophylline 100% bioavailability for non-SR orals; injectable doses equal to oral doses; TD forms used successfully in human neonates	4 mg/kg q 8 to 12 hr	4 mg/kg q 8 to 12 hr	4 mg/kg q 8 to 12 hr	Serum theophylline level in therapeutic range (those values are not firmly established for veterinary patients, but the human range is 10 to 20 µg/mL); evidence of controlled asthma	Tachycardia, arrhythmia, seizure, hyperthermia
Amitriptyline 48% oral bioavailability (humans); extensive first-pass hepatic extraction; accumulation after multiple doses; active metabolites must be conjugated with glucuronic acid to inactive (cats cannot do that)	5 to 10 mg/cat q 24 hr	NP	1.25 mg/cat q 24 hr; behaviorists who have used TD amitriptyline in cats advise careful monitoring to avoid accumulation	Cessation of undesirable behavior; cessation of cystitis; onset of action as early as 3 to 5 days after initiation of therapy	Dry mouth, gastric distress, constipation, ataxia, tachycardia, weakness, sedation, urinary retention
Amlodipine Oral bioavailability 75% in humans; undetermined in cats; slowly but extensively metabolized to inactive compounds in the liver	0.625 mg/cat q 24 hr	NP	0.625 mg/cat q 24 hr	Reduction in blood pressure	Headache is reported most commonly in humans, although it may be difficult to recognize in veterinary patients; hypotension
Amoxicillin clavulanate NR because doses > 50 mg are required and possibility of induction of bacterial resistance	0.625 mg/cat q 24 hr	NP	NR	NR	NR

Drug / Comments					
Atenolol 50% oral bioavailability; minimal (<50%) metabolism	0.625 mg/cat	NP	3.25 mg/cat q 24 hr	Reduction in pulse to 140 to 200 bpm	Hypotension, bradycardia, bronchospasm, cardiac failure, hypoglycemia
Azithromycin NR because doses > 50 mg are required and possibility of induction of bacterial resistance	7 to 15 mg/kg q 12 hr for 5 to 7 days, then every 5 days	NP	NR	Eradication of bacterial infection	Head tilt (otic toxicity), elevated hepatic enzymes
Buprenorphine Injectable form available; high degree of first-pass extraction with gut wall and liver metabolism, conjugation with glucuronide	0.01 to 0.03 mg/kg up to q 8 hr	0.005 to 0.015 mg/kg IM, IV	0.01 mg/kg q 8 hr	Apparent analgesia, animal benefiting from pain management	Respiratory depression
Buspirone NR until further studies available; extensive first-pass extraction (95% of oral dose removed by hepatic extraction)	2.5 mg/cat q 12 hr	NP	NR	Cessation of undesirable behavior or phobia	Sedation, anorexia, nausea, tachycardia
Butorphanol Extensive first-pass extraction (84% of oral dose removed by hepatic extraction)	1 mg/cat PO q 12 hr	0.4 mg/kg SQ q 6 hr	0.4 mg/kg q 6 hr	Apparent analgesia, animal benefiting from pain management	Oversedation, respiratory depression
Carboplatin NR. Cytotoxic agent; tissue necrosis occurs at concentrations > 0.5 mg/mL	NR	NR	NR	NR	NR
Chloramphenicol NR. Highly toxic to humans, bacterial resistance; large doses preclude TD dosing	NR	NR	NR	NR	NR

(continued)

TABLE 29-2 Veterinary Drugs Considered for Transdermal Therapy (Continued)

Drug and Pharmacokinetics	Dose in Cats[a]		Maximum Starting TD Dose[b]	Target for Efficacy	Symptoms of Toxicity
	Oral	Injectable			
Cisapride Oral bioavailability 35% to 40%; can be problematic to caregiver who may be taking drugs such as antihistamines and benzimidazole antibiotics, which may interact with cisapride	5 mg/cat q 8 to 12 hr	NP	2.5 mg/cat q 12 hr	Resolution of ileus, evidence of colonic motility with no constipation or obstruction	Diarrhea, abdominal pain and cramping, arrhythmia from drug interactions
Clomipramine Substantial first-pass hepatic extraction; oral bioavailability 50%; may accumulate in cats, which are very sensitive to TCADs	2.5 mg/cat q 24 hr	NP	1.25 mg/cat q 24 hr	Cessation of undesirable behavior	Excessive sedation, dry mouth, urinary retention
Cyclophosphamide NR. Cytotoxic agent	NR	NR	NR	NR	NR
Cyproheptadine Good oral bioavailability; extensive hepatic metabolism and conjugation with glucuronide; metabolites excreted in urine; accumulates in renal failure	2 mg/cat q 12 hr	NP	2 mg/cat q 12 hr; monitor for accumulation	Stimulation of appetite, relief of pruritus, cessation of undesirable behavior	Excessive sedation, dry mouth, urinary retention
Digoxin NR. Narrow therapeutic index; cats are very sensitive to digoxin; potential exposure by caregiver	0.007 to 0.015 mg/kg q 24 to 48 hr. Do not use in HCM in cats	NP	NR	Achievement of therapeutic serum levels: serum 0.9 to 2.0 ng/mL for cats	Cats very sensitive. Bradycardia, worsening of arrhythmia, serum levels > 2.0 ng/mL

Drug					
Diltiazem 10% TD bioavailability in cats (compared with IV administration); extensive first-pass hepatic extraction (50% to 80% oral bioavailability in cats)	7.5 mg/cat (non-SR) q 8 hr	0.25 mg/kg IV bolus up to 0.75 mg/kg	7.5 mg/cat q 12 hr to q 24 hr	Reduction in pulse rate to 140 to 200 bpm	Bradycardia, vomiting, heart block
Doxycycline Irritating to gastric and esophageal mucosa of cats; rubbing this chemical into ears is NR; also a potent photosensitizer; application to ears that might be exposed to sunlight is NR; bacterial or rickettsial resistance to this drug from subtherapeutic concentrations leaves few alternatives for treating tick-borne disease	5 mg/kg q 12 hr	5 mg/kg q 24 hr	NR	NR	NR
Enalapril Hepatically metabolized to active drug enalaprilat; 60% oral bioavailability	0.25 to 0.5 mg/kg q 24 hr	NP	0.25 mg/kg q 24 hr	Improvement of clinical signs of heart failure	GI distress, hypotension
Enrofloxacin NR. Risk of retinal toxicity in cats, risk of inducing bacterial resistance, risk of causing hallucinations in caregiver; raw chemical is FDA-targeted high-priority drug for regulatory action	2.5 mg/kg q 12 hr DO NOT EXCEED 5 mg/kg/day	2.5 mg/kg q 12 hr DO NOT EXCEED 5 mg/kg/day	NR	Eradication of bacterial infection	Pupillary dilation (early indicator of retinal toxicity), lameness (indicator of joint erosion in immature animals), seizure, behavior change (auditory and visual hallucinations commonly reported in human patients)

(continued)

TABLE 29-2 Veterinary Drugs Considered for Transdermal Therapy (Continued)

| Drug and Pharmacokinetics | Dose in Cats[a] | | | Target for Efficacy | Symptoms of Toxicity |
	Oral	Injectable	Maximum Starting TD Dose[b]		
Fluoxetine NR. Extremely long terminal half-life in cats (60+ hr), likely to accumulate	1 to 5 mg/cat q 24 hr, obtain baseline lab work, assess after 1 to 4 weeks of therapy	NP	NR	Cessation of undesirable behavior	Anxiety, irritability, sleep disturbance, anorexia, hepatotoxicity
Furosemide NR. Very unstable at acid pH	0.5 to 2.0 mg/ kg/day	Up to 4.4 mg/kg IV or IM to desired effect	NR	Improvement in respiratory rate and/or character; resolution of effusion or edema	Head tilt (ototoxicity), electrolyte imbalances, weakness, lethargy
Glipizide 100% oral bioavailability in humans	2.5 mg/cat q 12 hr	NP	2.5 mg/cat q 12 hr	Reduction in blood glucose < 200	GI distress, hypoglycemia, icterus, increased ALT, hyperglycemia from therapeutic failure
Insulin NR. Anecdotal reports of efficacy, but no sustained effect or documented blood glucose levels during treatment; possible increase in risk of lipodystrophy because of larger surface area exposed to insulin	NA	Variable	NR	Achievement of blood glucose value	Hypoglycemia (too much insulin delivered), hyperglycemia (therapeutic failure)
Methimazole Oral bioavailability 45% to 98% (hepatic metabolism); large interpatient variation in response; allow 1 to 3 weeks of therapy before assessment	5 mg/cat q 8 to 12 hr	NP	2.5 mg/cat q 12 hr	Reduction in serum T4 level, improvement in clinical symptoms	Worsening of vomiting, dermal excoriations, leukopenias, hepatopathies, thrombocytopenia

Drug					
Metoclopramide Large interpatient variability in oral bioavailability may be as low as 30% in some patients; not effective for centrally mediated vomiting in cats, as they lack dopamine-mediated vomiting receptors	0.2 to 0.4 mg/kg q 6 to 8 hr	0.2 to 0.4 mg/kg SQ q 6 to 8 hr	0.2 to 0.4 mg/kg q 8 hr	Cessation of vomiting, resolution of gastric stasis	Frenzied behavior, disorientation, constipation
Phenobarbital Oral bioavailability 90%; conjugation with glucuronide; very polar, very low lipid solubility, $t_{1/2}$ 34 to 43 hr in cats—drug may accumulate	2 mg/kg q 12 hr	2 to 5 mg/kg IV bolus for status epilepticus persisting after diazepam use	2 mg/kg q 12 hr	Seizure free, serum/plasma concentration of 10 to 30 µg/mL	Ataxia, oversedation, lethargy, bone marrow suppression, immune-mediated reactions, hepatotoxicity in dogs (cats are not as likely to experience hepatotoxicity)
Prednisolone NR. Great risk of epidermal atrophy	1 to 2 mg/kg q 12 to 24 hr	1 to 3 mg/kg IV or IM (prednisolone sodium succinate)	NR	Cessation of inflammatory signs	Atrophy of epidermis and/or cartilage, signs of hyperadrenocorticism from chronic use, signs of diabetes mellitus

SR = sustained release, TD = transdermal, NP = none published, NR = not recommended, bpm = beats per minute, IM = intramuscular, IV = intravenous, PO = by mouth, SQ = subcutaneous, TCADs = tricyclic antidepressants, HCM = hypertrophic cardiomyopathy, GI = gastrointestinal, FDA = U.S. Food and Drug Administration, ALT = alanine transaminase, NA = not available, $t_{1/2}$ = half-life.

[a]Oral and injectable doses are given for reference.

[b]Until scientific studies or clinical experience indicate otherwise, the dosages in this table are suggested as the maximum starting dosage for the drugs listed. These suggested dosages do not guarantee the safety or efficacy of the medication in any patient. Future scientific studies may completely invalidate these recommendations, which are meant only as guidelines for the prevention of possible toxicity.

Source: Reprinted with permission from reference 6.

Mastitis syringes are used to insert a drug formulation directly into the mammary gland through the teat canal.

Jet injectors contain orifices through which a liquid can be administered under extremely high pressure onto or near the skin of the animal.

Projectile delivery systems include arrows and darts that can be propelled by bows or blowguns. The drug can be placed on the tip of the arrow or dart or in a special syringe that will expel the contents on contact with the animal.

Implants are sterile dosage forms designed so that a depot of drug can be placed at a site in the body for prolonged release of the drug.

Implanting devices are used to insert pellets, balls, and molten and ballistic types of implants at the chosen site in the body.

Intrauterine drug dispensers are designed to stay in the uterine cavity for a period of days, weeks, or months to deliver a sustained-release drug. Some of these devices will even self-destruct at the end of the drug delivery period.

Vaginal drug dispensers are used to deliver drug-containing sponges and suppositories.

The BioBullet represents a new technology developed by veterinarians and pharmacists. The BioBullet is fired from a special rifle using compressed air. It consists of a measured amount of a drug contained within a 5/8-inch long, 1/4-inch diameter biodegradable bullet that travels at a speed of 900 feet per second. It pierces the animal's skin and lodges 1 to 3 cm into the animal's muscle. The medication is released as the casing, composed of hydroxypropyl cellulose, dissolves within 12 to 24 hours.

Nasal Administration

Nasal administration of drugs results in an onset of action almost as fast as the onset after intravenous injection. Nasal administration does not involve piercing and avoids some of the problems associated with parenteral administration. Vaccines for a number of diseases, including Newcastle disease and infectious bronchitis, and antibiotics are often administered through the nasal passageways. The following types of dispensers are used most often to administer these agents to animals.

Dropper dispensers are generally used to deliver a single dose of a medication. This type of dispenser can be as simple as a plastic dropper attached to a rubber bulb; the dropper must be properly calibrated to deliver the required dose. A syringe without a needle or a syringe with a plastic tip can also be used. These types of syringes will not cause injury to mucosal membranes.

Spray dispensers are used to immunize small chicks against a number of poultry viral pathogens. The chicks pass through a closed chamber and inhale vaccine solutions that are dispensed as an aerosol spray. These devices can also dispense a vaccine as a powder mist. Metered-spray dispensers are also available.

Pharmacological Considerations

Variations among animal species cause differences in systemic availability of drugs, accessibility to the site of action, and the rate of elimination.

Pharmacokinetics

As in humans, the effect of a drug on an animal depends on the drug's movement throughout the body and the concentration that builds up at the specific site of action. The extent of response of the individual animal's receptors is important. Factors that influence the concentration of a drug in the plasma include the size of the dose, formulation of the drug, route of administration, extent of distribution and plasma protein binding, and rate of

TABLE 29-3 Pharmacokinetic Parameters of Diazepam in the Human, Dog, and Rat

Pharmacokinetic Variable	Human	Dog	Rat
Half-life (hours)	32.9	7.6	1.1
Body clearance (mL/kg/minute)	0.35	18.9	81.6
Plasma protein binding (%)	96.81	6.0	86.3
Blood clearance (mL/kg/minute)	0.64	35.0	214.7
Hepatic extraction ratio	0.029	0.81	6.31
Fraction of free drug	0.032	0.04	0.14

Source: Adapted from reference 5.

elimination. The pharmacokinetics of a drug vary among animals; for example, the differing pharmacokinetics of diazepam in humans, dogs, and rats are illustrated in Table 29-3. In all animals, however, pharmacokinetics involves the same four basic processes—absorption, distribution, metabolism, and excretion.

Absorption

Gastric emptying is an important physiologic factor controlling the rate of drug absorption. Some animals, such as the horse, are continuous feeders, and their stomachs are seldom empty. The emptying rate of multistomach animals can vary as greatly as the consistency of the material in each of the stomachs.

Distribution

Distribution of drugs to the various tissues and organs will differ among animals because they have different body compositions. Table 29-4 provides a comparison of the body composition of humans and several animals.

TABLE 29-4 Variations in Body Composition among Animals

| Anatomical Component | % of Live Weight | | | |
	Horse	Dog	Goat	Human
Blood	8.6	—	—	7.8
Brain	0.2	0.5	0.3	2.0
Heart	0.7	0.8	0.5	0.5
Lung	0.9	0.9	0.9	1.4
Liver	1.3	2.3	2.0	2.6
Kidney	0.4	0.6	0.4	0.4
Gastrointestinal tract	12.7	0.7	13.9	1.4
Skin	7.4	9.3	9.2	3.7
Muscle	40.1	54.5	45.5	40.0
Bone	14.6	8.7	6.3	14.0
Adipose tissue	5.1	—	—	18.1
Total weight (kg)	308	16	39	70

— = Not available.
Source: Adapted from reference 5.

TABLE 29-5 Half-Lives of Selected Drugs in Various Animals

Drug	Half-life (hours)				
	Horse	Dog	Cat	Pig	Ruminant
Amphetamine	1.4	4.5	6.5	1.1	0.6
Ampicillin	1.6	0.8	—	—	1.2
Chloramphenicol	0.9	4.2	5.1	1.3	2.0
Kanamycin	1.5	1.0	—	—	1.9
Oxytetracycline	10.5	6.0	—	—	9.1
Penicillin G	0.9	0.5	—	—	0.7
Pentobarbital	1.5	4.5	4.9	—	0.8
Salicylate	1.0	8.6	37.6	5.9	0.8
Sulfadimethoxine	11.3	13.2	10.2	15.5	12.5
Sulfadoxine	14.0	—	—	8.2	11.7
Trimethoprim	3.2	3.0	—	2.3	0.8

— = Not available.
Source: Adapted from reference 5.

Metabolism

The rate at which drugs are metabolized differs from animal to animal. For example, cats have a slow rate of glucuronide synthesis, acetylation is absent in the dog, and sulfate conjugation is present in the pig only to a limited extent. The slow rate of glucuronide conjugation in cats means that compounds such as aspirin and phenols, which undergo glucuronide formation, appear to be relatively more toxic in cats. Veterinary caregivers should minimize the amount of benzene-containing agents given to cats. In the case of metronidazole, however, the benzoate ester offers a less stressful, more palatable dosage form for short-term therapy. Because stress can be as detrimental as any infectious disease, increasing the palatability of medication can improve acceptance of therapy, decrease the length of treatment, and improve therapeutic outcome. Veterinarians can be reassured that metronidazole, when indicated for short-term use in hepatocompetent cats, is a relatively safe choice.[7]

Excretion

The urinary pH of herbivores is alkaline (pH 7–8), but the urinary pH of carnivores is acidic (pH 5.5–7). This difference obviously can affect the excretion rate of drug products, especially those with pK_a values in the close vicinity of these ranges. The half-lives of drugs vary among animals, as is shown in Table 29-5. The drug preparation to be used must be selected and administered at a dosage that is appropriate for a particular species of animal. For example, Table 29-6 shows how dosages of two drugs differ for various animals.

TABLE 29-6 Drug Dosage Variations in Different Animals

Drug	Route	Dose (mg/kg)			
		Ruminant	Horse	Dog	Cat
Xylazine	IM	0.2	2.0	2.0	2.0
Succinylcholine	IV	0.02	0.1	0.3	1.0

IM = intramuscular; IV = intravenous.
Source: Reference 5.

Pharmaceutical Preparations

There are numerous dosage forms that can be compounded for veterinary patients. These includes boluses, capsules, drenches and tubing products, drinking water medication, feed additives (Type A Medicated Articles, Type B Medicated Feeds, Type C Medicated Feeds), intramammary infusions, oral pastes and gels, parenteral dosage forms, premixes, topical dosage forms (dips [plunge dips, shower dips], dust bags, flea and tick collars, pour-on/spot-on applications, transdermal gels), and tablets. Each dosage form has its own characteristics, advantages, and disadvantages.

Variables that modify the rate and extent of absorption, thus changing the response to a drug, include the crystal habit of the drug, polymorphism, the specific salt used, the state of solvation or hydration, excipients and adjuvants, processing variations, and the formation of complexes. Choosing a flavoring for a drug can be a challenge, because different animals prefer different flavors. Table 29-7 suggests flavors for use with various animals.

TABLE 29-7 Suggested Flavors for Veterinary Medications

Animal	Comment	Flavor
Pets		
Avian	Birds prefer sweet and fruity flavors; use gels for birds that like to bite, or add fresh juice or flavored vehicle to bread balls or stuffing.	Banana, grape, honey/millet, molasses/millet, nectar, orange, orange juice, piña colada, raspberry, tangerine, tutti-frutti (and mixtures of these)
Canine	Dogs prefer meats, sweets, fixed oils, or a syringe of processed cheese spread as a vehicle. Use a mini ice cube tray for larger troches or make a milk bone for larger doses.	Bacon, beef, liver, chicken, turkey, cheese, chocolate (artificial), peanut butter, cod liver oil, honey, malt, molasses, caramel, anise, marshmallow, raspberry, strawberry
Feline	Cats usually do not like too much sweetness but hate bitter tastes. Flavored troches work, but make treats with square corners, not round. Flavored paste to the paw as an alternative is acceptable, but, if appropriate, consider transdermal administration.	Fish, fish and liver, tuna, cod liver oil, sardine, mackerel, salmon, beef, liver, chicken, cheese, cheese with fish, bacon, molasses, peanut butter, butter, butterscotch, marshmallow
Ferret	In the wild, they prefer fish and meat, but if domesticated, they can develop a sweet tooth.	Chocolate, peanut butter, molasses, honey, fish, beef, liver, bacon, raspberry, fruit punch, tutti-frutti, apple, strawberry, peas
Gerbil	As a rule, they like sweet and fruity flavors.	Banana cream, orange, peach, tangerine, tutti-frutti
Guinea pig	Flavor a paste, and spread it on their favorite vegetable.	Carrot, celery, lettuce, pumpkin
Iguana	Make the preparation smell good.	Banana, cantaloupe, kiwi, orange, tangerine, watermelon and other melons,
Parrot		Hot and spicy flavors (cayenne pepper)
Rabbit	Find their favorite vegetable or fruit, and use it.	Banana cream, carrot, celery, lettuce, parsley, pineapple, vanilla butternut
Reptile	Smell can be more important than taste. (Snakes are the exception; administer drug by dropper.)	Banana cream, lemon custard, melon, tutti-frutti

(continued)

TABLE 29-7 Suggested Flavors for Veterinary Medications *(Continued)*

Animal	Comment	Flavor
Rodent	Use a flavored paste or jelly.	Banana cream, cheese, lemon custard, peanut butter, vanilla butternut
Tropical bird		Banana, piña colada, tutti-frutti (and mixtures)
Farm Animals		
Cattle		Alfalfa, anise, anise and licorice, blue-grass, clover, eggnog, forage, honey, maple, meal, molasses
Emu	These birds are attracted to bright colors, especially yellow.	Cantaloupe, kiwi, honeydew, strawberry, tutti-frutti, watermelon
Equine	Horses need large amounts in reasonable volumes. Use thick suspensions or pastes.	Alfalfa, apple, apple and caramel, blue-grass, butterscotch, caramel, cherry, clover, forage, honey, maple, molasses
Goat	The statement that they will eat anything is not true.	Apple, caramel, cherry, honey, molasses
Poultry		Cantaloupe, corn, meal, milk, vanilla butternut, watermelon,
Swine	Mix the drug with peanut butter, and roll it in corn flakes.	Anise, anisette, cherry, corn, honey, licorice, meal, milk, peanut butter, sarsaparilla
Exotics and Zoo Animals		
Armadillo		Bacon, canned dog food
Bear		Honey, licorice
Chinchilla		Banana, tutti-frutti
Coyote		Meat flavors, watermelon
Elephant	They differ in what they like, so check with the handler. Flavor and inject suspension into a favorite food. To neutralize the bitterness, use lots of stevia if needed. Avoid shots, which can easily cause abscesses. Check what handlers are able to do. Can they shoot the liquid in the mouth? If not, an option is to put nonbitter liquid on bread and cover with vegetables.	Apple, apple and peanut butter, cantaloupe, chewing tobacco orange, pumpkin, raspberry, watermelon
Baby monkey		Apple, banana, carrot
Colobus monkey		Apple, banana, carrot, leafy vegetables (lettuce, spinach), sweet potato
Orangutan		Apricot nectar
Ostrich	These birds are attracted to bright colors, especially green.	Raspberry, strawberry, tutti-frutti
Primate	Hide the bitterness; numerous flavors will work.	Apricot, banana, chocolate, orange, peach, raspberry
Rhinoceros		Apple
Sea lion	Captive (inland) sea lions need sodium chloride supplementation. Place drug into a fish.	Whole fish
Tiger, lion		Beef, chicken, liver, turkey bacon, other meats (preferably freshly killed or live)
Zebra		Apple, apple and caramel

Physiology

Physiologic considerations that affect drug response include drug sensitivity, age, sex, pregnancy, drug interactions in vivo, and disease states. The normal or distinctive habits of animals must be considered. For example, because cats are constantly grooming themselves, any drug placed on them topically is likely to be ingested.

Compounded Veterinary Formulations

Bases

Oral Paste Formulations (100 g)

	Formula 1	Formula 2	Formula 3	Formula 4	
Polyethylene glycol 300	65 g	25 g			Vehicle
Polyethylene glycol 3350	35 g	25 g	25 g		Vehicle
Propylene glycol		50 g	25 g		Humectant
Peanut butter				65 g	Vehicle/ Flavor
Hydrogenated vegetable oil				35 g	Vehicle
Molasses			50 g		Flavor/ Sweetener

1. Calculate the required quantity of each ingredient for the total amount to be prepared.
2. Accurately weigh or measure each ingredient.
3. Generally, the polyethylene glycol formulas are prepared by heating the ingredients to a temperature of about 70°C, followed by cooling and stirring (formula 1).
4. In formula 2, the propylene glycol is added while the preparation is hot, followed by cooling and stirring.
5. In formula 3, the polyethylene glycol 3350 and propylene glycol are prepared by heating the ingredients to a temperature of about 70°C, followed by cooling and stirring, and then the molasses is added as the preparation is cooling.
6. Formula 4 can be prepared by simply mixing the ingredients.
7. Package and label the product.

Nonaqueous Nonoleaginous Paste Base

Active drug	qs	Active
Carbomer 934	1.0–1.5 g	Thickener
Triethanolamine	0.23–0.35 g	Alkalizer
Flavoring	qs	Flavoring
Propylene glycol	qs 100 g	Vehicle

(Note: The consistency of this paste can be modified by altering the quantities of carbomer 934 or triethanolamine, or both, or by replacing up to half the propylene glycol with glycerin.)

For drugs soluble in propylene glycol:

1. Calculate the required quantity of each ingredient for the total amount to be prepared.
2. Accurately weigh or measure each ingredient.
3. Place the propylene glycol in a suitable mixer, and dissolve the active drug and flavoring.
4. Add the carbomer 934, and mix until dissolved.
5. Slowly add the triethanolamine, and mix well; blend until smooth and homogeneous.
6. Package and label the product.

For drugs insoluble in propylene glycol:

1. Calculate the required quantity of each ingredient for the total amount to be prepared.
2. Accurately weigh or measure each ingredient.
3. Dissolve the flavoring in the propylene glycol.
4. Add the carbomer 934, and mix until dissolved.
5. Slowly add the triethanolamine, and mix well; blend until smooth and homogenous.
6. Slowly add the active drug, as a fine powder, and mix until uniform.
7. Package and label the product.

Ophthalmics

℞ Veterinary Dexamethasone 0.1% Ophthalmic Ointment

Dexamethasone sodium phosphate	39.6 mg (equivalent to about 30 mg of dexamethasone)	Active
Bacteriostatic water for injection	0.4 mL	Solvent
Polysorbate 80	0.3 mL	Surfactant
Lacri-Lube	qs 30 g	Vehicle

(Note: This preparation should be prepared in a laminar-airflow hood by a validated aseptic compounding pharmacist, using aseptic techniques.)

1. Sterilize all equipment to be used before proceeding to the laminar-airflow hood.
2. Calculate the quantity of each ingredient required for the prescription.
3. Accurately weigh or measure each ingredient.
4. Mix the dexamethasone sodium phosphate with the bacteriostatic water for injection.
5. Add the polysorbate 80, and mix well.
6. Aspirate the liquid into a syringe, attach a sterilizing filter, and filter into a sterile syringe.
7. Remove the barrel from a second sterile syringe, and add the Lacri-Lube.
8. Connect the two syringes by using a sterile connector.
9. Thoroughly mix the product by alternately forcing the contents of one syringe into the other syringe.
10. Package and label the product.

Ointments, Creams, and Gels

℞ Dimethyl Sulfoxide 50% Cream, Veterinary

Dimethyl sulfoxide	50 g	Active
Cetyl alcohol	6 g	Emulsifier/Oil Phase
Stearyl alcohol	6 g	Emulsifier/Oil Phase
Polysorbate 80	6 mL	Emulsifier
Imidurea	100 mg	Preservative
Preserved water (parabens)	qs 100 g	Vehicle

1. Calculate the quantity of each ingredient required for the prescription.
2. Accurately weigh or measure each ingredient.
3. Mix the dimethyl sulfoxide, polysorbate 80, and about 32 mL of preserved water.
4. Add the imidurea, and heat to about 60°C while stirring.
5. In a separate container, heat the cetyl alcohol and stearyl alcohol until a clear melt is obtained.
6. Add the aqueous solution (step 4) to the oil solution (step 5) with stirring.
7. Remove the mixture from heat, and mix until cooled.
8. If necessary, add sufficient preserved water to make 100 g, and mix well.
9. Package the product in glass containers and label.

℞ Antifungal Preparation for Animals

Coal tar solution	5 mL	Active
Resorcinol	2.5 g	Active
Lanolin	6.5 g	Vehicle/Emulsifier/Water Absorber
Liquefied phenol	1.5 mL	Active/Preservative
Hydrophilic petrolatum	15 g	Vehicle
White petrolatum	qs 100 g	Vehicle

1. Calculate the quantity of each ingredient required for the prescription.
2. Accurately weigh or measure each ingredient.
3. Place the resorcinol powder on a pill tile.
4. Add 1 to 2 mL of coal tar solution at a time until the resorcinol powder is dissolved.
5. Add this mixture to about half of the hydrophilic petrolatum (Aquaphor or Aquabase can also be used). Using a spatula, incorporate the petrolatum until the mixture is smooth.
6. Add the lanolin and the remaining hydrophilic petrolatum until all these ingredients are incorporated.
7. Add the liquefied phenol, and mix until uniform.
8. Incorporate the white petrolatum, and mix until homogenous.
9. Package and label the product.

℞ Hair Moisturizer and Conditioner for Horses and Other Animals

| Mineral oil, light | 20 g | Vehicle/Active |
| Hydrophilic petrolatum | 80 g | Vehicle |

1. Calculate the quantity of each ingredient required for the prescription.
2. Accurately weigh or measure each ingredient.
3. Using low heat, heat the light mineral oil.
4. Add the hydrophilic petrolatum (Aquaphor or Aquabase), and thoroughly mix.
5. Remove the mixture from heat and cool, with intermittent stirring.
6. Package and label the product.

℞ Sulfur and Peruvian Balsam Ointment for Mange and Ringworm in Animals

Peruvian balsam	12 g	Active
Castor oil	12 g	Compounding Aid
Sulfur ointment	76 g	Active/Vehicle

1. Calculate the quantity of each ingredient required for the prescription.
2. Accurately weigh or measure each ingredient.
3. Mix the Peruvian balsam with the castor oil.
4. Incorporate the sulfur ointment.
5. Mix the ointment until uniform.
6. Package and label the product.

℞ Sulfur Ointment

Precipitated sulfur	10 g	Active
Liquid petrolatum	10 g	Vehicle
White ointment	80 g	Vehicle

1. Calculate the quantity of each ingredient required for the prescription.
2. Accurately weigh or measure each ingredient.
3. Levigate the precipitated sulfur with the liquid petrolatum until a smooth paste is formed.
4. Incorporate the white ointment, and mix until uniform.
5. Package and label the product.

℞ Fleabite Gel

Dexamethasone sodium phosphate	50 mg	Active
Quinine sulfate dihydrate	100 mg	Active
Diphenhydramine hydrochloride	1 g	Active
Methylcellulose 1500 cP	3 g	Thickener
Purified water	qs 100 mL	Vehicle

1. Calculate the quantity of each ingredient required for the prescription.
2. Accurately weigh or measure each ingredient.
3. Dissolve the diphenhydramine hydrochloride and dexamethasone sodium phosphate in about 40 mL of purified water.
4. Heat about 50 mL of purified water until steaming.
5. With rapid stirring, slowly sprinkle the methylcellulose 1500 cP onto the heated water until thoroughly dispersed.
6. Remove the mixture from heat, and pour in the diphenhydramine hydrochloride–dexamethasone sodium phosphate drug solution (step 3).
7. Add sufficient purified water to volume, followed by the quinine sulfate dihydrate, and mix well.
8. Store the gel in the refrigerator for about 2 hours until gelling is complete.
9. Package and label the product.

℞ Methimazole 5 mg/0.1 mL in Pluronic Lecithin Organogel

Methimazole	150 mg	Active
Lecithin:isopropyl palmitate 1:1 solution	0.66 mL	Emulsifier
Pluronic F-127 20% gel	qs 3 mL	Vehicle

(Note: The lecithin:isopropyl palmitate 1:1 solution can be prepared by mixing 0.2 g of sorbic acid, 50 g of soy lecithin, and 50 g of isopropyl palmitate. The Pluronic F-127 20% gel can be prepared by mixing 0.2 g of sorbic acid, 20 g of Pluronic F-127, and sufficient purified water to make 100 mL.)

1. Calculate the quantity of each ingredient required for the prescription.
2. Accurately weigh or measure each ingredient.
3. Remove the plunger from a 3-mL Luer-Lok syringe (or appropriate size depending on quantity to be prepared), and attach a tip cap.
4. Pour the methimazole powder carefully into a syringe barrel.
5. Add the lecithin:isopropyl palmitate 1:1 solution, and replace the plunger.
6. In a second syringe, measure 2 mL of the Pluronic F-127 20% gel.
7. Attach a Luer-Lok/Luer-Lok Adapter to fit the two syringes together, and mix the contents back and forth between the two syringes.
8. Carefully (so as not to entrap air), force all the preparation into one syringe, and measure the volume.
9. Remove the other syringe, and obtain sufficient Pluronic F-127 20% gel to volume.
10. Reattach the syringes, and mix the preparation back and forth until it is thoroughly mixed.
11. Package and label the product.

℞ Veterinary Antiseptic Emollient

Hydroxyquinoline	300 mg	Active
Liquefied phenol	2 mL	Active
Methyl salicylate	1 mL	Aromatic
Lanolin	32 g	Vehicle
Petrolatum (white or yellow)	65 g	Vehicle

1. Calculate the quantity of each ingredient required for the prescription.
2. Accurately weigh or measure each ingredient.
3. Levigate the hydroxyquinoline into a small quantity of petrolatum, and mix until smooth.
4. Gradually incorporate the remainder of the petrolatum into the mixture.
5. Incorporate the liquefied phenol and methyl salicylate into the mixture.
6. Incorporate the lanolin, and mix well.
7. Package and label the product.

℞ Sulfur and Tar Ointment for Dogs

Precipitated sulfur	25 g	Active
Pine tar	25 g	Active
Zinc oxide ointment	50 g	Vehicle

1. Calculate the quantity of each ingredient required for the prescription.
2. Accurately weigh or measure each ingredient.
3. Mix the precipitated sulfur, pine tar, and zinc oxide ointment geometrically until uniform.
4. Package and label the product.

℞ Pine Tar Wound Dressing with Allantoin and Benzocaine, Veterinary

Allantoin	1.25 g	Active
Benzocaine	2 g	Active
Pine tar	1 g	Active
Propylene glycol monostearate	47.63 g	Emulsifier
White petrolatum	47.63 g	Vehicle

1. Calculate the quantity of each ingredient required for the prescription.
2. Accurately weigh or measure each ingredient.
3. Melt the propylene glycol monostearate and white petrolatum together at 55°C–60°C, and allow to cool to room temperature.
4. In a separate container, triturate the allantoin and benzocaine powders together.
5. Add to the melted base geometrically.
6. Incorporate the pine tar, and mix well.
7. Package and label the product.

Otics

℞ Silver Sulfadiazine 1% Otic Lotion

Silver sulfadiazine 1% cream	18 g	Active
Silver sulfadiazine powder	315 mg	Active
Propylene glycol	qs	Levigating Agent
Bacteriostatic water for injection	24 mL	Vehicle

1. Calculate the quantity of each ingredient required for the prescription.
2. Accurately weigh or measure each ingredient.
3. Wet the silver sulfadiazine powder with a few drops of propylene glycol to make a paste.
4. Add the silver sulfadiazine 1% cream, and mix well.
5. Add the bacteriostatic water for injection, and mix well to make a lotion.
6. Package and label the product.

℞ **Gentamicin Sulfate, Polymyxin B Sulfate, Neomycin Sulfate, and Hydrocortisone Otic Drops**

Gentamicin sulfate activity	150 mg	Active
Polymyxin B sulfate	150 mg	Active
Neomycin sulfate	500 mg	Active
Hydrocortisone	1 g	Active
Propylene glycol	50 mL	Vehicle
Polysorbate 80	0.25 mL	Surfactant/Solubilizer
Sodium bisulfite	100 mg	Antioxidant
Purified water	30 mL	Vehicle
Glycerin	qs 100 mL	Vehicle

1. Calculate the quantity of each ingredient required for the prescription. The quantity of gentamicin sulfate will be calculated from the activity labeled on the bulk container.
2. Accurately weigh or measure each ingredient.
3. Combine the hydrocortisone with the polysorbate 80 in a beaker, and mix well.
4. Slowly, with stirring, add the propylene glycol. A small quantity of heat may be required to dissolve the hydrocortisone.
5. In a separate container, dissolve the gentamicin sulfate, polymyxin B sulfate, neomycin sulfate, and sodium bisulfite in the purified water.
6. Add about 10 mL of glycerin, and mix well.
7. Add the glycerin solution (step 6) to the cooled propylene glycol solution (step 4), and mix well.
8. Add sufficient glycerin to volume. and mix well.
9. Package and label the product.

℞ **EDTA-THAM Otic Solution**

Ethylenediaminetetraacetic acid (EDTA)	20 mg	Active
Tris (hydroxymethyl) aminomethane (THAM)	605 mg	Active
Sodium lauryl sulfate	190 mg	Surfactant
Sodium hydroxide 20% solution (fresh)	To adjust pH	Alkalizer
Sterile water for irrigation	qs 100 mL	Vehicle

1. Calculate the quantity of each ingredient required for the prescription.
2. Accurately weigh or measure each ingredient.
3. Dissolve the THAM in 90 mL of the sterile water for irrigation.
4. Dissolve the EDTA and sodium lauryl sulfate into the solution by using low heat and minimal stirring to avoid foaming.
5. Add sterile water for irrigation to a volume of about 98 mL.
6. Add sufficient sodium hydroxide 20% solution to obtain a pH of 8. (Note: Prepare the sodium hydroxide 20% solution by dissolving 2 g of sodium hydroxide in sufficient purified water to make 10 mL. Use within 5 days.)
7. Add sufficient sterile water for irrigation to volume, and mix well.
8. Sterilize by autoclaving or sterile filtration (0.22-μm filter).
9. Package and label the product.

℞ Veterinary Antibiotic, Antifungal, Anti-inflammatory, and Anesthetic Otic Drops

Gentamicin sulfate	300 mg (as gentamicin)	Active
Betamethasone valerate	100 mg	Active
Miconazole nitrate	1 g	Active
Tetracaine hydrochloride	1 g	Active
Propylene glycol	qs 100 mL	Vehicle

1. Calculate the quantity of each ingredient required for the prescription. For the gentamicin sulfate, calculate the quantity according to the labeled potency of the drug.
2. Accurately weigh or measure each ingredient.
3. Reduce the particle sizes of the gentamicin sulfate, betamethasone valerate, miconazole nitrate, and tetracaine hydrochloride powders, if necessary, and blend in a mortar with a pestle.
4. Add a small portion of the propylene glycol, and form a smooth paste.
5. Add the propylene glycol geometrically, and mix until uniform.
6. Package and label the product.

Injections

℞ Iodine 2% in Oil Injection

Iodine, resublimed	2 g	Active
Almond oil, sweet	qs 100 mL	Vehicle

(Note: This preparation should be prepared in a laminar-airflow hood in a clean room by a validated aseptic compounding pharmacist, using strict aseptic technique.)

1. Calculate the quantity of each ingredient required for the prescription.
2. Accurately weigh or measure each ingredient.
3. Place the resublimed iodine and sufficient sweet almond oil to make 100 mL in a beaker.
4. Stir by using a magnetic stirrer and gentle heat until the iodine is dissolved, which can take several hours.
5. Filter the solution through a 0.22-μm sterile filter into sterile vials.
6. Package and label the product.

℞ Canine Methylpyrazole Intravenous Solution for Ethylene Glycol Poisoning

4-Methylpyrazole	1 g	Active
Polyethylene glycol 300	9 mL	Thickener/Solvent
Bacteriostatic water for injection	qs 20 mL	Vehicle

1. Calculate the quantity of each ingredient required for the prescription.
2. Accurately weigh or measure each ingredient.
3. Place the 4-methylpyrazole and the polyethylene glycol 300 in a clean container, and mix well.
4. Add sufficient bacteriostatic water for injection to make 20 mL, and mix well.
5. Filter through a sterile 0.22-μm filter into a sterile container.
6. Package and label the product.

℞ Veterinary Electrolyte Injection

Sodium acetate trihydrate	4.333 g	Active
Potassium chloride	467 mg	Active
Calcium chloride dihydrate	200 mg	Active
Magnesium chloride	133 mg	Active
Benzyl alcohol	0.1 mL	Preservative
5% Dextrose injection	50 mL	Vehicle
Sterile water for injection	qs 100 mL	Vehicle

(Note: This product should be prepared in a laminar-airflow hood in a clean room by a validated aseptic compounding pharmacist, using strict aseptic technique.)

1. Calculate the quantity of each ingredient required for the prescription.
2. Accurately weigh or measure each ingredient.
3. Dissolve the sodium acetate trihydrate, potassium chloride, calcium chloride dihydrate, magnesium chloride, and benzyl alcohol in the 5% dextrose injection.
4. Add sufficient sterile water for injection to volume.
5. Filter through a sterile 0.22-μm filter into a sterile container *or* package in clean vials and autoclave at 121°C, 15 psi, for 20 minutes.
6. Package and label the product.

℞ Sterile Vehicle for a Mastitis Preparation for Animals

Aluminum monosterate	2 g	Emulsion Stabilizer/Gelling Agent
Methylparaben	200 mg	Preservative
Propylparaben	40 mg	Preservative
Sesame oil	100 mL	Vehicle
Active drug	qs	Active

1. Calculate the quantity of each ingredient required for the prescription.
2. Accurately weigh or measure each ingredient.
3. Using moderate agitation, dissolve the methylparaben and propylparaben in about 100 mL of the sesame oil. Ensure that the ingredients are at room temperature.
4. Place mixture in a container that, when closed, allows almost no headspace.
5. Add the aluminum monostearate, and stir rapidly until dispersion is complete.
6. Replace the container cap with a piece of aluminum foil, and, using dry heat, sterilize the mixture at 140°C for 2 hours.
7. Remove the mixture from the heat source, and allow mixture to cool to 100°C without agitation.
8. When the temperature of the mixture reaches 100°C, resume slow agitation; continue this action until the formulation reaches room temperature.
9. Using a clean air environment, add the active ingredient, which has been previously sterilized.
10. Package the product in a sterile container, and label.

Topical Sprays

℞ Sucrose Octaacetate and Capsicum Spray for Pets

Sucrose octaacetate	1 g	Active
Capsicum oleoresin	1 g	Active
Polysorbate 60	2 mL	Surfactant
Propylene glycol	10 mL	Cosolvent
Isopropyl alcohol 70%	31.4 mL	Cosolvent
Preserved water	qs 100 mL	Vehicle

1. Calculate the quantity of each ingredient required for the prescription.
2. Accurately weigh or measure each ingredient.
3. Dissolve the sucrose octaacetate, polysorbate 60, and propylene glycol in the isopropyl alcohol 70%.
4. Disperse the capsicum oleoresin in the solution.
5. Add sufficient preserved water to volume, and stir until a homogenous mixture is obtained.
6. Package and label the product.

Oral Liquids and Gels

℞ Amitriptyline Hydrochloride 1 mg/mL Oral Liquid and Gel

	Liquid	Gel	
Amitriptyline hydrochloride	100 mg	100 mg	Active
Glycerin	2 mL	10 mL	Levigating Agent
Flavoring	qs	qs	Flavoring
Simple syrup	qs 100 mL		Vehicle
Methylcellulose 4000 cP		4 g	Thickener
Sodium benzoate		200 mg	Preservative
Citric acid		200 mg	Acidifier
Purified water		qs 100 mL	Vehicle

Oral Liquid
1. Calculate the quantity of each ingredient required for the prescription.
2. Accurately weigh or measure each ingredient.
3. Mix the amitriptyline hydrochloride and the flavoring with the glycerin.
4. Add sufficient simple syrup to volume, and mix well.
5. Package and label the product.

Oral Gel
1. Calculate the quantity of each ingredient required for the prescription.
2. Accurately weigh or measure each ingredient.
3. Mix the amitriptyline hydrochloride, flavoring, sodium benzoate, citric acid, and methylcellulose 4000 cP with the glycerin.
4. Add sufficient purified water to volume, and mix well.
5. Package and label the product.

℞ Veterinary Phenobarbital 22 mg/mL Oral Liquid

Phenobarbital	2.2 g	Active
Propylene glycol	3.2 mL	Cosolvent
Xanthan gum	200 mg	Thickener
Aspartame	500 mg	Sweetener
Sodium saccharin	100 mg	Sweetener
Stevia powder	100 mg	Sweetener
Raspberry concentrate	3.33 mL	Flavoring
Peppermint spirit	13 drops	Flavoring
Simple syrup	qs 100 mL	Vehicle

1. Calculate the quantity of each ingredient required for the prescription.
2. Accurately weigh or measure each ingredient.
3. In a mortar, combine the phenobarbital, xanthan gum, aspartame, sodium saccharin, and stevia powder.
4. Add the propylene glycol, and mix until a smooth paste is formed.
5. Add the flavorings, and mix well.
6. Add sufficient simple syrup to volume, and mix well.
7. Package and label the product.

℞ Potassium Bromide 500 mg/mL Oral Solution

Potassium bromide	50 g	Active
Purified water	qs 100 mL	Vehicle

1. Calculate the quantity of each ingredient required for the prescription.
2. Accurately weigh the potassium bromide.
3. Add sufficient purified water to volume, and mix until dissolved.
4. Package and label the product.

℞ Sulfadiazine Sodium 333 mg/mL and Pyrimethamine 16.7 mg/mL Oral Liquid

Sulfadiazine sodium	33.3 g	Active
Pyrimethamine	1.67 g	Active
Diethanolamine	1.033 mL	Alkalizer
Polysorbate 80	0.1 mL	Surfactant
Xanthan gum	100 mg	Thickener
Hydroxyethylcellulose 5000 cP	0.925 g	Thickener
Sodium saccharin	100 mg	Sweetener
Appleade flavor (or other)	1.5 mL	Flavoring
Potassium sorbate	200 mg	Preservative
Sodium metabisulfite	99 mg	Antioxidant
Propylene glycol	1.5 g	Levigating Agent
Purified water	qs 100 mL	Vehicle

1. Calculate the quantity of each ingredient required for the prescription.
2. Accurately weigh or measure each ingredient.
3. On a magnetic stirrer, add the sodium metabisulfite to about 40 mL of purified water in a beaker.
4. Slowly add the sulfadiazine sodium until dissolved. (Note: This task can take 30 minutes; a small amount of sodium hydroxide can be used if needed.)
5. Add the diethanolamine, polysorbate 80, and flavoring with continued stirring.
6. Dissolve the sodium saccharin and potassium sorbate in a small quantity of purified water, and add to the mixture.
7. Mix propylene glycol with xanthan gum; add to the mixture, and mix well.
8. Add the pyrimethamine, and mix well.
9. Increase the speed of the stirrer, slowly add the hydroxyethylcellulose 5000 cP (sprinkle through a sieve), and stir until uniform.
10. Package and label the product.

Capsules

℞ Canine Diarrhea Capsules (#100)

Neomycin sulfate	1.44 g	Active
Sulfaguanidine	14.8 g	Active
Sulfadiazine	920 mg	Active
Sulfamerazine	920 mg	Active
Sulfathiazole	920 mg	Active
Kaolin	30 g	Active
Pectin	1 g	Active

1. Calculate the quantity of each ingredient required for the prescription.
2. Accurately weigh each ingredient.
3. Mix the sulfadiazine, sulfamerazine, and sulfathiazole together.
4. Add the pectin, followed by the neomycin sulfate, with mixing.
5. Geometrically, add the sulfaguanidine and then the kaolin.
6. Mix thoroughly.
7. Fill 100 capsules, size 0, with a tight pack.
8. Check for uniform capsule weights.
9. Package and label the product.

Chewable Treats and Troches

Gelatin Base

Gelatin	43.4 g	Vehicle
Glycerin	155 mL	Vehicle
Purified water	21.6 mL	Vehicle

1. Calculate the required quantity of each ingredient for the total amount to be prepared.
2. Accurately weigh or measure each ingredient.
3. Heat the glycerin using a boiling water bath.
4. Add the purified water, and continue heating for 5 minutes, while stirring.
5. Slowly add the gelatin over a 3-minute period, stirring until mixed thoroughly and free of lumps.
6. Continue to heat for 45 minutes only.
7. Remove the mixture from heat, and cool.

℞ Chewable Treat Base

Nugget-type animal food	65 g	Vehicle
Gelatin base, melted	qs 100 g	Binder
Active drug	qs	Active

1. Calculate the quantity of each ingredient required for the prescription.
2. Accurately weigh or measure each ingredient.
3. Pulverize a nugget-type animal food of choice.
4. Melt the gelatin base (see formula on page 520).
5. Incorporate the powdered animal food, and mix well.
6. Add the active drug, and mix well.
7. Pour the mixture into molds, and allow to set.
8. Package and label the product.

℞ Animal Treats for Drug Ingestion

Powdered animal food	13.2 g	Vehicle
Glycerin	2 mL	Levigating Agent
Flavoring (chicken, beef, etc.)	1 mL	Flavoring
Gelatin base	6.6 g	Binder
Active drug	qs	Active

1. Calculate the quantity of each ingredient required for the prescription.
2. Accurately weigh or measure each ingredient.
3. Cut the gelatin base (see formula on page 520) into small pieces, and put into a beaker in a water bath.
4. Mix the powdered animal food with the active drug powder.
5. Mix the flavoring with the glycerin, and add to the melted gelatin.
6. Incorporate the powdered animal food–active drug mixture (step 4).
7. Fill the desired molds, and allow to set until hardened. (Note: Blister molds, suppository molds, and the like will work.)
8. Package and label the product.

℞ Phenylpropanolamine Hydrochloride 10 mg Chewable Troches for Dogs

Phenylpropanolamine hydrochloride	240 mg	Active
Silica gel	240 mg	Suspending Agent
Acacia powder	480 mg	Demulcent/Texture
Peanut butter	14.4 g	Vehicle
Hydrogenated vegetable oil	9.6 g	Vehicle

1. Calculate the quantity of each ingredient required for the prescription.
2. Accurately weigh or measure each ingredient.
3. Mix the phenylpropanolamine hydrochloride, silica gel, and acacia powders together.
4. In a separate container, using low heat, mix the peanut butter and hydrogenated vegetable oil.
5. Incorporate the powders, and mix well.
6. Pour the mixture into troche molds, and allow to cool.
7. Package and label the product.

Other

℞ Implantable Pellet

2-Hydroxyethyl methacrylate	4200 parts	Vehicle
Ethylene glycol dimethacrylate	43 parts	Vehicle
Diisopropyl dicarbonate	750 parts	Vehicle
Active drug	750 parts (approximately)	Active

1. Calculate the quantity of each ingredient required for the prescription.
2. Accurately weigh or measure each ingredient.
3. Mix the 2-Hydroxyethyl methacrylate, ethylene glycol dimethacrylate, diisopropyl dicarbonate, and active drug thoroughly, and place into molds, preferably cylindrical.
4. Place molds in water bath maintained at 75°C for approximately 25 minutes to effect polymerization. The amount of cross-linking will determine the release rate: the more cross-linking, the longer the release rate. Cross-linking can be increased or decreased by altering the amount of diisopropyl dicarbonate present and the length of time the mold remains in the water bath.
5. Package and label the product.

References

1. Animal Health Institute. Animal drug compounding. Available at: www.ahi.org/issues-advocacy/animal-drug-compounding/. Accessed December 19, 2015.
2. American Veterinary Medical Association. Guidelines for veterinary prescription drugs: key points. Available at: https://www.avma.org/KB/Policies/Pages/Guidelines-for-Veterinary-Prescription-Drugs.aspx. Accessed December 19, 2015.
3. U.S. Food and Drug Administration. 2011 Revision of the Grade "A" Pasteurized Milk Ordinance. Available at: www.fda.gov/downloads/Food/GuidanceRegulation/UCM291757.pdf.
4. Comyn G. Extra-label drug use in veterinary medicine. Available at: www.fda.gov/AnimalVeterinary/NewsEvents/FDAVeterinarianNewsletter/ucm100268.htm. Accessed November 9, 2011.
5. Blodinger J. *Formulation of Veterinary Dosage Forms.* New York: Marcel Dekker; 1983.
6. Davidson G. Veterinary transdermal medications: A to Z. *Int J Pharm Compound.* 2003;7(2):106–13.
7. Davidson G. To benzoate or not to benzoate. Cats are the question. *Int J Pharm Compound.* 2001;5(2):89–90.

Additional Sources

Birchard SJ, Sherding RG. *Saunders Manual of Small Animal Practice.* 3rd ed. Philadelphia: Elsevier; 2005.

Davidson G. Submitting compelling case reports for drug therapy in veterinary patients. *Int J Pharm Compound.* 2007;11(4):390–5.

DeVeau I. USP Convention standards and clinical information for compounded medications used in veterinary medicine. *Int J Pharm Compound.* 2007;11(4):357–62.

Ettinger SJ, Feldman EC. *Textbook of Veterinary Internal Medicine Expert Consult.* Philadelphia: Elsevier; 2009.

Goodrum J. Survey of state veterinary compounding laws and regulations. *Int J Pharm Compound.* 2005;9(3):209–11.

Plumb DC. *Plumb's Veterinary Drug Handbook.* 7th ed. Hoboken, NJ: Wiley; 2011.

Chapter 30

Compounding for Clinical and Investigational Studies

In the medical and pharmaceutical literature, hundreds of clinical and investigational studies are reported annually comparing the effects of different drugs, dosage forms, and delivery systems. These studies may compare different products, or they may compare a product with a placebo. A compounding pharmacist is often the source of the products used in these drug studies.

Clinical and investigational drug studies for animals and humans can provide a critical understanding of a medication's safety profile (adverse drug reactions and drug interactions) and pharmacokinetic parameters (absorption, distribution, metabolism, and excretion). They can also provide some insight into early indications of therapeutic efficacy. A compounding pharmacist can often reduce the time needed to supply quality formulations for studies, which can be valuable in reducing late-stage dropouts or losses and being able to explore a less-confined dosing range, alternative formulations, and alternative routes of administration. Also, extemporaneous preparations are useful to rapidly screen alternative, unique formulation concepts to provide added value to a study.

Almost any dosage form can be used in investigational studies. For the best approach, the formulation should be as simple as is reasonable and should exclude any excipient that may negatively affect a patient's response to the drug. Pharmacies involved in compounding for clinical and investigational drug studies must be in compliance with all the appropriate *United States Pharmacopeia (USP)* general chapters and *United States Pharmacopeia/National Formulary (USP/NF)* standards pertaining to compounding.

Background

Studies may originate with an investigator or with a pharmaceutical company or a device or drug delivery company. For a pharmaceutical company, preparing small batches of drug products for clinical studies is not economical. Also, many of these studies are conducted at academic or research institutions and are not concerned with investigational new drug applications, new drug applications, or abbreviated new drug applications. Often, the study investigator must either prepare the drug product for the study or make arrangements with an outside entity (e.g., a pharmacy) to prepare it.

Appropriate controls must be followed during preparation of the study drug to ensure patient safety and appropriate record keeping and documentation. In the past, study drugs were required to be made in facilities with systems in place to meet Current Good Manufacturing Practices of the U.S. Food and Drug Administration. However, that has changed, as specified in 21 CFR Part 210 Section (c):

> An investigational drug for use in a phase 1 study, as described in § 312.21(a) of this chapter, is subject to the statutory requirements set forth in 21 U.S.C. 351(a)(2)(B). The production of such drug is exempt from compliance with the regulations in part 211 of this chapter. However, this exemption does not apply to an investigational drug for use in a phase 1 study once the investigational drug has been made available for use by or for the sponsor in a phase 2 or phase 3 study, as described in § 312.21(b) and (c) of this chapter, or the drug has been lawfully marketed. If the investigational drug has been made available in a phase 2 or phase 3 study or the drug has been lawfully marketed, the drug for use in the phase 1 study must comply with part 211.

An investigational drug study is a biomedical or health-related research study in humans or animals that follows a predefined protocol. Preclinical studies involve the testing of potential drugs in the laboratory setting or in animals and typically are conducted before a clinical study.

Clinical studies generally are conducted in four phases, and each phase has a different purpose, as follows:

- *Phase I:* An experimental drug or treatment is tested in a small group of people (20–80 generally healthy volunteers, but the study may include patients) for the first time to evaluate the drug's safety, determine a safe dosage range, and identify side effects.
- *Phase II:* The experimental study drug or treatment is administered to a larger group of people (100–300 patients with the specific disease state to be treated) to determine if the drug is effective and to further evaluate its safety.
- *Phase III:* The experimental study drug or treatment is administered to large groups of people (1000–3000 patients with the disease state of interest plus concomitant medical conditions) to confirm the drug's effectiveness, monitor side effects, compare the drug to commonly used treatments, and collect information that allows the experimental drug or treatment to be used safely.
- *Phase IV:* Postmarketing studies delineate additional information about the drug's risks, benefits, and optimal use.

Responsibility for all compounding and quality-related elements in an investigational study resides with both the sponsor and the compounding pharmacy. When delegated to a third party (individuals or contract research organizations) outside the sponsor's organization, written contractual documents should clearly specify the scope, roles, and responsibilities of work that will be performed by each party involved.

Even though Current Good Manufacturing Practices may not be required when extemporaneous compounding is used in preclinical and Phase I investigations, appropriate controls should be in place to ensure patient safety by means of appropriate record keeping and documentation. Local and state laws and regulations must also be observed.

In most clinical studies that eventually direct new and more effective therapies for human and veterinary diseases, the use of a placebo is required. However, the U.S. pharmaceutical industry is not equipped to prepare small quantities of placebos that cannot be visually distinguished from the active drugs against which they are evaluated. Although some placebo batches are prepared in smaller pilot-plant operations, compounding pharmacists' provision of capsules, creams, gels, inert tablets, injectables, or ointments for investigational drug studies is increasingly common.

In addition, the active drugs evaluated in clinical trials must often be modified from their manufactured dosage form. Compounding pharmacists can provide those customized medications; they may assist by developing a formulation (e.g., for intramuscular, intravenous, or subcutaneous administration if an injection is required) that meets the trial requirements.

Compounding for clinical and investigational drug studies may be addressed differently by different states. Some states may not specifically address the topic. In these studies, the patient's name is not always known for the labels, depending on the protocol design for the study. Also, investigational drugs used for animal studies may need to be handled differently from those used for some clinical studies.

Pharmacists who are interested in compounding drugs for clinical and investigational studies should be aware that extensive record keeping is required and stringent quality control programs must be in place. Compounding pharmacies that supply the study drugs must be fully equipped for preparation of the investigational drug (sometimes in a large volume) according to the exact specifications of the trial. Each step of the process must be addressed with appropriate standard operating procedures. These must be documented and the documentation available for review. For pharmacists willing to meet the rigorous requirements of compounding for clinical trials, personal and professional satisfaction more than compensates for the challenges.

All parties involved in clinical and investigational drug studies understand that pharmacies involved in compounding for these studies will be in compliance with all the appropriate *USP* general chapters and *USP/NF* standards; therefore, those will not be described in detail in this chapter. Several chapters in the *USP/NF* apply to this practice and should be consulted.

For the pharmaceutical industry, new drug product development is a priority. Companies must discover new drugs with fewer resources in faster time frames while maintaining the highest quality. Conducting clinical studies is costly but necessary. Generally, preparing relatively small batches of materials for clinical trials is not feasible or cost-effective for the pharmaceutical industry. Some companies have product development pharmacies and some do not. Companies may contract out the preparation of small batches of materials for clinical trials to compounding pharmacies.

When the preparation of study drugs is outsourced, the ultimate responsibility for all aspects of the clinical trial still resides with the sponsor. When responsibility is delegated to third parties (individuals or organizations) outside the sponsor's organization, typically there is a contract specifying the scope of work to be performed. Responsibility for the aspects of quality control or quality assurance being delegated must be clearly delineated in the primary contract. When possible, the principal aspects delegated and the identity of the individual third party or parties to whom the responsibility is designated should be itemized. Contract pharmacies must have (1) well-defined written procedures, (2) adequately controlled equipment and compounding environment, and (3) accurately and consistently recorded data.

Clinical and investigational studies often provide a critical understanding of a compound's safety and pharmacokinetic profile, and occasionally they provide insight into early indications of efficacy. Procedures that can shorten the time needed to supply quality formulations for studies can be critical in producing data that reduce later-stage attrition and lower the cost of new drug development. The clinical investigator may want to explore a broader dosing range or different formulations. Extemporaneous preparation by a compounding pharmacy may reduce production costs and shorten the time for product testing and release for clinical use. Extemporaneous preparations may also be useful for studying an alternative formulation or route of administration and for obtaining pharmacokinetic data or gaining insight into the drug's mechanisms of absorption, distribution, metabolism, and excretion. Finally, extemporaneous preparations may be used to rapidly screen concepts for innovative formulations to provide added value to patients and extend the life cycle of currently marketed medications.

Project Initiation and General Considerations

Processes and policies must be in place to ensure that investigational drugs are properly compounded. Standard operating procedures for the compounding of investigational drugs must be followed and their use documented. Processes should be in writing for reviewing, approving, supervising, and monitoring investigational medications; they should specify that when pharmacy services are provided, the pharmacy controls the acquisition, compounding, labeling, storage, dispensing, and distribution of the investigational medication.

For any clinical or investigational study to be valid, quality control must be built in from the beginning of the study to its conclusion. A study can be rendered invalid if the drug product is incorrectly prepared, labeled, stored, or administered. An effective quality control program must ensure that the product is prepared properly and is stable for the expected duration of its use. A pharmacist working with the study coordinator to ensure that the drug product is properly prepared, stored, labeled, administered, and disposed of (if any remains at the end of the study) is critical. Quality control testing can be done at a pharmacy or a contract analytical laboratory, or both.

Quality Control Variables

Five variables that must be addressed by a quality control program for clinical trial batches are the raw materials, in-process items, packaging materials, labels, and finished products.[1]

Raw materials include solvents and chemicals, whether active ingredients or inactive excipients. Raw materials must be of the appropriate quality (e.g., USP- or NF-grade substance) and be accompanied by valid certificates of analysis or other suitable documentation. For a large, critical study, having the raw materials tested and confirmed by an independent analytical laboratory is prudent. Physical, chemical, and microbiological procedures can be used in testing for identity, assay, quality, and purity.

In-process items include any item or product that is prepared and held during the compounding of the final product, such as gel components, premixes, primary emulsions, stock solutions, and triturations. These items may require testing, especially if held for any length of time before the final compounding steps.

Packaging materials include the immediate container, closure, and any other packaging materials. The packaging may include glass or plastic bottles, cans, metal or plastic caps, cardboard, drums, metal foil, jars, paper, plastic parts and film, tubes, or vials. Packaging materials should be accompanied by documentation of their composition and size specifications and should be selected because their physical and chemical characteristics contribute to the stability of the final product.

Labels include all written, printed, or graphic matter on the immediate container received by a patient. *Labeling* includes all the written, printed, or graphic matter accompanying the product. Information on the label and in the materials accompanying the product must be in complete agreement. The labeling includes the instructions to the clinicians involved in the study, patient package inserts, cartons, outer wrapping (if used), and any other materials accompanying the product. Label control is vitally important, and only the exact number of labels required should be printed. An example label should be affixed to the batch control record. An auxiliary label for supplying additional information may need to be affixed to individual drugs or to a bag that holds a supply of vials or containers. Such labels should supply information that is missing on the preparation label or information that is poorly visible on the label.

The *finished product* includes the dosage form, package, label, and any other necessary items. The final product must be analyzed for conformance to the specifications provided by the primary investigator. Sufficient checks and balances must be incorporated in the process to ensure that the actual yield matches the theoretical yield or that any difference is explained.

Dosage Forms

Virtually all known dosage forms may be used in clinical studies, but the most common are capsules, parenterals, liquids (solutions, suspensions, emulsions), semisolids (topical ointments, creams, gels), and suppositories. Keeping the formulation as simple as is reasonable and excluding any ingredient (excipient) that may alter the effect of or response to the drug are important.

Capsules

The capsule is probably the most versatile of all dosage forms; it is the form most commonly compounded for clinical studies. With capsules, one can easily adjust the dosage and prepare active and placebo products that look identical. Most capsules today are lockable, which hinders a patient in separating them to see their contents. Because most bulk drug substances, or active pharmaceutical ingredients, are white powders, the untrained eye cannot easily differentiate between an active and a placebo capsule. If the active pharmaceutical ingredient is colored, then a colored powder usually can be easily prepared as the placebo for encapsulation. Capsules for the study may be the standard powder-filled hard-gelatin capsule or special capsules for contents such as a liquid or a semisolid matrix.

Quality control for capsules used in clinical studies should address overall average weight, individual weight variation, dissolution of the capsule shell, disintegration of the capsule contents, active-drug assay results, physical appearance (color, uniformity, extent of fill, whether locked), and physical stability (discoloration or other changes).[2,3]

Parenterals

Many clinical studies require an injectable form of the drug. A pharmacy involved in compounding parenterals for clinical studies must have the facilities, equipment, trained personnel, and documentation program necessary to ensure that the finished product is free of microorganisms (sterile), bacterial endotoxins and pyrogens (nonpyrogenic), and extraneous insoluble materials.

Quality control for parenterals used in clinical studies should address weight or volume, physical observations (color, clarity, particulate matter), pH, specific gravity, osmolality, drug assay, sterility, and pyrogenicity.[4,5]

Liquids

Solutions, suspensions, and emulsions may be used in clinical studies. Oral liquids are the most common solution dosage form, but solutions may also be prepared for topical application. Preparation techniques for many of these liquid dosage forms are similar.

Solutions contain one or more drug substances molecularly dispersed in a suitable solvent or a mixture of mutually miscible solvents. Oral solutions contain one or more substances, with or without flavoring, sweetening, or coloring agents, dissolved in water or cosolvent–water mixtures. The excipients must be selected very carefully. Topical solutions are usually aqueous but may contain cosolvent systems such as various alcohols or other organic solvents with or without added active ingredients.

When components of a formula are not soluble, a suspension or an emulsion is often indicated. A suspension is a two-phase system consisting of a finely divided solid dispersed in a solid, liquid, or gas. Suspensions are appropriate when the drug to be incorporated is not sufficiently soluble in an ordinary solvent or cosolvent system. A good suspension ensures that the drug is uniformly dispersed throughout the vehicle.

In oral suspensions, solid particles of the active drug are dispersed in a sweetened, flavored, and sometimes viscous vehicle. Topical suspensions intended for application to the skin contain solid particles dispersed in a suitable liquid vehicle. A suitable vehicle for a suspension has the viscosity to keep the drug particles suspended separately from each other but is sufficiently fluid that the preparation can be poured from the container. The suspension dosage form can enhance the stability of a drug that is poorly stable in solution.

Emulsions are used whenever two immiscible liquids must be dispensed in the same preparation. Topical lotions are a popular form of emulsion. Emulsions for internal use are used to dispense oil and aqueous drugs together, to mask the taste of unpleasant oily drugs, and sometimes to enhance the absorption of selected drugs.

Quality control for liquid dosage forms may involve checking the final product for final volume or weight, physical observations (appearance, clarity, precipitation, mold or bacterial growth, odor, clarity), pH, specific gravity, active drug assay, particle or globule size range, and rheological properties or pourability.[6]

Semisolids

Ointments, semisolid preparations for application to the skin or mucous membranes, soften or melt at body temperature. They should spread easily and should not be gritty. Creams are opaque, soft solids or thick liquids for external application. They consist of medications dissolved or suspended in water-soluble or vanishing-cream bases and can be either water-in-oil (w/o) or oil-in-water (o/w) emulsions. The term *cream* is most frequently applied to soft, cosmetically acceptable types of preparations.

One of the most versatile delivery systems that can be compounded is the pharmaceutical gel. Gels are an excellent drug delivery system for various routes of administration and are compatible with many different drug substances. They are relatively easy to prepare and are very efficacious.

Quality control of ointments, creams, and gels involves checking the final product for final product weight, visual appearance, color, odor, viscosity, pH, homogeneity or phase separation, particle size distribution, rheological properties, and texture. A pharmacist should document the observations in a product record.[7]

Suppositories

Suppositories are solid dosage forms used to administer medicine through the rectum, vagina, or urethra. Rectal suppositories are cylindrical or conical and are tapered or pointed at one end. Usually they weigh approximately 2 g and are about 1 to 1.5 inches long. Infant rectal suppositories weigh about half as much as adult suppositories. Vaginal and urethral suppositories are called inserts. The drugs contained in suppositories and inserts can have either systemic or local effects. A suppository or insert base can help control the effect of the active drug and should be selected carefully; it should be stable, nonirritating, chemically and physiologically inert, compatible with a variety of drugs, stable during storage, and aesthetically acceptable.

Quality control of suppositories for clinical studies should address weight, specific gravity, active drug assay, physical observations (color, texture, appearance, feel), melting range, dissolution, and physical stability.[8]

Sources of Drug Substances

Precautions should be observed when using commercial dosage forms such as pure powders, tablets, capsules, liquids, or injectables in investigational studies. Pure powders, generally used in their original state, present the fewest complications and are the only source that should be used for injectables. Tablets should be finely comminuted before they can be incorporated into an oral liquid or capsule preparation. Generally, only immediate-release tablets should be used. Capsules also can be a source of the drug (i.e., opening the capsule shell and using the contents). Liquids can be evaporated to dryness by appropriate means, or they can be prepared with an adsorbent before incorporation into solid or semisolid dosage forms. Injectable preparations can be reconstituted, if required, and used. A pharmacist should analyze the content of commercial products for accuracy because some products have wide ranges in allowed strength.

Stability, Storage, and Distribution

Stability data are needed to support the proposed shelf life for the investigational drug. These data are used to establish a shelf life to ensure adequate strength and purity during storage under the labeled conditions. A stability study should be conducted using stability-indicating analytical methods, appropriate laboratory procedures, representative drug preparations, storage in the anticipated (or required) storage condition, and storage in the container–closure system that is ultimately used at the site of administration.

Storage

Storage temperatures throughout the entire study process must be carefully controlled, monitored, and documented. Any temperature deviations and their durations should be investigated and recorded. Electronic monitoring devices are recommended because they can provide a detailed record of storage conditions.

Distribution and Dispensing

Distribution and dispensing may be the least controllable part of the overall process from compounding to administration. If distribution and dispensing occur within the same facility, the potential problems should be minimal. However, if distribution and dispensing occur in different locations and common carriers are used, the potential problems can be substantial, especially if overnight delivery is required or distribution needs to be made during weather extremes in which proper packaging is required. In-package temperature monitoring devices should be used, and their information should be recorded immediately after the package is received at the study site, if required.

Quality Assurance

Overall responsibility for the development and execution of the quality program should be assigned to a qualified individual. Responsible quality personnel are essential in ensuring the safety, identity, strength, quality, and purity of investigational drugs and their components.

A quality assurance program (see *USP* Chapter <1163>, Quality Assurance in Pharmaceutical Compounding) should include at least the following integrated components: (1) training; (2) standard operating procedures (SOPs); (3) documentation; (4) verification; (5) testing; (6) cleaning, disinfecting, and safety; (7) containers, packaging, repackaging, labeling, and storage; (8) outsourcing, if used; and (9) responsible personnel.[9]

Sponsor companies or their vendors, including pharmacies or clinics, should conduct audits according to the protocol. As part of the inspection, a quality assurance auditor should verify that the pharmacist in charge (PIC) or the appropriate person is performing quality inspections.

Testing

A quality assurance program for compounded preparations should include in-process and finished compounded preparation testing as appropriate as described in the study protocol. Testing may involve physical, chemical, and microbiological testing. Acceptance criteria must be determined before testing. Investigative and corrective actions associated with the specific failure or discrepancy should be described. Regardless of the source, each drug substance and excipient should have predetermined acceptance criteria.

The PIC is responsible for either implementing an in-house testing program or working with a contract laboratory to confirm appropriate testing methods for the preparations. If testing is done at the compounding facility, appropriate equipment should be obtained and qualified. All personnel conducting in-house testing should be properly trained, skilled, and proficient in the procedure.

Appropriate SOPs must be developed and implemented to ensure that equipment and instruments are working properly and that preparations are properly compounded. Pharmacists can perform physical quality control tests to ensure the uniformity and accuracy of many small-scale compounded preparations. These tests address individual dosage unit weights; average individual dosage unit weights; total preparation weight; pH; and physical observations such as appearance, taste, and smell.

If testing is outsourced, the PIC and sponsor should determine what to outsource and how to select a laboratory and should develop an ongoing relationship with the selected laboratory. Contract laboratories must follow standards set forth in *USP* general chapters, as appropriate, and must be registered with the U.S. Food and Drug Administration or accredited by an appropriate agency, or both.

Documentation

Documentation for clinical study batches includes the original study specifications, the master formula record, the compounding record, test results, certificates of analysis, any documentation accompanying the ingredients and materials used in the product, and any calibration tests performed on the equipment being used.

Information on the product should consist of the product name, product or study identification number, dosage strength, dosage form, container and closure system, container size, beyond-use date, pharmacy name and address, date, and approval signatures. The master formula record should include the product name, product or study identification number, dosage strength, dosage form, ingredients by complete name and by theoretical quantity, total theoretical weight or volume of the dosage form, approval date, and approval signatures.

The compounding record should include the product identification, instructions, notations or precautions, and approvals. The identification consists of the product name, product or study identification number, dosage, dosage form, and master formula. Complete compounding instructions should be provided, covering all aspects of compounding (e.g., weight or measure of each raw material added, manufacturer and lot number of each raw material, order of addition, theoretical weight or volume at applicable phases, yield, equipment used, temperatures, mixing speeds, mixing times, drying times, storage conditions, and sampling points). Notations or precautions include any notes that are necessary for producing a successful product, avoiding loss of the product, or ensuring the safety and health of employees, together with any remedial measures to be taken in case of an adverse event.

Standard Operating Procedures

Compounding pharmacies must have appropriate SOPs to ensure that investigational materials are properly handled and compounded. SOPs for the handling, compounding, storage, and transport of investigational drugs should be clearly written and active, and they should be followed and documented. They may include policies for reviewing, approving, supervising, and monitoring investigational medications. These policies should be clearly written to ensure that when pharmacy services are provided, a pharmacy has the ultimate responsibility for the acquisition, compounding, labeling, storage, quality assurance, dispensing, and distribution of an investigational medication, as well as the destruction of any recalled, unused, or returned portions of that drug.

SOPs for pharmaceutical compounding are documents that describe how to perform routine and expected tasks in the compounding environment, including but not limited to procedures involving records of preparations, compendial standards, sponsor requirements, and testing, to ensure that quality, identity, purity, uniformity, and integrity have been achieved (see USP Chapters <51>, Antimicrobial Effectiveness Testing;[10] <71>, Sterility Tests;[11] and <85>, Bacterial Endotoxins Test;[12] see also USP Chapters <795>, Pharmaceutical Compounding—Nonsterile Preparations;[13] <797>, Pharmaceutical Compounding—Sterile Preparations;[14] and <1163>, Quality Assurance in Pharmaceutical Compounding[9]).

Safety Data Sheets

Safety data sheets must be available on-site or should be readily retrievable electronically. Appropriate personnel who are exposed to compounding materials must review them.

Certificates of Analysis

Certificates of analysis (COAs) should be obtained for every ingredient used in the compounding of investigational drugs, should be maintained throughout the study, and should be provided to the sponsor at the end of the study if requested. If the sponsor supplies all materials, the sponsor is responsible for maintaining the COAs for the ingredients and supplying these to the clinical site if requested.

Records

Documentation must include a record of all aspects of the compounding of investigational drugs. Information should be entered on appropriate record forms as the tasks are performed. Compounding records must be reviewed for accuracy and completeness (as appropriate) and must be approved by responsible quality assurance personnel before product release. After study termination, all records of the investigational study must be retained according to sponsor, United States Pharmacopeial Convention (USP), state, and local requirements.

Documentation for investigational drugs includes at least the original study specifications, the master formula record, the compounding record, test results, COA, any documentation accompanying the ingredients and materials used in the preparation, and any calibration tests performed on the equipment used.

Information about the preparation must consist of the preparation name, preparation or study identification number (protocol number or preparation number), dosage strength, dosage form, container–closure system, container size, beyond-use date, pharmacy name and address, date, and approval signatures.

Security

The area used for preparation, packaging, labeling, storage, and distribution of investigational drugs should be secure and should have restricted access. Appropriate SOPs should be in place and should be documented to facilitate traceability and recall.

Study Completion

After the study is completed, records of investigational drugs should be retained according to the sponsor's requirements, including records pertaining to the preparation, release, and disposition of each lot of material used, as well as source documentation and release testing, as appropriate, for raw materials. Pharmacists also should retain records pertaining to reference standards, if any, used to support investigational drugs.

Unused drug substances, excipients, placebo, or finished preparations should be disposed of in accordance with SOPs and sponsor requirements, and pharmacists should make an accounting for all investigational preparations received and dispensed and for those returned to the sponsor. Any discrepancies should be noted, e.g., preparation of doses that were not dispensed or any broken or breached containers.

At the completion of the study, the sponsor should visit the compounding pharmacy to account for all used and unused drug supplies. The sponsor can verify the accountability and note the quantity returned for reconciliation and destruction. The compounding pharmacy should verify the quantity returned for destruction and should complete and sign the necessary forms.

N-of-1 Studies

Single-patient trials are useful for assessing the effectiveness of a given treatment, determining tolerance of the therapy, and ultimately influencing decisions about continuing therapy over time.[15] These controlled trials in individual patients usually compare the proposed therapy and a placebo by using a series of scheduled switches between the active drug and the placebo over a period of weeks.

In addition to determining the effectiveness of a given drug or dosage form for the individual patient, a properly conducted single-subject trial can help establish the optimum dose for that patient. N-of-1 trials are evaluated clinically and statistically, and a pharmacist is indispensable in their conduct.

The strength of an N-of-1 study is dependent on an a priori strategy for analysis and interpretation of the results: how the results will be collected and analyzed and what will be the cutoff for deciding to continue or discontinue therapy. A pharmacist who provides professional services to support N-of-1 studies should be prepared to collaborate with the physician on the design, analysis, and interpretation of the results.

To begin a single-subject trial, a physician and a patient—perhaps with encouragement from a pharmacist—agree that an experimental therapy will be tried and evaluated. The physician and patient should understand the desired endpoint, which is usually to control the symptoms or signs of a chronic disease. An important ethical principle is that the patient must understand that the trial will involve both an active drug and a placebo and must agree that the identity of the active drug or placebo will be withheld from him or her during the trial.

The physician and the pharmacist should then confer about the design of the trial and the dose or doses to use. Thereafter, the pharmacist prepares the requisite treatment and placebo dosage forms and develops a randomization schedule that conforms to the chosen design. During the trial, the pharmacist does not divulge the identity of the treatment or placebo doses to either the physician or the patient, except in an emergency. Because the containers of the trial dosage forms are unlabeled, providing on the label the information an emergency room physician could use to contact someone who could break the code in case of accidental ingestion or overdose is important. Pharmacists participating in N-of-1 trials should be accessible at all times or should establish an alternative means for emergency disclosure of the true nature of the drug in a given container.

During the trial, the patient undergoes pairs of treatments in accordance with the randomization schedule. In some cases, as when the optimum dose is not known, triplets of treatments (two different doses of active drug compared with placebo) may be used. Typically, the patient records symptoms and the physician performs periodic physical examinations or laboratory studies, or both. At least one complete set of observations must be completed for each treatment period during the trial.

At the end of the trial, the data are analyzed to compare the results from each treatment arm, and then the pharmacist reveals the identity of each arm. According to the previously established criteria, the physician and the patient then decide whether to continue or discontinue treatment.

Conclusion

Compounding for clinical and investigational studies differs from routine pharmacy compounding primarily with respect to documentation and quality control. Compounding pharmacists have the opportunity to become involved in research and to contribute to new pharmaceutical and medical advancements. A pharmacist's ability to provide these services is a useful contribution to the delivery of pharmaceutical care. Pharmacists interested in compounding for investigational drug studies can obtain information about current and future studies from the research administration department of universities, government institutions, or private companies that conduct clinical trials.

References

1. Bryant R. *The Pharmaceutical Quality Control Handbook*. Eugene, OR: Aster Publishing; 1984:21–8.
2. Allen LV Jr. Standard operating procedure for performing physical quality assessment of powder-filled, hard-gelatin capsules. *Int J Pharm Compound*. 1999;3:232–3.
3. Allen LV Jr. Standard operating procedure for performing physical quality assessment of special hard-gelatin capsules. *Int J Pharm Compound*. 1999;3:312–3.
4. Allen LV Jr. Standard operating procedure for particulate testing for sterile products. *Int J Pharm Compound*. 1998;2:78.
5. Allen LV Jr. Standard operating procedure: quality assessment for injectable solutions. *Int J Pharm Compound*. 1999;3:406–7.
6. Allen LV Jr. Standard operating procedure for performing physical quality assessment of oral and topical liquids. *Int J Pharm Compound*. 1999;3:146–7.
7. Allen LV Jr. Standard operating procedure for performing physical quality assessment of ointments/creams/gels. *Int J Pharm Compound*. 1998;2:308–9.
8. Allen LV Jr. Standard operating procedure for performing physical quality assessment of suppositories, troches, lollipops and sticks. *Int J Pharm Compound*. 1999;3:56–7.
9. United States Pharmacopeial Convention. Chapter <1163>, Quality assurance in pharmaceutical compounding. In: *United States Pharmacopeia/National Formulary*. Rockville, MD: United States Pharmacopeial Convention; current edition.
10. United States Pharmacopeial Convention. Chapter <51>, Antimicrobial effectiveness testing. In: *United States Pharmacopeia/National Formulary*. Rockville, MD: United States Pharmacopeial Convention; current edition.
11. United States Pharmacopeial Convention. Chapter <71>, Sterility tests. In: *United States Pharmacopeia/National Formulary*. Rockville, MD: United States Pharmacopeial Convention; current edition.
12. United States Pharmacopeial Convention. Chapter <85>, Bacterial endotoxins test. In: *United States Pharmacopeia/National Formulary*. Rockville, MD: United States Pharmacopeial Convention; current edition.
13. United States Pharmacopeial Convention. Chapter <795>, Pharmaceutical compounding—nonsterile preparations. In: *United States Pharmacopeia/National Formulary*. Rockville, MD: United States Pharmacopeial Convention; current edition.
14. United States Pharmacopeial Convention. Chapter <797>, Pharmaceutical compounding—sterile preparations. In: *United States Pharmacopeia/National Formulary*. Rockville, MD: United States Pharmacopeial Convention; current edition.
15. Fassett WE. Single-patient trials, extemporaneously compounded products and pharmaceutical care. *Int J Pharm Compound*. 2003;7:441–7.

Chapter 31

Cosmetics for Special Populations and for Use as Vehicles

Pharmacists have been associated with cosmetics throughout history. Cosmetics have traditionally been used for beautifying, perfuming, cleansing, and ritual purposes. The 20th century brought progress in the diversification of these products and their functions, as well as in safety and protection for the consumer. Pharmacists' association with cosmetics had waned in recent years, but now pharmacists are receiving more requests to prepare cosmetics for two reasons: to address allergies or sensitivities to preservatives, dyes, and fragrances and to incorporate active medications into commercially available cosmetics.

Historical Use

The science of cosmetic preparations dates back at least to the beginning of recorded history. In the 15th to 17th centuries, literature on cosmetics consisted of "books of secrets" that were devoted not only to bodily embellishment, but also to medicine, care of the home, and other topics. Over the years, formulas for cosmetics were recorded in published books, but actual cosmetic compendia were not published in English until the 1940s.

The goals of cosmetics have always been essentially the same: enhance personal appeal through decoration of the body, camouflage flaws in the integument, and alter or improve on nature. Vases of alabaster and obsidian for cosmetics discovered by Flinders Petrie in 1949 illustrate that the ancient Egyptians were well versed in the use of eye and face paints, body oils, and ointments. Theophrastus (363–278 BC), a student of Aristotle, demonstrated considerable knowledge of the compounding of perfumes, and the Roman physician Galen of Pergamon (130–200 AD) is said to have innovated cold cream.

In the earliest times, cosmetics were associated with religious practices. The ancient Egyptians, Assyrians, Chaldeans, Babylonians, and others anointed both the living and the dead with aromatic incense, oils, and ointments. Early in the development of cosmetics, the

Jews carried these uses to unprecedented heights. In Egypt, many of the high priests were recognized as medical practitioners. Products for care of the body were closely associated with medicine for almost 5000 years, and the history of cosmetics can be traced through the history of medicine and pharmacy. Cosmetics were used in activities related to bathing and in the arts of makeup and hairdressing, hair dyeing and waving, and embalming. The writings of Dioscorides and Zosimos (known to students of pharmacy) explain many of the formulations used.

Hippocrates advanced the study of dermatology and advocated correct diet, exercise, sunlight, special baths, and massage as aids to good health and beauty. Cornelius Celsus, Pliny the Elder, Dioscorides, and Galen all contributed to the medical and cosmetic literature of their days. Cosmetics (when not made in the home) usually were prepared by pharmacists. Cosmetics as a specialty began separating from medicine during the period 1200–1500. Thereafter, cosmetics apparently branched into (1) products used for routine beautification of the skin and (2) those used for the correction of cosmetic disorders of the skin, hair, nails, and teeth (drawing on dermatology, pharmacology, dentistry, ophthalmology, dietetics, and other accepted medical arts).

The first pharmacopeia of London, published in 1618, showed that pharmacists had the necessary equipment and skill to make and sell cosmetic products, but the increasingly stringent regulations governing their work kept most of them occupied exclusively with the compounding of medications. During the 17th and 18th centuries, cosmetic products of all kinds were still made principally in the home, although the number of shops that sold such items increased steadily. Raw materials were purchased from pharmacists and "druggists" (a new term of German origin), but very few professional apothecaries sold anything other than assorted essences and "perfumed waters."

Sticks made from a base of oil and wax came into limited use before World War I as lipsticks, usually colored with carmine. These lipsticks simply applied a colored layer to the lips that, when removed, left the lips their natural color. Most dyes were water insoluble, but the incorporation of a water-soluble dye was found to actually dye the lips if they were premoistened before application of the lipstick. This was an early approach to the use of sticks containing a material that interacted with the skin. Some of these water-soluble dyes would develop an intense red color as the pH was lowered.

Today's cosmetics have resulted from cosmetic scientists introducing and improving products for various applications. Some cosmetic products, including gels, oils, ointments, pastes, powders, solutions, sticks, and suspensions, are still widely used in the pharmaceutical sciences.

Most recently, *active cosmetics* have been developed. In addition to improving the user's appearance or odor, they are intended to benefit their target (e.g., the skin, hair, mucous membranes, or teeth). Manufacturers are making a multitude of claims about their products' actions on the body, and the cosmetic market has greatly expanded. Many current cosmetic products focus on hydrating the skin, reducing or slowing the signs of aging skin, or protecting the skin against the usual daily environmental assaults.

The recent changes in cosmetic products and the constraints imposed on the manufacturers have given cosmetology greater credibility with scientists, physicians, and consumers. Cosmetology is now a science that combines various areas of expertise, including bioengineering, biology, chemistry, dermatology, microbiology, physics, statistics, and toxicology.

Definitions

The word "cosmetic" is derived from the Greek *kosmētikos,* meaning "having the power to arrange, skilled in decorating," from *kosmein,* "to adorn," and *kosmos,* "order, harmony." The true origin probably lies still further in antiquity; early cave paintings depict the use of body adornment in the rituals of mating and hunting.[1]

The U.S. Food and Drug Administration (FDA) defines cosmetics as articles intended to be applied to the human body for cleansing, beautifying, promoting attractiveness, or altering the appearance without affecting the body's structure or functions. This definition includes the following types of products, plus their component materials: baby products, bath oils, bubble baths, deodorants, eye and facial makeup, fingernail polishes, hair coloring, lipsticks, lotions, mouthwashes, perfumes, permanent waves, powders and sprays, and skin care creams.

Products that are intended to treat or prevent disease or otherwise affect structure or function of the human body are considered drugs. Any cosmetic that makes a therapeutic claim is treated as a drug *and* a cosmetic and must meet the labeling requirements for both. Such products can be identified by labels that list the "active ingredient." The manufacturer of such a product must have proof that the ingredient is safe for its intended use. In labeling, the active ingredient of these products is listed first. Examples include antiperspirant deodorants, dandruff shampoos, fluoride toothpastes, and foundations and tanning preparations that contain sunscreen. These products must have been proven to be safe and effective for their therapeutic claims.

The term "cosmeceutical" is not officially recognized by FDA, but the cosmetic industry uses it to refer to products that have medicinal or druglike benefits. Depending on their intended use, these products are regulated as cosmetics or drugs, or both.

Certain claims can cause a product to qualify as a drug even if the product is marketed as a cosmetic (e.g., claims to restore hair growth, reduce cellulite, treat varicose veins, or revitalize cells). The same is true for essential oils in fragrance products. A fragrance marketed for promoting attractiveness is a cosmetic. But a fragrance marketed with "aromatherapy" claims (e.g., that the scent will help the consumer sleep or quit smoking) meets the definition of a drug because of its intended use.

A product's intended use is established in several ways: by the claims stated on the product label, in advertising, on the Internet, or in other promotional materials; by consumer perception; and by the ingredients contained in the product.

Regulatory Framework

Section 201 (i) of the 1938 Food, Drug, and Cosmetic Act defines cosmetics as "(1) articles intended to be rubbed, poured, sprinkled, or sprayed on, introduced into, or otherwise applied to the human body or any part thereof for cleansing, beautifying, promoting attractiveness, or altering the appearance, and (2) articles intended for use as a component of any such articles; except that such term shall not include soap. . ."

FDA requirements governing the sale of cosmetics are not as stringent as those that apply to other FDA-regulated products. FDA is able to regulate cosmetics only after products are released to the marketplace.[2,3] Neither cosmetic products nor cosmetic ingredients are reviewed or approved by FDA before being sold to the public. FDA cannot require companies to test their cosmetic products for safety before marketing. If the safety of a cosmetic product has not been substantiated, however, the product's label must read: "Warning: The safety of this product has not been determined."

FDA can inspect cosmetics-manufacturing facilities, collect samples for examination, and take action through the U.S. Department of Justice to remove adulterated and misbranded cosmetics from the market. However, FDA does not have the authority to require manufacturers to register their cosmetic establishments, file data on ingredients, or report cosmetic-related injuries. The agency does maintain a voluntary data collection program; cosmetic companies that wish to participate forward data to FDA. Fortunately, serious injury from makeup is a rare event. Consumers can report adverse reactions to cosmetics to FDA.[4]

The regulatory category occupied by a product clearly has a great effect on the marketing of that product. As explained previously, intended use is determined principally, but not solely, by the claims that are made on product labeling.

Disallowed Ingredients

Distribution of cosmetics containing substances that are poisonous or that might injure users under normal conditions is illegal. Ingredients that are prohibited in cosmetics include bithionol, chloroform, halogenated salicylanilides, hexachlorophene, mercury compounds (except under certain conditions as preservatives in eye cosmetics), methylene chloride, methyl methacrylate monomer in nail products, vinyl chloride and zirconium salts in aerosol products, and zirconium complexes in aerosol cosmetics. Also, color additives must be tested for safety and FDA approval obtained for their intended use before they can be manufactured.

Labeling

Cosmetics sold to consumers must have labels that list ingredients in descending order of predominance, with the exception of trade secrets (as defined by FDA) and the ingredients of flavors and fragrances. The ingredient list is a consumer's only readily accessible source of information about what he or she is buying. Regulations concerning ingredient lists apply only to retail products intended for home use, not to those used exclusively by beauticians in salons. However, the product must state the distributor, list the content's quantity, and include all the necessary warning statements.

Expiration Dating and Beyond-Use Dating

There are no absolute dates for discarding various cosmetic products. Current U.S. law contains no requirement for cosmetic manufacturers to print expiration dates on the labels of their products. Nevertheless, manufacturers must determine the shelf life for products as a part of their overall responsibility to substantiate product safety. Products that contain so-called "all natural" ingredients that are plant-derived substances may be more conducive to microbial growth, so a shorter shelf life would be indicated. Expiration dates on cosmetics are simply "rules of thumb." However, if an active ingredient has been added during compounding, *United States Pharmacopeia (USP)* Chapter <795> guidelines should be followed.[5]

Categories of Cosmetics

FDA has classified cosmetics into 13 categories according to 21 CFR 720.4:

1. Skin care (creams, lotions, powders, sprays)
2. Fragrances
3. Eye makeup
4. Manicure products
5. Makeup other than for the eye (e.g., lipstick, foundation, blush)
6. Hair-coloring preparations
7. Shampoos, permanent waves, and other hair products
8. Deodorants
9. Shaving products
10. Baby products (e.g., shampoos, lotions, powders)
11. Bath oils and bubble baths
12. Mouthwashes
13. Tanning products

Of this list, pharmacists may be involved in compounding cosmetics for patients with specific needs or incorporating active drugs in deodorants, lipsticks or medication sticks, mouthwashes, shampoos, shaving products, and skin care preparations (creams, lotions, powders, and sprays). Some basic formulas for these preparations are provided later in this chapter; they can be easily modified to meet the needs of specific patients or to incorporate active drugs. When the formulas include preservatives or perfumes, a patient's sensitivities and requests should be considered. If a patient has a lanolin allergy, that ingredient can be omitted and possibly replaced by an equal quantity of hydrophilic petrolatum USP (Aquaphor, Aquabase). See Box 31-1 for suggestions for counseling patients about cosmetics.

Cosmetic Vehicles

Although a vehicle can be used to carry an active drug, in many cases it is used mainly for its effects on the skin: care, cleansing, decoration, hydration, or protection. Vehicles can be used as carriers for active cosmetics that, after application, are delivered to the specified target sites; however, this is usually allowed only if no systemic, physiological, or pharmacological effect is achieved and the product has been shown to be safe. Vehicles can include emulsions, gels, microemulsions, nanoemulsions or nanoparticles, solutions, and sticks.

BOX 31-1 Counseling about Cosmetics

Suggestions for counseling patients about cosmetics are as follows:

- Fragrances are the most common cause of allergic and irritant reactions to cosmetics.
- Preservatives are the second most common cause of allergic and irritant reactions to cosmetics.
- The term "hypoallergenic" can mean almost anything; there are no regulatory standards for use of the term.
- The labels "dermatologist tested," "sensitivity tested," "allergy tested," and "non-irritating" carry no guarantee that the product will not cause reactions.
- Like "hypoallergenic," the term "natural" can mean anything; there are no standards for its use. (If you've had poison ivy, you know that "natural" does not mean "hypoallergenic.")
- Never share cosmetics, not even with your best friend.
- Shared-use cosmetics (e.g., testers found at department store cosmetic counters) are more likely to become contaminated than the same products in an individual's home.
- At home, usually the preservatives have time to destroy bacteria that are inevitably introduced after each use; this is not the case with testers in department stores.
- Keep makeup containers tightly closed except when in use.
- Keep makeup out of sunlight, which can cause it to degrade.
- Do not use eye cosmetics if you have an eye infection, and throw away all products you were using when you first discovered the infection.
- Never add any liquid to a product to bring it back to its original consistency. Adding water or, even worse, saliva could introduce bacteria that could easily grow out of control.
- Throw away makeup if the color changes or an odor develops.
- Keep containers tightly closed when not in use.

Emulsions are probably the most widely used cosmetic vehicle. They offer important characteristics of skinfeel, consumer appeal, and ease of application. Emulsions are preferred to waterless oils and lipids. Oil-in-water emulsions feel light and are not greasy; they have good skin spreadability and penetration and provide active hydration by the external water phase. They cause a cooling effect as a result of evaporation of the external aqueous phase. Water-in-oil emulsions may be regarded as heavy, greasy, and sticky. However, they closely resemble the natural protective lipid layer in the stratum corneum, and they provide efficient skin protection, sustained moisturization, improved penetration, and a lowered risk of microbial growth. They are liquid at very low temperatures.

Gels are dispersed systems that do not include two immiscible phases of opposite lipophilicity. They are often transparent and have positive aesthetic characteristics. Hydrogels consist mainly (85% to 95%) of water or an aqueous–alcoholic mixture and the gelling agent. They have a cooling effect produced by evaporation of the solvent. A polymer residue may cause a sticky or tacky feel if inappropriate thickening agents have been used. Hydrophobic gels, including lipogels or oleogels, are prepared by adding a thickening agent to an oil or liquid lipid; colloidal silicone is often used.

Microemulsions are stable dispersions in the form of spherical droplets that have a diameter of 10 to 100 nm. Composition usually includes an oil, water, and surfactant and cosurfactant. Microemulsions have the disadvantage of containing a relatively high concentration of surfactants, which increases the risk of skin irritation and sensitization. Microemulsions can be used to incorporate or dissolve active substances and have been found to improve skin penetration and permeation.

Solutions used as vehicles remain physically stable. They are easily prepared by simple mixing, with heating if necessary. They are transparent, have a clean appearance, and are especially suitable for rinsing and cleaning body surfaces.

Sticks are a solid delivery vehicle prepared in an elongated form. They can be used for coloring agents, emollients, fragrances, and so on. Clear sticks are quite popular. One such formulation includes a gelling agent, dibenzylidene sorbitol, in propylene glycol or other related polyols.

Incorporation of Active Ingredients

The incorporation of any active ingredient into a cosmetic used as a vehicle must follow all the considerations of any compounded pharmaceutical, because the cosmetic is being converted to a drug preparation. Chemical and physical characteristics must be considered as well as stability. Chemical properties to consider include the structure, form, and reactivity of the active drug in the presence of the vehicle. Physical properties to consider include particle size, crystalline structure, melting point, and solubility. The active drug must be physically and chemically compatible with the cosmetic vehicle.

Pharmaceutical techniques such as solubilization, levigation, and pulverization by intervention can be used to thoroughly and uniformly incorporate the drug into the cosmetic. Knowledge of the composition of the particular cosmetic is important. For example, is it an emulsion, liposome, ointment, paste, solution, or suspension? Also, what ingredients are contained in the cosmetic? Sunscreens are becoming relatively common in cosmetics (Table 31-1).

Silicones

Silicones are used in all types of skin products for their sensory properties. Both during and after application, they tend to deliver greater emolliency values than many commonly used cosmetic ingredients. They are described as smooth and velvety and not greasy or oily, and they impart this feel to cosmetic and toiletry formulations, improving the negative feel associated with other

TABLE 31-1 Sunscreen Ingredients in Cosmetics

Name	Concentration (%)	Absorbance[a]
Aminobenzoic acid	≤ 15	UVB
Avobenzone	2–3	UVA I
Cinoxate	≤ 3	UVB
Dixoybenzone	≤ 3	UVB, UVA II
Homosalate	≤ 15	UVB
Menthyl anthranilate	≤ 5	UVA II
Octinoxate	≤ 7.5	UVB
Octisalate	≤ 5	UVB
Octocrylene	≤ 10	UVB
Oxybenzone	≤ 6	UVB, UVA II
Padimate O	≤ 8	UVB
Phenylbenzimidazole sulfonic acid	≤ 4	UVB
Sulisobenzone	≤ 10	UVB, UVA II
Titanium dioxide	2–25	Physical
Trolamine salicylate	≤ 12	UVB
Zinc oxide	2–20	Physical

[a]UVB = 290–320 nm; UVA = 320–400 nm; UVA I = 340–400 nm; UVA II (also called near UVA) = 320–340 nm.

ingredients. Silicone is a generic name for many classes of organosilicone polymers that consist of an inorganic siloxane (Si—O) backbone with pendant organic groups (usually methyl). This structure gives silicones their unique properties, particularly their surface properties.

Changes on Application

When a vehicle is applied to the skin, changes occur during and after application because of mechanical stress from being spread over the surface and evaporation of volatile ingredients. Mechanical stress and skin temperature may influence the viscosity of the vehicle and alter the release rate of any active ingredients. The uptake of water from the skin may also alter the composition of the vehicle, as can the loss of water resulting from evaporation. All these factors may cause phase inversion or phase separation. As a consequence, the thermodynamic activity of an active ingredient within the vehicle may change.

Quality Control

The same quality control procedures used for regular pharmaceutical dosage forms can be used in the preparation of cosmetics. Preparation of extra product that can be placed in storage for periodic observation over its expected use or life is useful; if adverse changes occur in the dosage form, a patient could be contacted and the remaining product recalled.

Storage and Labeling

Cosmetics should be packaged appropriately for the product, in either well-closed or tightly closed containers. They should be kept out of the reach of children; protected from heat and direct sunlight; and stored at either 5°C or 25°C, depending on the product.

Sample Formulations

Skin Care (Creams, Lotions, Powders)

 Hand Cream

Stearic acid	10 g	Thickener
Lanolin	4 g	Water Absorber
Glyceryl monostearate	4 g	Emulsifier
Sorbitol	4 g	Humectant
Span 60	4 g	Emulsifier
Tween 60	1 g	Emulsifier
Purified water	qs 100 g	Vehicle

1. Calculate the required quantity of each ingredient for the total amount to be prepared.
2. Accurately weigh or measure each ingredient.
3. Melt the stearic acid, lanolin, and glyceryl monostearate using low heat.
4. Add the sorbitol, Span 60, and Tween 80, and mix well.
5. Heat the purified water to the same temperature, add to the sorbitol mixture, and mix using mechanical agitation until a smooth cream forms.
6. Package and label the product.

Lotion

Stearic acid	4 g	Thickener
Lanolin	1 g	Water Absorber
Triethanolamine	1 g	Alkalizer
Mineral oil	6 g	Vehicle
Purified water	88 g	Vehicle

1. Calculate the required quantity of each ingredient for the total amount to be prepared.
2. Accurately weigh or measure each ingredient.
3. Melt the stearic acid and lanolin using low heat, and add the mineral oil.
4. Heat the purified water to the same temperature, and add the triethanolamine.
5. Pour the aqueous phase (step 4) into the melted oil phase (step 3) with stirring.
6. Stir the mixture until cool.
7. Package and label the product.

Dusting Powder

Kaolin	5 g	Active
Zinc stearate	2 g	Active
Zinc oxide	2 g	Active
Magnesium carbonate	10 g	Active
Menthol	0.05 g (optional)	Perfume
Talc	81 g	Vehicle

1. Calculate the required quantity of each ingredient for the total amount to be prepared.
2. Accurately weigh or measure each ingredient.
3. Using pulverization by intervention, dissolve the menthol in alcohol, spread over a pill tile or working surface, and allow to dry.
4. Separately, mix the kaolin, zinc stearate, zinc oxide, magnesium carbonate, and talc.
5. Sprinkle the powders over the menthol, and work the menthol into the powders by scraping it off the pill tile and blending it with the powders.
6. Mix the mixture until uniform.
7. Package and label the product.

Lipsticks and Medication Sticks

Stick Formulation 1

White wax	10 g	Thickener
White petrolatum	90 g	Vehicle

1. Calculate the required quantity of each ingredient for the total amount to be prepared.
2. Accurately weigh or measure each ingredient.
3. Melt the white wax in a beaker using low heat.
4. Add the white petrolatum, and mix thoroughly with stirring rod until uniform.
5. Cool the mixture until thick, and pour into ointment jar for storage at room temperature until used.
6. Package and label the product.

Stick Formulation 2

White wax	30 g	Thickener
Cetyl esters wax	30 g	Emulsifier
Mineral oil	40 g	Vehicle

1. Calculate the required quantity of each ingredient for the total amount to be prepared.
2. Accurately weigh or measure each ingredient.
3. Melt the white wax and cetyl esters wax in a beaker using low heat.
4. Add the mineral oil with stirring.
5. Cool the mixture until thickened.
6. Package and label the product.

Soft Stick Formulation (Clear Stick Base)

Sodium stearate	10 g	Vehicle
Alcohol	65 g	Vehicle
Propylene glycol	25 g	Vehicle

1. Calculate the required quantity of each ingredient for the total amount to be prepared.
2. Accurately weigh or measure each ingredient.
3. Melt the sodium stearate using low heat.
4. Mix the alcohol and propylene glycol, and add to the melted sodium stearate.
5. Mix the mixture well, cool slightly, and pour into stick molds.
6. Package and label the product.

 Blemish-Hiding Stick

Stearic acid	20	Thickener
Cetyl alcohol	25 g	Thickener/Emulsifier
Potassium hydroxide	1 g	Alkalizer
Purified water	3 g	Solvent
Preservative	0.1 g	Preservative
Titanium dioxide	14 g	Coloring Agent
Calamine	0–2 g	Coloring Agent
1% Sodium alginate solution	qs 100 g	Vehicle/Binding Agent

1. Calculate the required quantity of each ingredient for the total amount to be prepared.
2. Accurately weigh or measure each ingredient.
3. Melt the stearic acid and cetyl alcohol, and heat to 70°C.
4. Dissolve the potassium hydroxide in purified water, and warm to 70°C.
5. In a separate container, prepare the 1% sodium alginate solution and heat to same temperature.
6. Mix the titanium dioxide and calamine with the hot sodium alginate solution, and comminute the mixture.
7. Add the potassium hydroxide solution (step 4) to the stearic acid–cetyl alcohol melt (step 3) with mechanical agitation, and then immediately add the sodium alginate–coloring agent dispersion (step 6).
8. Continue stirring until the cream begins to thicken.
9. Pour the cream into molds as desired.
10. Package and label the product.

Classic Lipstick 1

	Gloss	Matte
Emollients	50%–70%	40%–55%
Waxes	10%–15%	8%–13%
Plasticizers	2%–5%	2%–4%
Colorants	0.5%–3%	3%–8%
Pearls	1%–4%	3%–6%
Actives	0%–2%	0%–2%
Fillers	1%–3%	4%–15%
Fragrance	0.05%–0.1%	0.05%–0.1%
Preservatives/antioxidants	0.5%	0.5%

1. Calculate the required quantity of each ingredient for the total amount to be prepared.
2. Accurately weigh or measure each ingredient.
3. Melt the waxes, emollients, and plasticizers together using low heat.
4. Add the colorants, pearls, preservatives, antioxidants, and fillers, followed by the actives and fragrance.
5. Pour the mixture into molds as appropriate.
6. Package and label the product.

 Solvent Lipstick 1

Solvents	25%–60%
Emollients	1%–30%
Waxes	10%–25%
Fixatives	1%–10%
Fillers	1%–15%
Colorants/pearls	1%–15%
Fragrance	0.05%–0.1%

1. Calculate the required quantity of each ingredient for the total amount to be prepared.
2. Accurately weigh or measure each ingredient.
3. Add the colorants to the emollients using a roller mill.
4. Add the waxes and fixatives, heat to 90°C–105°C, and mix until uniform.
5. Add the pearls, fillers, and solvents, and mix, with shear if necessary, until homogenous.
6. Add the fragrance, and mix until uniform.
7. Maintain a temperature just above the initial set point of the waxes, and fill the molds as appropriate.
8. Package and label the product.

Classic Lipstick 2

Carnauba wax	2.5%	Thickener
Beeswax, white	20%	Thickener
Ozokerite	10%	Vehicle/Base
Lanolin, anhydrous	5%	Emollient/Water Absorber
Cetyl alcohol	2%	Emulsifier
Liquid paraffin	3%	Vehicle/Base
Isopropyl myristate	3%	Emulsifier
Propylene glycol ricinoleate	4%	Emulsifier
Pigments	10%	Coloring Agent
Bromo acids	2.5%	Coloring Agent
Castor oil	qs 100%	Vehicle/Base

1. Calculate the required quantity of each ingredient for the total amount to be prepared.
2. Accurately weigh or measure each ingredient.
3. Melt the carnauba wax, white beeswax, ozokerite, anhydrous lanolin, cetyl alcohol, and liquid paraffin together using low heat.
4. Incorporate the isopropyl myristate, castor oil, propylene glycol ricinoleate, pigments, and bromo acids, and mix well.
5. Pour the mixture into appropriate molds.
6. Package and label the product.

Solvent Lipstick 2

Synthetic wax	6%	Thickener
Ceresin	4%	Thickener
Isododecane	10%	Solvent
Paraffin	3%	Thickener
Cetyl acetate/acetylated lanolin alcohol	5%	Emulsifier
Methylparaben	0.3%	Preservative
Propylparaben	0.1%	Preservative
Butylated hydroxyanisole	0.1%	Antioxidant
D&C Red No. 7 calcium lake	4%	Coloring Agent
FD&C Yellow No. 5 aluminum lake	3%	Coloring Agent
Titanium dioxide/mica	5%	Coloring Agent
Titanium dioxide/mica/iron oxides	3%	Coloring Agent
Bismuth oxychloride	10%	Coloring agent
Cyclomethicone	41.5%	Smoothing Agent
Isostearyl trimethylolpropane siloxy silicate	5%	Emollient

1. Calculate the required quantity of each ingredient for the total amount to be prepared.
2. Accurately weigh or measure each ingredient.
3. Mix the cetyl acetate/acetylated lanolin alcohol, methylparaben, propylparaben, butylated hydroxyanisole, D&C Red No. 7 calcium lake, FD&C Yellow No. 5 aluminum lake, titanium dioxide/mica, titanium dioxide/mica/iron oxides, bismuth oxychloride, and isostearyl trimethylolpropane siloxy silicate with the cyclomethicone.
4. Add the synthetic wax, ceresin, isododecane, and paraffin, with heating, and mix well.
6. While stirring, pour the mixture into molds, and allow to cool.
7. Package and label the product.

Shampoos

Clear Shampoo

Triethanolamine lauryl sulfate	50 g	Emulsifier
Polyoxyl 8 stearate	5 g	Emulsifier
Purified water	qs 100 g	Vehicle

1. Calculate the required quantity of each ingredient for the total amount to be prepared.
2. Accurately weigh or measure each ingredient.
3. Mix the triethanolamine lauryl sulfate and polyoxyl 8 stearate in sufficient warm purified water to volume, and mix well.
4. Package and label the product.

Cream Shampoo

Sodium lauryl sulfate	85 g	Emulsifier
Polyoxyl 8 stearate	5 g	Emulsifier
Magnesium stearate	2 g	Thickener
Purified water	68 g	Vehicle

1. Calculate the required quantity of each ingredient for the total amount to be prepared.
2. Accurately weigh or measure each ingredient.
3. Mix the sodium lauryl sulfate, polyoxyl 8 stearate, and magnesium stearate in warm purified water, and mix well.
4. Package and label the product.

Typical Shampoo Formulation

Ammonium lauryl sulfate	10%–20%	Cleanser
Lauramide DEA	3%–5%	Foam stabilizer
Methylparaben	0.08%	Preservative
Propylparaben	0.05%	Preservative
Sodium chloride	0.5–1.5%	Thickener
Disodium EDTA	0.2%	Sequestrant
Fragrance	0.5%	Fragrance
FD&C Yellow No. 5	0.001%	Coloring Agent
D&C Orange No. 4	0.002%	Coloring Agent
Purified water	qs 100%	Vehicle

1. Calculate the required quantity of each ingredient for the total amount to be prepared.
2. Accurately weigh or measure each ingredient.
3. Heat purified water, with agitation, to about 60°C–70°C.
4. Add the ammonium lauryl sulfate, lauramide DEA, methylparaben, propylparaben, sodium chloride, disodium EDTA, FD&C Yellow No. 5, and D&C Orange No. 4, and mix well.
5. Cool the mixture, add the fragrance, and mix until uniform.
6. Package and label the product.

Deodorants

Deodorant Stick

Alcohol	56 mL	Vehicle/Cosolvent
Purified water	4 mL	Vehicle
Propylene glycol	5 g	Vehicle/Cosolvent
Sodium stearate	4.25 g	Vehicle/Stiffener
Perfume	0.2 g	Perfume
Bacteriostatic agent	qs as appropriate	Preservative

1. Calculate the required quantity of each ingredient for the total amount to be prepared.
2. Accurately weigh or measure each ingredient.
3. Heat the propylene glycol and sodium stearate to low heat, and mix well.
4. Add the purified water and the alcohol (to which the perfume, if used, is added), and mix well.
5. The bacteriostatic agent can be dissolved in either the alcohol or water phase, as appropriate.
6. Pour the mixture into molds, and allow to cool.
7. Package and label the product.

Liquid Deodorant/Antiperspirant

Alcohol	14 g	Vehicle/Cosolvent
Purified water	71.75 g	Vehicle
Glycerin	6 g	Vehicle/Cosolvent
Aluminum chloride	8 g	Active
Perfume	qs as appropriate	Perfume
Antibacterial agent	qs	Preservative

1. Calculate the required quantity of each ingredient for the total amount to be prepared.
2. Accurately weigh or measure each ingredient.
3. Dissolve the aluminum chloride in the purified water.
4. Mix the alcohol, glycerin, and perfume together.
5. Add the aluminum chloride solution (step 3) to the alcohol solution (step 4) slowly with mixing.
6. The antibacterial agent can be added to the appropriate phase before mixing.
7. Mix well.
8. Package and label the product.

 Deodorant Stick—Alcohol Based

Purified water	16%	Vehicle/Solvent
Ethanol	75.5%	Vehicle/Cosolvent
Deodorizer	1%	Active
Sodium stearate	6.5%	Thickener
Fragrance	1%	Fragrance

1. Calculate the required quantity of each ingredient for the total amount to be prepared.
2. Accurately weigh or measure each ingredient.
3. Heat the purified water and ethanol, while stirring, to about 50°C–60°C.
4. Add the deodorizer and sodium stearate, and mix well.
5. Cool the mixture, add the fragrance while the mixture is still pourable, and mix until uniform.
6. Pour the mixture into molds, and allow to cool.
7. Package and label the product.

Deodorant Stick—Propylene Glycol Based

Purified water	3%	Vehicle/Solvent
Propylene glycol	10%	Vehicle/Cosolvent
Deodorizer	1%	Active
Sodium stearate	8%	Vehicle/Thickener
PPG-3 myristyl ether	77%	Emollient
Fragrance	1%	Fragrance

1. Calculate the required quantity of each ingredient for the total amount to be prepared.
2. Accurately weigh or measure each ingredient.
3. Heat the water and propylene glycol, while stirring, to about 60°C–70°C.
4. Add the deodorizer, sodium stearate, and PPG-3 myristyl ether, and mix well.
5. Cool the mixture, add the fragrance while the mixture is still pourable, and mix until uniform.
6. Pour the mixture into molds, and allow to cool.
7. Package and label the product.

Shaving Products

Shave Cream (Brushless) 1

Stearic acid	12 g	Thickener
Cetyl alcohol	2 g	Emulsifier
Castor oil	2 g	Emollient
Mineral oil, light	2 g	Vehicle/Emollient
Lanolin	3 g	Emollient
Tween 60	3 g	Emulsifier
Span 60	1 g	Emulsifier
Triethanolamine	1 g	Alkalizer
Purified water	qs 100 g	Vehicle

1. Calculate the required quantity of each ingredient for the total amount to be prepared.
2. Accurately weigh or measure each ingredient.
3. Melt the stearic acid, cetyl alcohol, Tween 60, and Span 60, using low heat, and incorporate the castor oil, light mineral oil, and lanolin.
4. Heat the purified water and triethanolamine to the same temperature.
5. Mix the purified water mixture (step 4) with the stearic acid mixture (step 3), using mechanical agitation, until a nice smooth cream forms.
6. Package and label the product.

Shave Cream (Brushless) 2

Stearic acid	16 g	Thickener
Lanolin	4 g	Emollient
Span 60	1 g	Emulsifier
Tween 60	3 g	Emulsifier
Propylene glycol monostearate	6 g	Emulsifier
Corn oil	2 g	Vehicle
Glycerin	2 g	Cosolvent
Triethanolamine	1 g	Alkalizer
Purified water	qs 100 g	Vehicle

1. Calculate the required quantity of each ingredient for the total amount to be prepared.
2. Accurately weigh or measure each ingredient.
3. Melt the stearic acid and lanolin together using low heat.
4. Incorporate the propylene glycol monostearate, corn oil, glycerin, and Span 60.
5. Heat the purified water, triethanolamine, and Tween 60 together to the same temperature.
6. Mix the stearic acid mixture (step 3) with the purified water mixture (step 4), and mix until a smooth cream forms.
7. Package and label the product.

Aerosol Shave Foam

Potassium hydroxide	0.44 g	pH Adjustment
Triethanolamine	2.98 g	pH Adjustment
Glycerin	5 g	Humectant
Polysorbate 20	1 g	Surfactant
Mineral oil	1.5 g	Emollient
Coconut acid	0.7 g	Surfactant
Stearic acid	8 g	Surfactant
Preservative	qs	Preservative
Fragrance	qs	Fragrance
Propane/butane/isobutene	4 g	Propellant
Purified water	qs 100 g	Solvent

1. Calculate the required quantity of each ingredient for the total amount to be prepared.
2. Accurately weigh or measure each ingredient.
3. Add the purified water, potassium hydroxide, triethanolamine, glycerin, and polysorbate 20 to a mixing vessel, mix well, and heat to 75°C.
4. In a separate vessel, add mineral oil, coconut acid, and stearic acid, heat to 75°C, and mix until uniform.
5. Add hot oil phase (step 4) to hot aqueous phase (step 3) while stirring.
6. Continue stirring, and cool the mixture to 45°C.
7. Add the preservative, and mix until dissolved.
8. Add the fragrance, stirring until uniformly dispersed.
9. Correct for water loss, fill the mixture into aerosol can, and secure valve.
10. Add propellant through valve.
11. Package and label the product.

Mouthwash

 ### Astringent Mouthwash

Sodium chloride	2.5 g	Tonicity Adjuster
Zinc chloride	0.5 g	Active
Menthol	0.05 g	Active
Alcohol	9.6 g	Solvent
Glycerin	10 g	Cosolvent
Cinnamon oil	0.1 g	Flavoring
Purified water	qs 100 g	Vehicle

1. Calculate the required quantity of each ingredient for the total amount to be prepared.
2. Accurately weigh or measure each ingredient.
3. Dissolve the zinc chloride and sodium chloride in the purified water.
4. Mix the alcohol, glycerin, menthol, and cinnamon oil together.
5. Add the aqueous solution (step 3) to the alcohol solution (step 4) slowly with mixing.
6. Package and label the product.

Eye Formulations

 ### Anhydrous Mascara Basic Formulation

Solvent(s)	40%–60%
Waxes	10%–20%
Resin(s)	3%–10%
Gellant	3%–7%
Colorant(s)	5%–15%
Filler(s)	2%–10%
Polar additive	qs

1. Calculate the required quantity of each ingredient for the total amount to be prepared.
2. Accurately weigh or measure each ingredient.
3. Heat the waxes, solvents, and resins in a jacketed kettle using low heat until uniform and clear.
4. Slowly add the colorants under high shear, and mill until a uniform dispersion is obtained.
5. Under high shear, add gellant, and mill until uniform.
6. Activate gellant with polar additive like propylene carbonate.
7. Under high shear, add fillers, and mill until uniform.
8. Cool the mixture to desired temperature.
9. Package and label the product.

Cream Eye Shadow Basic Formulation

Solvents	35%–55%
Gellant	1.5%–3.5%
Waxes	7%–12%
Emollients	3%–8%
Colorants/pearls	5%–20%
Fillers	10%–20%
Functional fillers	5%–15%
Polar additive	qs

1. Calculate the required quantity of each ingredient for the total amount to be prepared.
2. Accurately weigh or measure each ingredient.
3. Heat the waxes, solvents, and emollients in a jacketed kettle using low heat until uniform and clear.
4. Slowly add the colorants/pearls under high shear, and mill until a uniform dispersion is obtained.
5. Under high shear, add gellant, and mill until uniform.
6. Activate gellant with polar additive like propylene carbonate.
7. Under high shear, add fillers and functional fillers, and mill until uniform.
8. Cool the mixture to desired temperature.
9. Package and label the product.

 Eyeliner Basic Formulation

Purified water	50%–70%
Gellant	0.5%–1.5%
Wetting agent(s)	1%–3%
Polyol	4%–8%
Colorants	10%–20%
Alcohol	5%–10%
Film former	3%–8%

1. Calculate the required quantity of each ingredient for the total amount to be prepared.
2. Accurately weigh or measure each ingredient.
3. Mix the gellant with the polyol, and add to a heated water phase containing the wetting agent.
4. Disperse with a high shear until uniform.
5. Add colorants, and disperse until uniform.
6. Cool the mixture, and add alcohol and film former with low shear.
7. Package and label the product.

References

1. Butler H. Historical background. In: Butler H, ed. *Poucher's Perfumes, Cosmetics and Soaps.* 9th ed. London: Chapman & Hall; 1993:639–92.
2. U.S. Food and Drug Administration. FDA authority over cosmetics. August 3, 2013. Available at: www.fda.gov/Cosmetics/GuidanceRegulation/LawsRegulations/ucm074162.htm. Accessed October 17, 2015.
3. U.S. Food and Drug Administration. Is it a cosmetic, a drug, or both? (or is it soap?). Available at: www.fda.gov/Cosmetics/GuidanceRegulation/LawsRegulations/ucm074201.htm. Accessed October 17, 2015.
4. U.S. Food and Drug Administration. How to report problems with products regulated by FDA. December 18, 2006. Available at: www.cfsan.fda.gov/~dms/coscom00.html. Accessed November 9, 2011.
5. United States Pharmacopeial Convention. Chapter <795>, Pharmaceutical compounding—nonsterile preparations. In: *United States Pharmacopeia/National Formulary.* Rockville, MD: United States Pharmacopeial Convention; current edition.

Chapter 32

Compounding for Terrorist Attacks and Natural Disasters

As incidents of terrorism become more common, pharmacists and other health care professionals must plan for a possible domestic terrorist attack involving biological, chemical, or nuclear weapons. Federal, state, and local agencies must have the knowledge, intelligence, training, and supplies to counter this threat. Pharmacists have a unique role to perform in providing needed pharmaceuticals and information to their communities, and they should be involved in a community's planning for response to bioterrorist or terrorist attacks.

Preparedness

An effective response to bioterrorism will require prepared, well-trained local responders who can interact with state and federal agencies. Training for responders should cover the characteristics of biological and nonbiological agents that can be used in destruction. Pharmacists should be trained in their duties as responders, and they should be protected in the event of an attack so they can perform those duties. Security of the pharmacy may be a top concern, because break-ins to obtain medications may occur.

Although the threat of terrorist attacks has grown in recent years, natural disasters such as floods, hurricanes, and tornadoes are a recurring cause of mass destruction. For these situations, too, pharmacists should be involved in local disaster planning.

Even small communities must be prepared to handle a mass-casualty incident until state and federal assistance arrives. In such circumstances, health care providers must manage many patients who require urgent care, and pharmacists are likely to be pressed into action to deliver the medications needed to save lives; relieve pain; and limit potential damage from exposure to caustic, infectious, or other harmful agents. Pharmacists may be involved in treating not only patients suffering from exposure to nerve gas, biological weapons, or trauma, but also victims of a bombing.

Pharmacies' maintenance of just-in-time inventory works against an adequate response to disasters and terrorism. Competition for limited resources could challenge the ability to maintain civic order. Pharmacists involved in an emergency situation may find that providing information is relatively simple but providing pharmaceuticals is more difficult, because pharmacies routinely stock commercially available products in limited quantities only. Many pharmacists can compound some preparations to help fill the need until commercial stocks are replenished. Compounding pharmacists can provide various dosage forms to all types of patients.

Causative Agents

Terrorists may use chemical agents, including blistering agents (lewisite, mustard gas, phosgene oxime), choking agents, nerve agents (mustard gas, sarin gas, soman, tabun, VX), and cyanide. Biological agents used as weapons may include bacteria (e.g., those causing anthrax, brucellosis, plague, Q fever, and tularemia), toxins (e.g., botulinum toxin, ricin, and staphylococcal enterotoxin B), and viruses (e.g., those causing smallpox, Lassa fever, Rift Valley fever, and Venezuelan equine encephalomyelitis).

Genetic engineering is expanding the list of potential agents for use in terrorism. Novel forms of agents, including multidrug-resistant organisms, may be made available in vast quantities.

Biological agents may be disseminated through the use of conventional explosives or aerosol generators (aircraft, cruise missiles, mail) or through contamination of the food or water supply. Exposure may occur by the pulmonary (plague, Q fever, staphylococcal enterotoxin B) or systemic (botulinum toxin, viruses) route or through person-to-person (smallpox, pneumonic plague) or vector (plague, Rift Valley fever) contact.

Chemical Agents

The availability, extreme toxicity, and rapid onset of action of many chemical agents have made them desirable to terrorists. Agents of chemical warfare are commonly classified as blood agents (cyanogen chloride, hydrogen cyanide), nerve agents (sarin, soman, tabun), lung agents (diphosgene, phosgene), or blister agents (lewisite, mustard).

Blood Agents
Blood agents produce their effects by interfering with oxygen use at the cellular level. Certain types of cyanide are referred to as blood agents. Nitrite is the common ingredient used to displace cyanide from the oxygen that carries hemoglobin after contact with a blood agent has occurred. Other pharmaceuticals that serve as adjunctive therapy for cyanide poisoning are injectable sodium bicarbonate, which can correct metabolic acidosis, and benzodiazepines (e.g., diazepam or lorazepam), which are used as anticonvulsants. Formulations that counteract the effects of blood agents include (1) sodium nitrite 3% injection, (2) sodium thiosulfate 25% injection, (3) sodium bicarbonate 8.4% injection, (4) diazepam 5 mg/mL injection, and (5) lorazepam 2 mg sublingual tablets.

Nerve Agents
Nerve agents are organophosphorus cholinesterase inhibitors. They inhibit the enzyme acetylcholinesterase. Chemotherapeutic intervention consists of the use of three antidotal agents: atropine sulfate, which blocks muscarinic receptor sites; pralidoxime chloride, which regenerates cholinesterase activity; and diazepam or lorazepam, both of which are used as anticonvulsants. Topical ophthalmic homatropine or atropine can be used to relieve

dim vision, pain, and possible nausea. Formulations to counteract the effects of nerve agents include (1) pralidoxime chloride injection (1 g vial), (2) atropine sulfate 1 mg/mL injection, and (3) diazepam 5 mg/mL injection.

Lung Agents

Chemical agents that attack lung tissue are also referred to as pulmonary agents or choking agents. They inflict injury on the respiratory tract, including the nose, throat, and especially the lungs. Victims typically inhale these agents, which can all lead to pulmonary edema and respiratory failure. These agents include chlorine and phosgene, deadly and unpredictable gases that were used in World War I. Because they have many industrial applications, pulmonary agents are readily available to terrorists in large quantities. No specific antidotes exist for these lung and eye irritants, but supportive care may include the use of bronchodilators such as nebulized albuterol sulfate or sodium bicarbonate. Methylprednisolone acetate injection also has been used as supportive therapy to counteract the effects of these agents. Formulations that counteract the effects of pulmonary agents include (1) albuterol sulfate 0.5% inhalation solution, (2) sodium bicarbonate 3.75% inhalation solution, and (3) methylprednisolone acetate 40 mg/mL injection.

Blister Agents

Blister agents, or vesicants, are potent alkylating agents that produce scarring blisters, eye damage, and airway damage. They include lewisite, nitrogen mustard, and phosgene oxime. Treatment may include the application of topical silver sulfadiazine or topical mafenide acetate. Only one blister agent, lewisite, has an antidotal compound (dimercaprol), which acts as a chelating agent for arsenicals and other heavy metals. Dimercaprol skin and eye ointment applied to victims after decontamination may reduce the severity of lesions. Dimercaptosuccinic acid has been used successfully in animals for the treatment of lewisite exposure and lead ingestion. Available in 100 mg capsules, dimercaptosuccinic acid can be administered orally to treat multiple exposures to blister agents. Formulations that counteract the effects of blister agents include (1) silver sulfadiazine cream, (2) mafenide acetate cream, (3) dimercaprol injection, (4) dimercaprol ointment, and (5) dimercaptosuccinic acid 100 mg capsules.

Biological Agents

Biological terrorism could involve sophisticated or unsophisticated techniques (i.e., use of dried anthrax spores or botulinum toxins or use of *Salmonella* or other common bacteria, respectively). Unlike chemical nerve agents, which can cause immediate death or severe injury at the site of attack, biological agents cause delayed signs and symptoms because of their incubation periods. If used against unsuspecting, nonimmune civilian populations, biological weapons could enable terrorists to cause a large number of casualties and create international panic.

In the event of an attack, frontline clinicians and primary care practitioners will need to identify and manage exposed patients. Pharmacists will need to be knowledgeable about diseases caused by biological agents and about patient management, vaccines, and potential chemotherapeutic agents, so that they can educate the public and other health care practitioners.

Many oral and injectable medications, in extraordinarily large amounts, may be needed to treat an outbreak of illness caused by a biological weapon. Pharmaceutical needs will depend on the duration of illness, the virulence of an outbreak of disease, and the number of patients affected. Uncommonly used vaccines and antitoxins should be prepositioned with the assistance of federal government storage and distribution programs.

Nuclear Agents

Dirty bombs, conventional explosives used to spread hazardous radioactive material, might be involved in a terrorist attack. Radioactive materials can emit three types of harmful radiation: α (alpha), β (beta), and γ (gamma). Inhalation or ingestion of α or β particles poses the greatest hazard. The most harmful type overall, γ rays, can penetrate most sheltering material in a wide area.

Exposure to a harmful radiological agent may require treatment with a chelator or a radionuclide blocker. Some general radionuclide chelating agents are penicillamine (Cuprimine), edetate calcium disodium (Calcium Disodium Versenate), dimercaprol (British anti-Lewisite, or BAL), succimer (Chemet), and deferoxamine (Desferal). (Colony-stimulating factors may be considered in patients experiencing significant bone-marrow suppression.) Information about this specialized class of drugs can be obtained 24 hours a day from the Radiation Emergency Assistance Center/Training Site (http://orise.orau.gov/reacts/), telephone 865-576-3131, or 865-576-1005 for emergencies.

A variation of radionuclide chelation to entrap and remove the radioactive agent is the use of radionuclide-blocking agents. These agents saturate tissues with a nonradioactive element that reduces the uptake of radioactive iodine. The most commonly known radionuclide-blocking agents are potassium iodide tablets and Lugol's solution, both of which reduce the uptake of radioactive iodine by thyroid tissue.

Pharmacists' Involvement during the Emergency

Pharmacists' involvement in disaster planning is the first step in preparing for a terrorist attack. A formulary should be developed to include primary and secondary treatments for the effects of chemical, biological, and nuclear weapons. Variables in the dosing of antibiotics, antitoxins, vaccines, and prophylactic treatments for adolescent and pediatric patients should not be overlooked. The use of chemotherapeutics (and their respective teratogenic effects) in pregnant patients should be noted in each treatment protocol. Because a chemical, biological, or nuclear attack will create drug shortages, pharmacists should have preplanned procedures for rationing and agreements for support from a network of pharmacies.

Pharmacists can also provide valuable information when the agent used in an attack may not be clear, such as in an unusual outbreak of infections. Because they usually see hundreds of patients daily, pharmacists can help detect unusual occurrences that might be related to bioterrorism. For example, pharmacists might observe cases of a disease that is not endemic, unusual patterns of antibiotic resistance, atypical clinical presentations, case distribution in a certain geographic region, unusually high numbers of cases, and morbidity and mortality rates that deviate from the baseline.

After a terrorist incident occurs, pharmacists working with limited assets will be asked to provide medications in a very short time. In preparation for this situation, pharmacists should maintain current, accurate information on product procurement and manufacturing options. Self-reliant and adaptable, compounding pharmacists can provide drug treatment alternatives to lessen the damage from an attack. Formulations and procedures for extemporaneous compounding must be created, reviewed, and tested before an emergency occurs. Preestablished reference publications, bulk materials, source information, and pharmaceutical items (antibiotics, antidotes, antitoxins, other supportive-care agents) will facilitate hands-on training in the treatment of victims of biological, chemical, or nuclear attacks. In addition to providing pharmaceuticals, pharmacists can disseminate supplies such as gloves, gowns, masks, and respirators; provide information about dosages and vaccination schedules; and counsel patients.

Assistance is available from the federal government's Strategic National Stockpile, which has prepared "12-hour push packages" for immediate response. These caches of pharmaceuticals, antidotes, and medical supplies are designed to provide a broad range of items that may be needed in the early hours after an event. The packages are positioned in strategically located secure warehouses for deployment to designated sites within 12 hours of a federal decision to distribute these assets. The push packages contain bulk-packaged dosage forms such as tablets; there may be several hundred thousand in a drum, and they will need to be packaged into units for distribution to patients.

Critical Logistic Needs

A terrorist event might result in curtailment of travel and shipping, impeding the availability of pharmaceuticals and possibly leading to rationing. Plans should be in place for security of the pharmacy, pharmacists, and other personnel such as trained technicians. During a disaster, armed guards may need to be posted at pharmacies.

Disaster planning might include the following steps:

1. Determine the needs of your pharmacy and community (and your own family).
2. Ensure that the pharmacy is involved in planning with the local government and health care system.
3. Install a water purification system to provide an uninterrupted supply of water for the pharmacy.
4. Establish and maintain close communication with authorities.
5. Develop an emergency distribution system for pharmaceuticals within your service area.
6. Work in advance with the state board of pharmacy; certain state laws may need to be relaxed during the emergency.
7. Establish a reasonable stock of bulk drug substances and supplies for compounding. Bulk drug substances can be easily and rapidly formulated into various dosage forms for all age groups.
8. Make plans for the security of the pharmacy.

Compounded and Manufactured Treatments after a Disaster

Pharmaceuticals may be needed for decontamination, prophylaxis, or treatment, depending on the causative agents and the timing involved. Decontamination might involve a number of preparations (e.g., sodium hypochlorite solutions), depending on the agents used. Vaccines are available for anthrax, botulism, cholera, plague, Q fever, smallpox, tularemia, viral encephalitides, and the viral hemorrhagic fevers. Treatment is specific to the agent used. Treatment after attacks with chemical agents (poisons) might include (1) use of antagonists that compete with the poison for receptor sites, (2) use of compounds that inhibit the poison by reacting with it to form less active or inactive complexes or by interfering with its metabolism, (3) use of chelating agents, (4) use of agents that block essential receptors and thereby mediate the toxic effects, (5) use of compounds that reduce the rate of conversion of the poison to a more toxic compound, (6) induction of emesis, and (7) routine symptomatic treatment. Commonly used agents include BAL, dimercaptopropanesulfonate, dimercaptosuccinic acid, sodium nitrite, and sodium thiosulfate.

The ability to prepare a wide variety of dosage forms in response to an attack is important. All members of an affected community may need to be treated, and this will require various routes of administration and dosage forms, depending on the drugs involved. Preparation of enemas, nasal preparations (local and systemic), oral liquids, oral solids (capsules, tablets, troches), ophthalmics, parenterals, solutions for inhalation, suppositories, and topicals will be important.

Dosage forms that may be required for various age groups include the following:

- *Neonates:* Enemas, injections, oral inhalations, oral liquids, suppositories
- *Infants:* Enemas, injections, oral inhalations, oral liquids, suppositories
- *Young pediatric patients:* Enemas, injections, oral inhalations, oral liquids, suppositories, topicals
- *Older pediatric patients:* Enemas, injections, oral inhalations, oral liquids, oral solids, suppositories, topicals
- *Adults:* Enemas, injections, oral inhalations, oral liquids, oral solids, suppositories, topicals
- *Geriatric patients:* Enemas, injections, oral inhalations, oral liquids, oral solids, suppositories, topicals

Regulatory and Quality Control

An emergency situation may require the relaxation of certain restrictions on the practice of pharmacy, including pharmacy compounding. State boards of pharmacy may want to determine in advance which regulations can be eased immediately after an event to allow timely provision of pharmaceutical preparations and services.

Relatively simple standard quality control measures can still be performed during the crisis, including physical assessment (observations), weight, volume, pH, and specific gravity.

Stability Considerations

Stability must be considered even in an emergency situation when drug preparations are likely to be for immediate and short-term use. Stability is the extent to which a preparation retains, within specified limits, and throughout its period of storage and use, the same properties and characteristics that it possessed at the time of its preparation. Factors that affect the stability of drugs and dosage forms include pH, temperature, solvent, light, air (oxygen, carbon dioxide, moisture), humidity, and particle size.

Pharmacists should observe compounded drug preparations for signs of instability. Chemical, physical, microbiological, therapeutic, and toxicological stability should be addressed. A preparation is chemically stable if each active ingredient retains its chemical integrity and labeled potency within the specified limits. It is physically stable if the original physical properties, including appearance, palatability, uniformity, dissolution, and suspendability, are retained. It is microbiologically stable if sterility or resistance to microbial growth is retained according to the specific requirements; antimicrobial agents that are present retain their effectiveness within the specified limits. The preparation is therapeutically stable if its therapeutic effect remains unchanged and toxicologically stable if no significant increase in toxicity occurs.

The beyond-use date, or period during which a compounded preparation is usable after dispensing, should be based on available stability information and reasonable patient needs with respect to the intended drug therapy. When a commercial drug product is used as a source of active ingredient, its expiration date often can be used in determining the beyond-use date. Other factors to be considered include the nature of the drug and its degradation kinetics, the container in which it is packaged, the storage conditions to which it may be exposed, the expected length of therapy, the expiration dating of similar commercial products if the active ingredient is a *United States Pharmacopeia* or *National Formulary* product, and published and manufacturers' literature. (Chapter 6 of this book provides guidelines for assigning a beyond-use date to compounded medications.)

Suggested Formulations

Use against Biological Agents

℞ **Amoxicillin 250 mg Troches (#24)**

Amoxicillin trihydrate	6 g	Active
Citric acid	600 mg	Acidifier
Sodium saccharin	65 mg	Sweetener
Stevia powder	500 mg	Sweetener
Silica gel	240 mg	Suspending Agent
Acacia powder	400 mg	Demulcent/Texture
Polyethylene glycol 1450	18 g	Vehicle
Flavoring	qs	Flavoring

1. Calculate the quantity of each ingredient required for the prescription.
2. Accurately weigh the required quantity of each ingredient or obtain the required number of dosage units.
3. Blend the amoxicillin trihydrate, citric acid, sodium saccharin, stevia powder, silica gel, and acacia powder together until uniformly mixed.
4. Heat the polyethylene glycol 1450 until melted at approximately 70°C.
5. Add the powder mix (step 3) to the melted base (step 4), and blend thoroughly.
6. Cool the mixture to less than 55°C, add the flavoring, and mix well.
7. Pour the mixture into troche or cough drop molds, and allow to cool.
8. Package and label the product.

(Note: The quantity of polyethylene glycol may need to be adjusted, depending on the size of the mold used.)

℞ Amoxicillin 125 mg Suppositories (#12)

Amoxicillin trihydrate	1.5 g	Active
Isopropyl myristate	750 mg	Emulsifier/Wetting Agent
Silica gel	180 mg	Suspending Agent
Fatty acid base	qs	Active

1. Calculate the quantity of each ingredient required for the prescription.
2. Accurately weigh the required quantity of each ingredient or obtain the required number of dosage units.
3. Blend the amoxicillin trihydrate and silica gel together until uniformly mixed.
4. Carefully heat the fatty acid base to about 35°C–37°C, being careful not to overheat.
5. Add the isopropyl myristate, and mix well.
6. Sprinkle the amoxicillin trihydrate–silica gel powder blend (step 3) onto the melted base (step 5), and mix thoroughly.
7. Remove the mixture from heat, and pour into molds that are at room temperature, not chilled.
8. Once the pouring has started, do not stop. If reusable molds are used, allow a small quantity of the melt to bead up on the back of the suppository to allow for contraction.
9. Place the suppositories in a refrigerator to harden.
10. Remove the suppositories from refrigerator, and allow to set at room temperature for a few minutes.
11. Trim the suppositories, and package. If reusable molds are used, trim the suppositories, remove from molds, wrap if desired, and package.
12. Label the product.

℞ Chloramphenicol 250 mg Capsules (#100)

Chloramphenicol	25 g	Active
Lactose	11.4 g	Diluent/Vehicle

1. Calculate the quantity of each ingredient required for the prescription.
2. Accurately weigh the required quantity of each ingredient or obtain the required number of dosage units.
3. Reduce the particle size of the chloramphenicol and lactose, if necessary, and mix the powders well.
4. Fill each of 100 No. 1 capsules with 364 mg of the powder mix. (Note: The quantity of lactose per capsule may need to be altered, depending on the bulk density of the lactose being used.)
5. Check the weights of the capsules.
6. Package and label the product.

℞ Chloramphenicol 150 mg/5 mL Suspension

Chloramphenicol palmitate	5.22 g	Active
Glycerin	qs	Levigating Agent
Flavored syrup	50 mL	Vehicle
Methylcellulose 1% gel	qs 100 mL	Vehicle

1. Calculate the quantity of each ingredient required for the prescription.
2. Accurately weigh the required quantity of each ingredient or obtain the required number of dosage units.
3. Pulverize the chloramphenicol palmitate until uniform.
4. In a mortar, wet the powder with glycerin and mix to obtain a thick, smooth paste.
5. Add the flavored syrup, and mix well.
6. Slowly add the methylcellulose 1% solution geometrically to volume, with thorough mixing after each addition.
7. Package and label the product.

℞ Cidofovir Suppositories (#12)

Cidofovir	qs	Active
Isopropyl myristate	750 mg	Emulsifying/Wetting Agent
Silica gel	180 mg	Suspending Agent
Fatty acid base	qs	Vehicle

1. Calculate the quantity of each ingredient required for the prescription.
2. Accurately weigh the required quantity of each ingredient or obtain the required number of dosage units.
3. Blend the cidofovir and silica gel together until uniformly mixed.
4. Carefully heat the fatty acid base to about 35°C–37°C, being careful not to overheat.
5. Add the isopropyl myristate, and mix well.
6. Sprinkle the cidofovir–silica gel powder blend (step 3) onto the melted base (step 5), and mix thoroughly.
7. Remove the mixture from heat, and pour into molds that are at room temperature, not chilled.
8. Once the pouring has started, do not stop. If reusable molds are used, allow a small quantity of the melt to bead up on the back of the suppository to allow for contraction.
9. Place the suppositories in a refrigerator to harden.
10. Remove the suppositories from refrigerator, and allow to set at room temperature for a few minutes.
11. Trim the suppositories, and package. If reusable molds are used, trim the suppositories, remove from molds, wrap if desired, and package.
12. Label the product.

℞ Ciprofloxacin Oral Suspension

Ciprofloxacin tablets	qs	Active
Stevia powder	500 mg	Sweetener
Xanthan gum	500 mg	Thickening Agent
Glycerin	qs	Levigating Agent
Flavoring	qs	Flavoring
Simple syrup	qs 100 mL	Vehicle

1. Calculate the quantity of each ingredient required for the prescription.
2. Accurately weigh the required quantity of each ingredient or obtain the required number of dosage units.
3. If capsules are the source of the ciprofloxacin, empty the capsules and pulverize their contents and the stevia powder, dry flavoring (if used), and xanthan gum until uniform.
4. In a mortar, wet the powders with glycerin and mix to obtain a thick, smooth paste.
5. Slowly add the simple syrup and flavoring (if liquid), geometrically to volume, with thorough mixing after each addition.
6. Pour the mixture into a graduated cylinder.
7. Package and label the product.

℞ Clindamycin Hydrochloride 150 mg Capsules (#100)

Clindamycin hydrochloride	16.35 g	Active
Lactose	23.2 g	Diluent/Vehicle

1. Calculate the quantity of each ingredient required for the prescription.
2. Accurately weigh the required quantity of each ingredient or obtain the required number of dosage units.
3. Reduce the particle size of the clindamycin hydrochloride and lactose, if necessary, and mix the powders well.
4. Fill each of 100 No. 1 capsules with 396 mg of the powder mix. (Note: The quantity of lactose per capsule may need to be altered, depending on the bulk density of the lactose being used.)
5. Check the weights of the capsules.
6. Package and label the product.

℞ **Clindamycin 150 mg Capsules (#100)**

Clindamycin phosphate	18 g	Active
Lactose	17.5 g	Diluent/Vehicle

1. Calculate the quantity of each ingredient required for the prescription.
2. Accurately weigh the required quantity of each ingredient or obtain the required number of dosage units.
3. Reduce the particle size of the clindamycin phosphate and lactose, if necessary, and mix the powders well.
4. Fill each of 100 No. 1 capsules with 355 mg of the powder mix. (Note: The quantity of lactose per capsule may need to be altered, depending on the bulk density of the lactose being used.)
5. Check the weights of the capsules.
6. Package and label the product.

℞ **Clindamycin 10 mg/mL Oral Suspension**

Clindamycin palmitate	1.65 g	Active
Stevia powder	500 mg	Sweetener
Saccharin sodium	100 mg	Sweetener
Acesulfame potassium	500 mg	Sweetener
Purified water	40 mL	Vehicle
Chocolate syrup	qs 100 mL	Vehicle

1. Calculate the quantity of each ingredient required for the prescription.
2. Accurately weigh the required quantity of each ingredient or obtain the required number of dosage units.
3. If clindamycin capsules are the source of the drug, empty the capsules and pulverize the powder until uniform.
4. In a mortar, add the stevia powder, saccharin sodium, and acesulfame potassium, followed by the purified water, and mix to obtain a thick, smooth paste.
5. Slowly add the chocolate syrup, geometrically to volume, with thorough mixing after each addition.
6. Package and label the product.

℞ Doxycycline Hydrochloride 100 mg Capsules (#100)

Doxycycline hydrochloride	10 g	Active
Avicel	15.5 g	Diluent/Vehicle

1. Calculate the quantity of each ingredient required for the prescription.
2. Accurately weigh the required quantity of each ingredient or obtain the required number of dosage units.
3. Reduce the particle size of the doxycycline hydrochloride and Avicel, if necessary, and mix the powders well.
4. Fill each of 100 capsules with 255 mg of the powder mix. (Note: The quantity of lactose per capsule may need to be altered, depending on the bulk density of the lactose and the size of the capsule being used.)
5. Check the weights of the capsules.
6. Package and label the product.

℞ Erythromycin 200 mg Troches (#24)

Erythromycin	4.8 g	Active
Xanthan gum	400 mg	Demulcent/Texture
Silica gel	240 mg	Suspending Agent
Stevia powder	600 mg	Sweetener
Citric acid	600 mg	Acidifier
Polyethylene glycol 1450	22.3 g	Vehicle
Flavoring	qs	Flavoring

1. Calculate the quantity of each ingredient required for the prescription.
2. Accurately weigh the required quantity of each ingredient or obtain the required number of dosage units.
3. Blend the erythromycin, xanthan gum, silica gel, stevia powder, and citric acid together until uniformly mixed.
4. Heat the polyethylene glycol 1450 until melted at approximately 70°C.
5. Add the powder mix (step 3) to the melted base (step 4), and blend thoroughly.
6. Cool the mixture to less than 55°C, add the flavoring, and mix well.
7. Pour the mixture into troche or cough drop molds, and allow to cool.
8. Package and label the product.

(Note: The quantity of polyethylene glycol may need to be adjusted, depending on the size of the mold used.)

℞ Erythromycin 250 mg Suppositories (#12)

Erythromycin	3 g	Active
Silica gel	300 mg	Suspending Agent
Isopropyl myristate	750 mg	Emulsifier/Wetting Agent
Fatty acid base	qs	Base

1. Calculate the quantity of each ingredient required for the prescription.
2. Accurately weigh the required quantity of each ingredient or obtain the required number of dosage units.
3. Blend the erythromycin and silica gel together until uniformly mixed.
4. Carefully heat the fatty acid base to about 35°C–37°C, being careful not to overheat.
5. Add the isopropyl myristate, and mix well.
6. Sprinkle the erythromycin–silica gel powder mix (step 3) onto the melted base (step 5), and mix thoroughly.
7. Remove the mixture from heat, and pour into molds that are at room temperature, not chilled.
8. Once the pouring has started, do not stop. If reusable molds are used, allow a small quantity of the melt to bead up on the back of the suppository to allow for contraction.
9. Place the suppositories in a refrigerator to harden.
10. Remove the suppositories from refrigerator, and allow to set at room temperature for a few minutes.
11. Trim the suppositories, and package. If reusable molds are used, trim the suppositories, remove from molds, wrap if desired, and package.
12. Label the product.

℞ Penicillin G Potassium 20,000,000 units/100 mL Injection

Penicillin G potassium	12.821 g	Active
Sterile water for injection	qs 100 mL	Vehicle

1. Calculate the quantity of each ingredient required for the prescription.
2. Accurately weigh the required quantity of each ingredient or obtain the required number of dosage units.
3. Dissolve the penicillin G potassium in sufficient sterile water for injection to volume, and mix well.
4. Filter the mixture through 0.22-μm sterile filters into sterile containers.
5. Package and label the product.

(Note: This is a sterile preparation and requires strict adherence to aseptic technique and procedures.)

℞ Penicillin G Potassium 1,000,000 units/10 mL Injection

Penicillin G potassium	1,000,000 units	Active
Citric acid/sodium citrate buffer	1 mL	Buffer
Citric acid 50% solution	qs	Acidifier
Sterile water for injection	qs 10 mL	Vehicle

(Note: The citric acid/sodium citrate buffer can be prepared by adding 23.5 mg citric acid and 615 mg sodium citrate to sufficient sterile water for injection to make 25 mL.)

1. Calculate the quantity of each ingredient required for the prescription.
2. Accurately weigh the required quantity of each ingredient or obtain the required number of dosage units.
3. Dissolve the penicillin G potassium in the citric acid/sodium citrate buffer and sufficient sterile water for injection to 95% of volume, and mix well.
4. Adjust the pH to 6.0 to 8.5 with citric acid solution if necessary.
5. Add sufficient sterile water for injection to final volume, and mix well.
6. Filter the mixture through 0.22-µm sterile filters into sterile containers.
7. Package and label the product.

(Note: This is a sterile preparation and requires strict adherence to aseptic technique and procedures.)

℞ Ribavirin 33 mg/mL Injection

Ribavirin	3.3 g	Active
Sodium chloride	460 mg	Tonicity
Sterile water for injection	qs 100 mL	Vehicle

1. Calculate the quantity of each ingredient required for the prescription.
2. Accurately weigh the required quantity of each ingredient or obtain the required number of dosage units.
3. Dissolve the ribavirin and sodium chloride in sufficient sterile water for injection to volume, and mix well.
4. Filter the mixture through 0.22-µm sterile filters into sterile containers.
5. Package and label the product.

(Note: This is a sterile preparation and requires strict adherence to aseptic technique and procedures.)

℞ Rifampin 10 mg/mL Oral Suspension

Rifampin	1 g	Active
Glycerin	qs	Levigating Agent
Ascorbic acid	100 mg	Acidifier
Xanthan gum	200 mg	Thickener
Strawberry flavoring	qs	Flavoring
Simple syrup	qs 100 mL	Vehicle

1. Calculate the quantity of each ingredient required for the prescription.
2. Accurately weigh the required quantity of each ingredient or obtain the required number of dosage units.
3. If capsules are the source of the rifampin, empty the capsules, and pulverize the powder until uniform.
4. In a mortar, add the ascorbic acid and xanthan gum, wet with glycerin, and mix to obtain a thick, smooth paste.
5. Slowly add the strawberry flavoring and simple syrup geometrically to volume, with thorough mixing after each addition.
6. Package and label the product.

℞ Rifampin 150 mg Capsules (#100)

Rifampin	15 g	Active
Lactose	16 g	Diluent/Vehicle

1. Calculate the quantity of each ingredient required for the prescription.
2. Accurately weigh the required quantity of each ingredient or obtain the required number of dosage units.
3. Reduce the particle size of the rifampin and lactose, if necessary, and mix the powders well.
4. Fill each of 100 No. 1 capsules with 310 mg of the powder mix. (Note: The quantity of lactose per capsule may need to be altered, depending on the bulk density of the lactose being used.)
5. Check the weights of the capsules.
6. Package and label the product.

℞ Rifampin 3 mg/mL Intravenous Infusion

Rifampin	300 mg	Active
Propylene glycol	10 mL	Cosolvent
Benzyl alcohol	2 mL	Preservative
Poloxamer 188	1 g	Thickener
Sterile water for injection	qs 100 mL	Vehicle

1. Calculate the quantity of each ingredient required for the prescription.
2. Accurately weigh the required quantity of each ingredient or obtain the required number of dosage units.
3. Mix the propylene glycol and benzyl alcohol together.
4. Add the rifampin, and mix well.
5. Add the poloxamer 188, and mix well.
6. Add sufficient sterile water for injection to volume, and mix well.
7. Filter the mixture through 0.22-μm sterile filters into sterile containers.
8. Package and label the product.

(Note: This is a sterile preparation and requires strict adherence to aseptic technique and procedures.)

℞ Streptomycin Sulfate 400 mg/mL Injection

Streptomycin sulfate equivalent	40 g	Active
Sodium citrate, anhydrous	1 g	Buffer
Phenol	250 mg	Preservative
Sodium metabisulfite	200 mg	Antioxidant
1 N Hydrochloric acid or		Acidifier
1 N Sodium hydroxide solution	qs	Alkalizer
Sterile water for injection	qs 100 mL	Vehicle

1. Calculate the quantity of each ingredient required for the prescription.
2. Accurately weigh the required quantity of each ingredient or obtain the required number of dosage units.
3. Dissolve the streptomycin sulfate equivalent, anhydrous sodium citrate, phenol, and sodium metabisulfite in about 95 mL of sterile water for injection.
4. Adjust the pH using either 1 N hydrochloric acid or 1 N sodium hydroxide solution to the pH range of 5 to 8.
5. Add sufficient sterile water for injection to volume, and mix well.
6. Filter the mixture through 0.22-μm sterile filters into sterile containers.
7. Package and label the product.

(Note: This is a sterile preparation and requires strict adherence to aseptic technique and procedures.)

℞ Tetracycline 125 mg/5 mL Syrup

Tetracycline hydrochloride	2.5 g	Active
Citric acid	100 mg	Buffer
Sodium citrate	100 mg	Buffer
Polysorbate 60	1.5 g	Surfactant
Flavoring	qs	Flavoring
Simple syrup	qs 100 mL	Vehicle

1. Calculate the quantity of each ingredient required for the prescription.
2. Accurately weigh the required quantity of each ingredient or obtain the required number of dosage units.
3. Add the tetracycline hydrochloride, citric acid, and sodium citrate to a mortar, and mix well.
4. Add the polysorbate 60, and mix to form a smooth paste.
5. Add the flavoring, and mix well.
6. Add sufficient simple syrup geometrically to volume, with thorough mixing after each addition.
7. Package and label the product.

℞ Tetracycline Hydrochloride 20 mg/mL Intravenous Injection

Tetracycline hydrochloride	2 g	Active
Ascorbic acid	5 g	Acidifier
Sterile water for injection	qs 100 mL	Vehicle

1. Calculate the quantity of each ingredient required for the prescription.
2. Accurately weigh the required quantity of each ingredient or obtain the required number of dosage units.
3. Dissolve the tetracycline hydrochloride and ascorbic acid in sufficient sterile water for injection to volume, and mix well.
4. Filter the mixture through 0.22-μm sterile filters into sterile containers.
5. Package and label the product.

(Note: This is a sterile preparation and requires strict adherence to aseptic technique and procedures.)

℞ Tetracycline Hydrochloride 250 mg Capsules (#100)

| Tetracycline hydrochloride | 25 g | Active |
| Lactose | 30 g | Diluent/Vehicle |

1. Calculate the quantity of each ingredient required for the prescription.
2. Accurately weigh the required quantity of each ingredient or obtain the required number of dosage units.
3. Reduce the particle size of the tetracycline hydrochloride and lactose, if necessary, and mix the powders well.
4. Fill each of 100 No. 0 capsules with 550 mg of the powder mix. (Note: The quantity of lactose per capsule may need to be altered, depending on the bulk density of the lactose being used.)
5. Check the weights of the capsules.
6. Package and label the product.

℞ Tetracycline Hydrochloride 250 mg Suppositories (#12)

Tetracycline hydrochloride	3 g	Active
Silica gel	300 mg	Suspending Agent
Fatty acid base	qs	Vehicle

1. Calculate the quantity of each ingredient required for the prescription.
2. Accurately weigh the required quantity of each ingredient or obtain the required number of dosage units.
3. Blend the tetracycline hydrochloride and silica gel together until uniformly mixed.
4. Carefully heat the fatty acid base to about 35°C–37°C, being careful not to overheat.
5. Sprinkle the tetracycline hydrochloride–silica gel powder blend (step 3) onto the melted base (step 4), and mix thoroughly.
6. Remove the mixture from heat, and pour into molds that are at room temperature, not chilled.
7. Once the pouring has started, do not stop. If reusable molds are used, allow a small quantity of the melt to bead up on the back of the suppository to allow for contraction.
8. Place the suppositories in a refrigerator to harden.
9. Remove the suppositories from refrigerator, and allow to set at room temperature for a few minutes.
10. Trim the suppositories, and package. If reusable molds are used, trim the suppositories, remove from molds, wrap if desired, and package.
11. Label the product.

℞ Vancomycin Hydrochloride 250 mg Capsules (#100)

Vancomycin hydrochloride	25 g	Active
Avicel PH-105	7.5 g	Diluent/Vehicle

1. Calculate the quantity of each ingredient required for the prescription.
2. Accurately weigh the required quantity of each ingredient or obtain the required number of dosage units.
3. Reduce the particle size of the vancomycin hydrochloride, if necessary; add the Avicel PH-105; and mix the powders well.
4. Fill each of 100 No. 1 capsules with 325 mg of the powder mix. (Note: The quantity of lactose per capsule may need to be altered, depending on the bulk density of the lactose being used.)
5. Check the weights of the capsules.
6. Package and label the product.

Use against Chemical Agents

℞ Albuterol 0.5% Inhalation Solution

Albuterol sulfate	600 mg	Active
Benzalkonium chloride 50% solution	0.003 mL	Preservative
Citric acid	100 mg	Acidifier
Sodium chloride	760 mg	Tonicity
Sterile water for inhalation	qs 100 mL	Vehicle

1. Calculate the quantity of each ingredient required for the prescription.
2. Accurately weigh the required quantity of each ingredient or obtain the required number of dosage units.
3. Dissolve the albuterol sulfate, benzalkonium chloride 50% solution, citric acid, and sodium chloride in sufficient sterile water for inhalation to volume, and mix well.
4. Filter the mixture through 0.22-μm sterile filters into sterile containers.
5. Package and label the product.

(Note: This is a sterile preparation and requires strict adherence to aseptic technique and procedures.)

℞ Dimercaptosuccinic Acid 250 mg Capsules (#100)

| Dimercaptosuccinic acid | 25 g | Active |
| Avicel PH-105 | 5.037 g | Diluent/Vehicle |

1. Calculate the quantity of each ingredient required for the prescription.
2. Accurately weigh the required quantity of each ingredient or obtain the required number of dosage units.
3. Reduce the particle size of the dimercaptosuccinic acid and Avicel PH-105, if necessary, and mix the powders well.
4. Fill each of 100 No. 1 capsules with 301 mg of the powder mix. (Note: The quantity of lactose per capsule may need to be altered, depending on the bulk density of the lactose being used.)
5. Check the weights of the capsules.
6. Package and label the product.

℞ Sodium Thiosulfate–Sodium Nitrite Solution

Sodium thiosulfate	30 g	Active
Sodium nitrite	2 g	Active
Purified water	qs 100 mL	Vehicle

1. Calculate the quantity of each ingredient required for the prescription.
2. Accurately weigh the required quantity of each ingredient or obtain the required number of dosage units.
3. Dissolve the sodium thiosulfate and sodium nitrite in sufficient purified water to volume, and mix well.
4. Package and label the product.

Use against Radiological Agents

℞ Potassium Iodide Saturated Solution

Potassium iodide	100 g	Active
Sodium thiosulfate	50 mg	Stabilizer
Purified water	qs 100 mL	Vehicle

1. Calculate the quantity of each ingredient required for the prescription.
2. Accurately weigh the required quantity of each ingredient or obtain the required number of dosage units.
3. Dissolve the potassium iodide and sodium thiosulfate in sufficient purified water to volume, and mix well.
4. Package and label the product.

General

℞ Lorazepam 2 mg Gelatin Troches (#24)

Lorazepam	48 mg	Active
Gelatin base	28 g	Vehicle
Silica gel	240 mg	Suspending Agent
Stevia powder	500 mg	Sweetener
Acacia powder	400 mg	Demulcent/Texture
Citric acid	480 mg	Acidifier
Flavoring	qs	Flavoring

1. Calculate the quantity of each ingredient required for the prescription.
2. Accurately weigh the required quantity of each ingredient or obtain the required number of dosage units.
3. Blend the lorazepam, silica gel, stevia powder, acacia powder, and citric acid together until uniformly mixed.
4. Heat the gelatin base until melted.
5. Add the powder mix (step 3) to the melted base (step 4), and blend thoroughly.
6. Cool the mixture slightly, add the flavoring, and mix well.
7. Pour the mixture into troche or cough drop molds, and allow to cool.
8. Package and label the product.

(Note: The quantity of the gelatin base may need to be adjusted, depending on the size of the mold used.)

℞ Lorazepam 2 mg Polyethylene Glycol Troches (#24)

Lorazepam	48 mg	Active
Stevia powder	480 mg	Sweetener
Silica gel	240 mg	Suspending Agent
Acacia powder	400 mg	Demulcent/Texture
Polyethylene glycol 1450	23.2 g	Vehicle
Flavoring concentrate	qs	Flavoring

1. Calculate the quantity of each ingredient required for the prescription.
2. Accurately weigh the required quantity of each ingredient or obtain the required number of dosage units.
3. Blend the lorazepam, stevia powder, silica gel, and acacia powder together until uniformly mixed.
4. Heat the polyethylene glycol 1450 until melted at approximately 70°C.
5. Add the powder mix (step 3) to the melted base (step 4), and blend thoroughly.
6. Cool the mixture to less than 55°C, add the flavoring, and mix well.
7. Pour the mixture into troche or cough drop molds, and allow to cool.
8. Package and label the product.

(Note: The quantity of polyethylene glycol 1450 may need to be adjusted, depending on the size of the mold used.)

Oral Suspension Vehicle

Methylcellulose 1% gel	50 mL	Thickener
Flavored syrup	qs 100 mL	Vehicle

1. Calculate the required quantity of each ingredient for the total amount to be prepared.
2. Accurately measure the required quantity of each ingredient or obtain the required number of dosage units.
3. Mix the methylcellulose 1% solution and flavored syrup until uniform.
4. Package and label the product.

Chapter 33

Pharmaceutical Compounding Errors

An *error* is a belief, assertion, or act that unintentionally veers from what is correct or true. A medication error is "any preventable event that may cause or lead to inappropriate medication use or patient harm while the medication is in the control of the health care professional, patient, or consumer."[1]

There is no question that pharmacies that compound specific drugs for individual patients are an important part of health care today. Compounding pharmacies formulate therapeutic and diagnostic products for physicians in practice and those engaged in research. These pharmacies include hospital pharmacies, neighborhood pharmacies, chain pharmacies, nuclear pharmacies, specialty pharmacies, and others. These pharmacies are essential if the health care system is to serve populations with particular needs. Strict compliance with all the laws, regulations, and standards is vital to the provision of compounded preparations that are safe and effective.

However, the system is not perfect and problems can occur in the compounding of prescriptions with materials that are labeled incorrectly or are contaminated by microorganisms. This chapter discusses the compounding of preparations that do not meet the required standard of quality and the way they occur. One issue that sometimes occurs involves *errors* that may arise. Some errors are minimal with no adverse effects; however, some are serious and lead to patient harm and even death, as has been covered by the media. Table 33-1 has a summary of some illnesses and deaths associated with compounded medications (2001–12).

Classification, Description, and Prevention

Compounding errors can be divided into the following categories: (1) general errors, (2) incorrect ingredients, (3) incorrect concentration, (4) incorrect use of equipment, (5) physicochemical issues, (6) microbiological contamination, (7) analytical testing issues, (8) microbiological testing issues, and (9) miscellaneous errors. They are presented in the following format using groups under the headings of "Error Type," "Description," and "Avoiding the Error."[2]

TABLE 33-1 Adverse Events Related to Compounding Errors, 2001–12

Year	Number of Cases	Number of Deaths	Adverse Events	Error That Occurred	Preparation Involved
2001	4	—	Infection	Contamination	IV infusion
2001	11	3	Infection	Contamination	Spinal/joint injection
2002	5	1	Infection	Contamination	Spinal/joint injection
2004	64	—	Infection	Contamination	IV flush syringes
2004	2	—	Infection	Contamination	IV flush
2005	18	—	Infection	Contamination	IV solution
2005	5	3	Systemic Inflammatory Response Syndrome	Contamination	Cardioplegia
2005	6	—	Eye infection, loss of vision, loss of eye	Contamination	Ophthalmic Solution
2005	2	—	Infection	Contamination	IV flush
2004–06	80	—	Infection	Contamination	IV flush
2006	1	1	Overdose	Dose of zinc 1,000 times stronger than ordered	Neonatal PN solution
2006	1	1	Overdose	Dose of sodium chloride stronger than ordered	Chemotherapy infusion
2007	8	—	Infection	Contamination	IV solution
2007	3	3	Overdose	Dose of colchicine eight times stronger than labeled concentration	IV solution
2010	1	1	Overdose	Dose of sodium 60 times stronger than ordered	IV solution
2011	19	9	Infection	Contamination	PN solution
2011	5	—	Blindness	Unintended presence of another medication	Ophthalmic injection
2011	21	—	Infection, blindness, eye removal	Contamination	Ophthalmic injection
2012	33	—	Infection, vision loss	Contamination	Ophthalmic injection
2012	733	53	Infection	Contamination	Spinal injection
TOTALS	1022	75			

— = Not available; IV = Intravenous; PN = parenteral nutrition.
Source: Pew Charitable Trusts, American Society of Health-System Pharmacists, American Hospital Association. Summary of a stakeholder meeting. Pharmacy Sterile Compounding Summit, February 6, 2013, Washington, DC.

General Errors

Error Type	Description	Avoiding the Error
Receipt of the prescription	Incomplete and incorrect information is presented on the prescription.	On receipt of the prescription from either the patient or the health care provider, confirm the inclusion of complete information on the patient, the medication, and so on.
Interpretation of the prescription	The prescription can be misinterpreted with regard to legibility, misspellings, and so on.	Ask a second individual to confirm interpretation of the prescription.
Transcription errors	Following initial receipt and interpretation of the prescription, errors can occur when one enters the information into the computer. These errors can involve the names of the ingredients, the quantities, the units of weight and measurement, instructions for the patient, etc.	Ask a separate individual to check the information after computer entry.
Incorrect calculations	This is possibly the number one cause in compounding errors and includes misplaced decimals, incorrect calculations, lack of understanding of what needs to be done, and so on. Incorrect calculations can result in errors throughout the entire compounding process and have resulted in patients' deaths.	Routinely practice calculations and participate in continuing education. Also, ensure that the person checking the calculations does so without looking at the other person's work because doing so tends to influence the checker and the same mistake can be made. Checking must be done totally separately and then the answers compared and checked. A good practice is to use exact equivalents during the calculation process and round off at the end.
Labeling errors (e.g., colchicine 4 mg/mL labeled as 0.5 mg/mL)	Labeling errors are critical because the health care practitioner will use labeling information for administration to the patient.	Ensure that a second individual double-checks the label and compares it to the original prescription and calculations.
Error repetition	The same errors are being committed, and compounded preparations are not meeting required standards.	Maintain a file of all analytical and microbiological laboratory results and of standard operating procedure (SOP) variations and changes. Review these periodically with affected personnel so all will be aware of any issues that may be involved.

(continued)

Error Type	Description	Avoiding the Error
Expired drugs	When used in compounding, commercial products or bulk active ingredients must be in-date for the projected time of the use of the medication, i.e., stable throughout their beyond-use date.	Check the expiration dates of all ingredients, and consider the beyond-use date that will be assigned to the finished preparation.
Incorrect administration route	Incorrect interpretation of the original prescription has led to labeling errors and the incorrect route of administration. Also, for drugs packaged in containers for ease of removing the exact required dose (as in using a 1-cc tuberculin syringe for measuring creams, etc.), the labeling needs to state the exact route of administration with warnings of how it should *not* be administered.	Provide proper labeling and explanation to the patient and/or caregiver to help prevent this error. Also, the use of proper packaging for its intended use will be of benefit.
Improper beyond-use dates (BUDs)	This is a common error. BUD information may have been entered into the formulation record but not updated when new versions of *United States Pharmacopeia (USP)* Chapters <795>[3] and <797>[4] are provided. This can result in improper BUDs; the preparation's failure to retain its original physical, chemical, or microbiological characteristics; and the preparation's lack of efficacy and safety on administration to the patient.	To avoid a lack of understanding of the assignment of beyond-use dates, carefully read and reread *USP* Chapters <795>[3] and <797>,[4] which contain valuable information.
Confusion of two medications with similar names	This confusion can result in an improper drug being used for compounding for the patient. It can result from poor legibility of the original prescription or from lack of attention by the compounder.	Triple-check each ingredient used in compounding the preparation. First, check when it is removed from its shelf; second, when it is weighed or measured; and, third, when it is returned to the shelf. In each activity, compare the ingredient with the prescription order.

Error Type	Description	Avoiding the Error
Failure to consider overfill	Many injections are allowed a percentage of overfill in the container to enable the entire contents to be withdrawn. If not considered in the compounding process, it can result in the drug being diluted excessively in the case of overfill of a vehicle and a lower drug concentration, or, if an entire vial or ampul is used and placed into a defined volume, it may result in a concentration higher than that needed for the preparation.	Be aware of the overfill allowed in different containers, and make adjustments as required to ensure the quantity administered to the patient is correct.
Mismatched units	In a number of cases, hand-written "ug" or "μg" has been misinterpreted for "mg," resulting in a thousandfold increase in the concentration required for the prescription, and patient harm and even death. Another misinterpreted designation has been "u" when "units" was intended but "mg" or "μg" was used instead.	Double-check the original order. Also, check if the dosage the patient will receive is reasonable for the patient.

Incorrect Ingredients

Error Type	Description	Avoiding the Error
Use of incorrect active pharmaceutical ingredients (APIs)	A number of different occasions can arise involving an incorrect API. For example, the incorrect ingredient accidently is obtained; the incorrect salt form, ester form, hydrated form, particle size, or other form can be mistakenly used.	Double-check the *exact* name and form of the ingredient to be used for the prescription. If any questions arise, check with another compounder to confirm the exact name and form of the API to be used. If appropriate, check with the prescriber to confirm the exact form of the API that was ordered. For suspensions, confirm that the particle size is reduced appropriately.
Use of incorrect form of API	As above, the incorrect form can involve an incorrect salt, ester, or hydrate or even the particle or crystalline form to be used.	Confirm the *exact* form of the API that was prescribed, and if necessary, check with the prescriber. Also, check the *United States Pharmacopeia/National Formulary (USP/NF)* monographs or official product labeling for clarification on which form is to be used.

(continued)

Error Type	Description	Avoiding the Error
Use of incorrect excipients	Excipients can markedly alter the final preparation and its bioavailability and efficacy. In fact, numerous instances of incompatibility can occur between an excipient and an API and even between excipients.	Confirm the compatibility of each of the excipients with the API and with each of the other excipients to ensure their suitability for the preparation. When using levigating agents, confirm that they will be compatible or miscible with the finished preparation.
Use of incorrect supplies	The use of incorrect packaging, compounding personnel protective equipment (PPE), and so on can result in an altered preparation and potential harm to the compounder.	Confirm the appropriateness of the packaging and other supplies used in compounding the preparation. Also, confirm the proper use of PPE for the compounder.
Unintended presence of another medication	This generally involves the accidental use of another medication instead of the one prescribed. It can also result from interactions between ingredients and the degradation of ingredients to produce another ingredient with some untoward effects.	Confirm each and every ingredient that is to be used, and confirm there are no interactions involving chemical reactions that may occur.

Incorrect Concentration

Error Type	Description	Avoiding the Error
Drug quantity or concentration too high	A drug concentration that is too high can result from improper weights, incorrect form of the drug used, loss of vehicle during preparation (evaporation, loss from the weighing or measuring device or container during transfer, etc.), and improper packaging.	See comments above ("Incorrect Ingredients") for improper drug form, weighing, measuring, and so on. Proper storage and use of proper packaging is critical. When using an ointment mill with a cream or a gel, the exposure to the atmosphere will result in some water or solvent loss and an increase in the actual drug concentration; the loss needs to be corrected by adding it back into the formulation after milling. Use of excessive heat resulting in loss of vehicle can occur with some formulations, which results in an increased drug concentration. Lower heat, covers on beakers, and so on can help.

Error Type	Description	Avoiding the Error
Drug quantity or concentration too low	A drug concentration that is too low can result from improper weights, use of the incorrect form of the drug, improper vehicle measurement, use of hygroscopic or deliquescent powders during weighing, incomplete emptying of weighing devices during transfer of the active drug, sorption (adsorption and/or absorption) of the active drug to the container walls (syringe walls or plunger tip, etc.) and so on.	See comments above ("Incorrect Ingredients"). Also, when weighing hygroscopic or deliquescent powders, observe caution when performing the activity in a low humidity room in order to prevent the materials from taking up moisture from the air and increasing the weight while decreasing the actual amount of API obtained. Care in transferring chemicals (powders, semisolids, liquids, etc.) is of utmost importance to ensure all the material has been completely obtained. Sorption problems can generally be found in the literature; they mainly involve very potent, low concentration drugs. Also, when one mixes liquids and some semisolids, excessive air can become entrapped in the preparations, hampering efforts to qs to final volume. Mix the ingredients to minimize any incorporation of air into the preparation. An occasional issue occurs in the use of a nonsolvent to make a liquid dilution of a potent drug; confirming that the potent drug is soluble in the liquid used for the dilution can eliminate this issue. Also, the proper alcohol and solvent concentrations must be maintained for ensuring complete solubility of the API in a solution dosage form. When working with alcohol and water, maintain as high an alcohol concentration as possible by adding the water to the alcohol solution, not the reverse. When pipets and micropipets are used, insufficient volume will be delivered if the user is not aware of how to correctly use the pipet.
Drug concentration too high or too low	Analytical results from laboratories have reported out-of-specification (OOS) results when using manufactured drug products as the drug source.	Compounding pharmacists do not have access to the actual analyzed concentration or quantity of drug in a specific manufactured dosage form. Furthermore, with USP tolerances ranging up to 80% to 120% and even greater, a compounding pharmacist does not know the actual quantity of drug

(continued)

Error Type	Description	Avoiding the Error
		in the capsules, injections, and so on that are used as the drug source in compounding. Because compounding allows only a 90%–110% variation, one can easily understand that the finished compounded preparation may be outside the acceptable range through no fault of the compounding pharmacist.
Stratification and lack of uniform appearance	If heated semisolids are poured into containers while hot, they may tend to separate and stratify. Separation can also occur among particles that are different in size and density.	For semisolids, allow the mixture to cool to just above the congealing point before pouring it into containers. For powders, reduce them to the same particle size range before mixing.
Lack of uniformity of capsule weights	Improperly filled capsules will result in several capsules being outside the acceptable weight range.	When filling capsules at the powder incorporation stage, keep the spatula or plastic card in a vertical position as it is moved over the capsules holes to allow the powder to fall into the cavities, and tamp lightly. Then repeat until all capsules are uniformly filled. Do not slant the spatula or plastic card at an angle to force the powder in the holes because the filling will be nonuniform and result in weights that are outside the range. Allow the powder to simply fall into the capsule openings of its own weight.
Improperly filled or nonuniform suppositories or medication sticks	Contraction or dimpling of suppositories and medication sticks results in insufficient preparation for each dosage form.	Contraction or dimpling occurs when the melt is poured while too hot. Allow the melt to cool to just above its congealing point, and then pour it into the molds.
Missing drug	Occasionally, a drug product that has been analyzed has been reported to have no API in the prescription.	For each ingredient, exercise care in obtaining, weighing and measuring, and so on in order to eliminate this potential error. Generally, when weighing ingredients, observe good practice by placing the ingredients on one side of the balance and, as each is weighed, moving it to the opposite side or to a different location. Marking the weigh boats has also been useful.

Incorrect Use of Equipment

Error Type	Description	Avoiding the Error
Incorrect use of equipment	This results in preparations that are of less-than-desired quality and aesthetics, including improper mixture, insufficient particle size reduction, separation of phases, discoloration, precipitation, and so on. Electrostatic charges that may be present during weighing are problematic.	Confirm that each compounding pharmacist knows how to correctly use each piece of equipment involved in the formulation, including not only actual operation, but also actual maintenance and, in some cases, simple repair or replacement of disposable items. A number of techniques are available to minimize electrostatic charges, and devices can be purchased from suppliers to accomplish this.
Stirring rod in graduated cylinder while measuring	Improper volume of the required vehicle can result in a higher-than-desired concentration of the API.	Remove the stirring rod during final measuring of the volume of vehicle to be added to the compounded preparation.
Magnetic stir bar in measuring device while measuring	When using a calibrated beaker and so on, leaving a magnetic stir bar in the beaker will result in an improper volume of the vehicle and, in turn, a higher-than-desired concentration of the API; less vehicle will be present.	Remove the magnetic stir bar from the beaker or container when adding the vehicle to the calibrated volume line of the container.
pH meter not calibrated before use	An improper pH reading can result in a decrease in the stability of the drug as well as a decrease in the solubility of the drug, resulting in precipitation and so on.	Always calibrate the pH meter before using it each day and several times throughout the day. Clean or rinse the electrodes between each measurement.
Electronic balance not calibrated daily	Improper weighings result in too little or too much of an ingredient in the final compounded preparation.	Calibrate each balance at the beginning of each work shift and throughout the shift as required.

Physicochemical Issues

Error Type	Description	Avoiding the Error
Nonhomogeneous mixing	Large standard deviations in powdered dosage forms (capsules, creams, gels, ointments, papers, etc.) can occur because of mixing that does	Confirm the mixing procedures that are used in compounding for different types of preparations. Uniform use of equipment, mixing times, powder particle size, and so on are critical for homogeneous

(continued)

Error Type	Description	Avoiding the Error
	not result in a homogeneous blend of the API in the bulk of the prescription.	mixing. Dissolve salts in a minimum quantity of water before adding to a semisolid vehicle to prevent grittiness. Stir constantly when combining two liquids to prevent a layering effect and a potential incompatibility. The particle size may be too large and require comminution or levigation.
Solubility issues and precipitation	These issues result in too little API in some liquid doses and then excessive API in doses at other times.	Be aware that solvent, pH, cosolvents, temperature, and other factors can alter the solubility or precipitation of APIs in compounded preparations. Control these variables properly to prevent precipitation, haze formation, and so on.
Failure to follow instructions	This failure can even involve official labeling; in the reconstitution of manufactured antibiotics, failure to use the correct volume of water will result in an incorrect concentration of the API. An example was reported where the powder was not reconstituted and the patient measured and took the powder. This error also applies to lack of following precise instructions on the formulation record.	Follow steps exactly in the official labeling and the formulation record to compound a correct prescription.

Microbiological Contamination

Error Type	Description	Avoiding the Error
Nonsterile contamination	Bacterial, mold, and fungal growth have been reported in some nonsterile compounded preparations.	Confirm all equipment and supplies are clean, dry, and properly stored. Confirm preservatives are present and appropriately used or the preparation is self-preserved. If using commercial preserved vehicles, confirm that the vehicle has not been diluted to the point that the preservative effectiveness is no longer present. Clean and rinse the dispensing container to remove any potential microorganisms.

Error Type	Description	Avoiding the Error
Contamination	Nonsterile prescriptions (injections, ophthalmics, etc.) have been reported and have caused death and injury.	Maintain strict compliance with *all* aspects of *USP* Chapter <797>.[4] Reported errors have been traced back to noncompliance. Many state boards of pharmacy report lack of compliance during their inspections. Critical review of the SOPs, facility, equipment, chemicals, personnel training and performance, packaging, and quality control and assurance activities should be routinely performed.

Analytical Testing Issues

Error Type	Description	Avoiding the Error
Sample preparation and handling	Improper sample submission has led to OOS results.	Contact the analytical laboratory for the proper method of sampling (number of samples, packaging, storage, etc.) and shipping. Ship overnight if possible, and do not ship if the sample will be in transit over the weekend. Develop and implement SOPs for the different samples that are submitted. Use laboratories licensed and inspected by the U.S. Food and Drug Administration (FDA) that will work with you when you have OOS results.
Potential problems with laboratories	Some laboratories use improper sample handling methods, extraction procedures, and analytical methods for the analyses being done.	Provide the laboratory with the complete formulation of the sample so it can appropriately perform the extraction as required for the API. This is especially critical when cellulose derivatives, polymers, and so on are used that may entrap the API and prevent its complete extraction. Confirm that the analytical methods being used provide you the correct and complete information. If OOS results are received, contact the laboratory to help identify the problem and methods of correction. Occasionally, send duplicate samples to two different laboratories and compare results.
Improper BUDs	Some BUDs have been assigned by pharmacists using laboratories that perform only "potency over time" or "strength over time" testing.	BUDs must be determined using stability-indicating analytical methods. Confirm the laboratory is using the proper testing method. There can be a significant difference between a "potency/strength" method and a "stability-indicating" method.

Microbiological Testing Issues

Error Type	Description	Avoiding the Error
Sample preparation and handling	Some compounded preparations are not prepared or handled properly before testing for microbiological growth, sterility, or endotoxins.	Confirm the proper method of sampling, handling, and transporting the samples to the laboratory so they will be properly received. Ship them overnight, and do not ship them over the weekend.
Potential problems with laboratories	Some laboratories may actually contaminate the samples after they are received at the microbiological laboratory, resulting in reporting of incorrect results.	Check with the laboratory to confirm it is registered and inspected by FDA. Confirm its personnel are properly trained and follow strict SOPs. Occasionally, send duplicate samples to two different laboratories and compare results.

Miscellaneous Errors

Error Type	Description	Avoiding the Error
Brittle suppositories and medication sticks	Suppositories and medication sticks can be brittle and break easily, resulting in loss of the preparation.	Brittleness is often caused by excessive powder in the suppository or medication stick. In many cases, reduce the powder quantity or incorporate a liquid that is miscible with the base.
Oils floating on top of oral or topical liquids	Oils have been reported to be floating on top of liquids, both oral and topical. When used, there is a very strong flavor or odor.	Floating oil occurs when an oil is added to an aqueous preparation with no cosolvent or surfactant agent added to disperse it. Mix the oil with a solvent like propylene glycol or glycerin, or add a few drops of an oil-in-water surfactant.
Incorrect or insufficient cleaning of equipment	Improper cleaning technique can result in use of dirty and contaminated equipment.	Follow a strict SOP for cleaning different types of equipment. For example, clean items with water first, then with alcohol or suitable solvent. If alcohol is used first, it may precipitate proteins and so on that will be more difficult to move because they will tend to stick to surfaces.
Excess heating	When using a hot plate, initiating heat at too high a level can result in boilover and loss of preparation.	Calibrate the hot plate so a compounder knows the approximate temperature of the container contents at different dial settings on the hot plate. Microwaves should not be used unless the preparation has been demonstrated to be suitable. If used, a carousel type microwave should be used to minimize hot spots.

The New England Compounding Center Case

The New England Compounding Center (NECC) case[5] is discussed here because it has been a driving force for significant changes in the laws, regulations, and standards related to pharmaceutical compounding. NECC was breaking the law and was actually manufacturing drug products under the guise of compounding.

In 2012, an outbreak of fungal meningitis was traced to fungal contamination in three lots of methylprednisolone suspension for epidural steroid injections compounded by NECC. Doses from these three lots were administered to 14,000 patients. The NECC case is a tragedy for the 64 individuals who died, the hundreds who were sickened, and their families and loved ones.

In December 2014, the federal government issued an indictment against 14 NECC personnel, including the owners, supervising pharmacists, staff pharmacists, technicians, and the director of sales. The seriousness of the charges in the indictment is commensurate with the deaths and injuries allegedly caused by the lapses in compliance with law, quality assurance, and quality control at NECC. These charges include the following:

- Twenty-six charges of second-degree murder: Second-degree murder is defined as an intentional murder with malice aforethought, but is not premeditated or planned in advance.
- Mail fraud: Contaminated and mislabeled vials were sent by interstate courier.
- Criminal contempt: Defined as conduct that defies, disrespects, or insults the authority or dignity of a court, contempt often takes the form of actions seen as detrimental to a court's ability to administer justice. These charges stem from the fact that the owners of NECC transferred millions of dollars in assets after the court issued a restraining order prohibiting transfer of assets.
- Structuring: This is the practice of executing financial transactions in a specific pattern calculated to avoid the creation of certain records and reports required by law. These charges relate to the withdrawal of cash from certain accounts in a manner designed to avoid legal reporting requirements.
- Racketeering: This is the federal crime of conspiring to organize to commit crimes, especially on an ongoing basis as part of an organized crime operation.

The second-degree murder and racketeering charges are based on the allegation that NECC personnel purposely did not comply with applicable laws and United States Pharmacopeial Convention (USP) standards. Full compliance with USP standards and federal and state laws is a significant undertaking, even for the majority of compounding pharmacies that are committed to compliance. Lapses in compliance with standards designed to ensure the quality and safety of compounded medications, whether purposeful or unintentional, can result in patient harm or death.

The indictment states in part, "All compounding personnel were responsible for understanding the fundamental practices and procedures outlined in USP-797 for developing and implementing appropriate procedures, and for continually evaluating the procedures and quality of sterile drugs." This is a critical point in the indictment. The owners, pharmacist in charge, supervising pharmacists, pharmacists, and technicians were all indicted and cited regarding lapses in compliance with applicable law and USP standards. The indictment clearly states that in the interest of public safety, all personnel in the pharmacy are responsible for complying with quality and safety standards.

Two major charges relate to lapses in compliance with the laws and regulations of the Massachusetts Board of Registration in Pharmacy. These charges involve the failure to obtain patient-specific prescriptions and the preparation of sterile compounds by unlicensed personnel.

Lapse in Compounding for Patient-Specific Prescriptions

Medications were dispensed in bulk for office use without a patient-specific prescription. The indictment also notes that the pharmacy falsely claimed to be dispensing all medications on the basis of a patient-specific prescription in order to avoid registering as a manufacturer with FDA.

Pharmacies must comply with the laws of each state in which they do business. Although NECC may have shipped medications into states that permitted compounding for non-patient-specific office use, it was based in Massachusetts and was required to comply with Massachusetts law that prohibits non-patient-specific dispensing. Pharmacies do not get a choice of law; they must comply with *all* applicable laws and regulations in each state in which they do business.

The Drug Quality and Security Act (H.R. 3204, 113th Cong., 2013), a direct result of the NECC tragedy, specifically prohibits traditional compounding pharmacies from dispensing for non-patient-specific office use. Sterile compounding facilities that register as section 503B outsourcing facilities may dispense non-patient-specific medications provided they meet several requirements, including compliance with FDA's Current Good Manufacturing Practices.

The indictment also charges that although the pharmacy received prescription orders from prescribers, the dispensed medications were not actually labeled with the patient's name, so that they could be used for any patient.

Lapses in Compliance with USP Standards

Of note to compounding pharmacists is that many of the racketeering charges in the indictment relate to noncompliance with USP standards. In fact, the indictment explicitly recognizes that the USP sets standards for identity, quality, strength, and purity of medicines. It also notes that Massachusetts requires compliance with USP standards. As discussed earlier, the indictment notes that the responsibility for understanding the fundamental practices and procedures outlined in *USP* Chapter <797>[4] lies with NECC personnel and that "USP-797's standards were meant to prevent harm, including death, to patients that could result from non-sterility of drugs."

The tragic events associated with NECC are a stark lesson in the results of a failure to adhere to quality assurance, quality control, and legal requirements. The quality assurance and quality control requirements of *USP* Chapter <797>,[4] Chapter <71>,[6] and other applicable *USP* chapters are designed to establish systems that ensure sterile medications are safe and that verify their quality through sterility testing and other tests. These standards establish a redundant system of processes to ensure compounded sterile preparation quality. However, when these processes are not performed properly or their results are ignored, as is alleged in the NECC case, serious injury or death to patients can occur.

For many years, pharmacists have been reminded that *USP* Chapter <797> requirements are legally enforceable in all states. The prosecution of NECC personnel based on noncompliance with USP standards may set a precedent for future civil and criminal cases where a party can allege that patients were injured as a result of noncompliance with USP standards.

Conclusion

In all professions, errors occur occasionally. However, in pharmacy, an error can result in harm to the patient or the loss of life. Table 33-2 lists the general sources of error that have been discussed in detail in this chapter. These sources of error need to be addressed, beginning in the colleges of pharmacy. As an example, compounding errors have been observed in pharmacy student training.[7] Kadi and colleagues examined the accuracy of the compounding of two simple solutions by pharmacy students. For one of the solutions, only 54% of the students prepared the medications within 10% of the desired concentration. Errors for the remaining mixtures ranged from less than 75% to greater than 200% of the desired concentration. Although results for the second solution showed 78% of the students within +/− 10% of the desired concentration, the range of concentration errors was greater (−89% to 269%). Another study by Pignato and Birnie showed an error range of 0.6% to 140% with an average error of 23.7%.[8]

Clearly, insufficient time is spent studying both the sciences and the technology involved in pharmaceutical compounding and dispensing. The pharmaceutical sciences are the basis for pharmacy, especially pharmaceutical compounding. Student pharmacists need to devote more studies to this critical area of pharmacy. In turn, pharmacists need access to more quality continuing education programs related to compounding—both the basics and advanced topics. Quality control and assurance topics need to be covered in detail, as do the advantages of certification and advanced education. Pharmacists are taught to be extremely focused and careful, especially when preparing the actual medication—sterile or nonsterile—to be administered to a patient.

In summary, errors can and must be prevented. Doing so will be a process that begins at the colleges of pharmacy and progresses through the practice years by participation in continuing education programs, study of current literature, and sharing of experiences with colleagues. The process can, and must, be followed because patients put their trust in the pharmacists who serve them.

TABLE 33-2 General Causes of Compounding Errors

Lack of education and training of both pharmacists and technicians

Lack of available education and training by colleges and schools of pharmacy

Lack of complete, implemented standard operating procedures

Improper use of equipment or lack of maintenance and calibration

Improper chemicals and supplies

Calculation errors

Use of improper form of drug (salt/ester, hydrate form)

Incorrect potency calculations

Use of commercial products with unknown actual strength

Lack of proper documentation

Improper pH, buffers

Misinterpretation of orders or formula instructions

Lack of focus and/or attention

References

1. National Coordinating Council for Medication Error Reporting and Prevention. About medication errors. Available at: www.nccmerp.org/about-medication-errors.
2. Allen Jr LV. Pharmaceutical Compounding Errors. *Secundem Artem.* 2015;18(3).
3. United States Pharmacopeial Convention. Chapter <795>, Pharmaceutical compounding—nonsterile preparations. In: *United States Pharmacopeia/National Formulary.* Rockville, MD: United States Pharmacopeial Convention; current edition.
4. United States Pharmacopeial Convention. Chapter <797>, Pharmaceutical compounding—sterile preparations. In: *United States Pharmacopeia/National Formulary.* Rockville, MD: United States Pharmacopeial Convention; current edition.
5. Cabaleiro J. New England Compounding Center indictment. *Int J Pharm Compound.* 2015;19(2): 94–102.
6. United States Pharmacopeial Convention. Chapter <71>, Sterility tests. In: *United States Pharmacopeia/National Formulary.* Rockville, MD: United States Pharmacopeial Convention; current edition.
7. Kadi A, Francioni-Proffitt D, Hindle M, Soine W. Evaluation of basic compounding skills of pharmacy students. *Am J Pharm Educ.* 2005;69(4):Article 69.
8. Pignato A, Birnie CR. Analysis of compounded pharmaceutical products to teach the importance of quality in an applied pharmaceutics laboratory course. *Am J Pharm Educ.* 2014;78(3):61.

Drugs and Dosage Forms Not to Be Compounded (The FDA Negative List)

The U.S. Food and Drug Administration has compiled a list of drugs and dosage forms not to be compounded for safety reasons. In that list below, when a specific dosage form is noted, compounding may still be permitted for the drug in other dosage forms or for other indications. To view the most current list, which may change over time, visit www.accessdata.fda.gov/scripts/cdrh/cfdocs/cfcfr/cfrsearch.cfm?fr=216.24.
[Code of Federal Regulations]
[Title 21, Volume 4]
[Revised as of April 1, 2015]
[CITE: 21CFR216.24]

TITLE 21—FOOD AND DRUGS
CHAPTER I—FOOD AND DRUG ADMINISTRATION DEPARTMENT OF HEALTH AND HUMAN SERVICES
SUBCHAPTER C—DRUGS: GENERAL

Part 216—Pharmacy Compounding

Subpart B—Compounded Drug Products

Sec. 216.24 Drug products withdrawn or removed from the market for reasons of safety or effectiveness.

The following drug products were withdrawn or removed from the market because such drug products or components of such drug products were found to be unsafe or not effective. The following drug products may not be compounded under the exemptions provided by section 503A(a) of the Federal Food, Drug, and Cosmetic Act:

Adenosine phosphate	All drug products containing adenosine phosphate.
Adrenal cortex	All drug products containing adrenal cortex.
Azaribine	All drug products containing azaribine.
Benoxaprofen	All drug products containing benoxaprofen.
Bithionol	All drug products containing bithionol.
Bromfenac sodium	All drug products containing bromfenac sodium.
Butamben	All parenteral drug products containing butamben.
Camphorated oil	All drug products containing camphorated oil.
Carbetapentane citrate	All oral gel drug products containing carbetapentane citrate.
Casein, iodinated	All drug products containing iodinated casein.
Chlorhexidine gluconate	All tinctures of chlorhexidine gluconate formulated for use as a patient preoperative skin preparation.
Chlormadinone acetate	All drug products containing chlormadinone acetate.
Chloroform	All drug products containing chloroform.
Cobalt	All drug products containing cobalt salts (except radioactive forms of cobalt and its salts and cobalamin and its derivatives).
Dexfenfluramine hydrochloride	All drug products containing dexfenfluramine hydrochloride.
Diamthazole dihydrochloride	All drug products containing diamthazole dihydrochloride.
Dibromsalan	All drug products containing dibromsalan.
Diethylstilbestrol	All oral and parenteral drug products containing 25 milligrams or more of diethylstilbestrol per unit dose.
Dihydrostreptomycin sulfate	All drug products containing dihydrostreptomycin sulfate.
Dipyrone	All drug products containing dipyrone.
Encainide hydrochloride	All drug products containing encainide hydrochloride.
Fenfluramine hydrochloride	All drug products containing fenfluramine hydrochloride.
Flosequinan	All drug products containing flosequinan.
Gelatin	All intravenous drug products containing gelatin.
Glycerol, iodinated	All drug products containing iodinated glycerol.
Gonadotropin, chorionic	All drug products containing chorionic gonadotropins of animal origin.
Mepazine	All drug products containing mepazine hydrochloride or mepazine acetate.
Metabromsalan	All drug products containing metabromsalan.
Methamphetamine hydrochloride	All parenteral drug products containing methamphetamine hydrochloride.
Methapyrilene	All drug products containing methapyrilene.
Methopholine	All drug products containing methopholine.
Mibefradil dihydrochloride	All drug products containing mibefradil dihydrochloride.
Nitrofurazone	All drug products containing nitrofurazone (except topical drug products formulated for dermatalogic application).

Nomifensine maleate	All drug products containing nomifensine maleate.
Oxyphenisatin	All drug products containing oxyphenisatin.
Oxyphenisatin acetate	All drug products containing oxyphenisatin acetate.
Phenacetin	All drug products containing phenacetin.
Phenformin hydrochloride	All drug products containing phenformin hydrochloride.
Pipamazine	All drug products containing pipamazine.
Potassium arsenite	All drug products containing potassium arsenite.
Potassium chloride	All solid oral dosage form drug products containing potassium chloride that supply 100 milligrams or more of potassium per dosage unit (except for controlled-release dosage forms and those products formulated for preparation of solution prior to ingestion).
Povidone	All intravenous drug products containing povidone.
Reserpine	All oral dosage form drug products containing more than 1 milligram of reserpine.
Sparteine sulfate	All drug products containing sparteine sulfate.
Sulfadimethoxine	All drug products containing sulfadimethoxine.
Sulfathiazole	All drug products containing sulfathiazole (except those formulated for vaginal use).
Suprofen	All drug products containing suprofen (except ophthalmic solutions).
Sweet spirits of nitre	All drug products containing sweet spirits of nitre.
Temafloxacin hydrochloride	All drug products containing temafloxacin.
Terfenadine	All drug products containing terfenadine.
3,3',4',5-tetrachlorosalicylanilide	All drug products containing 3,3',4',5-tetrachlorosalicylanilide.
Tetracycline	All liquid oral drug products formulated for pediatric use containing tetracycline in a concentration greater than 25 milligrams/milliliter.
Ticrynafen	All drug products containing ticrynafen.
Tribromsalan	All drug products containing tribromsalan.
Trichloroethane	All aerosol drug products intended for inhalation containing trichloroethane.
Urethane	All drug products containing urethane.
Vinyl chloride	All aerosol drug products containing vinyl chloride.
Zirconium	All aerosol drug products containing zirconium.
Zomepirac sodium	All drug products containing zomepirac sodium.

Appendix II

Standard Operating Procedures

A compounding pharmacy should have a uniform standard operating procedure (SOP) for every repetitive process that is performed. The SOPs should be reviewed every year and updated as needed. Older SOPs that have been retired should be retained in the pharmacy for a period appropriate to meet the requirements of the state board of pharmacy and other agencies. An extensive collection of SOPs is available at: www.CompoundingToday.com.

SOPs can be numbered and categorized according to any method suitable for a pharmacy. For example, they might be organized as follows:

1.0 Administrative	8.0 Sterile Compounding Procedures
2.0 Personnel	9.0 Veterinary Compounding Procedures
3.0 Training	10.0 Inventory Control
4.0 Safety	11.0 Library and Reference Documents
5.0 Facility	12.0 Quality Assurance
6.0 Equipment	13.0 Miscellaneous
7.0 Nonsterile Compounding Procedures	

Ten SOPs are included here as examples of procedures that can be developed:

1. Basic Compounding Documentation—The Master Formula Form
2. Monitoring Air Temperature and Humidity
3. Use, Standardization, and Care of a pH Meter
4. Calibration of Hot Plates
5. Cleaning of Glassware
6. Physical Quality Assessment of Powder-Filled Hard-Gelatin Capsules
7. Quality Assessment of Oral and Topical Liquids
8. Quality Assessment of Gels
9. General Aseptic Procedures Used at a Laminar-Airflow Workbench
10. Maintenance of a Horizontal Laminar-Airflow Hood

Basic Compounding Documentation—The Master Formula Form

The purpose of this SOP is to establish a protocol for appropriately documenting procedures for preparing uniform formulations.

Equipment and Supplies Required

- Computer (optional but recommended)
- Copy of the standard operating procedure, "Length of Time to Keep Documents and Samples"
- Electronic or manual file system
- The Master Formula Form (referred to as the Formulation Record in the *United States Pharmacopeia/National Formulary*)

Responsibility

The pharmacist in charge is responsible for this procedure.

Procedure

The documentation of compounding procedures is equal in importance to the accurate measurement of active ingredients. A viable control system can be developed and updated on a computer or manual spreadsheet.

The development of written procedures that document the ingredients and methods used to compound a formulation need not be cumbersome or complicated. Ensuring that such procedures are in place to protect the public and comply with the United States Pharmacopeial Convention (USP) Good Compounding Practices is critical.

A. Use a Master Formula Form for any formulation routinely prepared by the pharmacy for dispensing.
B. Identify the following information on the Master Formula Form:
   1. Formula name
   2. Name, strength, and dosage form of all ingredients
   3. Formula number
   4. Quantity prepared
   5. Containers used for storage and dispensing
   6. Short proof of calculation (documenting the quantity calculation and including any explanatory comments, such as conversion factors) when appropriate
   7. Equipment required for the compounding procedure
   8. Step-by-step compounding instructions
C. Add levels of sophistication to the Master Formula Form, such as product description (e.g., color, texture, specific gravity, taste, odor), special handling instructions, sample labels for the finished formulation, and photographs that demonstrate any special techniques.
D. List the quality control tests that are to be conducted on the preparation.
E. Verify the accuracy and completeness of the form several times; preferably, more than one pharmacist should perform verification.
F. Keep the Master Formula Form on file electronically or manually, and retain the documentation according to the SOP, "Length of Time to Keep Documents and Samples."

Master Formula Form

Formula Title _____

Formula Number _____ Quantity Prepared _____

Strength of Formula _____ Dosage Form _____

Ingredient	Quantity	Unit	Calculation/Comment
_____	_____	_____	_____
_____	_____	_____	_____
_____	_____	_____	_____
_____	_____	_____	_____
_____	_____	_____	_____

Equipment Required:

_____

_____

_____

Compounding Instructions:

1. _____
2. _____
3. _____
4. _____
5. _____
6. _____
7. _____
8. _____
9. _____
10. _____

Written by _____ Checked by _____

Quality Control Tests:

Test	Results
_____	_____
_____	_____
_____	_____
_____	_____
_____	_____
_____	_____

Monitoring Air Temperature and Humidity

The purpose of this procedure is to ensure proper monitoring of room air temperature and humidity and to ensure good air quality in the pharmacy compounding laboratory.

Procedure

Monitoring Air Temperature

1. Maintain temperatures in the compounding pharmacy between 68°F (20°C) and 77°F (25°C) at all times. This temperature range is important for proper storage and stability of chemicals and products.
2. Determine the temperature of the room daily, using a suitable nonmobile thermometer located in the immediate vicinity of the compounding area. A digital centigrade thermometer reading to one decimal place is recommended.
3. Record the temperature on the Air Temperature and Humidity Log.
4. Place the form in a notebook.

Monitoring Air Humidity

1. Determine the humidity in the compounding pharmacy daily using a suitable nonmobile hygrometer located in the immediate vicinity of the compounding area. A digital hygrometer is recommended. Humidity control is important for proper storage and stability of chemicals and products. It is also important for compounding materials that are hygroscopic, deliquescent, or efflorescent or that contain water of hydration.
2. Record the humidity on the Air Temperature and Humidity Log.
3. Place the form in a notebook.

Maintaining Air Quality

Routinely cleaning reusable filters or installing new disposable filters in the air-handling system serving the compounding laboratory will ensure appropriately clean, filtered air. Filters should be checked on a scheduled basis, such as every 30 to 60 days, depending on the quality of the air in the laboratory.

The following procedures are suggested:

1. Using a nonlinting wiper moistened with 70% isopropanol, clean the outer surface of the air-handling unit.
2. Remove the fastening agents, and set aside the access panel.
3. Remove the soiled filter, gently slide it into a plastic bag, and tightly seal the bag.
4. Using a nonlinting wiper moistened with 70% isopropanol, clean the filter housing.
5. Install a new filter, noting the direction for proper airflow.
6. Clean the access panel with 70% isopropanol, replace the panel, and tighten the fastening agents firmly.
7. Attach a label to the exterior of the air-handling unit, noting the date the filter was changed and the next due date for changing the filter.
8. Properly discard the soiled filter, contained in the plastic bag, in the trash.
9. In the notebook of forms for monitoring air temperature and humidity, note when the next filter change is due.

Air Temperature and Humidity Log

Date	Time	Temperature	Humidity	Date	Time	Temperature	Humidity
____	____	_____	_____	____	____	_____	_____
____	____	_____	_____	____	____	_____	_____
____	____	_____	_____	____	____	_____	_____
____	____	_____	_____	____	____	_____	_____
____	____	_____	_____	____	____	_____	_____
____	____	_____	_____	____	____	_____	_____
____	____	_____	_____	____	____	_____	_____
____	____	_____	_____	____	____	_____	_____
____	____	_____	_____	____	____	_____	_____
____	____	_____	_____	____	____	_____	_____
____	____	_____	_____	____	____	_____	_____
____	____	_____	_____	____	____	_____	_____
____	____	_____	_____	____	____	_____	_____
____	____	_____	_____	____	____	_____	_____
____	____	_____	_____	____	____	_____	_____
____	____	_____	_____	____	____	_____	_____
____	____	_____	_____	____	____	_____	_____
____	____	_____	_____	____	____	_____	_____
____	____	_____	_____	____	____	_____	_____
____	____	_____	_____	____	____	_____	_____

Use, Standardization, and Care of a pH Meter

The purpose of this procedure is to provide for the use, standardization, and care of a pH meter. The meter should be standardized at each use and the results recorded on the pH Meter Standardization Log.

Procedure

Use of pH Meter
1. Use a pH meter with a readability of at least ±0.01 pH units.
2. Standardize the pH meter at each use.
3. Allow sufficient stabilization time for each measurement.
4. Ensure that the sample and buffer solution temperatures are the same.
5. Replace buffer solutions frequently to increase accuracy.
6. If sample pH values vary over a wide pH range, use a pH meter with a slope control to allow adjustment of the span for nonideal electrodes.

Buffer Solutions
1. Use commercially available pH buffer solutions whenever possible.
2. If commercially available buffer solutions are not available, prepare the following buffer solutions using water free of carbon dioxide (CO_2):
   - pH 4.01 buffer solution consisting of 0.05 M potassium hydrogen phthalate ($KHC_8H_4O_4$)

- pH 6.86 buffer consisting of 0.025 M potassium dihydrogen phosphate (KH_2PO_4) and 0.025 M disodium hydrogen phosphate (Na_2HPO_4)
- pH 9.18 buffer consisting of 0.01 M sodium tetraborate decahydrate ($Na_2B_4O_7 \cdot 10H_2O$)

Standardization of pH Meter

Two standardization methods can be used to standardize pH meters: the one-point method or the two-point method. If all sample pH values are close to the point of standardization (within 1–2 pH units), the one-point method can be used. However, if the pH values vary somewhat from the point of standardization (greater than 2 pH units) and a high degree of accuracy is required, the two-point method should be used.

The *one-point method* of standardization is as follows:

1. Measure the temperature of the standard buffer solution.
2. Set the temperature compensator (knob) on the pH meter to that measured temperature.
3. Rinse the electrode with a portion of distilled water or a portion of the standard buffer solution to be used.
4. Place the electrode in a fresh portion of the standard buffer solution, and activate the meter.
5. Allow the electrode to equilibrate with the standard buffer solution before setting the meter readout to the pH value for that temperature.
6. Set the meter readout to the standard buffer solution value.
7. Place the meter on "Standby," and rinse and blot the electrode.
8. Record the date of the calibration and the operator's initials on the pH Meter Standardization Log.

The *two-point method* requires a slope control adjustment:

1. Start the standardization using a pH 7 buffer.
2. Select a second standard buffer with a pH value close to the sample pH value.
3. Measure the temperature of the two standard buffer solutions. They should be similar.
4. Rinse the electrode with a portion of distilled water or a portion of the standard buffer solution to be used.
5. Place the electrode in a fresh portion of the pH 7 standard buffer solution, and activate the pH meter.
6. Allow the electrode to equilibrate with the standard buffer solution before setting the meter readout to the pH value of the standard buffer solution.
7. Set the meter readout to the standard buffer solution value.
8. Rinse and blot the electrode.
9. Repeat steps 6–8 with the second standard buffer solution.
10. Place the meter on "Standby."
11. To make a measurement, place the electrode in the sample and activate the pH meter.
12. Allow the electrode to equilibrate, and record the pH value.
13. Place the meter in the "Standby" position.
14. Rinse the electrode with distilled water, and blot.
15. Place the electrode in the storage solution.
16. Record the date of the calibration and the operator's initials on the pH Meter Standardization Log.

Measurement of pH
1. With the meter in a "Standby" position, remove the electrode from the storage buffer.
2. Rinse the electrode with distilled water or an aliquot of the sample.
3. Measure the sample temperature, and set the pH meter temperature compensator (knob) to that measured temperature.
4. Place the rinsed electrode in the sample, and activate the meter.
5. Allow the reading to stabilize before recording the pH value.
6. Place the meter in the "Standby" position.
7. Rinse the electrode with distilled water, and blot.
8. Repeat for additional samples, or place electrode in the storage solution.

Rinsing of the Electrode
1. To minimize carry-over contamination, rinse the electrode between measurements.
2. Use distilled water and a wiping tissue to blot, not rub, the electrode bulb, or, if a sufficient quantity of sample is available, rinse the electrode with the next sample before actually immersing the electrode in the sample for a reading. (Note: Rubbing the bulb can impart static electricity to the bulb, resulting in a slow equilibration time for the next reading.)

Care of the Electrode
1. Keep the electrode wet in a soaking or storage solution, preferably of pH 4 buffer.
2. Use a container for storage that fits around the electrode to provide a tight seal between the electrode and the cap for the container.

Rejuvenation of the Electrode
The response time to obtain a normal pH reading of a buffer solution should stabilize within 10 seconds to 98% of the final reading. If the electrode develops a long lag time (time to stabilize at the value) or slow response time (time the meter takes to respond), it may need to be rejuvenated:

1. If the electrode has been used with an organic material, use a suitable organic solvent to remove the material from the electrode bulb.
2. Remove the organic solvent from the electrode bulb by using an intermediate polarity solvent, such as alcohol.
3. Immerse the electrode bulb in 0.1 M hydrochloride (HCl) for 5 minutes, remove, rinse with distilled water, and blot dry.
4. Immerse the electrode bulb in 0.1 M sodium hydroxide (NaOH) for 5 minutes, remove, rinse with distilled water, and blot dry.
5. Immerse the electrode bulb in 0.1 M HCl for 5 minutes, remove, rinse with distilled water, and blot dry.
6. Check the electrode's response. The preceding measures should have made the electrode responsive. If the electrode is still unresponsive, it may need to be replaced.

pH Meter Standardization Log

pH Meter Model No. ─────────── Manufacturer ───────────────────────

Date	Initials	Date	Initials	Date	Initials
─────	─────	─────	─────	─────	─────
─────	─────	─────	─────	─────	─────
─────	─────	─────	─────	─────	─────
─────	─────	─────	─────	─────	─────
─────	─────	─────	─────	─────	─────
─────	─────	─────	─────	─────	─────
─────	─────	─────	─────	─────	─────
─────	─────	─────	─────	─────	─────
─────	─────	─────	─────	─────	─────
─────	─────	─────	─────	─────	─────
─────	─────	─────	─────	─────	─────
─────	─────	─────	─────	─────	─────
─────	─────	─────	─────	─────	─────
─────	─────	─────	─────	─────	─────
─────	─────	─────	─────	─────	─────
─────	─────	─────	─────	─────	─────
─────	─────	─────	─────	─────	─────
─────	─────	─────	─────	─────	─────
─────	─────	─────	─────	─────	─────

Calibration of Hot Plates

The purpose of this procedure is to document the actual temperatures of heated liquids at each dial setting of a particular hot plate. Variables such as the size of the container, the placement of the hot plate in an area where there may be drafts, and the heat conductivity of the liquid should be kept in mind. Different liquids may require different times to reach the desired temperature. A thermometer should always be used to determine the actual temperature in the liquid being heated.

Compounding Principle

To compound more efficiently, a compounding pharmacist or technician should know the approximate temperature indicated by a number on the adjustable dial. This can minimize long waits, which can occur if a desired temperature is approached too slowly, or unnecessary waits for the material to cool, which can occur from overshooting the temperature. As a hot plate ages, the efficiency of the heating elements may deteriorate and the calibration may not remain the same. Consequently, performance of this function at regularly scheduled intervals, such as quarterly, to monitor the performance of the hot plate is important.

Precautions for Use

The hot plate must be plugged into an outlet that provides the proper voltage so that a fire hazard is not created or circuit breakers are not tripped. If turning on a hot plate trips circuit breakers, a licensed electrician should be contacted. In addition, keeping the hot plate clean is important. If there is a chance of boilover, breakage, or other incidents, setting a flat-bottomed metal pan on the hot plate and setting the container to be heated inside the pan may be wise. This will prevent soiling the hot plate in case an accident occurs. Using a thermometer to check the temperature of the material as required and not depending completely on the calibration settings is a good practice.

Equipment and Materials

Only a few materials are needed to calibrate hot plates:

- Certified thermometer
- Beaker of purified water
- Beaker of suitable oil
- Marker or tape, or both

Procedure

1. Clean the hot plate.
2. Place the beaker of purified water on the hot plate, and turn the dial to the first incremental setting, usually 1.
3. Allow the water to warm to a constant temperature, periodically checking the temperature with a thermometer.
4. When the reading is obtained, record the setting on the Hot Plate Calibration Log.
5. Move the dial to the next incremental setting, and repeat steps 3 and 4.
6. Continue the process until a temperature of 90°C is reached. (Note: A reading cannot easily be made when water reaches the boiling point, because it remains at 100°C even though the dial setting may reflect a higher temperature.)
7. Replace the beaker of water with a beaker of oil, and repeat the process followed in steps 2 through 5.
8. Continue past the 90°C setting, and record the temperature of the oil at all the remaining incremental settings on the dial.
9. If the temperature readings at each dial setting are not the same for the water and the oil (for temperatures 90°C and less), then use the appropriate scale depending on the preparation being heated during the compounding process. (Note: The temperatures of the two liquids may not be exactly the same because of heat conductance and the rates of cooling from the sides and surface of the liquid in the containers.)
10. Using a marker or tape, or both, note the corresponding temperature readings labeled "water" and "oil" adjacent to the dial numbers. Also, affix a calibration date to the hot plate as a reminder of when to recalibrate.

Hot Plate Calibration Log

Hot Plate Brand Name _____

Model No. _____   Serial No. _____

		Temperature of Liquids	
Date	Dial Setting	Water	Oil
_____	_____	_____	_____
_____	_____	_____	_____
_____	_____	_____	_____
_____	_____	_____	_____
_____	_____	_____	_____
_____	_____	_____	_____
_____	_____	_____	_____
_____	_____	_____	_____
_____	_____	_____	_____

Cleaning of Glassware

The purpose of this procedure is to ensure the proper cleaning of all glass compounding equipment used in the pharmacy. The process of cleaning glass equipment used in compounding is crucial to providing a preparation that is free of contamination by materials used in previous compounding activities.

Equipment and Materials

The facility should have a sufficiently large sink with hot and cold running water, purified water USP, and a suitable draining rack for this activity. Commercial dishwashers generally will work for a portion of the cleaning process. Cleaning materials include the following:

- Detergent
- Potable water, hot and cold
- Purified water USP (distilled water, deionized water, reverse-osmosis water)
- Chromic acid cleaning mixture (optional)

Procedure

1. Remove any residual materials that remain in or on the glassware, as follows:
   - *Water-soluble materials:* Rinse any residual materials off the item using hot water so the waste flows down the sink. To avoid potentially contaminating the equipment being cleaned, do not place the materials into the washing water.
   - *Water-insoluble materials:* Using a paper towel or other disposable wipe, remove the materials from the item and discard appropriately. Wet a paper towel or other disposable wipe with alcohol or other suitable solvent for the material, remove any residual material from the item, and discard the waste appropriately.
2. Using an appropriate detergent and hot water, thoroughly wash the item. In the event of stains or difficult-to-remove discoloration, use the chromic acid cleaning mixture (described in the next section) before performing this step.

3. Rinse the item thoroughly with hot water to remove any residual detergent and the like.
4. Rinse the item thoroughly with purified water USP.
5. Place the item on a drain rack to dry.
6. Place the item in its storage unit.

Preparation of Chromic Acid Cleaning Mixture

Ingredients for the cleaning mixture include the following:

- Sodium dichromate 20 g
- Water 10 mL
- Sulfuric acid, concentrated 150 mL

The precautionary measures described in steps 1 and 2 should always be followed when preparing this mixture:

1. Use safety goggles.
2. Prepare this mixture in a hard, borosilicate glass beaker, because the heat produced may cause soft-glass containers to break.
3. Dissolve the sodium dichromate in the water.
4. Very slowly and cautiously, add the sulfuric acid, with stirring.
5. Package in a tightly closed, hard, borosilicate glass container.
6. Because the mixture is extremely corrosive and hygroscopic, store it in a glass-stoppered bottle in a safe place.
7. When mixture removed from the storage bottle acquires a green color, do not return it to the storage bottle; instead, discard the discolored mixture in accordance with hazardous materials procedures.

Glass tends to adsorb the chromic acid, which makes prolonged rinsing imperative. Alkaline cleansing agents such as trisodium phosphate and the synthetic detergents are highly useful but also require prolonged rinsing.

Physical Quality Assessment of Powder-Filled Hard-Gelatin Capsules

The purpose of this procedure is to provide a method of documenting physical quality assessment tests of and observations on powder-filled hard-gelatin capsules.

Equipment and Materials

The following items are used in one or more of the quality assessment tests:

- Balance
- Hot plate and stirrer
- 100-mL beaker
- Thermometer

Procedure

Conduct the necessary tests, and record the results and observations on the Physical Quality Assessment of Powder-Filled Hard-Gelatin Capsules worksheet.

Average Weight of Filled Capsules
1. Tare the balance with 10 empty capsules.
2. Select 10 filled capsules at random.
3. Place all 10 filled capsules on the balance, and record the weight on the worksheet.
4. Calculate the average weight of each capsule by dividing the weight of the 10 filled capsules by 10.

Individual Weight Variation of Capsule Contents and Active Ingredient
1. Tare the balance with a single empty capsule.
2. Weigh individually each of the 10 filled capsules used in the average weight test, and record the results on the worksheet.
3. Calculate the actual weight of the active ingredient in each capsule using the following proportional equation:

$$\frac{\text{Actual weight of filled capsule}}{\text{Theoretical weight of filled capsule}} = \frac{\text{Actual weight of active ingredient}}{\text{Theoretical weight of active ingredient}}$$

For example, a filled capsule is supposed to weigh 400 mg and contain 25 mg of active drug, but the actual weight of the filled capsule is 380 mg. The actual quantity of active drug per capsule is calculated as follows:

$$380 \text{ mg}/400 \text{ mg} = x/25 \text{ mg}$$
$$x = 23.75 \text{ mg of active drug}$$

4. To calculate the lower value for the theoretical weight of the active ingredient, multiply the theoretical weight by 85%. Calculate the upper value by multiplying the theoretical weight by 115%. Record the results on the worksheet.
5. To calculate the lower limit of the theoretical weight of the active ingredient, multiply the theoretical weight by 75%. Calculate the upper limit by multiplying the theoretical weight by 125%. Record the results on the worksheet.
6. Determine whether the weight variation of the active ingredient is within the range of 85.0% to 115.0% of label claim and whether any capsule is outside the range of 75.0% to 125.0% of label claim. If 2 or 3 capsules are outside the range of 85.0% to 115.0% of label claim, but not outside the range of 75.0% to 125.0% of label claim, test an additional 20 capsules. If more than 3 capsules are outside the range, discard the batch. The requirements are met if not more than 3 capsules of the 30 are outside the range of 85.0% to 115.0% of label claim and no capsule is outside the range of 75.0% to 125.0% of label claim. If any capsule is outside the range of 75.0% to 125.0% of label claim, the batch should be rejected.

Dissolution of Powder-Filled Capsule Shells
Place one capsule in a beaker of purified water USP maintained at 37°C with a stir bar rotating at about 30 revolutions per minute. The gelatin shell should be disrupted within about 20 to 30 minutes.

Disintegration of Powder-Filled Capsule Contents
Place one immediate-release capsule in a beaker of purified water USP maintained at 37°C with a stir bar rotating at about 30 revolutions per minute. The contents of the capsule should be broken apart or dispersed within 30 minutes.

Assay of Active Drug
As appropriate, depending on how many capsules are compounded, have representative samples of the capsules assayed for active drug content by a contract analytical laboratory. The initial assay is performed soon after preparation of the formulation. Assess stability by storing the product at room temperature and having the assay repeated on the stored samples.

Physical Appearance Tests
The following tests are important in ensuring that each capsule contains the desired quantity of ingredients:

- *Product color check:* Check the description on the master formula record. Use of a color chart for determining the actual color of the product may be advisable.
- *Uniformity test:* Check capsules for uniformity of appearance.
- *Extent of fill test:* Check capsules for uniformity of extent of fill for assurance that all capsules have been filled.
- *Locked-capsule test:* Check capsules for assurance that all have been tightly closed and locked.

Physical Stability Tests
1. Prepare an additional quantity of capsules, and package and label them (for physical stability observations).
2. Weekly, observe the product for signs of discoloration or change.
3. Record a descriptive observation on the form at each observation interval.

Physical Quality Assessment of Powder-Filled Hard-Gelatin Capsules

Product _____ Strength _____

Lot/Rx Number _____ Date _____

A. Weight: Overall Average Weight
   I. Weight of 10 filled capsules _____ g
   II. Average weight of each filled capsule _____ g
       (Divide weight of 10 filled capsules by 10.)
B. Weight: Individual Weight Variation
   I. Record the weight of each capsule in Column I.

Column I (Actual Capsule Weight)	Column II (Actual Active Ingredient Weight)
1. _____	_____
2. _____	_____
3. _____	_____
4. _____	_____
5. _____	_____
6. _____	_____
7. _____	_____
8. _____	_____
9. _____	_____
10. _____	_____

II. Calculate the actual active ingredient weight per capsule and record it in Column II, as follows:

On the basis of the *theoretical active ingredient weight* per *theoretical capsule weight,* calculate the *actual active ingredient weight per capsule.* For this calculation, use the actual capsule weight from part A, step II, above: _____ g.

Example: If the total theoretical capsule weight was 400 mg and was to contain 25 mg of active drug (actual active ingredient weight), but the actual capsule weight was 380 mg, the actual quantity of active drug per capsule (actual active ingredient weight) would be as follows:

Actual capsule weight/Theoretical capsule weight = Actual active ingredient weight/Theoretical active ingredient weight

$380/400 = x/25$

Thus, $x = 23.75$ mg, so 23.75 mg is the actual active ingredient weight per capsule.

III. Multiply the *theoretical active ingredient weight* per capsule by 85.0% and 115.0% and record the results:

Lower value (85%): _____ g   Upper value (115%): _____ g

IV. Multiply the *theoretical active ingredient weight* per capsule by 75.0% and 125.0% and record the results:

Lower limit (75%): _____ g   Upper limit (125%): _____ g

V. Do any of the 10 individual active drug weights fall outside the lower and upper values in part B, step III?

Yes ___   No ___

If yes, how many? (If 2 or 3, repeat the test.)

VI. If yes, do any of the 10 individual active drug weights fall outside the upper and lower limits in part B, step IV?   Yes ___ No ___

If yes, discard the batch.

C. Dissolution of Capsule Shell   Yes ___ No ___
    Immediate-Release Capsule   Yes ___ No ___

    Coated-Capsule
      0.1 N HCl   Yes ___ No ___
      0.1 N NaOH   Yes ___ No ___

D. Disintegration of Capsule Contents   Yes ___ No ___
    Immediate-Release Capsule   Yes ___ No ___
    Altered-Release Capsule   Yes ___ No ___

E. Active Drug Assay Results _____
    Initial Assay _____
    After Storage No. 1 _____
    After Storage No. 2 _____

F. Physical Observation:
   Color of Product _____
   Uniformity   Yes ___ No ___
   Extent of Fill   Yes ___ No ___
   Locked   Yes ___ No ___

G. Was sample set aside for physical observation?   Yes ___ No ___

   If yes, record results.   Date   Observation
                              _____   _____
                              _____   _____
                              _____   _____
                              _____   _____
                              _____   _____
                              _____   _____
                              _____   _____
                              _____   _____

Quality Assessment of Oral and Topical Liquids

The purpose of this procedure is to provide a method of documenting quality assessment tests of and observations on oral and topical solutions, suspensions, and emulsions.

Materials
The following equipment is used in one or more of the assessment tests:

- Balance
- Graduates
- pH meter
- Pycnometer (optional)

Procedure
Conduct the appropriate tests, and record the results or observations on the Quality Assessment Form for Oral and Topical Liquids.

Weight and Volume
Accurately weigh the product on a balance or measure the quantity in a graduate.

pH
Calibrate the pH meter, and then determine the apparent pH of the product.

Specific Gravity
   1. If a pycnometer is available, ensure it is clean and dry.
   2. Weigh the empty pycnometer (W_1), and then fill it with the prepared product, being careful not to entrap air bubbles.
   3. Weigh the pycnometer a second time (W_2).
   4. Subtract the first weight from the second weight to obtain the net weight of the product. Divide this weight (grams) by the volume (milliliters) of the pycnometer to obtain the density/specific gravity of the product:

$$SG = \frac{(W_2 - W_1)}{V}$$

Quality Assessment Form for Oral and Topical Liquids

Product _____ Date_____

Lot/Rx Number _____ Form: Solution _____ Suspension _____ Emulsion ____

	Theoretical	Actual	Normal Range
Weight/volume	_____	_____	_____
pH	_____	_____	_____
Specific gravity	_____	_____	_____
Active drug assay results	_____	_____	_____
Initial assay	_____	_____	_____
After storage No. 1	_____	_____	_____
After storage No. 2	_____	_____	_____
Color of product	_____	_____	_____

Clarity (solution)   Clear   1   2   3   4   5   Opaque

Globule size range (emulsion)
(estimated, mm) <1 1–2   2–3   3

Rheologic properties
(pourability, settling,
resuspendability)   Good   1   2   3   4   5   Poor

Sample set aside for physical stability observation?   Yes ___ No ___

   If yes, results   Date   Observation

Date	Observation
_____	_____
_____	_____
_____	_____
_____	_____
_____	_____
_____	_____
_____	_____
_____	_____
_____	_____

Active Drug Assay Results
As appropriate, have representative samples of the product assayed for active drug content by a contract analytical laboratory. Assess stability by storing the product at room, refrigerated, and/or frozen temperatures and having the assay repeated on the stored samples.

Color of Product
Use of a color chart for determining the actual color of the product may be advisable.

Clarity (solutions)
Evaluate clarity by a visual inspection. A light–dark background can be used. On the worksheet, 1 is the clearest and 5 is the least clear on the scale provided.

Globule Size Range
Place a drop of the product on a glass plate (microscope slide), and illuminate from the bottom. Estimate the globule size range of the product.

Rheologic Properties and Pourability
Visually determine whether the product pours easily or with difficulty (before and after it sits for a period of time).

Physical Observation
Describe the appearance and organoleptic qualities of the product.

Physical Stability
Prepare an additional quantity of the product, and package and label it (for physical stability observations). Weekly, observe the product for signs of discoloration, foreign materials, gas formation, mold growth, and so forth. Record a descriptive observation on the form at each observation interval. Sufficient lines are provided for 8 weeks of observations.

Quality Assessment of Gels

The purpose of this procedure is to provide a method of documenting quality assessment tests of and observations on gels.

Materials
The following items are used in one or more of the quality assessment tests:

- Balance
- pH meter
- Pycnometers (optional)
- Graduated cylinders or calibrated syringes

Procedure
Conduct the appropriate tests, and record the results and observations on the Quality Assessment Form for Gels.

Tests and Observations
Weight and Volume
Weigh the product on a balance, or measure the quantity in a graduated cylinder.

pH
Calibrate the pH meter, and then determine the pH of the product.

Specific Gravity
1. If a pycnometer is available, ensure it is clean and dry.
2. Weigh the empty pycnometer.
3. Fill it with the prepared product, being careful not to entrap air bubbles.
4. Weigh it a second time.
5. Subtract the first weight from the second weight to obtain the net weight of the product.

6. Divide this weight (grams) by the volume (milliliters) of the pycnometer to obtain the density/specific gravity of the product:

SG = W/V

Active Drug Assay Results
As appropriate, have representative samples of the product assayed for active drug content by a contract analytical laboratory. Assess stability by storing the product at room, refrigerated, and/or frozen temperatures and having the assay repeated on the stored samples.

Color of Product
Use of a color chart to determine the actual color of the product may be advisable.

Clarity
Evaluate clarity by visual inspection.

Surface Texture
1. Observe the product in a container.
2. Note the smoothness of the surface. (Refer to scale.)

Spatula Spread
1. Spread a small portion of the product on a pill tile or other flat surface.
2. Note the smoothness of the product. (Refer to scale.)

Appearance
Does the product appear dry or wet and oozing with liquid?

Feel
To the touch, is the product sticky (tacky) or hard (plastic)? Does it bounce back (elastic)?

Rheologic Properties
1. Place a small quantity of the product on a glass plate.
2. Lift one edge of the glass plate up to a 45° angle.
3. Does the product flow easily or remain stationary?

Physical Observation
Describe the appearance and organoleptic qualities of the product.

Physical Stability
1. Prepare a few additional dosage forms, and package them, adding the label "For Physical Stability Observations."
2. Weekly, observe the product for signs of discoloration, dryness, cracking, mottling, mold growth, and so forth.
3. Record a descriptive observation on the worksheet at each observation interval. Sufficient lines are provided for 8 weeks or approximately 60 days.

Quality Assessment Form for Gels

Product _____ Date_____

Lot/Rx Number _____ Form: Gel

	Theoretical	Actual	Normal Range
Weight/volume	_____	_____	_____
pH	_____	_____	_____
Specific gravity	_____	_____	_____
Active drug assay results	_____	_____	_____
Initial assay	_____	_____	_____
After storage No. 1	_____	_____	_____
After storage No. 2	_____	_____	_____
Color of product	_____	_____	

Clarity (solution)	Clear	1	2	3	4	5	Opaque
Surface texture	Smooth	1	2	3	4	5	Rough
Spatula spread	Smooth	1	2	3	4	5	Rough
Appears dry	Yes	1	2	3	4	5	No
Appears weeping	Yes	1	2	3	4	5	No
Feels tacky	Yes	1	2	3	4	5	No
Feels plastic	Yes	1	2	3	4	5	No
Feels elastic	Yes	1	2	3	4	5	No
Rheologic properties (ease of flow)	Easy	1	2	3	4	5	Resistant

Sample set aside for physical stability observation? Yes ___ No ___

If yes, results	Date	Observation
	_____	_____
	_____	_____
	_____	_____
	_____	_____
	_____	_____
	_____	_____
	_____	_____
	_____	_____
	_____	_____
	_____	_____

General Aseptic Procedures Used at a Laminar-Airflow Workbench

The purpose of the procedure is to provide guidelines for personnel working at a laminar-airflow workbench (LAFW).

Equipment and Supplies
The following items are used for this procedure:

- Laminar-airflow workbench
- Nonlinting gauze sponges
- Disinfectant (sterile 70% alcohol or other, as required by facility SOP)
- Materials for compounding

Procedure
1. Before beginning work, scrub and don a gown (including rescrubbing and regowning) according to the specific SOPs of the facility. This practice applies to all personnel. Wear clean apparel that is appropriate for the level of aseptic compounding to be done.
2. Operate the hood blower continuously if the hood is used on a daily basis. If the hood is not used daily, turn it off but start it at least 30 minutes before use.
3. Clean the entire interior surface of the LAFW, except for the filter grill, with a nonlinting gauze sponge dampened with distilled water; then clean the entire interior surface of the LAFW, except for the filter grill, with a nonlinting gauze sponge dampened with a suitable disinfectant. (Note: Disinfectants may be rotated, depending on the SOPs of the facility).
4. Do not spray disinfectant solutions at or on the filter or filter grill.
5. If any spills occur, immediately wash the area with sterile water for injection; then clean the area with a nonlinting gauze sponge dampened with the disinfectant.
6. Plan the work for a certain time period to minimize movement within the hood and in the immediate work area surrounding the hood.
7. Remove all supplies from their outer cartons, boxes, and the like before taking the supplies into the clean room or immediate work area.
8. Clean each vial or ampul to be placed in the LAFW by wiping the outer surface with a suitable disinfectant, such as sterile 70% alcohol.
9. Remove syringes, needles, and the like from their immediate wrapper, and place them in the aseptic work area.
10. Place only the necessary supplies for the immediate preparation in the LAFW at one time. (Do not use the LAFW to store items.)
11. Organize all materials to enhance efficiency of work and to maintain the integrity of the critical sites for all materials in accordance with the flow of air, horizontal or vertical.
12. All work shall be done at least 6 inches into the LAFW.
13. Be careful not to touch the critical sites of any of the items with gloved hands, because the hands are not sterile.
14. Periodically use an alcohol wipe on the gloved hands, as necessary.
15. Immediately before opening, clean the necks of ampuls with a nonlinting gauze sponge and a disinfectant (e.g., sterile 70% alcohol).

16. Clean all rubber stoppers of vials and other containers, before opening or penetrating with a needle, with a nonlinting gauze sponge and a disinfectant (e.g., sterile 70% alcohol).

17. Filter all solutions removed from glass ampuls to remove possible glass particles before adding the solutions to a vehicle or to another component.

18. During addition of drugs, gently swirl or rotate the solutions to speed mixing and minimize the occurrence of an incompatibility.

19. During compounding, constantly observe the preparation for precipitation, cloudiness, leakage, and gas formation as indicated by a stopper bulging outward, cracks in the container, and particulates.

20. As appropriate, filter products through a 0.22-μm filter into sterile containers.

21. After completion, observe the final product for any evidence of an incompatibility, and visually inspect for particulate matter.

22. Place a tamper-evident cap or seal on the finished product, as appropriate.

23. Label the product, remove it from the LAFW, and place it in an overwrap, if required, and seal.

24. Remove the empty containers, used syringes and needles, and other materials from the LAFW, and wipe area with a clean, nonlinting sponge dampened with a suitable disinfectant.

Maintenance of a Horizontal Laminar-Airflow Hood

The purpose of this procedure is to document the maintenance of a horizontal laminar-airflow (LAF) hood.

Principle
An aseptic working environment is required for any pharmacy preparing sterile products. Use of a class 100 horizontal LAF hood located within a class 10,000 clean room for aseptic processing is recommended. The procedure describes how to conduct nonroutine, thorough cleaning; filter replacement; and lubrication for the LAF.

Materials
The following items are used in one or more of the maintenance steps:

- Mild detergent or suitable disinfectant
- Prefilter
- Plastic bag
- High-efficiency particulate air (HEPA) filter
- Sticker
- Lubricant

Procedure
Cleaning
1. Clean the exterior surfaces of the LAF hood with a mild detergent or suitable disinfectant, according to the disinfectant rotation program. (Note: Do not use 70% isopropyl alcohol or any other liquid that may damage the hood's clear plastic surfaces. Check with the manufacturer to determine which substances should be used.)

2. Remove access panel(s), and clean all accessible interior surfaces with a suitable mild detergent or disinfectant solution. (Note: Do not touch the HEPA filter unit.)

3. Replace the access panel(s).
4. Document the required information on the Laminar-Airflow Hood Maintenance Log.

Prefilter Changes

1. Change the prefilter(s) every ___ months. (Change on a regular basis, depending on level of use.)
2. Clean exterior surfaces of the access panel with a mild detergent or suitable disinfectant.
3. Open the access panel to expose the filter and filter housing.
4. Clean the exterior of the filter housing with the detergent or disinfectant.
5. Remove the soiled prefilter, place it in a new plastic bag, and close tightly.
6. Clean the interior of the filter housing with the detergent or disinfectant.
7. Insert a new prefilter, observing the airflow direction indicator, and lock in place.
8. Close the access panel, and lock in place.
9. Document the required information on the Laminar-Airflow Hood Maintenance Log.

HEPA Filter Changes

1. Change the HEPA filter(s) every ___ months. (Change on a regular basis, depending on level of use.)
2. Ensure that a qualified contractor changes the HEPA filter.
3. Document the required information on the Laminar-Airflow Hood Maintenance Log.
4. Ensure that a qualified pharmacist conducts media fills to document hood performance.

Certification

1. Ensure that a qualified contractor certifies the LAF hood at least every 6 months, or when it is relocated, to safeguard operational efficiency and integrity.
2. Obtain a copy of the procedures used by the contractor, and place it in an SOP notebook.
3. Document the required information on the Laminar-Airflow Hood Maintenance Log.
4. Affix a sticker to the LAF hood indicating that service has been performed and giving a date when it should be repeated.
5. Ensure that a qualified pharmacist conducts settle plate or other appropriate tests and media fills to document hood performance.

Lubrication (if recommended by the manufacturer)

1. Clean the exterior surface of the hood containing the access panel(s) to the motor and blowers with a mild detergent or suitable disinfectant.
2. Remove the access panel(s), and clean the accessible surfaces.
3. Lubricate the motor and blower bearings if recommended by the manufacturer.
4. Replace the access panel(s).
5. Document the required information on the Laminar-Airflow Hood Maintenance Log.
6. Perform air velocity and other quality control checks as recommended.

Laminar-Airflow Hood Maintenance Log

Date	Procedure	Cleaning Agent	Initials

Procedures:	Filter	Filter replacement
	Cleaning	Nonroutine, thorough cleaning and disinfection
	Lube	Lubrication of motor and fan bearings
	Other	Describe

Specific Gravity Values of Selected Liquids

Liquid	Specific Gravity	Liquid	Specific Gravity
Acetic acid, glacial	1.05	Dimethicone 100	0.97
Acetic acid NF	1.04	Dimethicone 200	0.97
Acetone	0.79	Dimethicone 350	0.97
Acetyl tributyl citrate	1.05	Dimethicone 500	0.97
Acetyl triethyl citrate	1.14	Dimethicone 1000	0.97
Alcohol, ethyl	0.82	Dimethicone 30,000	0.97
Alkyl (C12–C15) benzoate	0.92	Dimethyl sulfoxide	1.10
Almond oil	0.91	Ethyl acetate	0.90
Alpha-tocopherol	0.95	Ethyl lactate	1.03
Ammonium solution, strong	0.90	Ethyl oleate	0.87
Amylene hydrate	0.81	Glucose, liquid	1.43
Benzoin tincture	0.85	Glycerin	1.25
Benzyl alcohol	1.05	Hexylene glycol	0.92
Benzyl benzoate	1.12	Hydrochloric acid	1.18
Canola oil	0.92	Hydrochloric acid, diluted	1.05
Castor oil	0.96	Isopropyl alcohol	0.78
Chloroform	1.48	Isopropyl myristate	0.85
Coal tar solution (LCD)	0.87	Isopropyl palmitate	0.85
Coconut oil	0.92	Lactic acid	1.20
Compound benzoin tincture	0.91	Oleic acid	0.90
Corn oil	0.92	Maltitol solution	1.36
Cottonseed oil	0.92	Medium-chain triglycerides	0.95
Cresol	1.03	Methylene chloride	1.32
Diethanolamine	1.09	Methyl salicylate	1.18
Diethylene glycol monoethyl ether	0.99	Mineral oil, heavy	0.88
Dimethicone 20	0.95	Mineral oil, light	0.85

(continued)

Liquid	Specific Gravity	Liquid	Specific Gravity
Mineral oil and lanolin alcohols	0.85	Polysorbate 80	1.08
Monoethanolamine	1.01	Propionic acid	0.99
Monothioglycerol	1.25	Propylene carbonate	1.21
Nitric acid	1.41	Propylene glycol	1.04
Octyldodecanol	0.84	2-Pyrrolidone	1.11
Oleic acid	0.90	Resorcinol monoacetate	1.20
Oleyl alcohol	0.85	Rose soluble	1.16
Olive oil	0.91	Safflower oil	0.92
Peanut oil	0.92	Sesame oil	0.92
Peppermint oil	0.91	Simethicone	0.97
Phenol, liquefied	1.06	Sodium lactate	1.33
Phenoxyethanol	1.11	Soybean oil	0.92
Phenylethyl alcohol	1.02	Squalane	0.80
Phosphoric acid	1.71	Sulfuric acid	1.84
Phosphoric acid, diluted	1.06	Sunflower oil	0.92
Polyethylene glycol 300	1.12	Triacetin	1.16
Polyethylene glycol 400	1.12	Tributyl citrate	1.04
Polyethylene glycol 600	1.12	Triethyl citrate	1.14
Polysorbate 20	1.10	Trolamine	1.12
Polysorbate 40	1.08	Water	1.00
Polysorbate 60	1.10	Witch hazel	0.98

Using Weight-Related Conversion Factors

In the performance of pharmaceutical calculations before compounding, some conversions are sometimes necessary. If these are not performed, the final drug concentration in the preparation may be out of the allowable range. Assay value, loss on drying, water of hydration, and base and salt or ester conversions are discussed in this appendix. These examples can be used to supplement the material presented in Chapter 2 of this book.

For *assay value* and *loss on drying,* conversions are not required generally. An exception is that assay values must be converted when the chemical manufacturer has provided a specific value. For example, the label of gentamicin sulfate lists a potency equivalent of not less than 590 µg of gentamicin per milligram, calculated on the dried basis; the actual value provided on the label is to be used in calculating the quantity for use in the prescription.

Assay Value in Certificate of Analysis

The certificate of analysis of a chemical will show both the assay value of that specific lot and the allowable range of values for that assay, which was established either by the official monograph or by the manufacturer of the chemical. If the assay value of that particular lot falls within the specified range, the chemical is considered to be within specifications, and no correction in concentration needs to be made. If the assay value is outside the specifications, the chemical is unacceptable and must be returned to the manufacturer. For example, if the assay range for dexchlorpheniramine maleate USP, established by the United States Pharmacopeial Convention (USP), is 98%–100.5% and the value is 100.2%, no correction is required.

Loss on Drying

Similarly, the description of the loss on drying in a chemical analysis should fall within the allowable range as described in that document. Upon receiving a chemical, a pharmacist must note if the value for loss on drying falls within the allowable specifications; if not, the pharmacist must return the chemical to the manufacturer. For example, if the loss on drying specification for dexchlorpheniramine maleate USP is up to 0.5%, a value of 0.04% is within the allowable range and no correction is needed.

Water of Hydration

Chemicals may have different degrees of hydration. For example, citric acid anhydrous contains no water molecule and citric acid monohydrate contains one water molecule. If a formula calls for citric acid anhydrous in a solution and a pharmacy has in stock citric acid monohydrate, a pharmacist must convert the weight of the chemical to account for the water weight.

However, analyzing each situation to determine if substitution of the chemical in that specific formula is appropriate is important. Not all chemicals in formulations may be exchanged; an improper substitution may cause a chemical reaction or shorten the preparation stability and beyond-use date.

To obtain the conversion factor for using citric acid monohydrate instead of the anhydrous form, divide the molecular weight (MW) of citric acid monohydrate by that of citric acid anhydrous:

$$\frac{210.14}{192.13} = 1.093$$

To substitute citric acid monohydrate in a formula for citric acid anhydrous, for each milligram of citric acid anhydrous, the pharmacist must weigh 1.093 mg of citric acid monohydrate instead.

Conversely, to obtain the conversion factor for using citric acid anhydrous instead of the monohydrate form, divide the MW of citric acid anhydrous by the MW of citric acid monohydrate:

$$\frac{192.13}{210.14} = 0.914$$

To substitute citric acid anhydrous in a formula for citric acid monohydrate, for each milligram of citric acid monohydrate, the pharmacist must weigh 0.914 mg of citric acid anhydrous instead.

Example problem

If a formula calls for 50 mg of citric acid anhydrous and the pharmacy has only citric acid monohydrate, the pharmacist must calculate:

50 mg × 1.093 = 54.65 mg

The pharmacist must weigh out 54.65 mg of citric acid monohydrate.

Base–Salt–Ester Conversion

For some drugs, the active pharmaceutical ingredient is marketed in different chemical forms, i.e., in the base form and different salt or ester forms. A pharmacist must determine on which form of the drug the dosage is based. Once this is known, calculations can be made to adjust the quantity of drug used in compounding the preparation for a patient.

If a drug product in some form is commercially available, a pharmacist must refer to the commercially available product of that drug to determine how it is expressed (i.e., as the base or salt or ester) before performing calculations and compounding a prescription. For example, albuterol sulfate is available in an inhalation solution labeled as 1.25 mg/3 mL as albuterol (equivalent to 1.50 mg albuterol sulfate); therefore, it contains 1.50 mg albuterol sulfate per 3 mL, which is equivalent to 1.25 mg of the albuterol base per 3 mL. Determining whether the drug concentration is expressed as the base, salt, or ester form is very important.

Three examples of different types of conversions are as follows:

1. The commercially available product is expressed in terms of the base of the drug (e.g., fluoxetine):
   - The commercially available product uses fluoxetine, not fluoxetine hydrochloride, as its reference. Before compounding preparations with fluoxetine, a pharmacist must calculate and convert the weight to the correct weight of fluoxetine hydrochloride.
   - To obtain the conversion factor to weigh fluoxetine hydrochloride before compounding prescriptions for fluoxetine, divide the MW of fluoxetine hydrochloride by the MW of fluoxetine:

   $$\frac{345.79}{309.29} = 1.12$$

   - For each milligram of fluoxetine, use 1.12 mg of fluoxetine hydrochloride in your formula.
   - If a prescription calls for fluoxetine 25 mg capsules, find the amount of fluoxetine hydrochloride per capsule needed to make 25 mg capsules of fluoxetine as follows:

   25 mg × 1.12 = 28 mg of fluoxetine hydrochloride must be weighed.

2. The commercially available product is expressed in terms of the salt or ester of the drug (e.g., phenylpropanolamine):
   - The commercially available products with phenylpropanolamine are expressed in terms of phenylpropanolamine hydrochloride, not phenylpropanolamine. To prepare formulas of phenylpropanolamine, a pharmacist must use phenylpropanolamine hydrochloride. No conversion is needed.

3. The commercially available product is expressed in terms of a salt or ester of the drug, and conversion of a different salt or ester of the drug to the referenced salt is necessary (e.g., propoxyphene):
   - The commercially available product is expressed in terms of propoxyphene hydrochloride. When using propoxyphene napsylate in a prescription, a pharmacist must first convert the amount to reflect propoxyphene hydrochloride.
   - To obtain the conversion factor to weigh propoxyphene napsylate before compounding prescriptions for propoxyphene, divide the MW of propoxyphene napsylate by the MW of propoxyphene hydrochloride:

   $$\frac{565.72}{375.93} = 1.50$$

- For each milligram of propoxyphene, use 1.50 mg of propoxyphene napsylate in your formula.
- If a prescription is for propoxyphene hydrochloride 65 mg capsules and a pharmacy has only propoxyphene napsylate in stock, a pharmacist must find the amount of propoxyphene napsylate needed to make 65 mg capsules of propoxyphene hydrochloride by converting the amount to propoxyphene hydrochloride, as follows:

65 mg × 1.50 = 97.5 mg of propoxyphene napsylate must be weighed.

Appendix V

Sodium Chloride Equivalent Values of Selected Agents

Substance	NaCl E1%[a]
A	
Acetrizoate methylglucamine	0.08
Acetrizoate sodium	0.10
Acetylcysteine	0.20
Acriflavine	0.10
Adenosine phosphate	0.41
Alcohol, 95%	0.65
Alcohol, 100%	0.70
Alphaprodine hydrochloride	0.19
Alum (potassium)	0.18
Amantadine hydrochloride	0.31
Aminacrine hydrochloride	0.17
Aminoacetic acid	0.41
Aminocaproic acid	0.26
Aminohippuric acid	0.13
Aminophylline	0.17
p-Aminosalicylate sodium	0.29
Ammonium carbonate	0.70
Ammonium chloride	1.08
Ammonium lactate	0.33
Ammonium nitrate	0.69
Ammonium phosphate, dibasic	0.55
Ammonium sulfate	0.55
Amobarbital sodium	0.25
Amphetamine phosphate	0.34
Amphetamine sulfate	0.22
Amylcaine hydrochloride	0.22

Substance	NaCl E1%[a]
Anileridine hydrochloride	0.19
Antimony potassium tartrate	0.18
Antipyrine	0.17
Antistine hydrochloride	0.18
Apomorphine hydrochloride	0.14
Arecoline hydrobromide	0.27
Arginine glutamate	0.17
L-Arginine hydrochloride	0.30
Arsenic trioxide	0.30
Ascorbic acid	0.18
Atropine methylbromide	0.14
Atropine sulfate	0.13
Aurothioglucose	0.03
B	
Bacitracin	0.05
Baclofen	0.27
Barbital sodium	0.29
Benoxinate hydrochloride	0.18
Benzalkonium chloride	0.16
Benzethonium chloride	0.05
Benztropine mesylate	0.21
Benzyl alcohol	0.17
Bethanechol chloride	0.39
Bismuth potassium tartrate	0.09
Bismuth sodium tartrate	0.13
Boric acid	0.50

(continued)

Substance	NaCl E1%[a]
Brompheniramine maleate	0.09
Bupivacaine hydrochloride	0.17
Butabarbital sodium	0.27
Butacaine sulfate	0.20

C

Substance	NaCl E1%[a]
Caffeine	0.08
Caffeine and sodium benzoate	0.25
Caffeine and sodium salicylate	0.12
Calcium aminosalicylate	0.27
Calcium chloride	0.51
Calcium chloride (6 H_2O)	0.35
Calcium chloride, anhydrous	0.68
Calcium chloride, dihydrate	0.51
Calcium disodium edetate	0.21
Calcium gluconate	0.16
Calcium lactate	0.23
Calcium lactate pentahydrate	0.23
Calcium lactobionate	0.08
Calcium levulinate	0.27
Camphor	0.20
Capreomycin sulfate	0.04
Carbenicillin sodium	0.20
Carboxymethylcellulose sodium	0.03
Cephaloridine	0.07
Chloramine-T	0.23
Chloramphenicol	0.10
Chloramphenicol sodium succinate	0.14
Chlordiazepoxide hydrochloride	0.22
Chlorobutanol	0.24
Chlorobutanol (hydrated)	0.24
Chloroprocaine hydrochloride	0.20
Chloroquine phosphate	0.14
Chloroquine sulfate	0.09
Chlorpheniramine maleate	0.15
Chlortetracycline hydrochloride	0.11
Chlortetracycline sulfate	0.13
Citric acid	0.18
Clindamycin phosphate	0.08
Clonidine hydrochloride	0.22

Substance	NaCl E1%[a]
Cocaine hydrochloride	0.16
Codeine phosphate	0.14
Colistimethate sodium	0.15
Congo red	0.05
Cromolyn sodium	0.14
Cupric sulfate	0.18
Cupric sulfate, anhydrous	0.27
Cupric sulfate, pentahydrate	0.18
Cyclophosphamide	0.10
Cytarabine	0.11

D

Substance	NaCl E1%[a]
Deferoxamine mesylate	0.09
Demecarium bromide	0.12
Dexamethasone sodium phosphate	0.17
Dextroamphetamine hydrochloride	0.34
Dextroamphetamine phosphate	0.25
Dextroamphetamine sulfate	0.23
Dextrose	0.16
Dextrose (anhydrous)	0.18
Dextrose, monohydrate	0.16
Diatrizoate sodium	0.09
Dibucaine hydrochloride	0.13
Dicloxacillin sodium (1 H_2O)	0.10
Diethanolamine	0.31
Dihydrostreptomycin sulfate	0.06
Dimethpyrindene maleate	0.12
Dimethyl sulfoxide	0.42
Diperodon hydrochloride	0.14
Diphenhydramine hydrochloride	0.20
Diphenidol hydrochloride	0.16
Disodium edetate	0.23
Dopamine hydrochloride	0.30
Doxapram hydrochloride	0.12
Doxycycline hyclate	0.12
Dyphylline	0.10

E

Substance	NaCl E1%[a]
Echothiophate iodide	0.16
Edetate disodium	0.23

Substance	NaCl E1%[a]	Substance	NaCl E1%[a]
Edetate trisodium monohydrate	0.29	Hexamethonium tartrate	0.16
Emetine hydrochloride	0.10	Hexamethylene sodium acetaminosalicylate	0.18
Ephedrine hydrochloride	0.30	Histamine phosphate	0.25
Ephedrine sulfate	0.23	Histamine 2 hydrochloride	0.40
Epinephrine bitartrate	0.18	L-Histidine monohydro-chloride	0.29
Epinephrine hydrochloride	0.29		
Ergonovine maleate	0.16	Holocaine hydrochloride	0.20
Erythromycin lactobionate	0.07	Homatropine hydrobromide	0.17
Ethylenediamine	0.44	Homatropine methylbromide	0.19
Ethylhydrocupreine hydrochloride	0.17	Hyaluronidase	0.01
		Hydromorphone hydrochloride	0.22
Ethylmorphine hydrochloride	0.16	Hydroxyamphetamine hydrobromide	0.26
Eucatropine hydrochloride	0.18		
Evans blue	0.06	Hydroxystilbamidine isethionate	0.16

F

Substance	NaCl E1%[a]	Substance	NaCl E1%[a]
Fentanyl citrate	0.11	**I**	
Ferric ammonium citrate, green	0.17	Imipramine hydrochloride	0.20
Ferrous gluconate	0.15	Indigotindisulfonate sodium	0.30
Ferrous lactate	0.21	Iopamidol	0.03
Floxuridine	0.13	Isometheptene mucate	0.18
Fluorescein sodium	0.31	Isopropyl alcohol	0.53
Fluorouracil	0.13	Isoproterenol sulfate	0.14
Fluphenazine 2-hydrochloride	0.14		
D-Fructose	0.18	**K**	
Furtrethonium iodide	0.24	Kanamycin sulfate	0.07

G

Substance	NaCl E1%[a]	Substance	NaCl E1%[a]
Galactose, anhydrous	0.18	**L**	
Gentamicin sulfate	0.05	Lactic acid	0.41
D-Glucuronic acid	0.20	Lactose	0.07
L-Glutamic acid	0.25	Lactose, anhydrous	0.07
Glutathione	0.34	Levallorphan tartrate	0.13
Glycerin	0.34	Levorphanol tartrate	0.12
Glycine	0.41	Lircomycin hydrochloride	0.16
Glycopyrrolate	0.15	Lyapolate sodium	0.09
Gold sodium thiomalate	0.10		
Guanidine hydrochloride	0.65	**M**	
		Magnesium chloride	0.45

H

Substance	NaCl E1%[a]	Substance	NaCl E1%[a]
		Magnesium sulfate	0.17
		Magnesium sulfate, anhydrous	0.32
Heparin sodium	0.07	Magnesium sulfate, septahydrate	0.17
Hetacillin potassium	0.17		
Hexafluorenium bromide	0.11	Mannitol	0.17

(continued)

Substance	NaCl E1%[a]	Substance	NaCl E1%[a]
Maphenide hydrochloride	0.075	Naloxone hydrochloride	0.14
Menthol	0.20	Naphazoline hydrochloride	0.27
Meperidine hydrochloride	0.22	Neomycin sulfate	0.11
Mepivacaine hydrochloride	0.21	Neomycin sulfate pentahydrate	0.11
Merbromin	0.14	Neostigmine bromide	0.22
Mercuric chloride	0.13	Neostigmine methylsulfate	0.20
Mercuric cyanide	0.15	Nicotinamide	0.26
Mesoridazine besylate	0.07	Nicotinic acid	0.25
Metaraminol bitartrate	0.20	Novobiocin sodium	0.10
Methacholine bromide	0.28		
Methacholine chloride	0.32	**O**	
Methadone hydrochloride	0.17	Oleandomycin phosphate	0.08
Methamphetamine hydrochloride	0.37	Orphenadrine citrate	0.13
Methdilazine hydrochloride	0.10	Oxymetazoline hydrochloride	0.22
Methenamine	0.23	Oxyquinoline sulfate	0.21
Methiodal sodium	0.24		
Methionine	0.28	**P**	
Methitural sodium	0.25	*d*-Pantothenyl alcohol	0.18
Methocarbamol	0.10	Papaverine hydrochloride	0.10
Methotrimeprazine hydrochloride	0.10	Paraldehyde	0.25
Methoxyphenamine hydrochloride	0.26	Pargyline hydrochloride	0.29
p-Methylaminoethanolphenol tartrate	0.17	Penicillin G potassium	0.18
		Penicillin G procaine	0.10
Methyldopate hydrochloride	0.21	Penicillin G sodium	0.18
Methylergonovine maleate	0.10	Pentazocine lactate	0.15
N-Methylglucamine	0.20	Phenacaine hydrochloride	0.20
Methylphenidate hydrochloride	0.22	Phenobarbital sodium	0.24
Methylprednisolone sodium succinate	0.09	Phenol	0.35
		Phentolamine mesylate	0.17
Metycaine hydrochloride	0.20	Phenylephrine hydrochloride	0.32
Mild silver protein	0.18	Phenylethyl alcohol	0.25
Minocycline hydrochloride	0.10	Phenylpropanolamine hydrochloride	0.38
Monoethanolamine	0.53		
Morphine hydrochloride	0.15	Physostigmine salicylate	0.16
Morphine hydrochloride trihydrate	0.15	Pilocarpine hydrochloride	0.24
		Pilocarpine nitrate	0.23
Morphine nitrate	0.19	Piperocaine hydrochloride	0.21
Morphine sulfate	0.14	Polyethylene glycol 300	0.12
		Polyethylene glycol 400	0.08
N		Polyethylene glycol 1500	0.06
		Polyethylene glycol 1540	0.02
		Polyethylene glycol 4000	0.02
Nafcillin sodium	0.14	Polymyxin B sulfate	0.09
Nalbuphine hydrochloride	0.16	Polysorbate 80	0.02
Nalorphine hydrochloride	0.21	Polyvinyl alcohol (99% hydrol)	0.02

Substance	NaCl E1%[a]	Substance	NaCl E1%[a]
Polyvinylpyrrolidone	0.01	Silver nitrate	0.33
Potassium acetate	0.59	Silver protein, mild	0.17
Potassium chlorate	0.49	Sodium acetate	0.46
Potassium chloride	0.76	Sodium acetate, anhydrous	0.77
Potassium iodide	0.34	Sodium acetazolamide	0.23
Potassium nitrate	0.56	Sodium ampicillin	0.16
Potassium permanganate	0.39	Sodium antimonyl tartrate	0.13
Potassium phosphate	0.46	Sodium ascorbate	0.32
Potassium phosphate dibasic	0.46	Sodium benzoate	0.40
Potassium phosphate monobasic	0.44	Sodium bicarbonate	0.65
		Sodium biphosphate, anhydrous	0.46
Potassium sorbate	0.41	Sodium biphosphate (H_2O)	0.40
Potassium sulfate	0.44	Sodium biphosphate (2 H_2O)	0.36
Povidone	0.01	Sodium bismuth thioglycollate	0.19
Pralidoxime chloride	0.32	Sodium bisulfite	0.61
Prilocaine hydrochloride	0.22	Sodium borate	0.42
Procainamide hydrochloride	0.22	Sodium borate, decahydrate	0.42
Procaine hydrochloride	0.21	Sodium bromide	0.58
Prochlorperazine edisylate	0.06	Sodium cacodylate	0.32
Promazine hydrochloride	0.13	Sodium carbonate, anhydrous	0.70
Proparacaine hydrochloride	0.15	Sodium carbonate, monohydrated	0.60
Propiomazine hydrochloride	0.15		
Propylene glycol	0.43	Sodium carboxymethyl cellulose	0.03
Pyrathiazine hydrochloride	0.17		
Pyridostigmine bromide	0.22	Sodium cephalothin	0.17
Pyridoxine hydrochloride	0.36	Sodium chloride	1.00
		Sodium citrate	0.31
Q		Sodium colistimethate	0.15
Quinine bisulfate	0.09	Sodium folate	0.12
Quinine dihydrochloride	0.23	Sodium iodide	0.39
Quinine hydrochloride	0.14	Sodium lactate	0.55
Quinine and urea hydrochloride	0.23	Sodium lauryl sulfate	0.08
		Sodium metabisulfite	0.67
R		Sodium methicillin	0.18
Resorcinol	0.28	Sodium nafcillin	0.14
Riboflavin phosphate, sodium	0.08	Sodium nitrate	0.68
Rolitetracycline	0.11	Sodium nitrite	0.84
Rose Bengal	0.07	Sodium oxacillin	0.17
Rose Bengal B	0.08	Sodium phenylbutazone	0.18
		Sodium phosphate	0.29
S		Sodium phosphate, dibasic, anhydrous	0.53
Scopolamine hydrobromide	0.12		
Scopolamine methylnitrate	0.16	Sodium phosphate, dibasic, dodecahydrate	0.22
Secobarbital sodium	0.24		

(continued)

Substance	NaCl E1%[a]	Substance	NaCl E1%[a]
Sodium phosphate, dibasic, septahydrate	0.29	Thiopropazate dihydrochloride	0.16
		Thioridazine hydrochloride	0.05
Sodium phosphate, dibasic (2 H$_2$O)	0.42	Thiotepa	0.16
		Tridihexethyl chloride	0.16
Sodium phosphate, dibasic (12 H$_2$O)	0.22	Triethanolamine	0.21
		Trifluoperazine hydrochloride	0.18
Sodium phosphate, dihydrate	0.42	Triflupromazine hydrochloride	0.09
Sodium phosphate, monobasic	0.43	Trimeprazine tartrate	0.06
Sodium propionate	0.61	Trimethadione	0.23
Sodium ricinoleate	0.10	Trimethobenzamide hydrochloride	0.10
Sodium salicylate	0.36		
Sodium succinate	0.32	Tripelennamine hydrochloride	0.30
Sodium sulfate	0.26	Trisodium edetate, monohydrate	0.29
Sodium sulfate, anhydrous	0.58	Tromethamine	0.26
Sodium sulfite, exsiccated	0.65	Tropicamide	0.09
Sodium sulfobromophthalein	0.06	Trypan blue	0.26
Sodium tartrate	0.33	Tubocurarine chloride	0.13
Sodium thiosulfate	0.31		
Sodium warfarin	0.17	**U**	
Sorbitol hemihydrate	0.16	Urea	0.59
Sparteine sulfate	0.10	Uridine	0.12
Spectinomycin hydrochloride	0.16		
Streptomycin sulfate	0.07	**V**	
Strong silver protein	0.08	Valethamate bromide	0.15
Sucrose	0.08	Vancomycin sulfate	0.05
Sulfacetamide sodium	0.23	Viomycin sulfate	0.08
Sulfadiazine sodium	0.24		
Sulfamerazine sodium	0.23	**W**	
Sulfanilamide	0.22	Warfarin sodium	0.17
Sulfapyridine sodium	0.23		
Sulfathiazole sodium	0.22	**X**	
		Xylometazoline hydrochloride	0.21
T			
Tannic acid	0.03	**Z**	
Tartaric acid	0.25	Zinc chloride	0.62
Tetracaine hydrochloride	0.18	Zinc phenolsulfonate	0.18
Tetracycline hydrochloride	0.14	Zinc sulfate	0.15
Thiamine hydrochloride	0.25	Zinc sulfate (dried)	0.23
Thiethylperazine maleate	0.09	Zinc sulfate, septahydrate	0.15

[a]Sodium chloride equivalents based on a 1% solution.

Appendix VI

Buffers and Buffer Solutions

Buffer Selection

pH Range	Buffer
1–3	Hydrochloric acid
2.5–6.5	Citrate buffer
3.6–5.6	Acetate buffer
6–8	Sorenson's phosphate buffer
8–9	Sodium bicarbonate
9–11	Sodium bicarbonate/sodium carbonate
11–13	Sodium hydroxide

Buffers and Buffer Solutions

Boric Acid Buffer (pH 5)

Boric acid	19 g
Purified water	qs 1000 mL

Boric Acid–Sodium Borate Buffer

Boric acid	0.43 g
Sodium borate	4.2 g
Purified water	qs 1000 mL

Sorensen's Modified Phosphate

Acid stock solution (1/15 M sodium biphosphate)

Sodium biphosphate, anhydrous	8.006 g
Purified water	qs 1000 mL

Alkaline stock solution (1/15 M sodium phosphate)

Sodium phosphate, anhydrous	9.473 g
Purified water	qs 1000 mL

Preparation of Sorensen's Modified Phosphate Buffer with Specific pH

| pH | Required Volume of Stock Solutions | | Grams of Sodium Chloride Required for Tonicity |
	mL of Acid Stock Solution	mL of Alkaline Stock Solution	
5.9	90	10	0.52
6.2	80	20	0.51
6.5	70	30	0.50
6.6	60	40	0.49
6.8	50	50	0.48
7.0	40	60	0.46
7.2	30	70	0.45
7.4	20	80	0.44
7.7	10	90	0.43
8.0	5	95	0.42

 ## Gilford Ophthalmic Buffer

Acid stock solution

Boric acid	12.4 g
Potassium chloride	7.4 g
Purified water	qs 1000 mL

Alkaline stock solution

| Sodium carbonate, monohydrate | 24.8 g |
| Purified water | qs 1000 mL |

Preparation of Gilford Ophthalmic Buffer with Specific pH

| pH | Required Volume of Stock Solutions | |
	mL of Acid Stock Solution	mL of Alkaline Stock Solution
6.0	30	0.05
6.2	30	0.1
6.6	30	0.2
6.8	30	0.3
6.9	30	0.5
7.0	30	0.6
7.2	30	1.0
7.4	30	1.5
7.6	30	2.0
7.8	30	3.0
8.0	30	4.0
8.5	30	8.0

Palitzsch Buffer

Acid stock solution (0.2 M boric acid solution)
Boric acid   12.404 g
Purified water   qs 1000 mL

Alkaline stock solution (0.05 M sodium borate solution)
Sodium borate, decahydrate   19.108 g
Purified water   qs 1000 mL

Preparation of Palitzsch Buffer with Specific pH

pH	Required Volume of Stock Solutions	
	mL of Acid Stock Solution	mL of Alkaline Stock Solution
6.8	97	3
7.1	94	6
7.4	90	10
7.6	85	15
7.8	80	20
7.9	75	25
8.1	70	30
8.2	65	35
8.4	55	45
8.6	45	55
8.7	40	60
8.8	30	70
9.0	20	80
9.1	10	90

Sodium Acetate–Boric Acid Stock Solution

Acid stock solution (pH 5)
Boric acid crystals   19 g
Purified water   qs 1000 mL

Alkaline stock solution (pH approx. 7.6)
Sodium acetate, trihydrate   20 g
Purified water   qs 1000 mL

Preparation of Sodium Acetate–Boric Acid Stock Solution with Specific pH

| pH | Required Volume of Stock Solutions | |
	mL of Acid Stock Solution (pH 7.6)	mL of Alkaline Stock Solution (pH 5)
5.0	100	—
5.7	95	5
6.05	90	10
6.3	80	20
6.5	70	30
6.65	60	40
6.75	50	50
6.85	40	60
6.95	30	70
7.1	20	80
7.25	10	90
7.4	5	100
7.6	0	100

Atkins and Pantin Buffer Solution

Acid stock solution (0.2 M boric acid solution)
Boric acid   12.405 g
Sodium chloride   7.5 g
Purified water   qs 1000 mL

Alkaline stock solution (0.2 M sodium carbonate solution)
Sodium carbonate, anhydrous   21.2 g
Purified water   qs 1000 mL

Preparation of Atkins and Pantin Buffer Solution with Specific pH

pH	Required Volume of Stock Solutions	
	mL of Acid Stock Solution	mL of Alkaline Stock Solution
7.6	93.8	6.2
7.8	91.7	8.3
8.0	88.8	11.2
8.2	85.0	15.0
8.4	80.7	19.3
8.6	75.7	24.3
8.8	69.5	30.5
9.0	63.0	37.0
9.2	56.4	43.6
9.4	49.7	50.3
9.6	42.9	57.1
9.8	36.0	64.0
10.0	29.1	70.9
10.2	22.1	77.9
10.4	15.4	84.6
10.6	9.8	90.2
10.8	5.7	94.3
11.0	3.5	96.5

Feldman Buffer

Acid stock solution

Boric acid	12.368 g
Sodium chloride	2.925 g
Purified water	qs 1000 mL

Alkaline stock solution

Sodium borate, decahydrate	19.07 g
Purified water	qs 1000 mL

Preparation of Feldman Buffer with Specific pH

pH	Required Volume of Stock Solutions	
	mL of Acid Stock Solution	mL of Alkaline Stock Solution
5.0	100	0
6.0	100	0.4
7.0	95	5
7.1	94	6
7.2	93	7
7.3	91	9
7.4	89	11
7.5	87	13
7.6	85	15
7.7	82	18
7.8	80	20
7.9	76	24
8.0	73	27
8.1	69	31
8.2	65	35

Preparation of Modified Walpole Acetate Buffer

pH	Acetic Acid 99% (mL/100 mL)	Sodium Acetate, Anhydrous (g/100 mL)	NaCl to make Isotonic (g/100 mL)
3.6	1.11	0.123	0.28
3.8	1.06	0.197	0.28
4.0	0.98	0.295	0.27
4.2	0.88	0.435	0.26
4.4	0.76	0.607	0.24
4.6	0.61	0.804	0.22
4.8	0.48	0.984	0.21
5.0	0.35	1.156	0.19
5.2	0.25	1.296	0.18
5.4	0.17	1.402	0.17
5.6	0.11	1.484	0.16

Citrate Buffer

Acid stock solution
M/3 Citric acid
| Citric acid, monohydrate | 70 g |
| Purified water | qs 1000 mL |

Alkaline stock solution
M/3 Sodium citrate
| Sodium citrate, dihydrate | 98 g |
| Purified water | qs 1000 mL |

Preparation of Citrate Buffer

| | Required Volume of Stock Solutions | |
	mL of Acid Stock Solution	mL of Alkaline Stock Solution
pH		
2.5	92	8
3.0	82	18
3.5	68	32
4.0	58	42
4.5	44	56
5.0	28	72
5.5	14	86
6.0	6	94
6.5	2	98

Compendial Requirements for Bacterial Endotoxins in Sterile Preparations

Official Monograph Name	Maximum Endotoxin Units[a-c]
Acetazolamide for Injection	0.5 per mg
Acetic Acid Irrigation	0.5 per mL
Acyclovir for Injection	0.174 per mg
Adenosine Injection–Continuous Peripheral Intravenous	5.95 per mg
Adenosine Injection–Rapid Intravenous	11.62 per mg
Alcohol in Dextrose Injection	0.5 mg/mL
Alfentanil Injection	10.0 per mL
Alprostadil Injection	5.0 per 100 µg
Alteplase (for Injection)	1.0 per mg
Amifostine for Injection	0.2 per mg
Amikacin Sulfate Injection	0.33 per mg of amikacin
Aminocaproic Acid Injection	0.05 per mg
Aminohippurate Sodium Injection	0.04 per mg
Aminopentamide Sulfate Injection	25.0 per mg
Aminophylline Injection	1.0 per mg
Ammonium Chloride Injection	1.72 per mEq chloride
Amobarbital Sodium for Injection	0.4 per mg
Amoxicillin for Injectable Suspension	0.25 per mg
Amphotericin B for Injection	5.0 per mg
Ampicillin	0.15 per mg
Ampicillin and Sulbactam for Injection	0.17 per 1 mg of mixture (0.67 mg ampicillin and 0.33 mg sulbactam)

(continued)

Official Monograph Name	Maximum Endotoxin Units[a–c]
Ampicillin for Injectable Suspension	0.15 per mg
Ampicillin for Injection	0.15 units per mg
Anileridine Injection	7.2 per mg
Anticoagulant Citrate Dextrose Solution	5.56 per mL
Anticoagulant Citrate Phosphate Dextrose Adenine Solution	5.56 per mL
Anticoagulant Citrate Phosphate Dextrose Solution	5.56 per mL
Anticoagulant Heparin Solution	2.5 per mL
Anticoagulant Sodium Citrate Solution	5.56 per mL
Arginine Hydrochloride Injection	0.01 per mg
Ascorbic Acid Injection	1.2 per mg
Atenolol Injection	33.3 per mg
Atracurium Besylate Injection	5.56 per mg
Atropine Sulfate Injection	55.6 per mg
Azathioprine Sodium for Injection	1.0 per mg
Aztreonam (for Injection)	0.17 per mg
Bacitracin for Injection	0.01 per bacitracin unit
Bacteriostatic Sodium Chloride Injection	1.0 per mL
Bacteriostatic Water for Injection	0.5 per mL
Benztropine Mesylate Injection	55.6 per mg
Benzylpenicilloyl Polylysine Injection	5833.0 per mL
Betamethasone Sodium Phosphate and Betamethasone Acetate Injectable Suspension	29.2 per mg betamethasone
Betamethasone Sodium Phosphate Injection	29.2 per mg betamethasone
Bethanechol Chloride Injection	25.0 per mg
Biperiden Lactate Injection	83.3 per mg
Bleomycin for Injection	10.0 per bleomycin unit
Bretylium Tosylate in Dextrose Injection	0.20 per mg
Bretylium Tosylate Injection	0.20 per mg
Brompheniramine Maleate Injection	35.7 per mg
Bumetanide Injection	350.0 per mg
Bupivacaine Hydrochloride and Epinephrine Injection	1.6 per mg bupivacaine hydrochloride
Bupivacaine Hydrochloride in Dextrose Injection	1.8 per mg bupivacaine hydrochloride
Bupivacaine Hydrochloride Injection	2.5 per mg bupivacaine hydrochloride
Butorphanol Tartrate Injection	88.0 per mg
Caffeine and Sodium Benzoate Injection	0.7 per mg caffeine and sodium benzoate total
Calcium Chloride Injection	0.2 per mg
Calcium Gluceptate Injection	0.32 per mg
Calcium Gluconate Injection	0.17 per mg
Calcium Levulinate Injection	35.70 per mg
Capreomycin for Injection	0.35 per mg

Official Monograph Name	Maximum Endotoxin Units[a–c]
Carbenicillin for Injection	0.05 per mg
Carboplatin for Injection	0.54 per mg
Carboprost Tromethamine Injection	714.3 per mg
Cefamandole Nafate for Injection	0.15 per mg cefamandole
Cefazolin Injection (for Injection)	0.15 per mg
Cefepime for Injection	0.06 per mg
Cefepime Hydrochloride	0.04 per mg
Cefmetazole Injection (for Injection)	0.2 per mg
Cefonicid for Injection	0.35 per mg
Cefoperazone (for Injection)	0.20 per mg
Ceforanide (for Injection)	0.25 per mg
Cefotaxime Injection (for Injection)	0.20 per mg
Cefotetan Injection (for Injection)	0.17 per mg
Cefoxitin Injection (for Injection)	0.13 per mg
Ceftazidime for Injection	0.1 per mg
Ceftizoxime Injection (for Injection)	0.10 per mg
Ceftriaxone for Injection	0.20 per mg
Cefuroxime for Injection	0.10 per mg
Cephalothin Injection (for Injection)	0.13 per mg
Cephapirin for Injection	0.17 per mg
Cephradine for Injection	0.20 per mg
Chloramphenicol (Injection)	0.2 per mg
Chloramphenicol Sodium Succinate for Injection	0.2 per mg chloramphenicol
Chlordiazepoxide Hydrochloride for Injection	3.57 per mg
Chloroquine Hydrochloride Injection	0.7 per mg
Chlorothiazide Sodium for Injection	0.3 per mg
Chlorpheniramine Maleate Injection	8.8 per mg
Chlorpromazine Hydrochloride Injection	6.9 per mg
Chorionic Gonadotropin (for Injection)	0.03 per unit
Chromic Chloride Injection	16.70 per µg chromium
Cilastatin Sodium	0.17 per mg cilastatin
Cimetidine Injection	0.5 per mg cimetidine hydrochloride
Cimetidine in Sodium Chloride Injection	0.5 per mg cimetidine hydrochloride
Cisplatin for Injection	2.0 per mg
Citric Acid, Magnesium Oxide, and Sodium Carbonate Irrigation	2.80 per mL
Clavulanate Potassium	0.03 per mg
Clindamycin Injection (for Injection)	0.58 per mg
Codeine Phosphate Injection	5.8 per mg
Colchicine Injection	166.7 per mg
Colistimethate for Injection	2.0 per mg colistin

(continued)

Official Monograph Name	Maximum Endotoxin Units[a–c]
Corticotropin Injection (for Injection)	3.1 per unit
Corticotropin Zinc Hydroxide Injectable Suspension	3.1 per unit
Cupric Chloride Injection	250.0 per mg copper
Cupric Sulfate Injection	250.0 per mg copper
Cyanocobalamin Injection	0.4 per μg
Cyclophosphamide for Injection	0.20 per mg
Cyclosporine Injection	0.84 per mg
Cysteine Hydrochloride Injection	0.7 per mg
Cytarabine for Injection	0.07 per mg
Dacarbazine for Injection	0.52 per mg
Dactinomycin (for Injection)	100.0 per mg
Daunorubicin Hydrochloride for Injection	4.3 per mg daunorubicin
Deferoxamine Mesylate for Injection	0.33 per mg
Desoxycorticosterone Acetate Injection	71.4 per mg
Desoxycorticosterone Pivalate Injectable Suspension	2.78 per mg
Dexamethasone Acetate Injectable Suspension	21.7 per mg
Dexamethasone Injection	21.0 per mg
Dexamethasone Sodium Phosphate Injection	31.3 per mg dexamethasone phosphate
Dextran 1	25.0 per g
Dextran 40	1.0 per mL (tested in Sodium Chloride Injection)
Dextran 40 in Dextrose Injection	1.0 per mL
Dextran 40 in Sodium Chloride Injection	1.0 per mL
Dextran 70	0.5 per mL (tested in Sodium Chloride Injection)
Dextran 70 in Dextrose Injection	0.5 per mL
Dextran 70 in Sodium Chloride Injection	0.5 per mL
Dextrose and Sodium Chloride Injection	10.0 per g dextrose
Dextrose Injection	0.5 per mL for less than 5% dextrose; 10.0 per g for 5%–70% dextrose
Diatrizoate Meglumine and Diatrizoate Sodium Injection	1.8 per mL for < 60% diatrizoate meglumine; 3.6 per mL for ≥ 60% diatrizoate meglumine
Diatrizoate Meglumine Injection	1.1 per mL for < 50% diatrizoate meglumine; 5.0 per mL for ≥ 50% diatrizoate meglumine
Diatrizoate Sodium Injection	5.6 per mL for 20% diatrizoate sodium; 1.3 per mL for 25% diatrizoate sodium; 5.0 per mL for 50% diatrizoate sodium
Diazepam Injection	11.6 per mg
Diazoxide Injection	0.5 per mg

Official Monograph Name	Maximum Endotoxin Units[a–c]
Dibucaine Hydrochloride Injection	35.7 per mg dibucaine
Dicyclomine Hydrochloride Injection	17.2 per mg
Diethylstilbestrol Diphosphate Injection	0.7 per mg
Diethylstilbestrol Injection	0.7 per mg
Digitoxin Injection	111.0 per mg
Digoxin Injection	200.0 per mg
Dihydroergotamine Mesylate Injection	175.0 per mg
Dihydrostreptomycin Injection	0.5 per mg
Dimethyl Sulfoxide Irrigation	0.5 per mL
Diphenhydramine Hydrochloride Injection	3.4 per mg
Dipyridamole Injection	8.8 per mg
Dobutamine for Injection	5.56 per mg
Dobutamine in Dextrose Injection	5.56 per mg
Dobutamine Injection	2.08 per mg
Dolasetron Mesylate Injection	2.7 per mg
Dopamine Hydrochloride and Dextrose Injection	16.67 per mg dopamine hydrochloride
Dopamine Hydrochloride Injection	16.67 per mg
Doxapram Hydrochloride Injection	3.3 per mg
Doxorubicin Hydrochloride for Injection	2.2 per mg
Doxorubicin Hydrochloride Injection	2.2 per mg
Doxycycline for Injection	1.14 per mg doxycycline
Droperidol Injection	35.7 per mg
Dyphylline Injection	0.7 per mg
Edetate Calcium Disodium Injection	0.01 per mg
Edetate Disodium Injection	0.2 per mg
Edrophonium Chloride Injection	8.33 per mg
Emetine Hydrochloride Injection	5.4 per mg
Ephedrine Sulfate Injection	1.7 per mg
Epinephrine Injection	357.0 per mg
Ergonovine Maleate Injection	700.0 per mg
Ergotamine Tartrate Injection	357.0 per mg
Erythromycin Lactobionate for Injection	1.0 per mg erythromycin
Estradiol Injectable Suspension	250.0 per mg
Estrone Injectable Suspension	88.0 per mg
Ethacrynate Sodium for Injection	5.0 per mg
Etoposide Injection	2.0 per mg
Extended Insulin Human Zinc Suspension	80.0 per 100 units
Extended Insulin Zinc Suspension	80.0 per 100 units
Fenoldopam Mesylate Injection	84.0 per mg
Fentanyl Citrate Injection	50.0 per mg
Ferumoxides Injection	12.5 per mL

(continued)

Official Monograph Name	Maximum Endotoxin Units[a–c]
Fludarabine Phosphate for Injection	7.7 per mg
Flunixin Meglumine Injection	4.54 per mg flunixin
Fluorouracil Injection	0.33 per mg
Fluphenazine Hydrochloride Injection	166.7 per mg
Folic Acid Injection	357.1 per mg
Fosphenytoin Sodium Injection	14.0 per mL
Fructose and Sodium Chloride Injection	0.5 per mL
Fructose Injection	0.5 per mL
Furosemide Injection	3.6 per mg
Gadodiamide	3.5 per g
Gadodiamide Injection	0.029 per mg
Gadopentetate Dimeglumine Injection	25.0 per mL
Gadoteridol Injection	8.3 per mL
Gadoversetamide	15.0 per g
Gadoversetamide Injection	5.0 per mL
Gallamine Triethiodide Injection	5.0 per mg
Ganciclovir for Injection	0.84 per mg
Gemcitabine for Injection	0.05 per mg
Gentamicin Injection	0.71 per mg gentamicin
Glucagon for Injection	125.0 per mg
Glycine Irrigation	0.5 per mL
Glycopyrrolate Injection	555.5 per mg
Gonadorelin for Injection	3.60 per µg
Guaifenesin for Injection	0.05 per mg
Half-Strength Lactated Ringer's and Dextrose Injection	0.5 per mL
Haloperidol Injection	71.4 per mg
Heparin Calcium	0.03 per unit
Heparin Calcium Injection	0.03 per unit
Heparin Lock Flush Solution	0.5 per mL
Heparin Sodium (Injection)	0.03 per unit
Histamine Phosphate Injection	125.0 per mg
Hyaluronidase Injection (for Injection)	2.30 per unit
Hydralazine Hydrochloride Injection	1.45 per mg
Hydrocortisone Injectable Suspension	1.25 per mg
Hydrocortisone Sodium Phosphate Injection	1.25 per mg hydrocortisone
Hydrocortisone Sodium Succinate for Injection	1.25 per mg hydrocortisone
Hydromorphone Hydrochloride Injection	88.0 per mg
Hydroxocobalamin Injection	0.4 per µg
Hydroxyzine Hydrochloride Injection	3.6 per mg
Hyoscyamine Sulfate Injection	714.3 per mg
Idarubicin Hydrochloride for Injection	8.9 per mg
Ifosfamide for Injection	0.125 per mg
Imipenem	0.17 per mg

Official Monograph Name	Maximum Endotoxin Units[a–c]
Imipenem and Cilastatin for Injectable Suspension	0.23 per mg imipenem and 0.23 per mg cilastatin
Imipenem and Cilastatin for Injection	0.17 per mg imipenem and 0.17 per mg of cilastatin
Imipramine Hydrochloride Injection	5.0 per mg
Inamrinone Injection	0.5 per mg
Indigotindisulfonate Sodium Injection	5.0 per mg
Indocyanine Green for Injection	7.1 per mg
Indomethacin for Injection	20.0 per mg
Insulin	10.0 per mg
Insulin Human	10.0 per mg
Insulin Human Injection	80.0 per 100 units
Insulin Human Zinc Suspension	80.0 per 100 units
Insulin Injection	80 per 100 units
Insulin Lispro	10.0 per mg
Insulin Lispro Injection	80.0 per 100 units
Insulin Zinc Suspension	80.0 per 100 units
Inulin in Sodium Chloride Injection	0.1 per mg
Invert Sugar Injection	0.5 per mL
Iodipamide Meglumine Injection	3.6 per mL
Iodixanol Injection	0.2 per 50 mg iodine
Iohexol Injection	0.2 per 50 mg iodine
Iopamidol Injection	0.6 per mg iodine
Iophendylate Injection	0.9 per mg
Iopromide Injection	1.25 per mL
Iothalamate Meglumine and Iothalamate Sodium Injection	3.35 per mL
Iothalamate Meglumine Injection	0.9 per mL
Iothalamate Sodium Injection	3.35 per mL
Ioversol Injection	1.4 per mL
Ioxilan (Injection)	0.2 per 50 mg iodine
Iron Dextran Injection	0.50 per mg iron
Iron Sorbitex Injection	10.0 per mL
Iron Sucrose Injection	3.7 per mg iron
Isoflupredone Acetate	125.0 per mg
Isoflupredone Acetate Injectable Suspension	125.0 per mg
Isoniazid Injection	0.3 per mg
Isophane Insulin Human Suspension	80.0 per 100 units
Isophane Insulin Suspension	80.0 per 100 units
Isoproterenol Hydrochloride Injection	1250.0 per mg
Isoxsuprine Hydrochloride Injection	35.70 per mg
Kanamycin Injection	0.67 per mg kanamycin
Ketamine Hydrochloride Injection	0.4 per mg
Ketorolac Tromethamine Injection	5.8 per mg

(continued)

Official Monograph Name	Maximum Endotoxin Units[a–c]
Labetalol Hydrochloride Injection	1.2 per mg
Lactated Ringer's and Dextrose Injection	0.5 per mL
Lactated Ringer's Injection	0.5 per mL
Leucovorin Calcium Injection	1.95 per mg
Levocarnitine Injection	0.1 per mg
Levorphanol Tartrate Injection	125.0 per mg
Lidocaine Hydrochloride and Dextrose Injection	1.1 per mg
Lidocaine Hydrochloride and Epinephrine Injection	0.7 per mg lidocaine hydrochloride
Lidocaine Hydrochloride Injection	1.1 per mg lidocaine hydrochloride
Lincomycin Injection	0.5 per mg lincomycin
Lorazepam Injection	100.0 per mg
Magnesium Sulfate in Dextrose Injection	0.039 per mg magnesium sulfate
Magnesium Sulfate Injection	0.09 per mg
Mangafodipir Trisodium	0.13 per mg
Mangafodipir Trisodium Injection	0.66 per mg
Manganese Chloride Injection	0.45 per μg manganese
Manganese Sulfate Injection	0.45 per μg manganese
Mannitol Injection	0.04 per mg if 10% mannitol; 2.5 per g if > 10% mannitol
Mannitol in Sodium Chloride Injection	0.04 per mg mannitol
Mechlorethamine Hydrochloride for Injection	12.5 per mg
Menadiol Sodium Diphosphate Injection	25.0 per mg
Menadione Injection	58.3 per mg
Menotropins (for Injection)	2.5 per unit
Meperidine Hydrochloride Injection	2.4 per mg
Mepivacaine Hydrochloride and Levonordefrin Injection	0.8 per mg mepivacaine hydrochloride
Mepivacaine Hydrochloride Injection	0.8 per mg
Meropenem for Injection	0.125 per mg
Mesoridazine Besylate Injection	7.0 per mg
Metaraminol Bitartrate Injection	3.5 per mg metaraminol
Methadone Hydrochloride Injection	8.8 per mg
Methocarbamol Injection	0.2 per mg
Methohexital Sodium for Injection	0.5 per mg
Methotrexate Injection (for Injection)	0.4 per mg methotrexate sodium
Methotrimeprazine Injection	17.9 per mg
Methyldopate Hydrochloride Injection	0.5 per mg
Methylene Blue Injection	2.5 per mL
Methylergonovine Maleate Injection	1.7 per μg
Methylprednisolone Sodium Succinate for Injection	0.17 per mg methylprednisolone

Official Monograph Name	Maximum Endotoxin Units[a–c]
Metoclopramide Injection	2.5 per mg metoclopramide
Metoprolol Tartrate Injection	25.0 per mg
Metronidazole Injection	0.35 per mg
Mezlocillin for Injection	0.06 per mg
Miconazole Injection	0.10 per mg
Minocycline for Injection	1.25 per mg minocycline
Mitomycin for Injection	10.0 per mg
Mitoxantrone Injection	5.0 per mg mitoxantrone
Modified Lactated Ringer's and Dextrose Injection	0.5 per mL
Morphine Sulfate Injection	17.0 per mg
Morrhuate Sodium Injection	1.4 per mg
Multiple Electrolytes and Dextrose Injection Types 1, 2, 3, & 4	0.5 per mL
Multiple Electrolytes Injection Types 1 & 2	0.5 per mL
Nafcillin Injection (for Injection)	0.13 per mg nafcillin
Nalorphine Hydrochloride Injection	11.6 per mg
Naloxone Hydrochloride Injection	500.0 per mg
Neomycin for Injection	1.30 per mg neomycin
Netilmicin Sulfate Injection	1.25 per mg netilmicin
Niacinamide Injection	3.5 per mg
Niacin Injection	3.5 per mg niacin
Nitroglycerin Injection	0.1 per μg
Norepinephrine Bitartrate Injection	83.4 per mg norepinephrine
Ondansetron Injection	9.9 per mg
Orphenadrine Citrate Injection	5.8 per mg
Oxacillin for Injection	0.2 per mg oxacillin
Oxymorphone Hydrochloride Injection	238.1 per mg
Oxytetracycline Injection (for Injection)	0.4 per mg oxytetracycline
Oxytocin Injection	35.7 per unit
Paclitaxel	0.4 per mg
Paclitaxel Injection	0.67 per mg
Papaverine Hydrochloride Injection	2.9 per mg
Paricalcitol Injection	10.0 per μg
Penicillin G Benzathine (Injectable Suspension)	0.01 per 100 units
Penicillin G Potassium Injection (for Injection)	0.01 per 100 units
Penicillin G Procaine and Dihydrostreptomycin Sulfate Injectable Suspension	0.01 per 100 units
Penicillin G Procaine, Dihydrostreptomycin Sulfate and Prednisolone Injectable Suspension	0.01 per 100 units
Penicillin G Procaine, Dihydrostreptomycin Sulfate, Chlorpheniramine Maleate, and Dexamethasone Injectable Suspension	0.01 per 100 units
Penicillin G Procaine (Injectable Suspension)	0.01 per 100 units
Penicillin G Sodium for Injection	0.01 per 100 units

(continued)

Official Monograph Name	Maximum Endotoxin Units[a–c]
Pentazocine Injection	5.8 per mg
Pentazocine Lactate Injection	5.8 per mg pentazocine
Pentobarbital Sodium Injection	0.8 per mg
Perflutren Protein-Type A Microspheres for Injection (Injectable Suspension)	0.5 per mL
Perphenazine Injection	35.7 per mg
Phenobarbital Sodium for Injection	0.8 per mg
Phenobarbital Sodium Injection	0.3 per mg
Phentolamine Mesylate for Injection	5.8 per mg
Phenylbutazone Injection	1.1 per mg
Phenylephrine Hydrochloride Injection	25.0 per mg
Phenytoin Sodium Injection	0.3 per mg
Physostigmine Salicylate Injection	83.4 per mg
Phytonadione Injection (Injectable Emulsion)	14.0 per mg
Piperacillin for Injection	0.07 per mg
Plicamycin for Injection	100.0 per mg
Potassium Acetate Injection	8.80 per mEq
Potassium Chloride for Injection Concentrate	8.80 per mEq
Potassium Chloride in Dextrose and Sodium Chloride Injection	0.5 per mL
Potassium Chloride in Dextrose Injection	0.5 per mL
Potassium Chloride in Lactated Ringer's and Dextrose Injection	0.5 per mL
Potassium Chloride in Sodium Chloride Injection	0.5 per mL
Potassium Phosphates Injection	1.10 per mg
Pralidoxime Chloride for Injection	0.10 per mg
Prednisolone Sodium Phosphate Injection	5.0 per mg prednisolone phosphate
Prednisolone Sodium Succinate for Injection	5.8 per mg prednisolone
Prednisolone Tebutate Injectable Suspension	8.8 per mg
Prednisone Injectable Suspension	2.27 per mg prednisone
Prilocaine and Epinephrine Injection	0.9 per mg prilocaine hydrochloride
Prilocaine Hydrochloride Injection	0.9 per mg
Procainamide Hydrochloride Injection	0.35 per mg
Procaine and Tetracaine Hydrochlorides and Levonordefrin Injection	0.6 per mg procaine hydrochloride
Procaine Hydrochloride and Epinephrine Injection	0.6 per mg procaine hydrochloride
Procaine Hydrochloride (Injection)	0.6 per mg
Prochlorperazine Edisylate Injection	17.9 per mg prochlorperazine
Promazine Hydrochloride Injection	1.8 per mg
Promethazine Hydrochloride Injection	5.0 per mg
Prompt Insulin Zinc Suspension	80.0 per 100 units

Official Monograph Name	Maximum Endotoxin Units[a–c]
Propoxycaine and Procaine Hydrochlorides and Levonordefrin Injection	0.8 per mg propoxycaine hydrochloride
Propoxycaine and Procaine Hydrochlorides and Norepinephrine Bitartrate Injection	0.8 per mg propoxycaine hydrochloride
Propranolol Hydrochloride Injection	55.6 per mg
Protamine Sulfate Injection (for Injection)	7.0 per mg
Protein Hydrolysate Injection	0.5 per mg
Pyridostigmine Bromide Injection	17.0 per mg
Pyridoxine Hydrochloride Injection	0.4 per mg
Quinidine Gluconate Injection	0.6 per mg
Ranitidine Injection	7.00 per mg
Ranitidine in Sodium Chloride Injection	7.0 per mg
Repository Corticotropin Injection	3.1 per unit
Reserpine Injection	71.5 per mg
Riboflavin Injection	7.1 per mg
Rifampin for Injection	0.5 per mg
Ringer's and Dextrose Injection	0.5 per mL
Ringer's Injection	0.5 per mL
Ringer's Irrigation	0.5 per mL
Ritodrine Hydrochloride Injection	0.5 per mg
Sargramostim	5.0 per mg
Sargramostim for Injection	50.0 per mg
Scopolamine Hydrobromide Injection	555.0 per mg
Secobarbital Sodium Injection (for Injection)	0.9 per mg
Selenious Acid Injection	3.5 per µg
Sincalide for Injection	83.3 per µg
Sisomicin Sulfate Injection	0.5 per mg sisomicin
Sodium Acetate Injection	3.90 per mEq
Sodium Bicarbonate Injection	5.0 per mEq
Sodium Chloride Injection	0.5 per mL if 0.5%–0.9%; 3.6 per mL if 3.0%–24.3%
Sodium Chloride Irrigation	0.5 per mL
Sodium Lactate Injection	2.0 per mEq
Sodium Nitrite Injection	0.33 per mg
Sodium Nitroprusside for Injection	0.05 per µg
Sodium Phosphates Injection	1.10 per mg
Sodium Thiosulfate Injection	0.03 per mg
Spectinomycin Hydrochloride	0.09 per mg spectinomycin
Sterile Erythromycin Gluceptate	1.0 per mg erythromycin
Sterile Erythromycin Lactobionate	1.0 per mg erythromycin
Sterile Vancomycin Hydrochloride	0.33 per mg
Sterile Water for Inhalation	0.5 per mL
Sterile Water for Injection	0.25 per mL

(continued)

Official Monograph Name	Maximum Endotoxin Units[a–c]
Sterile Water for Irrigation	0.25 per mL
Streptomycin Injection (for Injection)	0.25 per mg streptomycin
Succinylcholine Chloride Injection (for Injection)	2.0 per mg
Sufentanil Citrate Injection	6.25 per mL
Sulbactam Sodium	0.17 per mg
Sulfadiazine Sodium Injection	0.1 per mg
Terbutaline Sulfate Injection	1250.0 per mg
Testosterone Injectable Suspension	3.5 per mg
Tetracaine Hydrochloride in Dextrose Injection	1.0 per mg tetracaine hydrochloride
Tetracaine Hydrochloride Injection (for Injection)	0.7 per mg
Tetracycline Hydrochloride for Injection	0.5 per mg
Theophylline in Dextrose Injection	1.0 per mg
Thiamine Hydrochloride Injection	3.5 per mg
Thiopental Sodium for Injection	1.0 per mg
Thiotepa for Injection	6.25 per mg
Thiothixene Hydrochloride Injection (for Injection)	88.0 per mg thiothixene
Ticarcillin and Clavulanic Acid Injection (for Injection)	0.07 per mg ticarcillin
Ticarcillin for Injection	0.05 per mg
Tiletamine and Zolazepam for Injection	0.07 per mg of combined tiletamine and zolazepam equivalents
Tiletamine Hydrochloride	0.07 per mg tiletamine
Tilmicosin Injection	0.5 per mg
Tobramycin Inhalation Solution	60.0 per mL
Tobramycin Injection (for Injection)	2.00 per mg tobramycin
Tolazoline Hydrochloride Injection	0.8 per mg
Tolbutamide for Injection	0.35 per mg tolbutamide sodium
Triamcinolone Acetonide Injectable Suspension	4.4 per mg
Triamcinolone Diacetate Injectable Suspension	7.1 per mg
Triamcinolone Hexacetonide Injectable Suspension	17.2 per mg
Trifluoperazine Hydrochloride Injection	172.0 per mg
Triflupromazine Hydrochloride Injection	5.8 per mg
Trimethobenzamide Hydrochloride Injection	1.80 per mg
Tripelennamine Hydrochloride Injection	4.6 per mg
Tromethamine for Injection	0.03 per mg
Tubocurarine Chloride Injection	10.0 per mg
Urea for Injection	0.003 per mg
Valrubicin Intravesical Solution	0.14 per mg
Vancomycin Hydrochloride for Injection	0.33 per mg vancomycin
Vancomycin Injection	0.33 per mg vancomycin
Vasopressin Injection	17.0 per unit
Verapamil Hydrochloride Injection	16.7 per mg

Official Monograph Name	Maximum Endotoxin Units[a–c]
Verteporfin	0.5 per mg
Vidarabine	0.5 per mg
Vinblastine Sulfate for Injection	10.0 per mg
Vincristine Sulfate for Injection	100.0 per mg
Vincristine Sulfate Injection	62.5 per mg
Warfarin Sodium for Injection	24.0 per mg
Water for Hemodialysis	2.0 per mL
Water for Injection	0.25 per mL
Xylazine Injection	1.7 per mg
Yohimbine Injection	45.5 per mg
Zidovudine Injection	1.0 per mg
Zinc Chloride Injection	25.0 per mg zinc
Zinc Sulfate Injection	25.0 per mg zinc
Zolazepam Hydrochloride	0.07 per mg zolazepam

[a]Refer to the current edition of *United States Pharmacopeia/National Formulary (USP/NF)* before calculating and determining endotoxin levels for the methods used.
[b]Where "unit" is used for the amounts in this column, refer to *USP/NF* to determine what type of unit is indicated.
[c]1 USP endotoxin unit (EU) is equal to 1 international unit (IU) of endotoxin.

Viscosity-Increasing Agents for Aqueous and Nonaqueous Systems

Properties of Commonly Used Viscosity-Increasing Agents

Substance	Solubility Water (1 g in _ mL)	Alcohol (1 g in _ mL)	Glycerin (1 g in _ mL)	Usual Suspension Concentration (%)	pH of Aqueous Solution (% Solution)	Most Effective pH Range	Recommended Preservatives
Acacia NF	2.7	PrIn	20	5.0–10.0	4.5–5 (5%)	—	Benzoic acid 0.1%, sodium benzoate 0.1%, methylparaben 0.17% with propylparaben 0.03%
Agar NF	Swells	IS	—	<1.0	—	—	—
Alginic acid NF	Swells	PrIn	—	—	1.5–3.5 (3%)	—	Benzoic acid 0.1%–0.2%, sodium benzoate 0.1%–0.2%, sorbic acid 0.1%–0.2%, parabens
Ammonium alginate	Swells	PrIn	—	—	1.5–3.5 (3%)	—	Benzoic acid 0.1%–0.2%, sodium benzoate 0.1%–0.2%, sorbic acid 0.1%–0.2%
Attapulgite colloidal/activated	PrIn	PrIn	—	—	7.5–9 (5%)	6–8.5	—
Bentonite NF	PrIn	PrIn	PrIn	0.5–5.0	9.5–10.5 (2%)	>6	—
Calcium alginate	PrIn	PrIn	—	—	—	—	—
Carbomer 910, 934, 934P, 940, 941, 1342 NF	Sol	Sol (after neutralization)	—	0.5–1.0	2.5–3 (1%)	6–11	Chlorocresol 0.1%, methylparaben 0.1%, thimerosal 0.1%
Carboxymethylcellulose calcium NF	IS	PrIn	—	0.25–5.0	4.5–6 (1%)	2–10	—
Carboxymethylcellulose sodium USP	Sol	PrIn	—	0.25–5.0	6.5–8.5 (1%)	2–10	—
Carrageenan NF	100[a]	—	—	—	—	—	—

Cellulose, microcrystalline NF	PrIn	—	—	0.5–5.0	5–7	0.5–5.0	—
Microcrystalline cellulose and carboxymethyl-cellulose sodium NF	PartSol	—	—	—	6–8 (1.2%)	—	—
Ceratonia	Sol[a]	IS	IS	—	5.3 (1%)	—	—
Cetostearyl alcohol	IS	Sol	Sol	—		—	—
Chitosan	IS	IS	—	—	4–6 (1%)	—	—
Cyclomethicone	IS	Sol	Sol	—	—	—	—
Dextrin NF	Sol	PrIn	PrIn	—	—	—	—
Ethylcellulose	IS	FS	FS	—	—	—	—
Ethylene glycol palmito-stearate	IS	Sol	Sol	—	—	—	—
Gelatin NF	Sol	Sol	PrIn	—	3.8–6 (type A), 5–7.4 (type B)	—	—
Glycerin	Sol	Sol	Sol	—	—	—	—
Glyceryl behenate	IS	—	PrIn	—	—	—	—
Guar gum NF	FS	—	PrIn	2.5	5–7 (1%)	4–10.5	Methylparaben 0.15% with propylparaben 0.02%
Hydroxyethyl cellulose NF	Sol	—	PrIn	1.0–5.0	5.5–8.5 (1%)	2–12	—
Hydroxyethyl methyl-cellulose	Sol	—	PrIn	—	5.5–8.0 (2% w/v)	—	—
Hydroxypropyl cellulose NF	2	PrIn	2.5	—	5–8 (1%)	6–8	—
Hydroxypropyl methyl-cellulose USP (Hypromellose)	Sol	—	PrIn	0.5–5.0	5.5–8 (1%)	3–11	—
Hydroxypropyl starch	IS	—	IS	—	4.5–7 (10%)	3–9	—

(continued)

Properties of Commonly Used Viscosity-Increasing Agents (*Continued*)

Substance	Solubility Water (1 g in __ mL)	Solubility Alcohol (1 g in __ mL)	Solubility Glycerin (1 g in __ mL)	Usual Suspension Concentration (%)	pH of Aqueous Solution (% Solution)	Most Effective pH Range	Recommended Preservatives
Magnesium aluminum silicate NF	PrIn	PrIn	—	0.5–10.0	9–10 (5%)	—	—
Maltodextrin	FS	SlS	—	—	—	—	—
Methylcellulose USP	Sol	PrIn	—	—	5.5–8 (1%)	3–11	—
Octyldodecanol	IS	Sol	—	—	—	—	—
Pectin USP	20	PrIn	—	—	5% acidic	—	—
Poloxamer NF	Varies	Varies	—	10.0–40.0	6–7.4 (2.5%)	—	—
Polycarbophil	Swells	—	—	<1	2.5–3.0 (1%)	—	—
Polydextrose	Sol	Sol	PartSol	—	>2.5 (10%)	—	—
Polyethylene glycol	Sol	Sol	Sol	—	—	—	—
Polyethylene oxide	Sol	IS	—	—	—	—	—
Polyethylene oxide NF	Sol	IS	—	1.0	—	—	—
Polyvinyl acetate phthalate	IS	Sol	—	—	—	4.5–5	—
Polyvinyl alcohol USP	FS	—	—	0.5–3.0	5–8 (4%)	—	—
Potassium alginate	Sol	IS	—	—	—	4–10	—
Povidone USP	FS	FS	—	2.0–10.0	3–7 (5%)	—	—
Propylene glycol alginate NF	Sol	—	—	1.0–5.0	3–6	—	—
Saponite	Swells	—	—	—	—	—	—

Silicon dioxide NF, colloidal	PrIn	IS	—	2.0–10.0	3.5–4.4 (4%)	1–7.5	—
Sodium alginate NF	Sol (slowly)	PrIn	—	1.0–5.0	7.2 (1%)	4–10	Chlorocresol 0.1%, chloroxylenol 0.1%, parabens, benzoic acid (if acidic)
Stearyl alcohol	PrIn	Sol	—	—	—	—	—
Sulfobutylether-β-cyclodextrin	Sol	PrIn	—	50	—	—	—
Tragacanth NF	PrIn	PrIn	—	5–6	4–8 (1%)	—	Benzoic acid 0.1%, sodium benzoate 0.1%, methylparaben 0.17% with propylparaben 0.03%
Trehalose	Sol	VSS	—	—	4.5–6.5 (30%)	—	—
Vegetable oil, hydrogenated	PrIn	—	—	1–4	—	—	—
Xanthan gum NF	Sol	PrIn	—	1.0–2.0	6–8 (1%)	3–12	—
Zinc stearate	PrIn	PrIn	—	Up to 1.5%	—	—	—

— = Not available.
[a] Hot water.

Appendix IX

Disinfecting Agents Used in Compounding Pharmacies

Surfaces in a compounding pharmacy that require cleaning and disinfection, especially when sterile preparations are compounded, include working surfaces (e.g., laminar-airflow hoods, countertops), ceilings, equipment, floors, walls, and the skin of pharmacists and technicians.

Antiseptics and disinfectants are similar in that they kill microorganisms or inhibit their growth on contact. Antiseptics are applied to living tissues, and disinfectants are applied to inanimate objects; the same agent may be used for both, but in different concentrations.

The ideal disinfectant would exert a rapidly lethal action against all potentially pathogenic microorganisms and spores, have good penetrating power into organic matter, be compatible with organic compounds, not be inactivated by living tissue, be noncorrosive, and be aesthetically acceptable (nonstaining, odorless).

Antiseptics and disinfectants are generally categorized by chemical category. Agents in various categories are described in the following sections and summarized in Table IX-1.

Oxidizing Agents

Hydrogen peroxide solution (H_2O_2, MW 34.01) occurs as a clear, colorless liquid and is odorless or has a slight odor resembling that of ozone. It is acidic to taste and to litmus testing. It decomposes rapidly on contact with many oxidizing and reducing substances. It should be packaged in tight, light-resistant containers and kept at controlled room temperature.

Sodium hypochlorite solution (NaClO, MW 74.44, antiformin) occurs as a clear, pale greenish-yellow liquid with the odor of chlorine. It is affected by light. It should be preserved in tight, light-resistant containers at a temperature not exceeding 25°C.

Phenols and Related Compounds

Chlorocresol (C_7H_7ClO, MW 142.58) occurs as colorless or practically colorless crystals or crystalline powder, with a characteristic nontarry, phenolic odor. It is slightly soluble in water and more soluble in hot water. It is very soluble in alcohol and soluble in fixed oils. Incompatibilities include strong alkalis, calcium chloride, codeine phosphate, and iron salts,

TABLE IX-1 Disinfecting Agents Used in Compounding Pharmacies

Agent	Usual % Concentration	Solubility Water	Solubility Alcohol	pH of Aqueous Solution	Specific Gravity	Boiling Point (°C)	Melting Point (°C)
Oxidizing Agents							
Hydrogen peroxide solution	3	Misc	Misc	—	1.01	—	—
Sodium hypochlorite solution	5	Misc	Misc	—	—	—	—
Phenols and Related Compounds							
Chlorocresol	—	SlS	VS	—	—	235	55–65
Cresol	—	SpS	Misc	Neutral	1.030–1.038	—	—
Hexachlorophene	2–3	IS	FS	—	—	—	—
Phenol	5	Sol	VS	6 (Sat sol)	1.071 (Liq)	181.8	43
Heavy Metals							
Iodine	2–5	VSS	Sol	—	—	—	—
Povidone iodine	—	Sol	Sol	—	—	—	—
Surface-Active Agents							
Benzalkonium chloride	1:750 to 1:5000	VS	VS	5–8 (10%)	0.98	—	40
Benzethonium chloride	1:750 to 1:5000	Sol	Sol	—	—	—	—
Cetrimide	—	FS	FS	5–7.5 (1%)	—	—	232–247
Chlorhexidine gluconate	—	Misc	—	—	—	—	—
Alcohol, Glycol, Aldehyde, and Acids							
Alcohol (ethanol)	60–95	Misc	—	—	0.812–0.816	78.15	—
Benzyl alcohol	10	SpS	FS (50% Alco)	Neutral	1.043–1.049	204.7	−15.2
Formaldehyde	—	Misc	Misc	—	—	—	—
Glutaraldehyde	2	Misc	—	—	—	—	—
Isopropyl alcohol	>70	Misc	Misc	—	0.783–0.787	82.4	−88.5

— = Not available; Alco = alcohol; Liq = liquid; Sat sol = saturated solution.

and it binds to rubber, certain plastics, and nonionic surfactants. It is most effective in acidic solutions and is inactive above pH 9. It has synergistic effectiveness with other antimicrobial preservatives, such as 2-phenylethanol. Its aqueous solutions can be sterilized by autoclaving.

Cresol (C_7H_8O, MW 108.14) occurs as a highly refractive liquid that is colorless, yellowish to brownish-yellow, or pinkish, becoming darker with age and on exposure to light. It has a phenol-like, sometimes empyreumatic odor. A saturated solution of cresol is neutral or only slightly acid to litmus. Cresol is sparingly soluble in water and dissolves in solutions of fixed alkali hydroxides. It is miscible with alcohol and glycerin. Incompatibilities include chlorpromazine and nonionic surfactants. Cresol is active below pH 9, with optimum activity in acidic media.

Hexachlorophene ($C_{13}H_6Cl_6O_2$, MW 406.90) occurs as a white to light tan, crystalline powder. It is odorless or has a slight phenolic odor. It is insoluble in water but is freely soluble in acetone and alcohol. It is generally used in a 2% to 3% concentration.

Phenol (C_6H_6O, MW 94.11, carbolic acid, hydroxybenzene, phenylic acid) occurs as colorless to light pink, interlaced or separate needle-shaped crystals or as a white to light pink, crystalline mass. It has a characteristic odor. When exposed to air, phenol turns red or brown. It is soluble in water and very soluble in alcohol and glycerin. Incompatibilities include acetaminophen, albumin, camphor, chloral hydrate, ethyl aminobenzoate, gelatin, menthol, methenamine, phenacetin, phenazone, phenyl salicylate, resorcinol, sodium phosphate, terpin hydrate, and thymol. The bulk material should be stored in a well-closed container at a temperature not exceeding 15°C. Phenol is very corrosive and toxic; it should be handled with caution. Protective polyvinyl chloride or rubber clothing is recommended, together with gloves, eye protection, and a respirator. Spills onto the skin or into the eyes should be washed with copious amounts of water; for affected skin areas, this should be followed by an application of a vegetable oil. Medical attention should be sought.

Heavy Metals

Iodine (I_2, MW 253.81) occurs as heavy, grayish black plates or granules having a metallic luster and a characteristic odor. It is very slightly soluble in water and soluble in alcohol and in solutions of iodides. It is sparingly soluble in glycerin.

Povidone iodine [$(C_6H_9NO)_n \cdot xI$] occurs as a yellowish-brown to reddish-brown, amorphous powder having a slight characteristic odor. Its solution is acid to litmus. It is soluble in water and in alcohol.

Surface-Active Agents

Benzalkonium chloride is a mixture of alkylbenzyldimethylammonium chlorides of the general formula [$C_6H_5CH_2N(CH_3)_2R$]Cl, where R represents a mixture of alkyls, from n-C_8H_{17} through n-$C_{12}H_{25}$, with the major portion consisting of n-$C_{14}H_{29}$ and n-$C_{16}H_{33}$. The average molecular weight of benzalkonium chloride is 360. The quaternary ammonium compound occurs as a white or yellowish-white thick gel or gelatinous pieces. It usually has a mild aromatic odor, and its aqueous solutions have a bitter taste and foam strongly when shaken. It is slightly alkaline in aqueous solution. It is very soluble in water and in alcohol. Benzalkonium chloride solution occurs as a clear liquid, colorless or slightly yellow unless a color has been added. It has an aromatic odor and a bitter taste. It is stable over wide pH and temperature ranges. Its solutions can be autoclaved. Incompatibilities include aluminum, anionic surfactants, citrates, cotton, fluorescein, H_2O_2, hydroxypropyl methylcellulose, iodides, kaolin, lanolin, nitrates, nonionic surfactants in high concentration, permanganates, protein, salicylates, silver salts, soaps, sulfonamides, tartrates, zinc oxide, and zinc sulfate. Its activity is increased when combined with benzyl alcohol, disodium edetate, phenylethanol, or phenylpropanol. Its maximum inhibitory activity occurs between pH 4 and 10. It is hygroscopic and may be affected by light, air, and metals.

Benzethonium chloride ($C_{27}H_{42}ClNO_2$, MW 448.08) occurs as white crystals with a mild odor. It is slightly alkaline (1 in 100 aqueous solution). It is soluble in water (1 g in 750 mL) and in alcohol (1 g in 5000 mL).

Cetrimide consists of a mixture of tetradecyltrimethylammonium bromide with smaller amounts of dodecyltrimethylammonium bromide and hexadecyltrimethylammonium bromide. This quaternary ammonium compound occurs as a white to creamy-white free-flowing powder with a faint but characteristic odor and a bitter, soapy taste. Cetrimide is freely soluble in alcohol and water. Incompatibilities include acid dyes, alkali hydroxides, anionic surfactants, bentonite, iodine, high concentrations of nonionic surfactants, phenylmercuric nitrate, and soaps. In aqueous solution, it will react with metals. It is most effective at neutral or slightly alkaline pH, with activity reduced in acidic media and in the presence of organic matter. The presence of alcohols can enhance its activity. It should be stored in a well-closed container in a cool, dry place.

Chlorhexidine gluconate ($C_{22}H_{30}Cl_2N_{10} \cdot 2C_6H_{12}O_7$, MW 897.77) solution is an almost colorless or pale-yellow clear liquid. It is miscible with glacial acetic acid and with water.

Alcohol, Glycol, Aldehyde, and Acids

Alcohol (ethanol) (C_2H_6O, MW 46.07, ethyl alcohol, ethyl hydroxide, grain alcohol, methyl carbinol) refers to 96.0% to 96.6% volume per volume (v/v) ethanol. If other strengths are intended, the term *alcohol* or *ethanol* is used with the statement of the intended strength. Ethanol is a clear, colorless, mobile, volatile liquid that has a characteristic odor and produces a burning sensation on the tongue. It is readily volatilized and boils at about 78°C. It is flammable. It is miscible with water and with practically all organic solvents. Ethanol is bactericidal in aqueous mixtures at 60%–95% v/v, with an optimum concentration of about 70% v/v. Edetic acid or edetate salts will enhance the antimicrobial activity. Ethanol can be sterilized by autoclaving or filtration. It should be stored in airtight containers in a cool place. Ethanol is incompatible with oxidizing materials. Mixtures containing alkali may darken because of reaction with residual amounts of aldehyde. Ethanol is incompatible with aluminum containers and may interact with some drugs. Solutions of ethanol can be sterilized by autoclaving or by filtration and should be stored in airtight containers in a cool place.

Benzyl alcohol (C_7H_8O, MW 108.14) occurs as a clear, colorless, oily liquid that boils at about 205°C. It is sparingly soluble in water, freely soluble in 50% alcohol, and miscible with alcohol. Incompatibilities include oxidizing agents, strong acids, and methylcellulose. In addition, it can be sorbed by closures of butyl rubber, natural rubber, and neoprene, and it can damage polystyrene syringes. In aqueous solution, benzyl alcohol can be sterilized by filtration or autoclaving. Generally, it should be stored in metal or glass containers. Plastic containers should not be used, with the exception of polypropylene or vessels coated with inert fluorinated polymers such as Teflon. Benzyl alcohol should be stored in airtight containers, protected from light in a cool, dry place.

Formaldehyde solution (CH_2O, MW 30.03) occurs as a clear, colorless, or practically colorless liquid with a pungent odor. The vapor is irritating to the mucous membranes of the throat and nose. It may become cloudy upon standing, especially in the cold, but the cloudiness disappears with warming. Formaldehyde solution is miscible with water and with alcohol.

Glutaraldehyde (glutaral) disinfectant solution ($C_5H_8O_2$, MW 100.12) concentrate occurs as a clear, colorless, or faintly yellow liquid with a characteristic irritating odor. It is used in a 2% solution buffered to a pH between 7.5 and 8.0. Nonbuffered solutions are not stable and lose about 44% of their activity after 15 days; buffered solutions retain 86% of their original activity up to 30 days after preparation.

Isopropyl alcohol (C_3H_8O, MW 60.10, IPA, 2-propanol) occurs as a transparent, colorless, mobile, volatile liquid with a characteristic odor and a slightly bitter taste. It is flammable. It is miscible with alcohol, chloroform, ether, and water. Incompatibilities include oxidizing agents such as hydrogen peroxide and nitric acid. Isopropanol can be salted out by the addition of sodium chloride, sodium sulfate, and other salts or by the addition of sodium hydroxide. It is bactericidal and is more effective than alcohol at concentrations greater than 70% v/v. Its activity increases steadily as the concentration approaches 100% v/v. It should be stored in an airtight container in a cool, dry place.

Index

Note: Page numbers followed by *b*, *f*, and *t* indicate boxes, figures, and tables, respectively.